C000112426

Molecular Interventions and
Local Drug Delivery

Frontiers in Cardiology

Series Advisors:
MICHEL BERTRAND
JOHN CAMM
DESMOND JULIAN
NORMAN KAPLAN
ULRICH SIGWART

Published

Management of Acute Myocardial Infarction
Edited by Desmond G. Julian and Eugene Braunwald

Forthcoming

Noninvasive Electrocardiology: Clinical Aspects of Holter Monitoring
Edited by Arthur J. Moss and Shlomo Stern

Endoluminal Stenting
Edited by Ulrich Sigwart

Molecular Interventions and Local Drug Delivery

Edited by

Elazer R. Edelman

Hermann Von Helmholtz Associate Professor, Cardiovascular Division, Brigham and Women's Hospital, Harvard Medical School and Harvard/MIT Division of Health Sciences and Technology, Boston, USA

Electrophysiology Section Edited by

Robert J. Levy

Professor of Pediatrics, Communicable Diseases and Pharmaceutics, The University of Michigan Medical School, Ann Arbor, USA

W. B. Saunders Company Ltd
London • Philadelphia • Toronto • Sydney • Tokyo

W. B. Saunders Company Ltd   24–28 Oval Road
London NW1 7DX, UK

The Curtis Center
Independence Square West
Philadelphia, PA 19106-3399, USA

Harcourt Brace & Company
55 Horner Avenue
Toronto, Ontario M8Z 4X6, Canada

Harcourt Brace & Company, Australia
30–52 Smidmore Street
Marrickville, NSW 2204, Australia

Harcourt Brace & Company, Japan
Ichibancho Central Building, 22-1 Ichibancho
Chiyoda-ku, Tokyo 102, Japan

© 1995 W. B. Saunders Company Ltd, except for Chapter 8, which is an official contribution of the National Institutes of Health, not subject to copyright in the United States.

This book is printed on acid free paper

All rights reserved. No part of this publication may be reproduced, stored in a retrieval system or transmitted, in any form or by any means, electronic, mechanical, photocopying or otherwise, without the prior permission of W. B. Saunders Company Ltd, 24–28 Oval Road, London NW1 7DX, England

A catalogue record for this book is available from the British Library

ISBN 0-7020-1910-0

Typeset by Paston Press Ltd, Loddon, Norfolk
Printed in Great Britain by The University Press, Cambridge

Contents

Contributors   *vii*

Preface   *ix*

Proliferative Vascular Disease

1   Restenosis – an accelerated arteriopathy: pathophysiology, preventive strategies   *1*
    and research horizons
    K.-W. Lau and U. Sigwart

2   Local interventions for vasculoproliferative diseases   *29*
    A. Nathan and E. R. Edelman

3   Targeted therapies for accelerated arteriopathies   *53*
    A. D. Johnson and S. W. Casscells

4   Accelerated arteriopathies: molecular approach   *79*
    M. Simons

Thrombotic Heart Disease and myocardial infarction

5   Introduction and contemporary therapies   *107*
    D. I. Simon and C. R. Meckel

6   Local therapy   *131*
    C. Rogers

7   Antibody-targeted thrombolytic and antithrombotic agents   *149*
    E. Haber

8   Molecular approaches to the therapy of ischemic heart disease   *171*
    S. W. Lee and D. A. Dichek

Vasoreactive Disease

9   Endothelium and vasoreactive diseases   *203*
    A. P. Selwyn and P. Ganz

10 Vasoreactive diseases: molecular approach   *213*
    D. Marks and J. Loscalzo

11 Molecular basis of vasoreactive diseases: angiotensin II as a paradigm   *233*
    G. H. Gibbons

12 Pulmonary vasoreactive diseases: inhaled nitric oxide   *249*
    W. E. Hurford and W. M. Zapol

Congestive Heart Failure

13   Secondary molecular alterations in failing human myocardium   *267*
         W. S. Colucci

14   Congestive heart failure: molecular approach and transplantation   *283*
         J. A. Jarcho

15   Gene and cell-based therapies for myocardial dysfunction   *313*
         M. W. Chang and *J. M. Leiden*

Electrophysiology – Edited by R. J. Levy

16   Electrophysiologic disorders   *327*
         J. K. Gibson and *R. J. Levy*

17   The molecular biology of the long QT syndrome   *353*
         M. W. Russell and *L. C. Brody*

18   Iontophoresis for modulating cardiac delivery of antiarrhythmic agents   *383*
         V. Labhasetwar, S. P. Schwendeman, T. Nguyen, T. Underwood and *R. J. Levy*

19   Feedback control of antiarrythmic agents   *399*
         J. C. Wood, M. Telting-Diaz, D. R. Bloem, T. Nguyen, M. Meyerhoff, R. Arzbaecher,
         A. Sintov and *R. J. Levy*

         Index   *473*

Contributors

Robert Arzbaecher
Pritzker Institute of Medical Engineering, Illinois Institute of Technology, Chicago, IL, USA

David R. Bloem
Pritzker Institute of Medical Engineering, Illinois Institute of Technology, Chicago, IL, USA

Lawrence C. Brody
National Institutes of Health, Bethesda, MD, USA

S. Ward Casscells
Cardiology Research, Texas Heart Institute, Houston, TX, USA

Mark W. Chang
Department of Medicine, University of Chicago, Chicago, IL, USA

Wilson S. Colucci
Cardiovascular Division, Brigham and Women's Hospital, Boston, MA, USA

David A. Dichek
Gladstone Institute of Cardiovascular Disease, University of California, San Francisco, USA

Elazer R. Edelman
Cardiovascular Division, Brigham and Women's Hospital, Harvard Medical School and Harvard/MIT Division of Health Sciences and Technology, Boston, USA

Peter Ganz
Cardiac Catheterization Laboratory, Harvard Medical School, Cardiovascular Division, Brigham and Women's Hospital, Boston, MA, USA

Gary H. Gibbons
Stanford University School of Medicine, Falk Cardiovascular Research Center, Stanford, CA, USA

J. Kenneth Gibson
Upjohn Laboratories, Cardiovascular Diseases Research, Kalamazoo, MI, USA

Edgar Haber
Center for Prevention of Cardiovascular Disease, Harvard School of Public Health, Boston, MA, USA

William E. Hurford
Department of Anesthesia, Massachusetts General Hospital, Boston, MA, USA

John A. Jarcho
Cardiovascular Division, Brigham and Women's Hospital, Harvard Medical School, Boston, MA, USA

A. Daniel Johnson
Vascular Cell Biology Laboratory, Texas Heart Institute, Houston, TX, USA

Vinod Labhasetwar
Pediatrics, Communicable Diseases and Pharmaceutics, University of Michigan, Ann Arbor, MI, USA

Kean-Wah Lau
Department of Cardiology, Singapore General Hospital, Singapore

Sung W. Lee
Division of Cardiology, George Washington University School of Medicine, Washington, DC, USA

Jeffrey M. Leiden
University of Chicago, Cardiovascular Division, Chicago, IL, USA

Robert J. Levy
Pediatrics, Communicable Diseases and Pharmaceutics, University of Michigan, Ann Arbor, MI, USA

Joseph Loscalzo
Cardiovascular Division, Boston University Hospital, Boston, MA, USA

David Marks
Department of Medicine, Brigham and Women's Hospital, Harvard Medical School, Boston, MA, USA

Clyde R. Meckel
Cardiovascular Division, Brigham and Women's Hospital, Harvard Medical School, Boston, MA, USA

Mark Meyerhoff
Chemistry Department, University of Michigan, Ann Arbor, MI, USA

Aruna Nathan
Harvard/MIT Division of Health Sciences and Technology, MIT, Cambridge, MA, USA

Tam Nguyen
Pediatrics, Communicable Diseases and Pharmaceutics, University of Michigan, Ann Arbor, MI, USA

Campbell Rogers
Cardiovascular Division, Brigham and Women's Hospital, Harvard Medical School, Boston, MA, USA

Mark W. Russell
National Institutes of Health, Bethesda, MD, USA

Steven P. Schwendeman
University of Michigan Medical Center, Ann Arbor, MI, USA

Andrew P. Selwyn
Cardiac Catheterization Laboratory, Harvard Medical School, Cardiovascular Division, Brigham and Women's Hospital, Boston, MA, USA

Ulrich Sigwart
Department of Invasive Cardiology, Royal Brompton National Heart and Lung Hospital, London, UK

Daniel I. Simon
Harvard Medical School, Cardiovascular Division, Brigham and Women's Hospital, Boston, MA, USA

Michael Simons
Harvard Medical School, Cardiovascular Division, Beth Israel Hospital, Boston, MA, USA

Amnon Sintov
Agis Industries, Yeruchem, Israel

Marten Telting-Diaz
Department of Chemistry, University of Michigan, Ann Arbor, MI, USA

Thomas Underwood
University of Michigan Medical Center, Ann Arbor, MI, USA

John C. Wood
Yale Children's Hospital Pediatric Programme, Newhaven, CT, USA

Warren M. Zapol
Department of Anesthesia, Massachusetts General Hospital, Boston, MA, USA.

Preface

Motivation

Issues related to drug delivery are important everyday concerns to the practicing cardiologist and the cardiovascular research scientist. The greatest debates currently raging in every area of clinical cardiology revolve about pharmacologic therapy. Similarly, issues of pharmacokinetics and pharmacodynamics are assuming an ever increasing role in the scientific laboratory. This has arisen both as a response to the clinical imperatives and because of direct research needs to deal with novel compounds that have short half lives, are active in minute quantities and may have variable effects dependent on dose and mode of administration.

The people and technologies that address these concerns are from widely disparate fields. Cardiovascular therapeutics and research now requires an interdisciplinary approach and a full appreciation of the relationship between pharmacology, pharmacokinetics, biochemistry, biomaterials, controlled drug delivery, polymer science, chemical engineering, cell and molecular biology, physiology and toxicology among others. No one forum provides an adequate venue for discussing these issues. We hope that this book will provide such a medium by presenting topics related to cardiovascular drug delivery in an organized and related fashion. The book presents contemporary issues related to the treatment and investigation of five major disease areas: proliferative vascular diseases, thrombotic heart disease and myocardial infarction, vasoreactive disease, congestive heart failure and electrophysiologic disorders. Each section contains an overview chapter describing basic pathophysiology and existing clinical imperatives and research obstacles, followed by discussions of how innovations in targeted, local or controlled drug delivery have been applied to breakthroughs in molecular and cell biology to create new classes of therapies and new avenues for research.

Summary of book chapters

Drs Lau and Sigwart review the cellular mechanisms that govern the development and progression of the accelerated arteriopathies that follow balloon angioplasty, vascular bypass surgery and organ transplantation. They describe how an understanding of these processes can be used to design novel curative strategies and set the tone for the chapters that follow. Dr Simons discusses the molecular pathology of the accelerated arteriopathies and then shows how an understanding of these pathways can be used to suggest new therapies for the prevention and treatment of these diseases. In particular, he has focused on the use of antisense oligonucleotides in this regard. Drs Nathan and Edelman detail the power of local drug delivery, the biologic basis for its efficacy and the range of techniques that are in place to provide for practical delivery at this level. In a similar chapter, Drs Johnson and Casscells describe targeted therapy for these diseases; discussing control of cell growth through toxin conjugates that link peptide growth factor receptor ligands to potent cell poisons, modulation of adhesion molecules and manipulation of the extracellular matrix.

Drs Simon and Meckel introduce the contemporary management of thrombotic heart disease and myocardial infarction by discussing the pathology, pathophysiology and state-of-the-art management of myocardial infarction. Background and rationale for future therapeutic strategies that employ principles of molecular biology and local drug delivery are provided as well. Dr Rogers subsequently shows how local therapy permits the precise, focal treatment of thrombotic heart disease. His chapter outlines the attributes needed for effective antithrombotic drug delivery and the technical and logistical limitations of existing methodologies. In following on Dr Rogers' discussion of local therapy, Dr Haber describes a body of work that includes the development of plasminogen activators that are based on the concept of antibody targeting to a specific component of the thrombus and the use of bivalent antibodies and fusion conjugates. In the ultimate extension of local therapy Drs Lee and Dichek review the status of gene transfer as a therapeutic approach to ischemic heart disease. The techniques and limitations of gene transfer are discussed including indirect, cell-based, *ex vivo* gene transfer and direct, vector-based *in vivo* gene transfer. A number of examples are presented, including vascular gene transfer to combat thrombosis, hepatic gene transfer to correct hypercholesterolemia, and intramyocardial gene transfer for enhancement of collateral formation.

The next set of diseases include alterations in vasomotor tone. Drs Ganz and Selwyn describe the classic history of vasoreactive disorders and the central role of the endothelium in this regard. They discuss the means by which this cell balances control of vasomotion, anticoagulation and growth, and the cascade of pathologic events that follow disruption of the endothelium. Dr Gibbons follows further with an in-depth discussion of the molecular mechanisms involved in this control and shows how innovative delivery schemes can be harnessed to control this regulation. Drs Marks and Loscalzo review remaining vascular factors that are candidates for molecular interventions at the local level and describe progress to date with use of vasoactive agents. Their discussion makes good use of the previous chapters and sets the tone for the chapter by Drs Hurford and Zapol on the use of inhaled nitric oxide in pulmonary vasoreactive diseases. Drug inhalation allows for rapid absorption and specific delivery. In particular the authors cite exciting data with the use of nitric oxide to treat disease states such as pulmonary hypertension of the adult and newborn, and acute respiratory distress syndromes (ARDS).

Dr Colucci begins the section on congestive heart failure describing the secondary molecular alterations in failing human myocardium and the morphologic changes associated with alterations in excitation–contraction coupling. He details the accompanying changes in contractile and regulatory proteins, growth factors and signaling pathways that lead to progressive abnormalities of heart function. The implications for therapy is provided. Dr Jarcho follows with a full discussion of the molecular and immunologic basis of allograft rejection. In some sense organ transplantation represents the ultimate in local therapy as a donor tissue is inserted within a specific site in the host. This chapter details how an understanding of the immunobiology of transplantation can be used to propose novel molecular controls to enhance the acceptance of foreign tissues. Drs Chang and Leiden summarize the recent progress in cardiovascular gene therapy and cellular transplantation with an emphasis on assessing the feasibility of these approaches for the treatment of congestive heart failure. Because cardiomyocytes are terminally differentiated cells that lack the ability to proliferate, they pose a unique series of problems for gene transfer not confronted within the vascular wall. Methodological advances concerning gene transfer in the heart are discussed along with a delineation of specific candidate genes for the prevention and treatment of congestive heart failure, and the potential of cardiomyocyte transplantation as a novel cell-based therapy for congestive heart failure.

The final section, edited by Dr Levy, extends the general discussion to include disorders of electrical impulse generation and conduction. While Drs Gibson and Levy provide an introductory chapter which highlights contemporary therapies in this field, Drs Russel and Brody describe the molecular basis of these disorders, in particular the long QT syndrome. Dr Labhasetwar and colleagues describe the innovative use of iontophoresis for enhancement of drug delivery to treat the dysrhythmias and Dr Wood and his co-workers detail how feedback and control systems can be used to regulate drug delivery and match it to specific disorders.

These topics are not meant to be all-inclusive and the discussions are not encyclopedic. We have simply tried to show the range and breadth of these topics and the way in which innovative drug delivery can enhance the power of break-throughs in medical science.

Cautionary note

The technologic advancements that permit continuous controlled release, targeted therapy and local drug administration will certainly change the treatment of cardiovascular disease. The toxicity, expense and disparity between the absolute dose of drug infused and the effective amount of drug delivered seen with more traditional modes of administration can be circumvented. Novel compounds that are rapidly denatured or degraded in the systemic circulation may now be used with much lessened concern for the physicochemical alterations that might significantly alter binding and bioactivity. Yet, it is important to end this discussion on a cautionary note. Just as no one would suggest that a single technique in cell or molecular biology could be applied to all pathologic conditions or every research problem, no single mode of drug delivery can be utilized for every disease.

Continuous exposure of cells and tissues to heightened local concentrations of compounds can be achieved in a variety of ways but it has not been demonstrated that this establishes optimal control. Constant exposure to excessive levels may lead to receptor downregulation, drug resistance, and even the potential for drug sequestration and recirculation with increased toxicity. Continuous infusion may be an absolute necessity for highly soluble, rapidly cleared compounds, but not for drugs with prolonged half-lives. Local therapy may limit systemic toxicity but may not control all disease states. Drug delivery must be directed by a coupled understanding of the pathophysiology of the disease and pharmacology of the compound. Complex diseases that involve interaction of circulating cells with primed surfaces, for example activated platelets or monocytes that adhere to denuded arterial walls with appropriate selectin expression, might benefit from systemic administration in one instance and local therapy in another. Local therapy is fine when the drug used is directed against and applied to the activated surface, but may fail if the compound is to act against the circulating cell. The latter case is simply overwhelming for the amount of drug that can be infused locally. The dose of drug capable of being administered would probably be insufficient to handle all of the cells that pass over or through the treated tissue, and the duration of exposure to the drug when released locally would probably be insufficient to block binding sites or physical processes before binding or activation occurs.

It is also important to remember that local administration of a drug is not local therapy, it is only local infusion. Local effects require adequate exposure to active drug. Rapid local release and clearance can dilute concentrations such that systemic infusion might achieve a more favorable equilibrium because of the increased amount of drug that can be administered. Moreover, site-specific infusions can still have profound global effects, and when complications extend systemically therapy is by definition no longer local. Disruption of local tissue integrity that activates circulating cells, releases growth or proinflammatory factors, elicits systemic inflammatory reactions, or dislocates intravascular debris only to have it embolize distally, all violate the local mandate.

Thus, while continuous, local or site-specific therapies are appealing in that they might produce heightened local concentrations of drug at limited systemic toxicities they may not be applicable to all drugs and all disease states. Further work at the interface of materials science and device engineering, pharmaceutics and cell biology, molecular biology and integrated physiology may provide additional insight into the pathology of specific diseases and the best way to treat them.

In closing I must acknowledge the tremendous efforts of the staff of W. B. Saunders and in particular the gentle, insightful and persistent guidance of Ms Gill Robinson. Finally, with the greatest humility, I wish to dedicate this book to my teachers in life and mentors in science, Professors Robert Langer and Morris J. Karnovsky.

Elazer R. Edelman

Restenosis – an Accelerated Arteriopathy: Pathophysiology, Preventive Strategies and Research Horizons

Kean-Wah Lau
Ulrich Sigwart

Introduction

Percutaneous transluminal coronary angioplasty (PTCA) is an accepted and well-established nonsurgical treatment modality for patients with underlying coronary artery disease, surpassing the number of coronary bypass grafting procedures performed.[1,2] However, despite substantial improvements in the acute success rate and safety profile of PTCA as a result of recent advances in catheter design and enhanced operator experience,[3] there has been, in contrast, much less progress in containing the problem of restenosis. Restenosis has thus emerged as the dominant limitation factor in the long-term effectiveness of the procedure and is truly the Achilles' heel of PTCA.

The incidence of restenosis varies widely depending on patient-lesion selection, the definition criterion for restenosis and the completeness of angiographic restudy.[2] On the average, it occurs in about 30–40% of patients and does so usually within 3–6 months after the procedure.[2]

Because of this unacceptable high restenosis rate and its profound health-cost implications, not surprisingly, there has been intense experimental research attempting to elucidate the pathophysiologic mechanisms and extensive clinical trials carried out to identify ways of reducing restenosis. This chapter will focus on the mechanisms of restenosis and provide an update on the strategies in circumventing this problem. The ideal strategy in the prevention of restenosis is not so much how to inhibit but to modulate and control the neointimal response. This response is treatable but when it progresses beyond control, it culminates in restenosis. Current clinical treatment modalities to prevent restenosis include the administration of drugs and the application of new intracoronary interventional devices, and these will be discussed.

Pathophysiology of restenosis

It has been more than a decade since the first documentation of intimal proliferation after PTCA causing restenosis by Essed *et al.*[4] At this stage, what is overtly clear from animal[5,6] and human pathological (autopsy, surgical resection and atherectomy specimens) studies[7–13] is that exuberant smooth-muscle cell (SMC) proliferation together with the large volume of extracellular matrix generated by these cells represents the final common pathway and the pivotal cause of restenosis; a small amount of neointimal growth, however, is essential for proper arterial repair and is clearly desirable. Less well defined and understood are the early events and major triggering factors causing this excessive reparative response to arterial injury. Information pertaining to this area remains scant and is derived principally from the animal injury model rather than from human studies. The prevailing paradigm for the genesis of restenosis is that of an accelerated version of atherosclerosis; it appears both spontaneous atherosclerosis and restenosis share many striking similarities in key events which are really a stereotypic response to injury.[14,15] This response, however, seems to progress at a much faster pace in restenosis. The current postulated mechanisms of restenosis (Figure 1.1) may be arbitrarily categorized into an early phase consisting of platelet activation and thrombus formation occurring within minutes to hours after injury, an intermediate phase of cellular recruitment (hours to days) and the late proliferative phase (days to months).

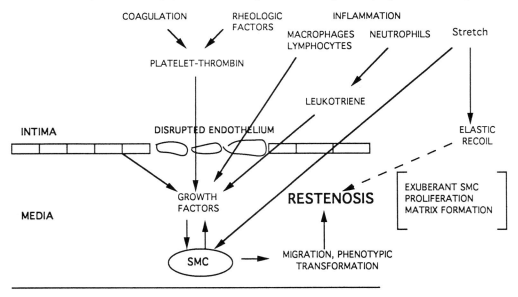

SMC=smooth muscle cells

Figure 1.1   Schematic representation of the postulated pathogenesis of restenosis after vessel wall injury.

Endothelium denudation, platelet activation and thrombus formation

Acutely, PTCA leads to endothelium denudation, plaque fracture and medial dissection. This damage, in turn, exposes the highly thrombogenic subintimal tissues to serum components and leukocytes. Within minutes after injury, there is aggressive platelet adhesion and aggregation that persists for hours, and thrombus formation, proportionate to the severity of injury and the degree of unfavorable rheologic factors present at the site of the lesion.[16–20] Activation of platelets then leads to secretion of various products which include platelet-derived growth factor (PDGF), 5-hydroxytryptamine (5-HT), transforming growth factor-β_1 (TGF-β_1), thromboxane A_2 (TXA$_2$) and ADP. 5-HT and ADP together with thrombin cause vasospasm in areas deficient in endothelium-derived relaxing factor (EDRF). 5-HT, in addition, stimulates vascular SMC migration and proliferation, and promotes the synthesis of collagen and proteoglycans in the extracellular matrix as does the multifunctional peptide TGF-β_1. Moreover, this platelet-derived growth factor also effects a positive feedback stimulation of platelets, enhancing further platelet aggregation. Platelets also activate leukocytes to release vasoconstrictor leukotrienes. These platelet-induced effects appear to be thromboxane-mediated as inhibition of thromboxane reduces leukocyte activation.[21,22] Although platelets and their secretory factors appear to contribute to exuberant intimal proliferation by two different mechanisms, namely those of induction of thrombosis and vasospasm in the early phase and increments in SMC proliferation later on, they alone are insufficient to cause restenosis which can be induced even in thrombocytopenic animals.[23] Thus, other cellular and secretory factors (such as endothelin and insulin-like growth factor) are also likely to be involved in restenosis.[21,22]

Injured and proliferating endothelial cells also secrete proteoglycans and peptides such as basic fibroblast growth factor (bFGF) which are mitogenic to SMCs. This is in contrast to intact quiescent endothelial cells which are vital in maintaining the low proliferative state of SMCs under normal vascular conditions as they have an inhibitory effect on SMC migration and proliferation.[22] Thrombus, rich in platelets, fibrin strands and fibronectin, and an invariable consequence of balloon injury, is mitogenic to SMCs and stimulates PDGF expression and release.[22] The magnitude of the exact role thrombus plays in SMC migration and proliferation is unclear, but there is evidence both from animal and human studies suggesting it may be important in the pathogenesis of restenosis.[22] The tissue renin–angiotensin autocrine system has also been implicated in neointimal thickening.[24–26] Angiotensin II affects SMC growth by inducing SMCs to express PDGF-like factors, bFGF and TGF-β into the media.[27–30]

Balloon dilatation causes arterial-wall stretch which in turn has the following direct and indirect effects on SMCs: (1) modulation of SMC DNA synthesis; (2) provocation of the autocrine synthesis and release of mitogens from SMCs themselves; (3) rupture of the internal elastic lamina and separation of SMCs causing loss of contact inhibition and allowing the permeation of mitogens from various sources through the medial SMCs; resulting (4) in subsequent SMC growth.[22] Additionally, there is significant elastic recoil following arterial stretch. In fact, various studies have documented a 30–50% recoil of the arterial cross-sectional area after conventional PTCA.[31–33] This may account for a significant incidence of restenosis, within the first 24 hours post-PTCA.[34–36]

Cellular recruitment phase

Attracted by the thrombus and damaged endothelium, leukocytes from blood are recruited. These cells then migrate into the degenerating thrombus and release growth factors and cytokines that affect SMC migration and proliferation.[19] These growth factors include platelet-derived growth factors, FGF, endothelial growth factor, TGF-β_1 and TGF-α_1.[37,38] Monocytes also elaborate fibrinolytic enzymes responsible for the dissolution of the thrombus.[39] Meanwhile, there is neoendothelialization of the thrombus usually within a few days after balloon injury, thereby preventing further platelet and fresh thrombus deposition.[19]

Late SMC proliferative phase

This final phase of healing involves SMC proliferation and extracellular matrix formation as the key event. When the reparative response is exuberant and uncontrolled, the end result is restenosis. Histologically, late restenotic lesions less than 6 months old consist of excessive neointimal volume of SMCs and a bulky extracellular matrix produced by the neointimal cells as the prime ingredients.[9–12] It is postulated that medial SMCs from the site of injury (and possibly also from the adjacent area) once stimulated by the numerous heterogeneous potential triggering factors mentioned earlier, migrate through breaks in the internal elastic lamina, proliferate and colonize the degenerating thrombus. Also, once activated, participating SMCs undergo a characteristic phenotypic transformation, from a predominantly 'contractile' into a predominantly 'synthetic' form.[10] It is these synthetic cells which are responsible for the production of the abundance of extracellular matrix seen in the relatively early stages (under 6 months) after balloon injury. Interestingly, these cells themselves have self-stimulatory capability, elaborating and secreting growth factors independent of exogenous factors and mitogens, and can thus replicate after platelet and leukocyte activation has ceased weeks after vascular injury.[15,40]

From the above description of the postulated model of restenosis, although pronounced SMC proliferation and the associated synthesis of copious amounts of extracellular matrix is undoubtedly the central cause of restenosis, the exact underlying mechanisms leading to it have not been clearly identified and remain nebulous. It is likely a multifactorial process involving numerous stimuli interacting with each other, frequently in a synergistic manner.

Pharmacologic approaches to prevent restenosis

These are outlined in Table 1.1.

Calcium antagonists

Theoretically, at least, vasodilators such as calcium antagonists may reduce restenosis. Increased vasomotor activity has been identified as a powerful risk determinant of restenosis.[41,42] Coronary segments with enhanced coronary vasomotor responses as in variant angina or stenotic sites which develop severe occlusion when exposed to vasoconstrictive stimuli (ergonovine, hyperventilation) are predisposed to high rates of restenosis when dilated.[41] Also, the damaged coronary artery itself is associated with an exaggerated vasoconstrictive response to factors such as serotonin and platelet aggregation.[43,44]

Unfortunately, several randomized trials testing the potential antirestenotic effects of calcium antagonists have not produced positive results. Whitworth et al.,[45] Corcos et al.[46] and more recently, Hoberg and coworkers[47] using nifedipine, diltiazem and verapamil, respectively, failed to attenuate the risk of restenosis.

Antiplatelet agents and anticoagulants

The rationale behind the use of antiplatelet agents and anticoagulants is to render less platelet-thrombus formation, and thus less available substrate for subsequent organization and a lower risk of late restenosis.

Aspirin and ticlopidine. To date, at least five prospective clinical trials have explored the role of these antiplatelet agents in the prevention of restenosis.[48–52] Schwartz et al.[48] in a randomized trial involving 376 patients failed to show any long-term protection against restenosis despite a combination of aspirin and dipyridamole started 24 hours before PTCA and continued until follow-up angiography. Similarly, in a study by Chesebro et al.[49] in which 207 patients were assigned to either aspirin and dipyridamole or placebo from 1 day before to 6 months after PTCA, no difference in restenosis was found between the two patient groups. Thornton et al.[50] compared the prophylactic effects of aspirin and therapeutic doses of warfarin in 248 patients undergoing PTCA. Neither treatment groups prevented restenosis in this study.

Bertrand and colleagues[51] studied 266 patients, randomized to receive either ticlopidine or placebo. Again, as was seen with aspirin–dipyridamole combination therapy, there was no mitigating effect on restenosis. In another prospective trial, White and coworkers[52] assigned ticlopidine to one group of patients, aspirin–dipyridamole to another and tested these drugs against placebo. The restenosis rate was similar in all three groups.

Thus, it is amply clear from all these well-controlled randomized trials that antiplatelet agents do not favorably affect the incidence of restenosis. They do, however, have a strong positive influence on the acute complication rate, in particular, a protection against acute vessel closure.

PDGF inhibitor. Trapidil (triazolopyrimidine) is a potent inhibitor of PDGF. Since PDGF may be a crucial factor in SMC proliferation, administering this drug should logically reduce restenosis. Indeed, two recent randomized trials suggest this

Table 1.1 Postulated effects and results of randomized clinical drug trials in the prevention of restenosis defined angiographically

Reference	Number of patients	Agents/dose	Rate of restenosis (%)	P value	Postulated mechanisms
Whitworth et al.[45]	241	Nifedipine 40 mg day⁻¹ vs placebo	28 / 29.5	NS	Vasodilatation
Corcos et al.[46]	92	Diltiazem 270 mg day⁻¹ vs placebo	15	NS	
Hoberg[47]	196	Verapamil 480 mg day⁻¹ vs placebo	48.3 / 62.7 } in UAP; 56 / 62 }; 38 / 63 } in CSA	0.059; NS; 0.038	
Schwartz et al.[48]	376	ASA 990 mg day⁻¹ plus DIP 225 mg day⁻¹ vs placebo	37.7 / 38.6	NS	Inhibition platelet aggregation and thrombus formation
Chesebro et al.[49]	207	ASA 990 mg day⁻¹ plus DIP 225 mg day⁻¹ vs placebo	–* / –	NS**	
Bertrand et al.[51]	226	Ticlopidine 500 mg day⁻¹ vs placebo	49.6 / 40.7	NS	
White et al.[52]	236	Ticlopidine 750 mg day⁻¹ vs ASA 650 mg day⁻¹ plus DIP 225 mg day⁻¹ vs placebo	39 / 33 / 25	NS	
Okamoto et al.[53]	72	Trapidil 600 mg day⁻¹ vs placebo (ASA plus DIP)	19 / 42	<0.05	Blocks PDGF
STARC[54]	305	Trapidil 300 mg day⁻¹ vs placebo (ASA)	24 / 40	0.01	
Serruys et al.[55]	707	GR32191B 80 mg day⁻¹ vs placebo	21 / 19	NS	Inhibits platelet aggregation and vasodilatation
Bove et al.[56]	755	Sulotroban 3200 μg day⁻¹ vs placebo	–	NS	
Knudtson et al.[57]	270	i.v. Prostacyclin 5 μg kg⁻¹ min⁻¹ plus ASA plus DIP vs placebo (ASA+DIP)	27	NS	Platelet inhibition and vasodilatation
Raizner et al.[58]	311	Ciprostene i.c./i.v. 120 μg kg⁻¹ min⁻¹ vs placebo	32 / 26	0.055	Platelet inhibition and vasodilatation
Thornton et al.[50]	248	ASA 325 mg day⁻¹ vs therapeutic warfarin	38 / 27 / 36	NS	Inhibits platelet-thrombus formation

	N	Treatment			
Urban et al.[60]	110	Therapeutic warfarin plus verapamil	29	NS	Inhibition of thrombus formation
		vs verapamil	37		
Ellis et al.[61]	416	i.v. therapeutic heparin	41	NS	Inhibition thrombus formation
		vs placebo	37		
Lehmann et al.[62]	23	Heparin s.c. 10 000 u day^{-1}	82	<0.05	
		vs placebo	33		
Stone et al.[68]	102	i.m. methylprednisolone plus prednisolone 60 mg day^{-1}	42	NS***	Anti-inflammatory and antiproliferative actions
		vs placebo	48		
Pepine et al.[69]	722	i.v. methylprednisolone 1 g before PTCA	43	NS	
		vs placebo	43		
MERCATOR[70]	693	Cilazapril 10 mg day^{-1}	28	NS	Antiproliferative and vasodilatory actions
		vs placebo	28		
Desmet et al.[71]	304	Fosinopril 40 mg day^{-1}	39.4	NS	
		vs placebo	37.2		
O'Keefe et al.[73]	197	Colchicine 1.2 mg day^{-1}	41	NS	Antiproliferative, antifibrotic and anti-inflammatory actions
		vs placebo	45		
Kent et al.[74]	1246	Angiopeptin at 190 µg day^{-1}	38.0	NS	Inhibits growth hormone and antiproliferative action
		at 750 µg day^{-1}	35.6		
		at 3000 µg day^{-1}	37.8		
		vs placebo	38.6		
Eriksen et al.[75]	112	Angiopeptin 750 µg day^{-1}	7.5	<0.001	
		vs placebo	37.8		
Serruys et al.[76]	658	Ketanserin 40 mg day^{-1}	32	NS	Inhibits SMC proliferation and platelet aggregation
		vs placebo	32		
Heik et al.[77]	97	Ketanserin 40 mg day^{-1}	22	NS	
		vs placebo	38		
Sachn et al.[82]	157	Lovastatin 20–40 mg day^{-1}	12	<0.001	Reduces serum lipids and inhibits SMC proliferation
		vs placebo	45		
Dehmer et al.[84]	82	Omega-3 FA 3.2 g day^{-1}	19	0.007	Inhibits platelet aggregation and SMC proliferation
		vs placebo	46		
Grigg et al.[85]	108	Omega-3 FA 3.0 g day^{-1}	34	NS	
		vs placebo	33		
Reis et al.[86]	186	Omega-3 FA 6.0 g day^{-1}	34	NS	
		vs placebo	23		
Nye et al.[87]	108	Omega-3 FA 2.16 g day^{-1}	11 }	<0.05 compared with placebo	
		vs ASA plus DIP	30 }		
			17		
Bairati et al.[88]	205	Omega-3 FA 15 g day^{-1}	30.5	0.05	
		vs placebo	48.3		

ASA, aspirin; CSA, chronic stable angina; DIP, dipyridamole; FA, fatty acids; i.c., intracoronary; i.v., intravenous; NS, not significant; PDGF, platelet-derived growth factor; s.c., subcutaneous; UAP, unstable angina pectoris.
*–, no data available. **Based on the mean late minimum luminal diameter using a linear model. ***Based on angiographic and clinical criteria.

positive effect on intimal hyperplasia. Data from a study by Okamoto *et al.*[53] showed a significant difference in the rate of restenosis between patients given trapidil and those who were on aspirin–dipyridamole therapy (19% vs 42%; $P < 0.05$). The multicenter STARC study[54] also demonstrated a lower restenosis rate with trapidil compared with placebo treatment (24% vs 40%; $P = 0.01$).

Thromboxane A$_2$-receptor blocker. Early platelet aggregation appears to play a central role in early thrombosis and subsequent restenosis. Thromboxane A$_2$ (TXA$_2$) is a potent platelet aggregatory factor and a vasoconstrictor released from activated platelets. In addition, it stimulates SMC proliferation directly.[55]

Based on these animal results, the CARPORT study[55] was initiated and randomized 707 patients to TXA$_2$-receptor blocker GR32191B and placebo; the drug, however, failed to reduce the lesion recurrence rate. Likewise, sulotroban, another TXA$_2$-receptor blocker, did not manage to lower the restenosis rate in a large randomized trial (M-HEART II).[56] There are two possible explanations for this failure of TXA$_2$ antagonists to substantially reduce SMC proliferation. First, prevention of platelet adhesion rather than platelet aggregation may perhaps be a more efficacious means of diminishing restenosis. Second, the pivotal role of platelets in restenosis may have been overemphasized and antiplatelet therapy as the sole treatment modality may be inherently deficient in controlling the restenosis phenomenon.

Prostacyclin. Prostacyclin is a naturally occurring platelet inhibitor and vasodilator. In a Canadian randomized study,[57] 270 patients were allocated to intravenous prostacyclin started just before PTCA and continued up to 48 hours and to placebo. All patients received aspirin and dipyridamole. There was no significant difference in the restenosis rate at six-month follow-up angiography (27% in the treated group compared with 32% in placebo group).

Ciprostene is a stable prostacyclin analog. To study its influence on restenosis, Raizner *et al.*[58] randomized 311 patients to intracoronary application of ciprostene before PTCA and intravenously for 48 hours subsequently and to placebo. Although a trend towards a lower rate of angiographic restenosis was noted in the treated group of patients, the difference was not significant (26% vs 38%; $P = 0.055$).

Platelet glycoprotein IIb/IIIa inhibitor. Glycoprotein IIb/IIIa and von Willebrand factor are both platelet membrane receptors and are essential for platelet adhesion–aggregation. Thus, theoretically, specific antagonists to these receptors should be able to decrease thrombosis and possibly restenosis. In the multicenter IMPACT trial,[59] therapy with integrelin, a platelet glycoprotein IIb/IIIa inhibitor, was compared with placebo in 150 patients. All patients received aspirin and heparin. Patients on integrelin sustained fewer cardiac events while in hospital and up to 30 days post-PTCA compared with placebo. The data on the restenosis rate are pending.

Warfarin. Apart from the study by Thornton *et al.*,[50] there was another more recent randomized study[60] looking into the potential preventive effect of warfarin on restenosis. Again, no demonstrable protection by warfarin against restenosis was evident in the study.

Heparin. Unfractionated heparin has both anticoagulant and antiproliferative components. In Atlanta, Georgia (USA), Ellis and colleagues[61] conducted a trial of conventional heparin in patients who did not have a major dissection following successful PTCA. These patients were randomly assigned to treatment with either intravenous heparin for 18–24 hours post-PTCA or an intravenous dextrose placebo. All patients were on aspirin. Six-month follow-up angiography in 60% of these patients revealed no difference in the incidence of restenosis, which was 41% in the heparin recipients and 37% in the placebo group.

In a subsequent small-scale prospective study,[62] patients were randomized to receive either chronic subcutaneous heparin 10 000 u daily or standard treatment after PTCA. The trial was terminated prematurely when the investigators observed a markedly higher restenosis rate in the heparin-treated group than in the placebo (82% and 33%, respectively; $P < 0.05$).

In contrast to regular heparin, low-molecular-weight heparin affects anticoagulation to a lesser extent but may be as, if not more, effective than regular heparin in inhibiting SMCs in experimental studies.[63,64] Although promising, there are no published clinical data on the effect of this heparin subfraction on restenosis. A large multicenter trial[65] to determine if low-molecular-weight heparin can successfully reduce restenosis is currently in progress in the USA.

Specific antithrombin agent. Hirudin is a very potent and specific antithrombin agent and has been shown to be more effective in preventing thrombosis than heparin in an animal model.[66] This experimental finding was confirmed in a recent human study by van den Bos *et al.*;[67] treatment with hirudin reduced the number of acute occlusions and engendered better forward flow immediately and at 24 hours after PTCA compared with placebo-treated patients in the study. However, whether this acute benefit will lead to less intimal thickening in a human model remains to be seen although, theoretically, less thrombus could result in less SMC proliferation.

Anti-inflammatory drugs

Clinically, steroids and nonsteroidal anti-inflammatory agents have not been shown to be successful in inhibiting neointimal proliferation.

Corticosteroids

These drugs are potent inhibitors of SMC proliferation and the associated production of collagen and matrix by retarding protein synthesis. In addition, they inhibit leukocyte migration and degranulation, and decrease the release of PDGF and macrophage-derived growth factors.[38] The two prospective randomized clinical trials,[68,69] however, have not been able to duplicate these experimental benefits.

Stone *et al.*[68] in Kansas, USA, administered high-dose intramuscular methylprednisolone prior to PTCA and after the procedure maintained these patients in the treatment group on oral prednisolone 60 mg day^{-1} for 7 days. The restenosis outcome was, however, similar between the treated and control cohort of patients (42% and 48%, respectively).

Another much larger trial, the multicenter prospective M-HEART,[69] which enrolled more than 900 patients to receive intravenous methylprednisolone or placebo 2–24 hours before PTCA, again found no difference in the overall restenosis rate between the two groups (43% each). These trials obviously showed that administration of corticosteroids has no influence on restenosis.

Antiproliferative agents

Angiotensin-converting enzyme (ACE) inhibitors. Despite the potential role of the renin–angiotensin system in neointimal proliferation, clinical studies[70,71] involving ACE inhibitors which block the conversion of angiotensin I to II have yielded inconclusive evidence of benefits.

In the recent MERCATOR trial,[70] 693 patients were randomized to cilazapril and placebo; there was no difference in the restenosis rate between the two cohorts. Identical restenosis outcome was obtained in the large single-center fosinopril trial[71] involving 304 patients; significant angiographic lesion recurrence (based on the binary definition) occurred in 39% of patients assigned to 40 mg of fosinopril daily and 37% of those in the control group (P = NS). These results indicate that perhaps angiotensin II has only a minor role in the very complex restenosis process.

Colchicine. This drug has antimitotic, anti-inflammatory and antifibrotic actions. Furthermore, it also inhibits platelet aggregation and the release of secretory products, and reduces neointimal proliferation in animals.[72] In contrast, in the randomized study by O'Keefe *et al.*,[73] only a neutral outcome was obtained with colchicine; the restenosis rate was similar between the colchicine and placebo group (41% and 45%, respectively; P = NS).

Somatostatin analog. Somatostatin is an endogenous growth hormone inhibitor. Angiopeptin, a synthetic analog of somatostatin has been shown to be able to inhibit SMC replication experimentally although its exact inhibitory mechanism is not known.[21] Inconclusive preliminary data from two studies[74,75] have been published. In a randomized study[74] of 1246 patients, angiopeptin in various graduated doses failed to reflect the experimental beneficial effects; the restenosis rate for all three doses of angiopeptin was similar to that of placebo in the study. On the other hand, in a much smaller multicenter Scandinavian randomized study,[75] 750 μg day^{-1} of angiopeptin was able to reduce the restenosis rate after PTCA (7.5% compared to 37.8% for the placebo group; P < 0.001). The restenosis rate using an identical dose of angiopeptin in the aforementioned trial by Kent *et al.*[74] was 35.6%. The reason for this large disparity in restenosis rates between the two studies is not clear.

Serotonin antagonist. Endogenous serotonin affects the restenosis process in several ways. It is a vasoconstrictor, a stimulus to platelet aggregation, and provokes

SMC proliferation. Therefore, administering a serotonin antagonist such as ketanserin may reduce restenosis. In the PARK trial[76] which had 658 patients recruited, the experimental benefits were, however, not demonstrated; equal restenosis rate of 32% was documented in the ketanserin-treated and placebo group. Heik *et al.*[77] in a similar study arrived at the same conclusion that ketanserin does not avert restenosis.

Hypolipidemic agents

Cholesterol-lowering agents. The role of lipids in the pathogenesis of restenosis is controversial. Experimental studies have indicated that hyperlipidemia seems to cause and perpetuate a progressive fibrocellular response, as opposed to the self-limiting pattern seen in the absence of an elevated cholesterol level. Oxidized/modified low-density lipoprotein (LDL) is chemotactic for monocytes, toxic to the endothelium causing cell injury and necrosis, and promotes foam cell formation.[15] Although it has been shown that modification of lipoprotein profile can halt the progression and even induce regression of coronary atherosclerosis,[78] whether it can similarly decrease the restenosis rate is unclear. There are conflicting reports on the relationship between lipids and restenosis.[79–81]

Sachni *et al.*[82] recently randomized 79 patients to lovastatin (a HMG CoA reductase inhibitor which has been shown experimentally to inhibit cell growth by blocking DNA synthesis and to reduce restenosis) and 78 patients to placebo. The restenosis rate was 12% in the treatment group vs 45% in the control ($P < 0.001$). These encouraging results, however, were not supported by the findings from the multicenter Lovastatin Restenosis Trial.[83] In a preliminary report from the investigators of the study, 80 mg day^{-1} of lovastatin administered to patients with serum cholesterol level >200 mg dl^{-1} failed to reduce the restenosis rate (39% vs 38% in the placebo group).

Omega-3 fatty acids. Eicosapentaenoic acid and docosahexaenoic acid could retard neointimal thickening in several ways: they decrease platelet aggregation, decrease blood viscosity resulting in improved rheology, alter monocyte function, inhibit PDGF-like production by endothelial cells and lower lipid levels. The several medium-sized randomized trials[84–88] involving the administration of omega-3 fatty acids have yielded conflicting results based on six-month angiographic determination of lesion renarrowing. A significant reduction in restenosis was observed in three studies,[84,87,88] whereas in two others,[85,86] only a neutral effect was noted. In a recent meta-analysis[89] of the major fish-oil trials, a statistically significant effect of this agent in reducing restenosis was found but the effect was minimal. Perhaps, to be of any benefit, the fish-oil supplement needs to be started about a week or so before intervention and at high doses.

Mechanical approaches to prevent restenosis

No drug regimen has convincingly succeeded in overcoming restenosis. Therefore, in an effort to limit this recalcitrant problem, attention is now directed to other newer second-generation nonballoon intracoronary devices (Table 1.2).

As alluded to earlier, elastic recoil is a major and ubiquitous problem of conventional balloon dilatation, particularly for eccentric lesions. It contributes to suboptimal results and early restenosis following balloon dilatation. Furthermore, because PTCA causes plaque fracture, intima–media dissection and arterial stretch, and does not reduce atheromatous mass, there is often a substantial residual lesion. Several investigators in the past have identified a close link between the severity of residual stenosis post-PTCA and the risk of subsequent restenosis.[90–92] Also, small arterial lumen size predisposes to restenosis. All this makes intuitive sense in terms of basic geometry: a narrow lumen, particularly in a small-caliber vessel allows less room for intimal hyperplasia before the lumen becomes significantly compromised. More recent data from the Beth Israel group have confirmed this direct association.[93,94] Furthermore, restenosis was shown to be dependent only on the acute gain (defined as the difference in the minimal lumen diameter before and immediately after the procedure) and reference vessel diameter and not on the type of device used. Of the various new devices currently available, stents followed by directional coronary atherectomy produce the largest luminal diameters, thereby making them potentially useful tools in overcoming the problem of restenosis, particularly in large vessels such as vein grafts or in lesions with adverse morphologies where the restenosis risk is high with conventional PTCA.[93–95]

Intracoronary stent

Currently, there are six major stents in clinical use. All have proved extremely effective in treating PTCA-related acute vessel closures, obviating the need for emergency bypass surgery in most patients and markedly reducing the extent of potential myocardial damage.[95] Stenting, in addition, may reduce restenosis by restoring vessel integrity by a number of ways. First, it provides a stable scaffolding, thus counteracting elastic recoil. Second, it limits exposure of deep tissue to blood components and ensures high antegrade flow through a smooth-contoured lumen, thereby diminishing unfavorable rheologic factors. Moreover, this high flow has an opposite effect to the barotrauma-induced stimulation of SMC proliferation and may contribute in the prevention of restenosis.[22] Third, it creates a wide lumen by achieving maximal acute gain, often larger than any other interventional device. However, unlike the other second-generation debulking interventional devices such as atherectomy catheters and laser, stents improve upon the luminal size by compressing the plaque in a radial fashion and thereby redistributing the plaque mass circumferentially without tissue removal.[96]

Observational studies[97–101] involving the Wallstent (Schneider Inc., Plymouth, MN, USA) have revealed a stent-related restenosis rate of between 12 and 47%. These restenosis rates appear more favorable than those of PTCA despite stenting lesions with adverse morphologies conventionally associated with a high restenosis risk in the majority of patients in these studies. The predictors of restenosis were stent implantation in bypass vein grafts, gross stent oversizing, inadequate poststent luminal dimensions, multiple overlapping stents and suboptimal stent placement

(Table 1.2). When optimally deployed in native coronary arteries, the restenosis was as low as 12% in one study.[101]

The Palmaz–Schatz stent (Johnson & Johnson Interventional Systems, Warren, NY, USA) has also been extensively studied. The restenosis rate observed for this stent design ranges from 13 to 57%.[93,102–115] A number of studies comparing the outcome of this stent model with other treatment modalities have been made. In two recent retrospective comparative studies by Kuntz *et al.*[94] and Kimura *et al.*,[113] the acute gain was substantially larger and the restenosis rate was significantly lower following Palmaz–Schatz stenting than after PTCA (Table 1.2). However, compared with PTCA, the stented arterial segment suffered from greater late loss (defined as the loss in postprocedure minimal lumen diameter during follow-up compared with the minimal lumen diameter immediately after the procedure), reflecting more intimal hyperplasia. However, because of the larger immediate gain in lumen diameter achieved, it could accommodate more loss before significant luminal encroachment resulting in restenosis occurred. These results have recently been confirmed by two moderate-sized landmark randomized trials comparing the two treatment modalities (single stent implantation vs PTCA) in *de novo* native coronary lesions.[114,115]

In both the Benestent trial[114] and Stent Restenosis Study (STRESS)[115] although the larger acute gain in luminal size after stent implantation was offset by a larger late loss, the net gain remained larger in the stent group of patients compared with PTCA. This luminal benefit was translated into a lower restenosis rate (22% vs 32%; $P = 0.02$ in the Benestent trial and 30% vs 43%; $P = 0.016$ in the STRESS) and a significantly reduced incidence of repeat intervention for ischemia-related restenosis of the treated lesion in the stent group. Of note, there was no difference in the acute success and in-hospital ischemic complication rate between the two treatment groups in both trials.

Several risk factors for this stent model have been identified in relation to increased restenosis. A few are in common with those of the Wallstent. These include the use of multiple overlapping stents, suboptimal poststent luminal size, stent implantation in an acute or threatened closure situation, in vessels with small reference diameter, in chronically occluded or restenotic lesions and the presence of diabetes (Table 1.2).

Compared to the Wallstent and Palmaz–Schatz stent, there is less published long-term data on the Gianturco–Roubin (Cook Inc., Bloomington, IN, USA)[116–119] and Wiktor stents (Medtronic Inc., Minneapolis, MN, USA).[120,121] In native coronary arteries, the restenosis rate after Wiktor stent placement has been reported to be between 29 and 37%.[120,121] Preliminary reports on the long-term overall restenosis rate after deployment of the Gianturco–Roubin stent in a threatened or acute closure scenario indicate between 39 and 52%.[116–118] In a small study[119] in which 66 patients with significant early loss of vessel lumen size after PTCA were randomized to receive either elective implantation of the Gianturco–Roubin stent or to serve as controls, the restenosis rate for those patients who received the stent was significantly less than those who did not (21.2% vs 75.7%; $P < 0.001$). The preliminary observations with the Advanced Cardiovascular Systems stent have yielded promising results.[122] There are no long-term data available for the Cordis stent.

Table 1.2 Angiographic restenosis data on second-generation intracoronary devices

Reference	Number of patients/lesions	Vessel type	Treatment modality	Success	F-U (months)	Rate of restenosis (%)	Significant rate of restenosis predictors
Urban et al.[97]	13	SVG	WS			20	
Strauss et al.[98]	176	NCA/SVG	WS		6.6	35	Multiple stents SVG, oversized stents, residual DS > 20% SVG (RS = 39%)
Strauss et al.[99]	265	NCA/SVG	WS		6.6	27	
Scheerder et al.[100]	69	SVG	WS		5	47	Suboptimal stent placement
Lau et al.[101]	84	NCA/SVG	WS	–	8	16	Multiple stents
Schatz et al.[102]	247	NCA	PS	99	6	20	
Carrozza et al.[103]	220	NCA/SVG	PS	98	6	25	LAD, small vessels, DM stent in AC (RS = 43%)
Herrmann et al.[104]	56	NCA/SVG	PS	98	6	23	
Colombo et al.[105]	100	NCA/SVG	PS	98	5	27	
Ellis et al.[106]	200	NCA	PS		5.8	36	Overlapping stents, CTO, restenotic lesions, residual DS > 0%
Foley et al.[109]	99	NCA/SVG	PS	99	6.3	32	Restenotic lesions
Colombo et al.[110]	56	NCA A/T close	PS		5	36	
Baim et al.[111] (Registry)	1189	NCA/SVG	PS		6	30	
Kastrati et al.[112]	82	NCA	PS		3, 6, 12	22, 32, 33	
Kimura et al.[113]	275	NCA	96 PS / 179 PTCA	97	3–6	13 / 39 } $P < 0.001$	
Serruys et al.[114]†	520	NCA	PS / PTCA	93 / 91	6	22 / 32 } $P = 0.02$	
Fishman et al.[115]†	410	NCA	PS / PTCA	96 / 89	6	30 / 43 } $P = 0.016$	Small initial gain, small NCA, LAD
Kuntz et al.[93]	223	NCA/SVG	87 PS / 125 DCA / 11 LBA		6	19 / 31 / 50 } $P = 0.02$	Small initial gain
Kuntz et al.[94]	524	NCA	PS / DCA / PTCA		6	26 $P < 0.01$ / 32 $P = 0.06$ / 42	Compared with PTCA / Compared with PTCA
Kuntz et al.[107]	290	NCA/SVG	102 PS / 134 DCA		6	26 / 32 } $P = 0.03$	
Pomerantz et al.[108]	97	SVG	69 PS / 28 DCA	99 / 94	6	25 / 28 } $P = NS$	
Roubin et al.[116]	115	NCA A/T close	G-R		6	41	

Study	n	Lesion/vessel	Device	Success (%)	Follow-up (months)	Restenosis (%)	Comments
Hearn et al.[117]	103	NCA/SVG A/T close	G-R	89	4	53	SVG, small NCA
George et al.[118] (Registry)	518	NCA/SVG A/T close	G-R	97	6	39	
Rodriguez et al.[119]†	66	–	G-R / Control	–	4	21.2 / 75.7 }$P < 0.001$	
Burger et al.[120]	119	NCA	Wiktor stent		6	37	
Jaegere et al.[121]	91	NCA	Wiktor stent		6	30	
Umans et al.[125]	174	NCA	87 DCA / 87 PTCA		6	27 / 29 }$P = $ NS	
Topol et al.[126]†	1012	NCA	512 DCA / 500 PTCA	89[a] / 80	6	50 / 57 }$P = 0.06$	
Adelman et al.[127]†	274	NCA (Posterior LAD)	138 DCA / 136 PTCA	98[b] / 88	6	44 / 39 }$P = 0.59$	
Garratt et al.[128]	158	134 NCA / 24 SVG	DCA	88	6	D56 RS62 / D69 RS88	$P < 0.05$ for RS** lesions / $P < 0.05$ for RS lesions
Hinohara et al.[129]	289	NCA/SVG	DCA	85	6	42	SVG, long lesions, small vessels
Popma et al.[130]	305	NCA/SVG	DCA	86	6	44	SVG, long lesions, male
Fishman et al.[131]	190	NCA/SVG	DCA		6	32	
Garratt et al.[132]	70	NCA/SVG	DCA	95	6	50	Deep cuts
Spears et al.[135]	58	NCA	LBA		5.5	51*	
Reis et al.[136]	21	NCA	LBA		6	56	
Karsh et al.[139]	60	NCA	ELCA	91	5.2	46***	
Bitt et al.[140]	200	NCA/SVG	ELCA	91	6	48	
Margolis and Mehta[141] (ELCA registry)	958	NCA/SVG	ELCA	93		51	
Bittl et al.[142] (ELCA registry)	764	NCA/SVG	ELCA	86	6	60	Long lesions, stand-alone ELCA
Estella et al.[143]	142	NCA/SVG	ELCA	95 (no ICT)	5.4	52	Long lesions
Teirstein et al.[145]	42	NCA/SVG	RA	76	6.2	59	
Bertrand et al.[146]	51	NCA	RA	86	3–6	31	
Bertrand et al.[147]	129	NCA	RA	95	4.6	38	
Safian et al.[148]	104	NCA	RA	91	5	51	
Safian et al.[149]	146	SVG	TEC	86	6	69	
Twidale et al.[150]	67	SVG	TEC		6	52	

A/T close, stent placement in acute/threatened closure setting; CTO, chronic total occlusion; D, *de novo* lesions; DCA, directional coronary atherectomy; DS, diameter stenosis; ELCA, excimer laser coronary angioplasty; G–R, Gianturco–Roubin stent; ICT, intracoronary thrombus; LAD, left anterior descending artery; LBA, laser balloon angioplasty; NCA, native coronary arteries; NS, not significant; –, no data available; PS, Palmaz–Schatz stent; RA, rotational atherectomy; RS, restenosis; SVG, saphenous vein grafts; WS, Wallstent.

†Randomized trials. [a]$P < 0.001$ and [b]$P = 0.06$ for difference in success rate between DCA and PTCA.

All RS definition based on the binary criterion except RS* defined on clinical criteria; RS** defined as increase of $\geq 30\%$ luminal diameter on late follow-up; RS*** defined as loss of $\geq 50\%$ initial gain in luminal diameter.

Directional coronary atherectomy (DCA)

Unlike PTCA, this treatment modality debulks atheroma and is associated with less vessel wall recoil and dissection.[123,124] The result is that the final lumen is much larger than after PTCA,[94,125,126] but usually smaller than after stent implantation.[93,94,107] The fundamental question of whether this larger luminal diameter imparted by DCA will ultimately translate into a lower restenosis rate was recently addressed by several studies.

Data from two nonrandomized studies have yielded contradictory results. Kuntz et al.[94] found that the acute gain following DCA was larger compared with PTCA (2.21 mm vs 1.14 mm; $P < 0.01$); this resulted in a lower restenosis rate after treatment with DCA (32% vs 42%; $P = 0.06$). In contrast, Umans et al.[125] failed to show any significant difference in the incidence of restenosis after DCA and PTCA (27% vs 29%, respectively). One possible explanation for this disparity in long-term outcome in the two studies is that the initial gain and final lumen following DCA were larger in the Beth Israel study[94] compared to the Thoraxcenter study,[125] thereby permitting more intimal thickening to occur before the onset of hemodynamically significant luminal narrowing (⩾50% luminal diameter).

The reports from two recent randomized trials[126,127] have not demonstrated the anticipated improved restenosis risk with DCA. The multicenter CAVEAT trial[126] which randomized 1012 patients to DCA ($n = 512$) and PTCA ($n = 500$) showed almost similar six-month angiographic restenosis rates for DCA and PTCA (50% and 57%, respectively; $P = 0.06$). Besides, a higher rate of early complications in the DCA group (11% vs 5% for PTCA; $P < 0.001$) was also observed. Subgroup analysis, however, showed that patients with stenosis in the proximal left anterior descending artery had a lower restenosis rate after DCA than after PTCA (51% vs 63%, respectively; $P = 0.04$). Thus, the marginal reduction in restenosis conferred by DCA was confined largely to the proximal left anterior descending artery.

In another randomized trial (CCAT)[127] comparing the two procedures in the treatment of proximal left anterior descending artery restenosis, the initial gain in minimal luminal diameter was larger with DCA than PTCA. However, there was a larger late loss nullifying the greater initial gain in those who received DCA treatment. This resulted in a similar luminal size in the two groups at six-month follow-up angiography. In contrast to the CAVEAT trial, there was no significant reduction in restenosis offered by DCA treatment over that of PTCA for proximal left anterior descending artery stenosis (DCA, 44% vs PTCA, 39%; $P = 0.59$).

Several investigators have found a higher restenosis rate after DCA for vein grafts than native coronary arteries;[128–130] others have not.[131] Most studies,[128–131] however, disclosed an unacceptably high restenosis rate for restenotic vein graft lesions treated with DCA (range 78–88%) compared to de novo graft lesions (up to 56%). Long lesions (>1 cm length)[130] and small vessels[129,132] have also been noted to predispose to restenosis.

This lack of hard evidence of a salutary effect on the restenosis process following DCA could be secondary to a combination of factors. The residual lumen after DCA is often smaller than after stenting and, hence, less tolerant of subsequent late loss and allows for a higher probability of restenosis. Furthermore, DCA often produces aggressive resection resulting in the retrieval of deep arterial-wall components, and subsequent coronary ectasia and aneurysms (about 10%);[133] medial and adventitial tissues have been demonstrated in about 60% and 30% of specimens, respectively.[8,131–134] This extensive injury stimulates a proportionately exaggerated intimal proliferative response resulting in restenosis. To overcome this shortcoming, modification is necessary of the DCA technique and catheter design or the application of intraprocedural intravascular ultrasound to optimize the results, by providing a guide and better control over the site and depth of tissue resection; this in turn may improve the long-term results. Until further data are available, whether there exists a profound impact of this new technology on restenosis remains controversial.

Laser balloon angioplasty (LBA)

Although associated with a high success rate and low complication risk and has proven itself extremely effective as a bailout device for post-PTCA acute closures, often re-establishing antegrade flow, salvaging myocardium and obviating the need for emergency bypass surgery, LBA has been rather disappointing and inadequate as a means for preventing restenosis. Its overall restenosis rate[93,135,136] is higher than that of conventional PTCA and is even higher if high laser energy is used.[135]

Excimer laser coronary angioplasty (ELCA)

ELCA produces a high success rate of about 90–95% in both native coronary arteries and saphenous vein grafts, but adjunct PTCA is required in about 70–90% of cases because the residual post-ELCA stenosis remains substantial (average 50%). PTCA further reduces the stenosis to about 25%. A 1–2% incidence of perforation has been reported with this device.[137,138] Long-term studies have identified a 30–50% restenosis rate, comparable with that of conventional PTCA.[139–143] Thus, as a tool to prevent restenosis, ELCA is not superior to PTCA. However, its advantage lies in the treatment of either heavily calcified, ostial or diffusely diseased lesions where the acute success rate and major complication rate following ELCA appear more favorable than those of PTCA.

Rotational atherectomy (RA)

High-speed RA pulverizes the atheromatous plaques into small microparticles and often creates a smooth luminal surface without deep cuts into the vessel wall.[137] It seems particularly well suited in the treatment of the 1–4% of lesions which have failed with conventional PTCA (e.g. balloon failing to cross or adequately dilate the lesion).[144] It is also useful in the ablation of heavily calcified or long lesions although a high incidence of vasospasm, and no-reflow phenomenon and non-Q wave myocardial infarction in lesions with large atheromatous burden have been encountered presumably secondary to blockage of the distal small vessels from the large amount of debris generated.[145] Adjunct PTCA to optimize the luminal result is frequently required (about 70%). The overall incidence of restenosis is between 30 and 50% and hence offers no advantage over PTCA in this respect.[145–148]

Transluminal extraction-endarterectomy catheter (TEC)

There are relatively sparse data on this particular device. Suffice to say, it is linked with a high success rate, usually in excess of 90%, for both native coronary and vein graft vessels.[137,149,150] However, the majority of TEC procedures require PTCA assistance to improve upon the often significant post-TEC residual luminal stenosis. Preliminary long-term results have identified a restenosis rate not different from PTCA.[137,149,150] Because its intrinsic debris aspiration mechanism potentially attenuates the risk of distal embolization, the current clinical utility of TEC might be in treating thrombus-laden vessels or degenerated vein grafts although even this niche is controversial because of conflicting results in the risk of distal embolization in such a scenario.[95,149]

Local delivery and new developments

Systemic application of drugs to limit lesional recurrence has largely been ineffective, perhaps in part because its inability to provide high drug concentrations at the target site. Local drug delivery, on the other hand, addresses this deficiency of systemic drug application by allowing for local drug treatment at high concentrations, many times higher than oral or intravenous dosing, without causing severe systemic side effects.[19] It is an attractive approach and offers an alternative therapeutic modality that may be more efficacious than systemic treatment in eventually curbing restenosis. Furthermore, potentially useful but toxic agents/products which would otherwise be unlikely to be used because of the hazards of such toxic therapy for a relatively benign though troublesome process may be applied via this route.[72]

There are a number of alternative methods of directly infusing drugs at the site of balloon-induced tissue disruption. One such method is with the use of perforated or infusion balloons. Several investigators working with this balloon system have found that this experimental technique of drug delivery causes significant local tissue damage and necrosis particularly when high delivery pressures and large volumes of infusate are utilized.[151–154] Wolinsky et al.[151,152] and Santoian et al.[153] demonstrated a positive correlation between perfusion pressure, depth of wall injury and duration of local drug action. Rasheed and co-investigators[154] found that local intramural delivery through an infusion balloon of ≤4 ml of aqueous solution infused at 4 atm. into diseased animal vessels after standard balloon angioplasty did not result in any worsening in arterial wall dissection either angiographically or histologically compared with balloon angioplasty alone.

Other local delivery techniques include implantation of polymer-coated metallic or biodegradable stents impregnated with various drugs,[155] or seeding stents and vascular prosthetic grafts with genetically-primed cellular elements.[156–158] Direct gene transfer into the injured vessel wall is also another possibility.[159,160] Polymeric stents, in addition to drug-eluting capability, have the potential to be biodegradable and possess high tensile strength. Initial experimental studies, however, have yielded discouraging results because of a high incidence of early thrombotic closure and high restenosis rate.[161,162] The intimal proliferation elicited by PET stents was associated with both a pronounced chronic foreign-body inflammatory reaction around the individual stent filaments and extensive SMC proliferation. Furthermore, polymeric implants are well known for their tendency to calcify with time.

In contrast, naturally occurring compounds like fibrin, phosphatidylcholine and collagen are not only potentially nonthrombogenic and have drug-eluting capability, they do not, in addition, seem to induce the same intense vessel-wall reaction seen with polymers.[163,164] Thus, stents made of, or coated with, these materials may offer an attractive bioresorbable alternative to polymers. They are, however, still in the experimental stages of development.

Other concepts which are currently being explored include strategies to target the various growth factors or their receptors for inhibition such as antibodies against such substances as PDGF and bFGF, and conjugating growth factors with cytotoxics.[21]

Even though such varied local delivery systems appear appealing, there are still many unresolved and confounding issues that need to be urgently researched and answered before commencement of clinical trials of this nature are feasible.

Conclusion

The failure to effectively circumvent the problem of restenosis, the Achilles' heel of PTCA, after a decade of research underscores the complexity of the restenosis phenomenon which, to date, has not been fully elucidated and is not well understood. Drugs which have been shown to reduce intimal hyperplasia in experimental preparations have proved to be disappointing in humans with no major positive results. The concept of delivering drugs and/or gene-transfer technology locally via either balloon-based method or drug-eluting stents is exciting, and may provide part of the solution in the search for a 'magic bullet' that can favorably modify intimal hyperplasia. However, major strides are still needed in this area of research before any conclusion regarding its clinical utility can be made.

Given the multimechanistic nature of restenosis, perhaps it is oversimplistic to expect a single therapy (drug or mechanical) will be completely effective in overcoming this problem. The solution will most likely be a multifactorial approach, possibly involving the use of drug therapy in conjunction with adjunctive second-generation interventional devices. Of these devices, the niche for intracoronary stenting in the prevention of restenosis certainly looks most promising, particularly as it confers the most optimal post-treatment luminal size in comparison to other devices, including DCA. This geometric benefit may ultimately be reflected in a lower restenosis risk in accordance with the 'bigger is better' (or perhaps more aptly termed 'normal is better') principle which emphasizes the close relationship between a bigger initial gain and a lower risk of restenosis. Indeed, there are data from observational and randomized studies to support this long-term favorable outcome after the placement of certain stent models. Finally, while it is ideal and certainly pleasing to the interventionalist to obtain the smallest residual stenosis and as large a postintervention lumen as possible, it cannot be overemphasized that this goal should be achieved safely.

References

1. Fanelli, C. and Aronoff, R. (1990) Restenosis following coronary angioplasty. *Am. Heart J.*, **119**, 357–68.
2. Lau, K. W. and Sigwart, U. (1992) Restenosis after PTCA: risk factors and pathophysiology. *J. Myocard. Ischemia*, **4**(6), 15–33.
3. Detre, K., Holubkov, R., Kelsey, S. *et al.* (1988) PTCA in 1985–1986 and 1977–1981. The NHLBI Registry. *N. Engl. J. Med.*, **318**, 265–70.
4. Essed, C. E., van der Brand, M. and Becker, A. E. (1983) Transluminal coronary angioplasty and early restenosis: fibrocellular occlusion after wall laceration. *Br. Heart J.*, **49**, 393–6.
5. Becker, A. E. (1992) The urge to prevent restenosis after PTCA. Scylla and Charybdis in disguise [Editorial]. *Circulation*, **85**, 1632–3.
6. Karas, S. P., Gravanis, M. B., Santoian, E. C. *et al.* (1992) Coronary intimal proliferation after balloon injury and stenting in swine: an animal model of restenosis. *J. Am. Coll. Cardiol.*, **20**, 467–74.
7. Austin, G. E., Ratliff, N. B., Hollman, J. *et al.* (1985) Intimal proliferation of smooth muscle cells as an explanation for recurrent coronary artery stenosis after PTCA. *J. Am. Coll. Cardiol.*, **6**, 369–75.
8. Safian, R. D., Gelbfish, J. S., Erny, R. E. *et al.* (1990) Coronary atherectomy: clinical, angiographic and histological findings and observations regarding potential mechanisms. *Circulation*, **82**, 69–79.
9. Ueda, M., Becker, A. E., Tsukada, T. *et al.* (1991) Fibrocellular tissue response after PTCA: an immunocytochemical analysis of the cellular composition. *Circulation*, **83**, 1327–32.
10. Nobuyoshi, M., Kimura, T., Ohishi, H. *et al.* (1991) Restenosis after PTCA: pathological observations in 20 patients. *J. Am. Coll. Cardiol.*, **17**, 433–9.
11. Garratt, K. N., Edwards, W. D., Kaufmann, U. P. *et al.* (1991) Differential histopathology of primary atherosclerotic and restenotic lesions in coronary arteries and saphenous vein bypass grafts: analysis of tissue obtained from 73 patients by directional atherectomy. *J. Am. Coll. Cardiol.*, **17**, 442–8.
12. van Beusekom, H. M. M., van der Giessen, W. J., van Suylen, R. J. *et al.* (1993) Histology after stenting of human saphenous vein bypass grafts: observations from surgically excised grafts 3 to 320 days after stent implantation. *J. Am. Coll. Cardiol.*, **21**, 45–54.
13. MacLeod, D. C., Strauss, B. H., de Jong, M. *et al.* (1994) Proliferation and extracellular matrix synthesis of smooth muscle cells cultured from human coronary atherosclerotic and restenotic lesions. *J. Am. Coll. Cardiol.*, **23**, 59–65.
14. Ross, R. (1986) The pathogenesis of atherosclerosis – an update. *N. Engl. J. Med.*, **314**, 488–500.
15. Ip, J. H., Fuster, V., Badimon, L., Badimon, J. *et al.* (1990) Syndromes of accelerated atherosclerosis: role of vascular injury and smooth muscle cell proliferation. *J. Am. Coll. Cardiol.*, **15**, 1667–87.
16. Steele, P. M., Chesebro, J. H., Stanson, A. W. *et al.* (1985) Balloon angioplasty. Natural history of the pathophysiological response to injury in a pig model. *Circ. Res.*, **57**, 105–12.
17. Wilentz, J. R., Sanborn, T. A., Haudenschild, C. C. *et al.* (1987) Platelet accumulation in experimental angioplasty: time course and relation to vascular injury. *Circulation*, **75**, 636–42.

18. Gasperetti, C. M., Gonias, S. L., Gimple, L. W. and Powers, E. R. (1993) Platelet activation during coronary angioplasty in humans. *Circulation*, **88**, 2728–34.
19. Schwartz, R. S., Edwards, W. D., Huber, K. C. *et al.* (1993) Coronary restenosis: prospects for solution and new perspectives from a porcine model. *Mayo Clin. Proc.*, **68**, 54–62.
20. Harker, L. A. (1987) Role of platelets and thrombus in mechanisms of acute occlusion and restenosis after angioplasty. *Am. J. Cardiol.*, **60**, 20B–28B.
21. Cooke, J. P. and Candipan, R. (1994) Vascular biology of restenosis: insights for therapeutic strategies. *J. Invas. Cardiol.*, **6**, 25–35.
22. Casscells, N. (1992) Migration of smooth muscle and endothelial cells. Critical events in restenosis. *Circulation*, **86**, 723–9.
23. Fingerle, J., Johnson, R., Clowes, A. W. *et al.* (1989) Role of platelets in smooth muscle cell proliferation and migration after vascular injury in rat carotid artery. *Proc. Natl Acad. Sci. USA*, **86**, 8412–16.
24. Daemen, M. J. A. P., Lombardi, D. M., Bosman, F. T. and Schwartz, S. M. (1991) Angiotensin II reduces smooth muscle cell proliferation in the normal and injured rat arterial wall. *Circ. Res.*, **68**, 450–6.
25. Powell, J. S., Clozel, J. P., Muller, R. K. M. *et al.* (1989) Inhibitors of angiotensin-converting enzyme prevent myointimal proliferation after vascular injury. *Science*, **245**, 186–8.
26. Powell, J. S., Muller, R. K. M. and Baumgartner, H. R. (1991) Suppression of the vascular response to injury: the role of angiotensin-converting enzyme inhibitors. *J. Am. Coll. Cardiol.*, **17**, 137B–142B.
27. Burden, T. S., Resink, T. J., Hahn, A. W. A. and Buhler, F. R. (1990) Induction of thrombospondin expression in vascular smooth muscle cells by angiotensin II. *J. Cardiovasc. Pharmacol.*, **16**(Supp. 7), 17–20.
28. Powell, J. S., Muller, R. K. M., Rouge, M. *et al.* (1990) The proliferative response to vascular injury is suppressed by angiotensin-converting enzyme inhibition. *J. Cardiovasc. Pharmacol.*, **16**(Supp. 4), 42–9.
29. Powell, J. S., Rouge, M., Muller, R. K. and Baumgartner, H. R. (1991) Cilazapril suppresses myointimal proliferation after vascular injury: effects on growth factor induction and vascular smooth muscle cells. *Basic Res. Cardiol.*, **86**(Supp. 1), 65–74.
30. Itoh, H., Pratt, R. E., Gibbons, G. H. and Dzau, V. J. (1991) Angiotensin II modulates proliferation of vascular smooth muscle cells via dual autocrine loops of transforming growth factor-beta and basic fibroblast growth factor. (Abstract) *Hypertension*, **18**, 22.
31. Rensing, B. J., Hermans, W. R., Beatt, K. J. *et al.* (1990) Quantitative angiographic assessment of elastic recoil after PTCA. *Am. J. Cardiol.*, **66**, 1039–44.
32. Hanet, C., Wijns, W., Michel, X. and Schroeder, E. (1991) Influence of balloon size and stenosis morphology on immediate and delayed elastic recoil after PTCA. *J. Am. Coll. Cardiol.*, **18**, 506–11.
33. Haude, M., Erbel, R., Issa, H. and Meyer, J. (1993) Quantitative analysis of elastic recoil after balloon angioplasty and after intracoronary implantation of balloon-expandable Palmaz–Schatz stents. *J. Am. Coll. Cardiol.*, **21**, 26–34.
34. Val, P. G., Bourassa, M. G., David, P. R. *et al.* (1987) Restenosis after successful PTCA: The Montreal Heart Institute experience. *Am. J. Cardiol.*, **60**, 50B–55B.
35. Serruys, P. W., Luitjen, H. E., Beatt, K. J. *et al.* (1988) Incidence of restenosis after successful coronary angioplasty: a time-related phenomenon. *Circulation*, **77**, 361–71.
36. Nobuyoshi, M., Kimura, T., Nosaka, H. *et al.* (1988) Restenosis after successful PTCA: serial angiographic follow-up of 229 patients. *J. Am. Coll. Cardiol.*, **12**, 616–23.
37. Libby, P. and Hansson, G. K. (1991) Involvement of the immune system in human atherogenesis. *Lab. Invest.*, **64**, 5–15.
38. Berk, B. C., Gordon, J. B. and Alexander, R. W. (1991) Pharmacologic roles of heparin and glucocorticoids to prevent restenosis after coronary angioplasty. *J. Am. Coll. Cardiol.*, **17**, 111B–117B.
39. Chapman, H. A., Varrin, Z. and Hibbs, J. B. (1982) Macrophage fibrinolytic activity: identification of two pathways of plasmin formation by intact cells and of a plasminogen activator inhibitor. *Cell*, **28**, 653–62.

40. Libby, P., Warner, S. J. C., Salomon, R. N. and Birinyi, L. K. (1988) Production of platelet-derived growth factor-like mitogen by smooth muscle cells from human atheroma. *N. Engl. J. Med.*, **318**, 1493–8.
41. Bertrand, M. E., Lablanche, J. M., Fourrier, J. L. *et al.* (1989) Relation of restenosis after PTCA to vasomotion of the dilated segment. *Am. J. Cardiol.*, **63**, 277–81.
42. Ardissimo, D., Barberis, P., de Servi, S. *et al.* (1991) Abnormal coronary vasomotion as a predictor of restenosis after successful coronary angioplasty in patients with unstable angina pectoris. *N. Engl. J. Med.*, **325**, 1053–7.
43. Shimokawa, H. and Vanhoutte, P. (1991) Angiographic demonstration of hyperconstriction induced by serotonin and aggregating platelets in porcine coronary arteries with regenerated endothelium. *J. Am. Coll. Cardiol.*, **17**, 1197–202.
44. McFadden, E. P., Bauters, C., Lablanche, J. M. *et al.* (1993) Response of human coronary arteries to serotonin after injury by coronary angioplasty. *Circulation*, **88**, 2076–85.
45. Whitworth, H. B., Roubin, G. S., Hollman, J. *et al.* (1986) Effects of nifedipine on recurrent stenosis after PTCA. *J. Am. Coll. Cardiol.*, **8**, 1271–6.
46. Corcos, T., David, P. R., Val, P. G. *et al.* (1985) Failure of diltiazem to prevent restenosis after PTCA. *Am. Heart. J.*, **109**, 926–31.
47. Hoberg, E., Dietz, R., Frees, U. *et al.* (1994) Verapamil treatment after coronary angioplasty in patients at high risk of recurrent stenosis. *Br. Heart J.*, **71**, 254–60.
48. Schwartz, L., Bourassa, M. G., Lesperance, J. *et al.* (1988) Aspirin and dipyridamole in the prevention of restenosis after PTCA. *N. Engl. J. Med.*, **318**, 1714–19.
49. Chesebro, J. H., Webster, M. W. I., Reeder, G. S. *et al.* (1989) Coronary angioplasty antiplatelet therapy reduces acute complications but not restenosis. (Abstract) *Circulation*, **80**(Supp. 2), 64.
50. Thornton, M. A., Gruentzig, A. R., Hollman, J. *et al.* (1984) Coumadin and aspirin in the prevention of recurrence after transluminal coronary angioplasty: a randomized study. *Circulation*, **69**, 721–7.
51. Bertrand, M. E., Allain, H. and Lablanche, J. M. (1990) Results of a randomized trial of ticlopidine vs placebo for prevention of acute closure and restenosis after coronary angioplasty. The TACT study. (Abstract) *Circulation*, **82**(Supp. 3), 190.
52. White, C. W., Knudson, M., Schmidt, D. *et al.* (1987) Neither ticlopidine nor aspirin–dipyridamole prevents restenosis post-PTCA: results from a randomized placebo-controlled multicenter trial. (Abstract) *Circulation*, **76**(Supp. 4), 213.
53. Okamoto, S., Inden, M., Setsuda, M. *et al.* (1992) Effects of trapidil (triazolopyrimidine), a platelet-derived growth factor antagonist, in preventing restenosis after PTCA. *Am. Heart J.*, **123**, 1439–44.
54. The Multicenter Italian Research Trial with trapidil in the prevention of restenosis after PTCA (STARC) (1993) Trapidil (PDGF) inhibitor prevents restenosis after PTCA: results of the STARC study. (Abstract) *Circulation*, **88**(Supp. 4), 595.
55. Serruys, P. W., Rutsch, W., Heyndrickx, G. R. *et al.* (1991) Prevention of restenosis after PTCA with thromboxane A_2-receptor blockade. A randomized double-blind placebo controlled trial. *Circulation*, **84**, 1568–80.
56. Bove, A., Savage, M., Deutsch, E. *et al.* (M-HEART investigators) (1992) Effects of selective and non-selective thromboxane A_2 blockade on restenosis after PTCA: M-HEART II. (Abstract) *J. Am. Coll. Cardiol.*, **19**, 259A.
57. Knudtson, M. L., Flintoft, V. F., Roth, D. L. *et al.* (1990) Effect of short-term prostacyclin administration on restenosis after PTCA. *J. Am. Coll. Cardiol.*, **15**, 691–7.
58. Raizner, A. E., Hollman, J., Abukhalil, J. and Demke, D. (1993) Ciprostene for restenosis revisited: quantitative analysis of angiograms. (Abstract) *J. Am. Coll. Cardiol.*, **21**, 321A.
59. Tcheng, J. E., Ellis, S., Kleiman, N. S. *et al.* (1993) Outcome of patients treated with the GPIIb/IIIa inhibitor integrelin during coronary angioplasty: results of the IMPACT study. (Abstract) *Circulation*, **88**(Supp. 2), 595.
60. Urban, P., Buller, N., Fox, K. *et al.* (1988) Lack of effect of warfarin on the restenosis rate or on clinical outcome after balloon angioplasty. *Br. Heart J.*, **60**, 485–8.

61. Ellis, S. G., Roubin, G. S., Wilentz, J. *et al.* (1989) Effect of 18 to 24 hour heparin administered for prevention of restenosis after uncomplicated coronary angioplasty. *Am. Heart J.*, **117**, 777–82.
62. Lehmann, K. G., Doria, R. J., Feuer, J. M. *et al.* (1991) Paradoxical increase in restenosis rate with chronic heparin use, final results of a randomized trial. (Abstract) *J. Am. Coll. Cardiol.*, **17**, 181A.
63. Currier, J. W., Pow, T. K., Haudenschild, C. C. *et al.* (1991) Low molecular weight heparin (enoxaparin) reduces restenosis after iliac angioplasty in the hypercholesterolemic rabbit. *J. Am. Coll. Cardiol.*, **17**, 118B–125B.
64. Hanke, H., Oberhoff, M., Hanke, S. *et al.* (1992) Inhibition of cellular proliferation after experimental balloon angioplasty by low-molecular-weight heparin. *Circulation*, **85**, 1548–56.
65. Faxon, D., Spiro, T., Minor, S. *et al.* (1992) Enozaparin, a low molecular weight heparin, in the prevention of restenosis after angioplasty: results of a double blind randomized trial. (Abstract) *J. Am. Coll. Cardiol.*, **19**, 258A.
66. Heras, M., Chesebro, J. H., Penny, W. J. *et al.* (1989) Effects of thrombin inhibition on the development of acute platelet-thrombus deposition during angioplasty in pigs. Heparin vs recombinant hirudin, a specific thrombin inhibitor. *Circulation*, **79**, 657–65.
67. van den Bos, A. A., Deckers, J. W., Heyndrickx, G. R. *et al.* (1993) Safety and efficacy of recombinant hirudin (CGP 39393) vs heparin in patients with stable angina undergoing coronary angioplasty. *Circulation*, **88**, 2058–66.
68. Stone, G. W., Rutherford, B. D., McConahay, D. R. *et al.* (1989) A randomized trial of corticosteroids for the prevention of restenosis in 102 patients undergoing repeat coronary angioplasty. *Cathet. Cardiovasc. Diagn.*, **18**, 227–31.
69. Pepine, C. J., Hirshfeld, J. W., Macdonald, R. G. *et al.* (M-HEART group) (1990) A controlled trial of corticosteroids to prevent restenosis after coronary angioplasty. *Circulation*, **81**, 1753–61.
70. The multicenter European research trial with cilazapril after angioplasty to prevent transluminal coronary obstruction and restenosis (MERCATOR) study group (1992) Does the new angiotensin converting enzyme inhibitor cilazapril prevent restenosis after PTCA? *Circulation*, **86**, 100–10.
71. Desmet, W. J., Vrolix, M. C., de Scheerder, I. K. *et al.* (1994) Angiotensin-converting enzyme inhibition with fosinopril sodium in the prevention of restenosis after coronary angioplasty. *Circulation*, **89**, 385–92.
72. Muller, D. W. M., Ellis, S. G. and Topol, E. J. (1991) Colchicine and antineoplastic therapy for the prevention of restenosis after percutaneous coronary interventions. *J. Am. Coll. Cardiol*, **17**, 126B–131B.
73. O'Keefe, J. H., McCalister, B. D., Baterman, T. M. *et al.* (1992) Ineffectiveness of colchicine for the prevention of restenosis after coronary angioplasty. *J. Am. Coll. Cardiol.*, **19**, 1597–600.
74. Kent, K. N., Williams, D. O., Cassagneau, B. *et al.* (1993) Double-blind, controlled trial of the effect of angiopeptin on coronary restenosis following coronary angioplasty. (Abstract) *Circulation*, **88**(Supp. 1), 506.
75. Eriksen, U. H., Amtorp, O., Bagger, J. P. *et al.* (Angiopeptin Study Group) (1993) Continuous angiopeptin infusion reduces coronary restenosis following balloon angioplasty. (Abstract) *Circulation*, **88**(Supp. 1), 594.
76. Serruys, P. W., Klein, W., Tijssen, J. P. G. *et al.* (1993) Evaluation of ketanserin in the prevention of restenosis after PTCA. *Circulation*, **88**, 1588–601.
77. Heik, S. C. W., Bracht, M., Benn, H. P. *et al.* (1992) No prevention of restenosis after PTCA with ketanserin: a controlled prospective randomized double blind study. (Abstract) *Circulation*, **86**(Supp. 1), 53.
78. Blankenhorn, D. H., Nessim, S. A., Johnson, R. L. *et al.* (1987) Beneficial effects of combined colestipol–niacin therapy on coronary atherosclerosis and coronary venous bypass grafts. *JAMA*, **257**, 3233–40.

79. Austin, G. E., Hollman, J., Lynn, M. J. and Meyer, N. (1989) Serum lipoprotein levels fail to predict postangioplasty recurrent coronary artery stenosis. *Clev. Clin. J. Med.*, **56**, 509–14.

80. Arora, R. R., Konrad, K., Badhwar, K. and Hollman, J. (1990) Restenosis after transluminal coronary angioplasty: a risk factor analysis. *Cathet. Cardiovasc. Diagn.*, **19**, 17–22.

81. Rozenman, Y., Gilon, D., Welber, S. *et al.* (1993) Plasma lipoproteins are not related to restenosis after successful coronary angioplasty. *Am. J. Cardiol.*, **72**, 1206–7.

82. Sahni, R., Maniet, A. R., Voci, G. and Banka, V. S. (1991) Prevention of restenosis after lovastatin after successful coronary angioplasty. *Am. Heart J.*, **121**, 1600–8.

83. Lovastatin Restenosis Trial Study Group (1994) Lovastatin Restenosis Trial: Results in patients with cholesterol over 200 mg dl^{-1}. (Abstract) *J. Am. Coll. Cardiol.*, 470A.

84. Dehmer, G. J., Popma, J. J., Egerton, K. *et al.* (1988) Reduction in the rate of early restenosis after coronary angioplasty by a diet supplemented with ω-3 fatty acids. *N. Engl. J. Med.*, **319**, 733–40.

85. Grigg, L. E., Kay, T. W. H., Valentine, P. A. *et al.* (1989) Determinants of restenosis and lack of effect of dietary supplementation with eicosapentaenoic acid on the incidence of coronary artery restenosis after angioplasty. *J. Am. Coll. Cardiol.*, **13**, 665–72.

86. Reis, G. J., Boucher, T. M., Slipperly, M. E. *et al.* (1989) Randomized trial of fish oil for the prevention of restenosis after coronary angioplasty. *Lancet*, **ii**, 177–81.

87. Nye, E. R., Ilsley, C. D. J., Ablett, M. B. *et al.* (1990) Effect of eicosapentaenoic acid on restenosis rate, clinical course and blood lipids in patients after PTCA. *Aust. NZ J. Med.*, **20**, 549–52.

88. Bairati, I., Roy, L. and Meyer, F. (1992) Double-blind, randomized controlled trial of fish oil supplements in prevention of recurrence of stenosis after coronary angioplasty. *Circulation*, **85**, 950–6.

89. Gapinski, J. P., van Ruiswyk, J. V., Heudebert, G. R. and Schectman, G. S. (1993) Preventing restenosis with fish oils following coronary angioplasty. A meta-analysis. *Arch. Intern. Med.*, **153**, 1595–601.

90. Levine, S., Ewels, C. J., Rosing, D. R. and Kent, K. M. (1985) Coronary angioplasty: clinical and angiographic follow-up. *Am. J. Cardiol.*, **55**, 673–6.

91. Leimgruber, P. P., Roubin, G. S., Hollman, J. *et al.* (1986) Restenosis after successful coronary angioplasty in patients with single vessel disease. *Circulation*, **73**, 710–17.

92. Rapold, H. J., Val, P. G., Mata, A. L. *et al.* (1987) Restenosis and its determinants in first and repeat coronary angioplasty. *Eur. Heart J.*, **8**, 575–86.

93. Kuntz, R. E., Safian, R. D., Levine, M. J. *et al.* (1992) Novel approach to the analysis of restenosis after the use of three new coronary devices. *J. Am. Coll. Cardiol.*, **19**, 1493–9.

94. Kuntz, R. E., Gibson, M., Nobuyoshi, M. and Baim, D. S. (1993) Generalized model of restenosis after conventional balloon angioplasty, stenting and directional atherectomy. *J. Am. Coll. Cardiol.*, **21**, 15–25.

95. Lau, K. W. and Sigwart, U. (1993) Angioplasty, stenting, atherectomy and laser treatment after coronary artery bypass grafting. *Curr. Opin. Cardiol.*, **8**, 951–62.

96. Laskey, W. K., Brady, S. T., Kussmaul, W. G. *et al.* (1993) Intravascular ultrasonographic assessment of the results of coronary artery stenting. *Am. Heart J.*, **125**, 1576–91.

97. Urban, P., Sigwart, U., Golf, S. *et al.* (1989) Intravascular stenting for stenosis of aortocoronary venous bypass grafts. *J. Am. Coll. Cardiol.*, **13**, 1085–91.

98. Strauss, B. H., Serruys, P. W., de Scheerder, I. K. *et al.* (1991) Relative risk analysis of angiographic predictors of restenosis within the coronary Wallstent. *Circulation*, **84**, 1636–43.

99. Strauss, B. H., Serruys, P. W., Bertrand, M. E. *et al.* (1992) Quantitative angiographic follow-up of the coronary Wallstent in native vessels and bypass grafts (European experience – March 1986 to March 1990). *Am. J. Cardiol.*, **69**, 475–81.

100. de Scheerder, I. K., Strauss, B. H., de Feyter, P. J. *et al.* (1992) Stenting of venous bypass grafts: a new treatment modality for patients who are poor candidates for reintervention. *Am. Heart J.*, **123**, 1046–54.
101. Lau, K. W., Gunnes, P., Williams, M. *et al.* (1992) Angiographic restenosis after successful Wallstent stent implantation: an analysis of risk predictors. *Am. Heart J.*, **124**, 1473–7.
102. Schatz, R. A., Goldberg, S., Leon, M. *et al.* (1991) Clinical experience with the Palmaz–Schatz coronary stent. *J. Am. Coll. Cardiol.*, **17**, 155B–159B.
103. Carrozza, J. P., Kuntz, R. E., Levine, M. J. *et al.* (1992) Angiographic and clinical outcome of intracoronary stenting: immediate and long-term results from a large single-center experience. *J. Am. Coll. Cardiol.*, **20**, 328–37.
104. Herrman, H. C., Buchbinder, M., Clemen, M. W. *et al.* (1992) Emergent use of balloon-expandable coronary artery stenting for failed PTCA. *Circulation*, **86**, 812–19.
105. Colombo, A., Maiello, L., Almagor, Y. *et al.* (1992) Coronary stenting: single institution experience with the initial 100 cases using the Palmaz–Schatz stent. *Cathet. Cardiovasc. Diagn.*, **26**, 171–6.
106. Ellis, S. G., Savage, M., Fischman, D. *et al.* (1992) Restenosis after placement of Palmaz–Schatz stents in native coronary arteries. *Circulation*, **86**, 1834–44.
107. Kuntz, R. E., Safian, R. D., Carrozza, J. P. *et al.* (1992) The importance of acute luminal diameter in determining restenosis after coronary atherectomy or stenting. *Circulation*, **86**, 1827–35.
108. Pomerantz, R. M., Kuntz, R. E., Carrozza, J. P. *et al.* (1992) Acute and long-term outcome of narrowed saphenous vein grafts treated by endoluminal stenting and directional atherectomy. *Am. J. Cardiol.*, **70**, 161–7.
109. Foley, J. B., Penn, I. M., Brown, R. I. G. *et al.* (1992) Safety, success and restenosis after elective coronary implantation of the Palmaz–Schatz stent in 100 patients at a single center. *Am. Heart J.*, **125**, 686–94.
110. Colombo, A., Goldberg, S. I., Almagor, Y. *et al.* (1993) A novel strategy for stent deployment in the treatment of acute or threatened closure complicating balloon coronary angioplasty. *J. Am. Coll. Cardiol.*, **22**, 1887–91.
111. Baim, D. S., Levine, M. J., Leon, M. B. *et al.* (1993) Management of restenosis in the Palmaz–Schatz coronary stent (The US Multicenter experience). *Am. J. Cardiol.*, **71**, 364–6.
112. Kastrati, A., Schomig, A., Dietz, R. *et al.* (1993) Time course of restenosis during the first year after emergency coronary stenting. *Circulation*, **87**, 1498–505.
113. Kimura, T., Nosaka, H., Yokoi, H. *et al.* (1993) Serial angiographic follow-up after Palmaz–Schatz stent implantation: comparison with conventional balloon angioplasty. *J. Am. Coll. Cardiol.*, **21**, 1557–63.
114. Serruys, P. W., de Jaegere, P., Kiemeneij, F. *et al.* (Benestent Study Group) (1994) A comparison of balloon-expandable-stent implantation with balloon in patients with coronary artery disease. *N. Engl. J. Med.*, **331**, 489–95.
115. Fischman, D. L., Leon, M. B., Baim, D. S. *et al.* (1994) (Stent Restenosis Study (STRESS) Investigators) (1994) A randomized comparison of coronary-stent placement and balloon angioplasty in the treatment of coronary artery disease. *N. Engl. J. Med.*, **331**, 496–501.
116. Roubin, G. S., Cannon, A. D., Agrawal, S. K. *et al.* (1992) Intracoronary stenting for acute and threatened closure complicating PTCA. *Circulation*, **85**, 916–27.
117. Hearn, J. A., King, III S. B., Douglas, J. S. *et al.* (1993) Clinical and angiographic outcomes after coronary artery stenting for acute or threatened closure after PTCA. *Circulation*, **88**, 2086–96.
118. George, B. S., Voorhees, III W. D., Roubin, G. S. *et al.* (1993) Multicenter investigation of coronary stenting to treat acute or threatened closure after PTCA: clinical and angiographic outcomes. *J. Am. Coll. Cardiol.*, **22**, 135–43.
119. Rodriguez, A., Santaera, O., Larribau, M. *et al.* (1994) Rational use of coronary stenting to prevent restenosis: a randomized study in lesions with early minimal luminal diameter loss after PTCA. (Abstract) *J. Am. Coll. Cardiol.*, (February, special issue), 118A.

120. Burger, W., Krieken, T., de Jaegere, P. *et al.* (1993) Mid-term follow-up after Wiktor-stent implantation for prevention of restenosis. (Abstract) *J. Am. Coll. Cardiol.*, **21**, 30A.
121. de Jaegere, P., Serruys, P. W., Bertrand, M. *et al.* (1993) Angiographic predictors of recurrence of restenosis after Wiktor stent implantation in native coronary arteries. *Am. J. Cardiol.*, **72**, 165–70.
122. Sigwart, U., Haber, R. H., Kowlachuk, G. J. *et al.* (1993) The new ACS metallic stent: experimental and clinical experience. (Abstract) *Circulation*, **88**, I-646.
123. Tanaglia, A. N., Buller, C. E., Kisslo, K. B. *et al.* (1992) Mechanisms of balloon angioplasty and directional atherectomy as assessed by intracoronary ultrasound. *J. Am. Coll. Cardiol.*, **20**, 685–91.
124. Kimball, B. P., Bui, S., Cohen, E. A. *et al.* (1992) Comparison of acute elastic recoil after directional coronary atherectomy vs standard balloon angioplasty. *Am. Heart J.*, **124**, 1459–66.
125. Umans, V. A., Hermans, W., Foley, D. P. *et al.* (1993) Restenosis after directional coronary atherectomy and balloon angioplasty: comparative analysis based on matched lesions. *J. Am. Coll. Cardiol.*, **21**, 1382–90.
126. Topol, E. J., Leya, F., Pinkerton, C. A. *et al.* (CAVEAT study group) (1993) A comparison of direct atherectomy with coronary angioplasty in patients with coronary artery disease. *N. Engl. J. Med.*, **329**, 221–7.
127. Adelman, A. G., Cohen, E. A., Kimball, B. P. *et al.* (1993) A comparison of directional atherectomy with balloon angioplasty for lesions of the left anterior descending coronary artery. *N. Engl. J. Med.*, **329**, 228–33.
128. Garratt, K. N., Holmes, D. R., Bell, M. R. *et al.* (1992) Results of directional atherectomy of primary atheromatous and restenosis lesions in coronary arteries and saphenous vein grafts. *Am. J. Cardiol.*, **70**, 449–54.
129. Hinohara, T., Robertson, G. C., Selmon, M. R. *et al.* (1992) Restenosis after directional coronary atherectomy. *J. Am. Coll. Cardiol.*, **20**, 623–32.
130. Popma, J. J., de Cesare, N. B., Pinkerton, C. A. *et al.* (1993) Quantitative analysis of factors influencing late lumen loss and restenosis after directional coronary atherectomy. *Am. J. Cardiol.*, **71**, 552–7.
131. Fishman, R. F., Kuntz, R. E., Carrozza, J. P. *et al.* (1992) Long-term results of directional coronary atherectomy: predictors of restenosis. *J. Am. Coll. Cardiol.*, **20**, 1101–10.
132. Garratt, K. N., Holmes, D. R., Bell, M. R. *et al.* (1990) Restenosis following directional coronary atherectomy: differences between primary atheromatous and restenotic lesions and influence of subintimal tissue resection. *J. Am. Coll. Cardiol.*, **16**, 1665–71.
133. Bell, M. R., Garratt, K. N., Bresnahan, J. F. *et al.* (1992) Relation of deep arterial resection and coronary artery aneurysms after directional coronary atherectomy. *J. Am. Coll. Cardiol.*, **20**, 1474–81.
134. de Cesare, N. B., Popma, J. J., Holmes, D. R. *et al.* (1992) Clinical angiographic and histologic correlates of ectasia after directional coronary atherectomy. *Am. J. Cardiol.*, **69**, 314–19.
135. Spears, J. R., Reyes, V. P., Wynne, J. *et al.* (1990) Percutaneous coronary laser balloon angioplasty: initial results of a multicenter experience. *J. Am. Coll. Cardiol.*, **16**, 293–303.
136. Reis, G. J., Pomerantz, R. M., Jenkins, R. D. *et al.* (1991) Laser balloon angioplasty: clinical, angiographic and histologic results. *J. Am. Coll. Cardiol.*, **18**, 193–202.
137. Lau, K. W. and Sigwart, U. (1992) Novel coronary interventional devices: an update. *Am. Heart J.*, **23**, 497–506.
138. Litvack, F., Eigler, N., Margolis, J. *et al.* (1994) Percutaneous excimer laser coronary angioplasty: results in the first consecutive 3000 patients. *J. Am. Coll. Cardiol.*, **23**, 323–9.
139. Karsh, K. R., Haase, K. K., Voelker, W. *et al.* (1990) Percutaneous coronary excimer laser angioplasty in patients with stable and unstable angina pectoris. *Circulation*, **81**, 1849–59.
140. Bittl, J. A. and Sanborn, T. A. (1992) Excimer laser-facilitated coronary angioplasty. Relative risk analysis of acute and follow-up results in 200 patients. *Circulation*, **86**, 71–80.
141. Margolis, J. R. and Mehta, S. (1992) Excimer laser coronary angioplasty. *Am. J. Cardiol.*, **69**, 3F–11F.

142. Bittl, J. A., Sanborn, T. A., Tcheng, J. E. *et al.* (1992) Clinical success, complications and restenosis rate with excimer laser coronary angioplasty. *Am. J. Cardiol.*, **70**, 1533–9

143. Estella, P., Ryan, T. J., Landzberg, J. S. and Bittle, J. A. (1993) Excimer laser-assisted coronary angioplasty for lesions containing thrombus. *J. Am. Coll. Cardiol.*, **21**, 1550–6.

144. Brogan, W. C., Popma, J. J., Pichard, A. D. *et al.* (1993) Rotational coronary atherectomy after unsuccessful coronary balloon angioplasty. *Am. J. Cardiol.*, **71**, 794–8.

145. Teirstein, P. S., Warth, D. C., Haq, H. *et al.* (1991) High speed rotational coronary atherectomy for patients with diffuse coronary artery disease. *J. Am. Coll. Cardiol.*, **18**, 1694–71.

146. Bertrand, M. E., Lablanche, J. M., Fourrier, J. L. *et al.* (1990) Percutaneous coronary rotary ablation. *Cardiovasc. Imag.*, **2**, 217–21.

147. Bertrand, M. E., Lablanche, J. M., Leroy, F. *et al.* (1992) Percutaneous transluminal coronary rotary ablation with Rotablator (European experience). *Am. J. Cardiol.*, **69**, 470–7.

148. Safian, R. D., Niazi, K. A., Strzelecki, M. *et al.* (1993) Detailed angiographic analysis of high-speed mechanical rotational atherectomy in human coronary arteries. *Circulation*, **88**, 961–8.

149. Safian, R. D., Grines, C. L., May, M. A. *et al.* (1994) Clinical and angiographic results of transluminal extraction coronary atherectomy in saphenous vein bypass grafts. *Circulation*, **89**, 302–12.

150. Twidale, N., Barth, C. W., Kipperman, R. M. *et al.* (1994) Acute results and long-term outcome of transluminal extraction catheter atherectomy for saphenous vein graft stenoses. *Cathet. Cardiovasc. Diagn.*, **31**, 187–91.

151. Wolinsky, H. and Thung, S. W. (1990) Use of a perforated balloon catheter to deliver concentrated heparin into the wall of the normal canine artery. *J. Am. Coll. Cardiol.*, **15**, 475–81.

152. Wolinsky, H. and Lin, C. S. (1991) Use of the perforated balloon catheter to infuse marker substances into diseased coronary artery walls after experimental postmortem angioplasty. *J. Am. Coll. Cardiol.*, **17**, 174B–178B.

153. Santoian, E. C., Gravanis, M. B., Schneider, J. E. *et al.* (1993) Use of the porous balloon in porcine coronary arteries. Rationale for low pressure and volume delivery. *Cathet. Cardiovasc. Diagn.*, **30**, 348–54.

154. Rasheed, Q., Cacchione, J. G., Berry, J. *et al.* (1994) Local intramural drug delivery using an infusion balloon following angioplasty in normal and atherosclerotic vessels. *Cathet. Cardiovasc. Diagn.*, **31**, 240–5.

155. Slepian, M. J. (1990) Polymeric endoluminal paving and sealing. Therapeutics at the crossroad of biomechanics and pharmacology. In: Topol, E. J. (ed.) *Textbook of Interventional Cardiology*, pp. 647–70. Philadelphia: W. B. Saunders.

156. Dichek, D. A., Neville, R. F., Zwiebel, J. A. *et al.* (1989) Seeding of intravascular stents with genetically engineered endothelial cells. *Circulation*, **80**, 1347–53.

157. Wilson, J. M., Birinyi, L. K., Salomon, R. N. *et al.* (1989) Implantation of vascular grafts lined with genetically modified cells. *Science* **244**, 1344–6.

158. Flugelman, M. Y., Virmani, R., Leon, M. B. *et al.* (1992) Genetically engineered endothelial cells remain adherent and viable after stent deployment and exposure to flow *in vivo*. *Circ. Res.*, **70**, 348–54.

159. Nabel, E. G., Plautz, G. and Nabel, G. J. (1991) Gene transfer into vascular cells. *J. Am. Coll. Cardiol.*, **17**, 189B–194B.

160. Lee, S. W., Trapnell, B. C., Rade, J. J. *et al.* (1993) *In vivo* adenoviral vector-mediated gene transfer into balloon-injured rat carotid arteries. *Circ. Res.*, **73**, 797–807.

161. Murphy, J. G., Schwartz, R. S., Edwards, W. D. *et al.* (1992) Percutaneous polymeric stents in porcine coronary artery. Initial experience with polyethylene terephthalate. *Circulation*, **86**, 1596–604.

162. van der Giessen, W. J., Slager, C. J., van Beusekom, H. M. M. *et al.* (1992) Development of a polymer endovascular prosthesis and its implantation in porcine arteries, *J. Interven. Cardiol.*, **5**, 175–85.

163. Bier, J. D., Zalesky, P., Li, S. T. *et al.* (1992) A new bioabsorbable intravascular stent. *In vitro* assessment of hemodynamic and morphometric characteristics. *J. Interven. Cardiol.*, **5**, 187–94.
164. Nordrehaug, J. E., Chronos, N. and Sigwart, U. (1994) A biocompatible phosphatidylcholine coating applied to metallic stents. (Abstract) *J. Am. Coll. Cardiol.*, 5A.

2

Local Interventions for Vasculoproliferative Diseases

Aruna Nathan
Elazer R. Edelman

Introduction

Almost two decades after the seminal work of Clowes and Karnovsky demonstrating the remarkable benefit of heparin as an antiproliferative agent in controlling vascular disease in laboratory rats[1] we are left with no clinically useful compound to combat these diseases in man. A multitude of potent agents have been directed against one or more of the cellular events thought to be involved in restenosis[1-22] and virtually all of them, true to form, suppress smooth-muscle cell growth in tissue culture. A large subset of these compounds even reduce proliferation in animal models of vascular disease, and yet the clinical paradox of proliferative vascular diseases is that no drug to date has yielded any demonstrable benefit against human disease. The list of failures includes the most promising classes of agents such as heparin and related compounds,[12,13,23] the angiotensin converting-enzyme inhibitors,[18,24] the calcium-channel blockers[6,16,20,25,26] and steroids.[11]

The implications of these findings are either that animal models of vascular disease do not adequately reflect the complexity of human lesions, and as a result provide positive results for agents that are simply not effective in man, or that the response of animal models can indeed predict activity against human disease but the dose or manner in which these drugs are administered is suboptimal. The melding of the technology of local drug delivery with the science of molecular and cell biology has provided a means by which to investigate this question, and in doing so provides a new perspective to understand the paradox of restenosis, and even a potential solution.

Rationale for continuous and local therapy

The dichotomy between experimental benefit and clinical futility is no more evident than with heparin. Heparin is the gold standard for inhibitors of cultured smooth-muscle cell growth, and is unique in that a natural heparin-like compound may be central to reparative processes that serve as a first-line mechanism in the body's attempt to limit accelerated arteriosclerosis.[1,27–32] Heparin markedly and rapidly inhibits DNA and RNA synthesis in growth arrested cells released from G_0 block.[28] Continuous intravenous infusion of heparin almost completely abolishes intimal smooth-muscle cell proliferation in the injured carotid artery.[1] However, studies initiated to determine whether the beneficial effects of heparin observed in laboratory animals and cell culture could be achieved in humans, paradoxically exhibited exacerbation of vascular injury. For example, when patients were randomized to heparin or dextrose infusion over the first 18–24 hours postangioplasty, 41.2% of the heparinized patients and only 36.7% of the dextrose infusion patients had evidence for restenosis.[12] Moreover, bleeding complications were twice as frequent in the heparinized group. Similarly, when heparin was administered as a single daily subcutaneous injection at 10 000 iu day^{-1}, patients faired so poorly that the trial was halted prematurely;[13] 82% of the patients who received heparin suffered restenosis, almost 2.5-fold more often than the 33% of the patients treated in standard fashion. Angina, myocardial infarction and bleeding complications were virtually nonexistent in the controls, but appeared in 76, 18 and 41% of the heparinized patients, respectively.

One interpretation of the results of these trials is that heparin is ineffective in treating accelerated arteriosclerosis in the human. Alternatively, the marked difference in the way in which drug was administered (continuous administration in rats versus intermittent therapy in humans) might explain the beneficial effect seen in animals and the deleterious effect produced in humans. To address this issue, we examined the effect of a range of heparin treatments on balloon denuding injury performed on the common carotid artery of Sprague–Dawley rats. A heparin preparation that inhibited smooth-muscle cell proliferation in culture[28,33–36] and neointimal hyperplasia in animal models of vascular injury[35–38] was administered as subcutaneous injections at a dose (55.5 iu, equivalent to $c.$ 1.0 mg kg^{-1}) calculated from clinical trials. Heparin injections given every other day or once a day made vascular injury worse (Figure 2.1). The intima:media area ratio was increased 22.5% with injections every other day, and 16.8% with daily injections. This mode of heparin administration was identical to that used in clinical trials, and as observed clinically, vascular injury was exacerbated by heparin. It was not until the drug was administered at 12-hour intervals that intimal hyperplasia and cell proliferation were lessened, and significant reduction in intimal hyperplasia was obtained only when heparin was administered continuously (Figure 2.1).

Continuous therapy, however, currently requires patient immobilization and hospitalization and chronic exposure to compounds with great potential for drug toxicity. The chemical modification of agents like heparin has prolonged their half-lives with the promise of less frequent dosing, but not the elimination of systemic side effects. The limited availability of these modified compounds and the expense of dosing to achieve effective systemic levels curtails their active use.[19,37,39,40] Thus, there is an increased interest in the development of local means of drug therapy. The remainder of this chapter reviews many approaches to local therapy, and attempts to categorize and evaluate them in the general context of vascular therapy.

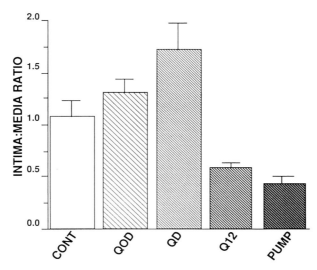

Figure 2.1 Heparin's effect on vascular injury depends on the mode of drug delivery (modified from Ref. 98). Control animals (CONT) exhibit such a significant amount of intimal hyperplasia that the area of the neointima approaches the area of the media. When heparin is delivered in a continuous fashion from osmotic minipumps neointimal hyperplasia is reduced over 60%. However, intermittent dosing is far less effective and as the dosing interval increases, the beneficial effect diminishes. When the drug is administered every day (QD) or even every other day (QOD), as was injected in clinical trials to date, intimal hyperplasia was exacerbated and not alleviated.

Pharmacologic interventions

Intravascular drug delivery via catheters

The most widely reported technique for drug delivery to the arterial wall involves direct intravascular deposition of therapeutic agents using intravascular catheters. Different catheter designs such as the porous balloon,[41] double balloon,[42,43] hydrogel[44,45] and iontophoresis catheters[46] have been suggested for the localized application of a multitude of potent agents (Table 2.1). Most catheter devices have been designed for a single-dose application of the drug at the time of angioplasty.

Porous balloon catheters

The porous balloon catheter was first used for the intravascular delivery of heparin,[41] and has since been used with a number of different compounds. Drug solutions delivered into a balloon under pressure are injected into the arterial wall through small perforations that typically measure 25 μm in diameter. The efficacy of this catheter design depends critically on the infusion pressure. A certain minimum pressure is necessary to fully inflate the balloon and position it against the arterial wall so that downstream distribution and dilution of the drug does not occur. The maximum pressure usually varies between 2 and 5 atm. and is related to the depth of penetration required to achieve transmural deposition of drug in the arterial wall.[47]

Fluorescent labeled heparin was detected throughout the media, and on occasion, to the inner aspect of the adventitia, of canine brachial arteries immediately

Table 2.1 Catheter-based local vascular drug release

Approach	Drug	Animal model	Biologic effect
Porous balloons	Standard heparin	Canine brachial arteries	Arterial retention of drug for up to 48 h at an infusion pressure of 500 mmHg. Higher pressures caused medial necrosis[41]
		Atherosclerotic rabbit femoral arteries	No reduction in restenosis[19]
	Low molecular-weight heparin	Atherosclerotic rabbit carotid arteries	Significant inhibition of smooth-muscle cell proliferation and intimal-wall thickness at early and late time periods[110]
	Angiopeptin	Rabbit abdominal aorta	Reduced proliferation only in area distal to local drug delivery site (downstream effect)[48]
	Methotrexate	Porcine carotid arteries	No reduction in restenosis[15]
	Colchicine	Rabbit femoral arteries	Arterial retention of <1 day. No reduction in restenosis[50]
	Thiol protease inhibitor SERP-1	Rabbit femoral arteries	Reduction in postangioplasty restenosis with preservation of the medial layer.[111] Significant decrease in intimal fatty cellular proliferation
	Polymeric microspheres with colchicine	Rabbit femoral arteries	Severe muscle atrophy and chronic inflammation. No reduction in restenosis[113]
Hydrogel balloons	PPACK	Dacron graft shunts in pigs	Effective inhibition of thrombosis[53]
Iontophoresis	Hirudin	Porcine carotid arteries	50-fold higher hirudin tissue levels than those obtained by passive diffusion or therapeutic systemic doses[112,114,115]
Photodynamic therapy	Chloroaluminum sulfonated phthalocyanine	Rat carotid arteries	Significant decrease in intimal hyperplasia in treated segments of arteries[107]
	8-Methoxypsoralen	Atherosclerotic rabbits	Reduction in smooth-muscle cell proliferation and cellularity in the neointima and media[108]

following catheter infusion.[41] However, when the animals were sacrificed 24–72 hours after infusion, nuclear fluorescence was confined only to the outer 20–25% of the media with marked necrosis of the inner media and prominent polymorpho-nuclear cell infiltration. The necrotic damage was observed when either commercial heparin or normal saline solution was infused, implying that the balloon and the high-pressure infusion caused significant damage to the blood vessel. A beneficial biologic effect has so far not been reported following intravascular delivery of standard heparin from balloon catheters. Gimple *et al.* found that while chronic subcutaneous delivery of heparin reduced intimal hyperplasia in denuded femoral arteries of hypercholesterolemic rabbits, intramural delivery of heparin showed no effect.[19]

Intramural delivery via porous balloon catheters has similarly been attempted for a host of other drugs including angiopeptin,[48] antineoplastic agents such as methotrexate[15] and doxorubicin,[49] and antimitotic agents such as colchicine[50] (Table 2.1). A significant decrease in intimal hyperplasia between drug-treated and control animals has, however, not been observed in any of these cases. Trauma caused by drug delivery using porous balloon catheters may mask any relative benefit resulting from the local administration of the drug itself. High infusion pressures and high-velocity fluid jets can lead to vessel perforations or dissection, increasing the stimulus for proliferation or creating a nidus for thrombus formation. In addition, large volumes of drug solution infused into the arterial wall will displace essential structures, alter vascular compliance and increase overall damage. The infusion of smaller volumes of more concentrated solutions may be less traumatic but expose the artery to greater potential for local drug toxicity. Non-uniform distribution of drug within the arterial wall and an inadequate duration of antiproliferative therapy could also have contributed to the inefficacy of intramural drug therapy.[47]

Several modifications of the single porous balloon have been designed to reduce tissue injury caused by fluid jets. Microporous balloons covered by a permeable polycarbonate membrane (pore size $0.8\,\mu$m) reduce jet-induced injury and channel balloons infuse drug through small perforated channels located on the surface of an angioplasty balloon.[51] A different system for the low-pressure infusion of drugs by use of an expandable stent within the balloon to position the balloon against the arterial wall has also been studied.[52] The optimal delivery protocol for each of these devices is, however, yet to be determined. The biggest challenge with the use of porous balloon catheters is to combine efficient drug delivery with minimal tissue damage so that the beneficial effects of local drug delivery outweigh the potentially negative consequences of the delivery procedure.[47]

Hydrogel-coated balloon catheters

Normal angioplasty balloon catheters can be coated with a hydrophilic polyacrylic acid polymer that can elute drug within a blood vessel with minimal trauma and without the need for special catheters.[44,45] The hydrogel coating has a thickness of only 5–20 mm when dry, and swells by a factor of three when exposed to an aqueous environment. A thin layer of therapeutic agent is applied to the gel-coated balloon and allowed to dry. Balloon inflation against the arterial intimal surface results in active diffusion of agents from the polymer into the vessel wall.

Heparin eluted from a hydrogel catheter was deposited in the arterial wall with a mean average depth of penetration of 1.4 ± 0.7 mm and mean maximal depth of penetration of 1.9 ± 0.9 mm independent of the time of contact or hydrogel thickness.[44] Local delivery of a specific antithrombin D-Phe-Pro-Arg chloromethylketone (PPACK) *in vivo* from such a hydrogel balloon was found to inhibit platelet-dependent thrombosis on thrombogenic Dacron porcine arteriovenous shunts.[53] The drug was dip-coat incorporated onto the balloon and *c.* 50% of it was transferred to the thrombus. Inhibition of radiolabeled platelet deposition was greater than that obtained when the same drug was infused intravenously at a 100-fold greater overall dose. The hydrogel system, however, has limited use. Because the drug is rapidly washed off the balloon after exposure to the bloodstream,[54] a protective sheath must be used, and the time between sheath removal and balloon inflation has to be minimized.

Iontophoresis catheters

Iontophoresis, electric current facilitated transport, has been used to enhance the penetration of drugs through skin, directly to myocardium, or into blood vessel walls.[114,115] Local delivery of ^{125}I-hirudin into normal pig carotid arteries[46] using this approach has been reported. Although vascular levels of hirudin after active iontophoresis (19 mA, 5 min) were 50-fold greater than those achieved by passive diffusion (without electricity), and homogeneously distributed through the arterial wall, the retention of hirudin in the vessel wall was found to decrease rapidly with time.

Drug release from stents

Indwelling devices may serve as endovascular scaffoldings for drug release over a more prolonged period of time than can be achieved with catheter-based systems alone. Endovascular stents have already been used to maintain luminal patency in the setting of abrupt closure of an angioplastied artery, and to combat restenosis in the six months that follow.[55–61] Despite the 95–100% success rate in stent place-ment,[55,57,61] long-term efficacy is limited by thrombosis and intimal hyperplasia. Aggressive antithrombotic regimens have reduced thrombosis within the first two weeks following implantation[59,62] but have not altered restenosis and are accom-panied by complications that include transfusion requiring hemorrhage,[55] thrombo-cytopenia, electrolyte and intravascular volume shifts, allergic reactions and the need for indwelling vascular access for drug infusion.

  The continuous release of antithrombotic or antiproliferative drugs can be effected from stents coated either directly with drugs or with drug-eluting biodegradable polymer materials. Two compositions of heparin coating applied to slotted tube stainless-steel stents reduced thrombosis when compared to uncoated stents after implantation in the left anterior descending (LAD) coronary artery of young pigs. Similarly, polymer-bound heparin $(0.28\,\mu\mathrm{g\,cm^{-2}})$ coated on Nitinol stents was shown to inhibit occlusive thrombosis to a greater extent than bare metal stents in a rabbit model of subacute thrombosis.[63] However, the elimination of thrombosis by heparin released from stents has not been accompanied by a decrease in neointimal hyperplasia. In a recent study, Cox *et al.* have reported no benefit from the local delivery of heparin and methotrexate on neointimal proliferation in a model involving oversized stenting of porcine coronary arteries.[64,65] Yet, like the perfusion balloon, stents can themselves induce such significant injury as to mask or dwarf the benefit for the drug they might deliver.

Local delivery of drugs using polymeric implants

The failure of catheter and stent-based drug release to achieve biologic benefit may derive in part from the limited residence time of these agents within the blood-vessel wall. Drugs delivered in this fashion are cleared rapidly from the arterial wall by both convection and diffusion. Heparin, for instance, has an intravascular half-life of 7–30 min, and when delivered intraluminally via a porous balloon catheter is cleared from the vessel wall within a few hours. To address this problem, the technology of polymer-based controlled drug delivery has been suggested. Polymer-based drug delivery systems offer the potential for quantifiable sustained and controlled release from minute devices that can be implanted adjacent to target tissues.[66–68] Such systems offer distinct advantages over the pumps that have been used to propel substances from a reservoir into the intravascular or extravascular spaces.[66–68] The pumps are large, complex, cumbersome and expensive, have limited storage capacity and require that the drug be stored as a liquid. Polymer-based systems can incorporate drug in dry form, dramatically reducing the size of the device and loss of drugs that are unstable in solution, rapidly degraded, prone to precipitation, or of limited solubility. As a result, polymer-based delivery systems retard release, dramatically decrease device size, prolong shelf-life and diminish drug degradation. We, and others, have used such systems in a variety of disparate systems, including maintenance of euglycemia in diabetic rats,[69] preservation and release of unstable growth factors,[70,71] inhibition or stimulation of tumor growth[72] and/or angiogenesis,[73] suppression of prosthetic heart valve calcification,[74] and induction and control of the immune response.[75]

Local release of heparin

In one set of experiments, we compared polymer-based delivery to the systemic infusion of both standard, anticoagulant and modified, nonanticoagulant heparin. Matrix release devices were prepared by solvent casting with ethylene-vinyl acetate copolymer (EVAc).[71,73] Release kinetics were tailored to provide rapid first-order release or more prolonged near zero-order release by varying the drug loading and by application of a polymer coating around the device (Figure 2.2). The devices were evaluated in a vascular injury model that involved balloon catheter rat common carotid artery endothelial denudation. The intravenous osmotic pump infusion ($0.3 \text{ mg kg}^{-1} \text{ h}^{-1}$) of standard anticoagulant heparin was used as control comparison for local therapy, as it is known to effectively inhibit intimal hyperplasia that follows such injury.[1] A systemic anticoagulated state was achieved with intravenous infusion and activated partial thromboplastin times (aPTT) were elevated 2.5 times the control value. At the same time, intimal hyperplasia from proliferating smooth-muscle cells was reduced by $67.8 \pm 4.3\%$ (Figure 2.3, AC, solid bar). When this same compound was released, at one-fifth the intravenous dose, from EVAc matrices implanted in the dorsal subcutaneous space of a rat subjected to balloon denuding injury, no effect on clotting was observed but the reduction in neointimal formation was maintained (Figure 2.3, AC, hatched bar). These results demonstrated that a potent smooth-muscle cell inhibitor, with profound systemic side effects, could be successfully delivered at a dose low enough to avoid systemic effects, but high enough to provide local protection against vascular disease. The same, however, was not observed with chemically modified antiproliferative nonanticoagulant

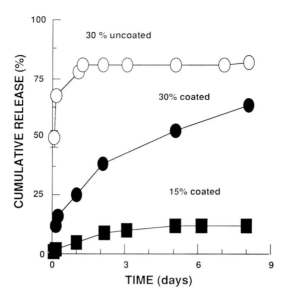

Figure 2.2 Heparin release from ethylene-vinyl acetate copolymer (EVAc) matrices can be modulated by alterations in drug loading, polymer material coating, and matrix geometry (after Ref. 37). Rapid first-order release was obtained from EVAc:heparin matrices (30% w/w). Release was prolonged and the surface drug burst removed when matrices were coated and release constrained to a single hole. If the loading was decreased to 15%, much of the heparin remained trapped within the matrix.

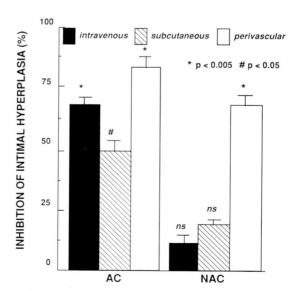

Figure 2.3 The ability of heparin to inhibit intimal hyperplasia is a function of the site of delivery and modification of compound rather than dose alone (modified from Ref. 37). Intravenous and subcutaneous anticoagulant heparin (AC) inhibited intimal hyperplasia, but neither mode was effective for nonanticoagulant heparin (NAC). Perivascular delivery, at 1:5 to 1:100 the dose infused systemically, was the only means where nonanticoagulant heparin inhibited intimal hyperplasia and the most efficient for anticoagulant heparin.

heparin. To avoid the potential for bleeding with increasing doses of the anticoagulant, standard heparin is subjected to periodate oxidation and borohydride reduction. This reduces the size of the polysaccharide, and modifies its chemical
structure so as to remove 90% of its anti-Xa and antithrombotic effect. In culture, this
compound was equipotent as regular heparin on a molar basis at inhibiting the
serum stimulated proliferation of smooth-muscle cells. Continuous intravenous
infusion or polymer matrix-controlled subcutaneous release of this nonanticoagulant heparin, however, had no effect on intimal hyperplasia (Figure 2.3, NAC, solid
and hatched bars).[37]

The truncated size of the nonanticoagulant heparin might increase drug clearance
so as to prevent contact of the drug with the target cells within the injured artery. We
therefore placed controlled-release matrices immediately adjacent to the injured
arteries to increase drug-to-vessel contact time and diminish clearance. Systemic
levels of drug were not detectable as perivascular heparin delivery did not elevate
aPTT, yet perivascular administration produced the greatest inhibition of intimal
hyperplasia. Controlled perivascular release reduced intimal hyperplasia
$83.0 \pm 2.6\%$ with anticoagulant heparin (Figure 2.3, AC, open bar), and $68.3 \pm 3.7\%$
with nonanticoagulant heparin (Figure 2.3, NAC, open bar). Perivascular release
was not only more efficient than the intravenous infusion of anticoagulant heparin,
but was the only means of observing a beneficial effect for nonanticoagulant
heparin. This benefit increased as the dose of nonanticoagulant heparin administered over the course of the two-week experiment was increased. At doses that could
not be administered with anticoagulant heparin because of uncontrolled bleeding,
nonanticoagulant heparin virtually suppressed intimal hyperplasia in its entirety.

Similar effects were noted in more severe forms of vascular injury. The implantation of endovascular stents discussed above induces a fourfold greater stimulus for
cell proliferation and intimal hyperplasia than balloon denudation alone.[76] The
systemic low-dose controlled release of heparin could not regulate this type of
vascular repair, and the endoluminal local release of heparin and/or methotrexate[64,77] did not reduce smooth muscle cell proliferation after 3–4 weeks. To some,
these studies raised the possibility that heparin was ineffective in stent-induced
arteriosclerosis. We wondered whether in fact the reported results were more a
reflection of the failure of systemic dosing for a potent local effect and the inability of
brief periods of release from local devices to control a prolonged form of injury. Intra-
arterial release does not provide heightened local concentration and the release rates
of heparin from the stents are so rapid that 99% of the drug is eluted within the first 2
hours. In addition, without a barrier overlying the release platform most of the drug
released would presumably be rapidly washed away into the bloodstream, and not
deposited within the arterial wall. Thus, we compared the effects of systemic
heparinization with local perivascular release, and two forms of local intraluminal
heparin therapy (Table 2.2). Stainless-steel stents, uncoated, coated with an inert
polymer, coated with immobilized bound heparin or coated with a polymer releasing heparin were balloon-expanded in de-endothelialized iliac arteries. The rate of
release of heparin from the polymer-coated stents was rapid and little heparin was
detectable 2 hours after implantation. Animals with uncoated stents were treated
with heparin via continuous pump infusion, continuous perivascular heparin

Table 2.2   Thrombosis and intimal hyperplasia of endovascular stents with inert or heparin coatings, and systemic or perivascular heparin release

Stent preparation	Thrombosis (%)			Intimal area (mm^2)			
Uncoated–untreated	42			1.2 ± 0.1			
Coated with							
inert polymer	8	$P = 0.004$	86% ↓	1.1 ± 0.1	NS		
immobilized heparin	8	$P = 0.004$	86% ↓	1.1 ± 0.1	NS		
polymer releasing heparin, 2 hours	13	$P = 0.02$	69% ↓	1.8 ± 0.2	$P = 0.02$	80% ↑	
Uncoated–heparin treated							
Perivascular matrix delivered							
3 days	0	$P = 0.007$	100% ↓	0.08 ± 0.1	$P = 0.04$	27% ↓	
14 days	0	$P = 0.04$	100% ↓	0.5 ± 0.1	$P = 0.03$	55% ↓	
Intravenous injection	0	$P = 0.04$	100% ↓	0.4 ± 0.1	$P = 0.002$	64% ↓	

release from a polymer matrix, or perivascular matrix release of heparin with first-order release kinetics completing release within the first three days of implantation. All forms of heparin therapy and all coatings reduced thrombosis 86–100% (Table 2.2). Neointimal thickening, and cell proliferation as determined by proliferating cell nuclear antigenicity (PCNA), were only reduced, however, after continuous heparin infusion or perivascular delivery, and the more prolonged the release, the more effective the inhibition. Perivascular release for the full 14 days of the experiment was twice as effective as release limited to three days. Inert coatings and heparin immobilized to the stent had no effect, and heparin rapidly and locally released from the stent actually increased intimal hyperplasia 80% as a result of an inflammatory reaction to the polymer:heparin complex (Table 2.2).

Further studies demonstrated that while thrombosis peaked early (hours) after stent implantation, intimal hyperplasia was prolonged and indices of cell proliferation remained elevated for an additional nine days. Thus, the examination of local vascular therapy requires a broad view of the responses not limited to one parameter alone, since the vascular response to injury is a multifactorial event involving waves and phases of cellular events that may require different forms of therapy.

In conclusion, local controlled release of heparin inhibited smooth-muscle cell proliferation following injury to vascular endothelium, for anticoagulant heparin without the need for systemic anticoagulation, for anticoagulant heparin when administered from a site distant from the injured vessel and in a manner more efficient than in systemic administration. Nonanticoagulant heparin, though equally effective as the anticoagulant heparin at suppressing smooth-muscle cell proliferation in tissue culture,[37] was virtually ineffective when administered intravenously or subcutaneously and only achieved a therapeutic response when delivered from matrices in the perivascular position. As the dose of perivascularly administered nonanticoagulant heparin was increased, the effect on smooth-muscle cell proliferation rose, such that at the highest dose tested, nonanticoagulant heparin inhibited smooth-muscle cell proliferation to an extent equal to that of anticoagulant heparin. Thus, in addition to demonstrating that subtoxic doses of potent drugs could be controlled released to inhibit smooth-muscle cell proliferation, the data support the hypothesis that it is possible to treat vascular injury as a local disease with local therapy. These results laid the groundwork for examining the local control of the vascular response to injury and for investigating site-specific means of modulating these processes.

Controlled release of basic fibroblast growth factor (bFGF): a biological imperative

In some cases, controlled release of drugs from polymeric devices seems to be the only means by which the vasoactive agents exert an effect. This was particularly the case for bFGF. One of the putative mechanisms by which antiproliferative agents such as heparin stabilize the blood-vessel wall after vascular injury involves their interactions with bFGF and other related growth factors. bFGF is carefully regulated within the local environment of the blood-vessel wall by basement membrane-bound heparin-like compounds such as the heparan sulfate proteoglycans.[78–82] bFGF has a remarkable heparin avidity and binds to these structures on the cell surface and within the extracellular matrix from which they may elute with time. Soluble heparin and heparan sulfate may interfere with this binding and alter the mitogenic effect of this and related compounds. The constantly changing balance between binding and release is required because bFGF has a serum half-life of <3 min[83] and no signal sequence, the genetic code necessary for establishing secretion from the cell. Injury elicits a prolonged, continuous release of sequestered bFGF making the growth factor available until repair is completed.[78–82] This complex and sophisticated release mechanism maintains heightened local concentrations of growth factor and provides a means for the rapid and sustained mobilization of this mitogen. Maciag and colleagues have recently noted that bFGF must be present in the culture media of smooth muscle cells for at least 12 hours before stimulation of growth is observed. If the growth factor is washed away prior to that time, no effect is seen. We have shown that bFGF is most active when controlled released to cells and arteries.[71,84]

A variety of investigators have used controlled administration to both sustain bFGF release and limit the amount of growth factor used.[85–89] Many of these attempts mimic natural release mechanisms by using some form of modified or synthetic extracellular matrix, and yet the retention of growth factor biological activity has been difficult and elusive. When we encapsulated ^{125}I-bFGF within the same EVAc matrices that successfully released heparin, the physical release of the radiolabeled growth factor followed expected kinetics (Figure 2.4A), but 99.97% of the biological activity was lost.

Subsequent studies demonstrated that bFGF is especially sensitive to the conditions necessary for fabrication of matrix release devices, such as, exposure to 50°C, liquid nitrogen or dichloromethane fumes. The presence of heparin in the bFGF solution prevented some of these losses, by protecting against denaturation and degradation.[90,91] Indeed heparin-like compounds appear to be an essential component of the extracellular matrix in binding and stabilizing bFGF *in vivo*.[91] Thus, we encapsulated heparin immobilized to a Sepharose carrier within alginate microspheres and incubated the spheres with bFGF. In this manner, the growth factor was

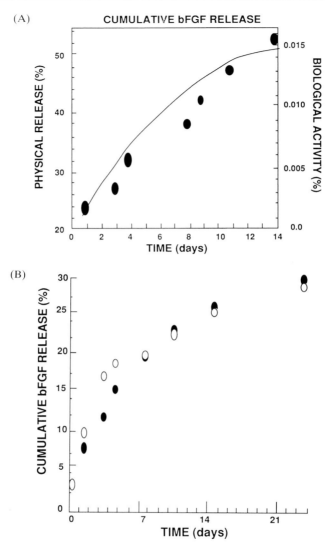

Figure 2.4   (A) Successful encapsulation and physical release of an agent within a drug-delivery device does not insure retention of biologic activity. When bFGF was incorporated within the EVAc matrices used for heparin release, virtually all of the biologic activiaty was lost. At 14 days, >50% of the growth factor was released but <0.02% of the expected biologic activity was retained. (After Ref. 71.) (B) Virtually all of the bFGF released from alginate microsphere incorporated heparin-Sepharose beads was biologically intact. The number of biologically active units of bFGF estimated from stimulation of 3T3 cell thymidine incorporation (○) was almost identical to the number of units estimated to have been released by following radioiodinated bFGF levels in the release buffer (●). (After Ref. 71.)

bound to the immobilized heparin and was released with kinetics similar to bFGF release from tissue-culture extracellular matrix (Figure 2.4B).[71] Release kinetics could be tailored[71] and prolonged by adjusting the amount of heparin present, or by co-encapsulating heparinase within the microspheres. More importantly, in stark

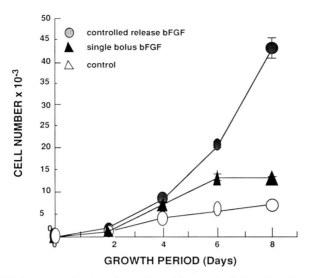

Figure 2.5 bFGF is far more effective when released in a controlled and continuous fashion. Release of bFGF with the kinetics depicted in Figure 2.4 stimulates smooth-muscle cells to a far greater extent than a bolus of an identical amount of bFGF.

contrast to the release of bFGF from EVAc matrices, >97% of the biologic activity was retained.

Effects in culture and in vivo

The devices described above were then used to study bFGF biology. The recognition that bFGF is mitogenic for a number of cells including vascular smooth muscle and endothelial cells stems from studies with the response of cells to a bolus of growth factor.[92,93] This is not how bFGF is released by natural mechanisms. To determine whether cells would respond differently if the growth factor were supplied with release kinetics resembling those documented for the interaction of bFGF at the extracellular matrix, we compared vascular smooth muscle and endothelial cells and fibroblast growth under the influence of a bolus of bFGF with growth under the influence of the controlled release of an equal amount of bFGF spaced out over the duration of the experiment. A single bolus injection of bFGF increased cell growth in the first four days but the effect dropped off subsequently. In contrast, the controlled release of the same amount of bFGF delivered over the course of the experiment at 33 ng day^{-1} stimulated the growth of cultured fibroblasts, smooth muscle and endothelial cells to a greater extent than a single bolus (Figure 2.5). Thus, cells in culture responded in a far different manner to the controlled release of bFGF compared to a single injection of the same amount of bFGF into the medium. The increased growth potential of cells under controlled-release conditions suggests that this mode of delivery may be more physiologic, i.e. more closely approximating the manner in which cells are exposed to bFGF *in vivo*.

To test whether controlled release of bFGF was an effective mitogenic stimulus *in vivo*, the bFGF controlled release devices were implanted into the perivascular space

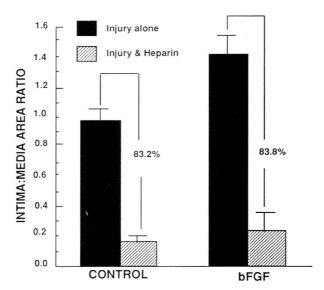

Figure 2.6 The controlled release of bFGF and heparin remain intact in *in vivo* models of vascular injury. Perivascular bFGF release increased intimal hyperplasia above control injury (solid bars) without altering the relative inhibitory effect of concomitant heparin (hatched bars). (Modified from Ref. 84.)

of rat carotid arteries.[84] Two weeks after denuding arterial injury, bFGF increased intimal mass (intima:media area ratio) 1.3-fold (solid bars, Figure 2.6), and the number of proliferating intimal cells 1.9-fold. With less arterial injury, intimal hyperplasia was increased 2.4-fold and the number of proliferating cells rose 4.0-fold. The relative ability of heparin to reduce smooth-muscle cell proliferation was not altered by the presence of bFGF (hatched bars, Figure 2.6). Concomitant perivascular heparin release inhibited intimal hyperplasia in the control state and after bFGF release to an identical 83%.

Thus, the perivascular release of bFGF enabled this potent mitogen to retain its biologic activity, and in addition, may have reproduced the physiologic means by which the growth factor is released and metabolized *in vivo*. For this and other reasons, continuous release into the perivascular space has proved to be the most efficient means of delivering this growth factor. Most recently, we have extended these experiments to other forms of cardiovascular injury and observed the same beneficial effects. Angiogenesis was stimulated by controlled release of bFGF in two models of wound repair,[94] and endothelial-dependent relaxation of the collateral-perfused porcine coronary microcirculation was enhanced.[95,96]

Antisense oligonucleotides

As discussed in Chapters 1 & 4, the resistance of restenosis to pharmacologic treatments has prompted investigation of genes involved in vascular smooth-muscle cell proliferation. Intracellular targeting to inhibit factors necessary for cell proliferation and migration could be achieved by molecular-based approaches using antisense strategies. Such strategies provide a theoretically simple means to inhibit

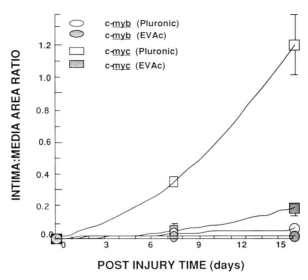

POST INJURY TIME (days)

Figure 2.7 The kinetics of drug release for vascular repair must be matched to the kinetics of gene expression following vascular injury. c-*myb* and c-*myc* are both expressed early after vascular injury. While the former rises transiently, the latter is expressed for a much larger period of time. Thus, both limited and prolonged release of antisense oligonucleotides to c-*myb* reduced intimal hyperplasia for the duration of the experiments, but only the continuous release of c-*myc* antisense oligomers achieved the same effect. When release was terminated at three days for c-*myc* intimal hyperplasia was increased 7 and 14 days after injury. Subsequent analyses revealed a second peak in c-*myc* expression long after the Pluronic® release was complete. (After Ref. 109.)

the expression of a specific gene. The biggest hurdle to the use of this technology is the mode of delivery. We had shown that antisense oligonucleotides to the late-G_1 gene, c-*myb*, inhibited smooth-muscle cell proliferation in culture, yet systemic administration of this compound had no demonstrable effect at the doses used, on the vascular response to injury.[97] Increased doses would most certainly increase potential toxicity and are prohibited by expense and limited availability. The release of this antisense sequence from a polymer gel (Pluronic®) in the perivascular space of injured arteries virtually obliterated intimal smooth-muscle cell accumulation following arterial injury in the rat (Figure 2.7).[97] It was assumed that this could serve as a means of releasing antisense oligomers to the full range of genes. Yet, when we used this system to study c-*myc*, the same effect was not observed. Antisense oligonucleotides to c-*myc* inhibited smooth-muscle cell proliferation in culture to an equal extent as the sequence to c-*myb*, but the release of this oligomer sequence from Pluronic® gels had no significant effect on intimal hyperplasia. These gels were especially effective in the first three days after injury. Arterial wall c-*myc* mRNA levels were reduced 2.5-fold, c-*myc* expression decreased 3.7-fold and the number of proliferating cells dropped 6.5-fold. Yet, by seven days postinjury, cell number within arteries exposed to Pluronic® gels releasing c-*myc* antisense was increased above that following administration of a scrambled oligonucleotide. The number of cells expressing c-*myc* increased 4.9-fold between days one and seven. Thus, early reduction in mRNA and protein levels decreased cell proliferation in the first few days after injury, but when this was not sustained, the end result was an intimal lesion no different than that observed in control untreated animals.

The release of antisense oligonucleotides from Pluronic® gels is very different from the release of heparin from EVAc matrices,[37,98,99] or bFGF from heparin-Sepharose beads encapsulated within alginate.[71,83,84] The Pluronic® polaxamer gels are hydrophilic and rapidly degrade in an aqueous environment resulting in complete release of drug within 72 hours. In contrast, hydrophobic EVAc matrices provide near zero-order release for well beyond the 14-day duration of the experiment. We therefore incorporated oligonucleotide sequences into both EVAc and Pluronic® gel formulations and examined the effects of these different forms of release _in vitro_ and _in vivo_. Though release of antisense oligonucleotides to both c-_myb_ and c-_myc_ suppressed _in vitro_ cell growth to an equal extent for both polymer systems (_c._ 50%), their effects _in vivo_ were discrepant. While both EVAc matrix and Pluronic® gel release of c-_myb_ antisense inhibited intimal hyperplasia two weeks after injury, only EVAc matrix release of antisense to c-_myc_ was effective. At one week, neointimal thickening in the animals treated with c-_myc_ antisense released from Pluronic® gels was 7.3-fold that seen in similar animals exposed to EVAc matrix release, and at two weeks this difference remained at 6.5-fold. Thus, single-dose suppression of some proto-oncogenes can forever prevent cell cycling[100–102] but other genes appear to require more prolonged inhibition to achieve the same effect. Continuous or periodic dosing in man would be logistically prohibitive. The technology of implantable devices has yet to reach the stage where prolonged, continuous delivery from these types of devices is possible, and repeated injections are doomed to noncompliance and failure. Moreover, the need for open field exposure for implantation of devices is problematic if these technologies are to be utilized in an adjunct fashion with percutaneous procedures.

Recent innovations with liposomal technology may provide for percutaneous administration of local release devices. For example, Morishita _et al._ studied oligonucleotides against cdk2 kinase,[102] a serine-threonine protein kinase, which interacts to form a complex with the cell-cycle progression regulating cyclins. The increase in cdk2 kinase mRNA levels one day after vascular injury was abolished by an intraluminal administration of antisense cdk2 kinase using hemagglutinating virus of Japan (HVJ)–liposome mediated transfer. The HVJ–liposome complex might increase the potential clinical utility of these agents by allowing for a shorter intraluminal incubation time, prolonging the duration of action and enhancing their specific activity. A single administration of this complex resulted in a significant reduction of neointima formation at two weeks after transfection, and a combination of antisense cdc2 and cdk2 kinase completely inhibited neointima formation. FITC-labeled oligonucleotide localized immediately to the medial layer and persisted up to two weeks after transfection.

Other drugs

In addition to heparin, heparin-binding growth factors and the antisense oligonucleotides, a number of other drugs have benefited from controlled local release

Table 2.3 Polymer-based drug delivery for cardiovascular applications

Drug	Animal model	Effect
Heparin	Rat carotid arteries	Up to 83% inhibition in intimal hyperplasia[36,37,98]
Heparin	Stented rabbit femoral arteries	Significant inhibition of thrombosis, monocyte adhesion and intimal hyperplasia over stented arterial segments[38]
Cyclosporine	Rat heterotopic heart transplant	Local immunosuppression with longer mean survival times[103]
Dexamethasone	Rabbit carotid arteries	Up to 76% inhibition in intimal hyperplasia[104]
Hirulog	Stented porcine carotid arteries	No difference in intima:media ratios of treated and nontreated segments[105]
bFGF	Rat carotid arteries	Up to 2.4-fold increase in intimal hyperplasia[84]
RGD peptides	Rat carotid arteries	92% reduction in hyperplasia[106]

(Table 2.3). The local delivery of cyclosporine following heart transplants is one such example.[103] While the use of this immunosuppressant has allowed the widespread application of heart transplantation as therapy for end stage heart failure, systemic cyclosporine immunosuppression is associated with severe side effects such as reduced renal function, cardiac toxicity, pericardial effusions, cardiomyopathy, hepatotoxicity and numerous other complications. Collagen matrices releasing cyclosporine at the rate of 0.2 or $1\,mg\,kg^{-1}\,day^{-1}$ were implanted around rat heterotopic heart transplants. Local immunosuppression with the higher dose significantly delayed transplant rejection, and the lower dose showed significant survival benefit with negligible drug levels in the blood and kidneys.

The local delivery of anti-inflammatory drugs like dexamethasone has similarly been investigated. Dexamethasone inhibits smooth-muscle cell proliferation *in vitro*. Systemic administration of this glucocorticoid causes severe side effects at high doses presumably through action on cytokine production by inflammatory cells present at the site of arterial injury and at low doses is ineffective.[104] Controlled drug release from silicone polymer matrices implanted around the denuded common carotid artery reduced the intima:media ratio by 75% compared to the control group.

The use of silicone polymers has been extended to other species and modes of injury. The local release of the potent antithrombotic hirulog, for example, inhibited thrombosis, but not intimal hyperplasia, following stent implantation.[105] The localized delivery of a cyclic integrin antagonist peptide on neointimal hyperplasia was assessed in a similar rat balloon injury model.[106] Pluronic® gel containing GPenGRGDSPCA (cRGD) (1 mM) applied at the adventitial surface of the artery reduced intimal hyperplasia 92%. Cell–matrix interactions mediated via cell surface integrins and matrix protein ligands are known to regulate cell phenotype and function. Thus cell integrin–matrix interactions may be an additional target for pharmacologic manipulation aimed at limiting restenosis following balloon injury.

The varied response of studies with the perivascular release of heparin, bFGF, antisense oligonucleotides, hirudin, dexamethasone and the integrins illustrate that the biologic response depends on the drug, the means of administration, site of drug delivery and extent of arterial injury. Different forms of injury may require different therapies, and complications of arterial intervention such as excessive neointimal hyperplasia and thrombosis may demand alternate therapeutic regimens. This, rather than frank resistance to therapy, may explain why experimentally effective antiproliferative and antithrombotic agents fail clinically.

Photodynamic therapy

Photodynamic therapy, currently under evaluation for cancer treatment, has been extended to the vascular system.[107] This technique uses high-intensity light in the presence of photosensitizers such as chloroaluminum-sulfonated phthalocyanine to regulate production of reactive oxygen species that cause cell injury and death. These photosensitizers have no cytotoxic biologic effect unless they are activated by the appropriate wavelength of light. Chloroaluminum-sulfonated phthalocyanine was selected as the photosensitizer since it does not produce skin sensitivity and has a high absorption peak of light at 675 nm, a wavelength with good tissue penetration. Preliminary studies indicated that administration of the drug with laser radiant exposure of $100 \, J \, cm^{-2}$ resulted in a homogeneous, circumferential effect on the whole artery.

Intimal hyperplasia following balloon injury of rat carotid arteries was reduced 65% by this therapy, whether the photosensitization and laser activation were performed two or seven days postinjury. Transmission electron microscopy showed early evidence of photosensitizer-mediated cytotoxic effects at 4 hours but no alterations in vascular collagen or elastic tissue.

The effect of a combination of 8-methoxypsoralen and ultraviolet-A (UVA) light on smooth-muscle cell proliferation after angioplasty has been studied as well.[108] The use of UVA light to activate 8-methoxypsoralen had previously been shown to be cytostatic in smooth-muscle cell culture. When atherosclerotic New Zealand White rabbits were subjected to balloon angioplasty, the combination of 8-methoxypsoralen and transcatheter UVA irradiation ($10 \, J \, cm^{-2}$) significantly lowered indices of smooth-muscle cell proliferation and cellularity in the neointima and media.

Conclusion

The continued evolution of thought and elucidation of mechanisms of arteriopathic diseases, coupled with the potential availability of novel compounds and interventions to combat these diseases has provided the impetus for consideration of local drug delivery. A wide range of techniques are becoming increasingly available by which to administer drugs directly to isolated segments of the blood-vessel wall. As noted in the introduction to this book it is important not to confuse local delivery with local therapy, and to avoid the temptation of extrapolating from one drug to all and from one model of a specific disease to every possible clinical scenario. Only continued investigation in the basic science laboratory and medical clinic will enable us to determine whether the promise of these techniques will bear scrutiny and succeed at limiting disease. For the time, however, these methods have helped immensely in the definition and characterization of a variety of diseases, identification of biologic phenomena, and the development of innovative device designs and therapeutic modalities.

Acknowledgments

This work was supported in part by grants from the National Institutes of Health (GM/HL 49039 and AG00294), the Burroughs-Wellcome Fund in Experimental Therapeutics, and the Whitaker Foundation for Biomedical Engineering.

References

1. Clowes, A. W. and Karnovsky, M. J. (1977) Suppression by heparin of smooth muscle cell proliferation in injured arteries. *Nature*, **265**, 625–6.
2. Clowes, A. W. and Karnovsky, M. J. (1977) Failure of certain antiplatelet drugs to affect myointimal thickening following arterial endothelial injury in the rat. *Lab. Invest.*, **36**, 452–64.
3. Bjornsson, T. D., Dryjski, M., Tluczek, J. *et al.* (1991) Acidic fibroblast growth factor promotes vascular repair. *Proc. Natl Acad. Sci. USA*, **88**, 8651–5.
4. Epstein, S. E., Siegall, C. B., Biro, S. *et al.* (1991) Cytotoxic effects of a recombinant chimeric toxin on rapidly proliferating vascular smooth muscle cells. *Circulation*, **84**, 778–87.
5. Ferns, G., Reidy, M. and Ross, R. (1990) Vascular effects of cyclosporine A *in vivo* and *in vitro*. *Am. J. Pathol.*, **137**, 403–13.
6. Hoberg, E., Schwarz, F., Schomig, A. *et al.* (1990) Prevention of restenosis by verapamil. The verapamil angioplasty study (VAS). *Circulation*, **82**, III-428.
7. Liu, M. W., Roubin, G. S., Robinson, K. A. *et al.* (1990) Trapadil in preventing restenosis after balloon angioplasty in the atherosclerotic rabbit. *Circulation*, **81**, 1089–93.
8. Okamoto, S., Inden, M., Setsuda, M. *et al.* (1990) Trapadil (triazolopyrimidine), a platelet derived growth factor (PDGF) antagonist in preventing restenosis after percutaneous coronary angioplasty. *Circulation*, **82**, III-428.
9. Ellis, S. G., Roubin, G. S., Wilentz, J. *et al.* (1987) Results of a randomized trial of heparin and aspirin versus aspirin alone for prevention of abrupt closure and restenosis after angioplasty. (Abstract) *Circulation*, **76**, 213.
10. Hettleman, B. D., Aplin, R. L., Sullivan, P. R. *et al.* (1990) Three days of heparin pretreatment reduces major complications of coronary angioplasty in patients with unstable angina. *J. Am. Coll. Cardiol.*, **15**, 154A.
11. Pepine, C. J., Hirshfeld, J. W., Macdonald, R. G. *et al.* (1990) A controlled trial of corticosteroids to prevent restenosis after coronary angioplasty. *Circulation*, **81**, 1753–61.
12. Ellis, S. G., Roubin, G. S., Wilentz, J. *et al.* (1989) Effect of 18- to 24-hour heparin administration for prevention of restenosis after uncomplicated coronary angioplasty. *Am. Heart J.*, **117**, 777–82.
13. Lehmann, K. G., Doria, R. J., Feuer, J. M. *et al.* (1991) Paradoxical increase in restenosis rate with chronic heparin use: final results of a randomized trial. *J. Am. Coll. Cardiol.*, **17**, 181A (Abstract).
14. Leung, W-H., Kaplan, A. V., Grant, G. W. *et al.* (1990) Local delivery of antithrombin agent reduces platelet deposition at the site of balloon angioplasty. *Circulation*, **82**, III-428 (Abstract).

15. Muller, D. W. M., Topol, E. J., Abrams, G. *et al.* (1990) Intramural methotrexate therapy for the prevention of intimal proliferation following porcine carotid balloon angioplasty. *Circulation*, **82**, III-429 (Abstract).
16. Whitworth, H. B., Roubin, G. S., Hollman, J. *et al.* (1986) Effect of nifedipine in recurrent stenosis after percutaneous coronary angioplasty. *J. Am. Coll. Cardiol.*, **8**, 1271–6.
17. Laskey, M. A., Deutsch, E., Hirshfeld, J. W. Jr *et al.* (1990) Influence of heparin therapy on percutaneous transluminal coronary angioplasty outcomes in patients with coronary arterial thrombus. *Am. J. Cardiol.*, **65**, 179–82.
18. Powell, J. S., Clozel, J-P., Muller, R. K. M. *et al.* (1989) Inhibitors of angiotensin-converting enzyme prevent myointimal proliferation after vascular injury. *Science*, **245**, 187–9.
19. Gimple, L. W., Owen, R. M., Lodge, V. P. *et al.* (1992) Reduction in angioplasty restenosis in rabbits by chronic subcutaneous heparin with or without intramural heparin delivery. *Circulation*, **82**, III-338 (Abstract).
20. Handley, D. A., van Valen, R. G., Melden, M. K. and Saunders, R. N. (1986) Suppression of rat carotid lesion development by the calcium channel blocker PN-200-110. *Am. J. Pathol.*, **124**, 88–93.
21. Jackson, C. L., Bush, R. C. and Bowyer, D. E. (1988) Inhibitory effect of calcium antagonists on balloon catheter-induced arterial smooth muscle cell proliferation and lesion size. *Atherosclerosis*, **69**, 115–22.
22. Lundergan, C. F., Foegh, M. L. and Ramwell, P. W. (1991) Peptide inhibition of myointimal proliferation by angiopeptin, a somatosatin analogue. *J. Am. Coll. Cardiol.*, **17**, 132B–136B.
23. Faxon, D., Spiro, T., Minor, S. *et al.* (1992) Enoxaprin, a low molecular weight heparin, in the prevention of restenosis after angioplasty: the results of a double blind randomized trial. *J. Am. Coll. Cardiol.*, **19**, 258A (Abstract).
24. MERCATOR (1992) Does the new angiotensin converting enzyme inhibitor cilazapril prevent restenosis after percutaneous transluminal coronary angioplasty? *Circulation*, **86**, 100–10.
25. Henry, P. D. and Bentley, K. I. (1981) Suppression of atherogenesis in cholesterol-fed rabbits treated with nifedipine. *J. Clin. Invest.*, **68**, 1366–9.
26. El-Sanadiki, M. N., Cross, K. S., Murray, J. J. *et al.* (1990) Reduction of intimal hyperplasia and enhanced reactivity of experimental vein bypass grafts with verapamil treatment. *Ann. Surg.*, **212**, 87–96.
27. Castellot, J. J. J., Addonizio, M. L., Rosenberg, R. D. and Karnovsky, M. J. (1981) Cultured endothelial cells produce a heparin-like inhibition of smooth muscle growth. *J. Cell Biol.*, **90**, 372–9.
28. Castellot, J. J. J., Cochran, D. L. and Karnovsky, M. J. (1985) Effect of heparin on vascular smooth muscle cells. I. Cell metabolism. *J. Cell. Physiol.*, **124**, 21–8.
29. Clowes, A. W. and Clowes, M. M. (1986) Kinetics of cellular proliferation after arterial injury. IV. Heparin inhibits rat smooth muscle mitogenesis and migration. *Circ. Res.*, **58**, 839–45.
30. Clowes, A. W., Clowes, M. M. and Reidy, M. A. (1986) Kinetics of cellular proliferation after arterial injury. III. Endothelial and smooth muscle growth in chronically denuded vessels. *Lab. Invest.*, **54**, 295–303.
31. Clowes, A. W., Clowes, M. M., Fingerle, J. and Reidy, M. A. (1989) Kinetics of cellular proliferation after arterial injury. V. Role of acute distension in the induction of smooth muscle proliferation. *Lab. Invest.*, **60**, 360–4.
32. Clowes, A. W. and Clowes, M. M. (1985) Kinetics of cellular proliferation after arterial injury. II. Inhibition of smooth muscle growth by heparin. *Lab. Invest.*, **52**, 611–16.
33. Castellot, J. J. Jr, Wright, T. C. and Karnovsky, M. J. (1987) Regulation of vascular smooth muscle cell growth by heparin and heparan sulfate. *Semin. Thromb. Hemost.*, **13**, 489–503.
34. Pukac, L. A., Hirsch, G. M., Lormeau, J-C. *et al.* (1991) Antiproliferative effects of novel nonanticoagulant heparin derivatives on vascular smooth muscle cells *in vitro* and *in vivo*. *Am. J. Pathol.*, **139**, 1501–9.

35. Hirsch, G. and Karnovsky, M. (1991) Heparin inhibits neointimal proliferation in rat arterio-venous interposition grafts. *Am. J. Pathol.*, **139**, 581–7.
36. Edelman, E. R., Pukac, L. and Karnovsky, M. J. (1993) Protamine and protamine insulins exacerbate vascular injury. *J. Clin. Invest.*, **91**, 2308–13.
37. Edelman, E. R., Adams, D. A. and Karnovsky, M. J. (1990) Effect of controlled adventitial heparin delivery on smooth muscle cell proliferation following endothelial injury. *Proc. Natl Acad. Sci. USA*, **87**, 3773–7.
38. Rogers, C., Karnovsky, M. J. and Edelman, E. R. (1993) Inhibition of experimental neointimal hyperplasia and thrombosis depends on the type of vascular injury and the site of drug administration. *Circulation*, **88**, 1215–21.
39. Buchwald, A., Unterberg, C., Nebendahl, K. *et al.* (1992) Low-molecular weight heparin reduces neointimal proliferation after coronary stent implantation in hypercholesterol-emic minipigs. *Circulation*, **86**, 531–7.
40. Clowes, A. (1992) Heparin: will it control intimal thickening after angioplasty? *Circulation*, **86**, 1657–8.
41. Wolinsky, H. and Thung, S. N. (1990) Use of a perforated balloon catheter to deliver concentrated heparin into the wall of the normal canine artery. *J. Am. Coll. Cardiol.*, **15**, 475–81.
42. Goldman, B., Blanke, H. and Wolinsky, H. (1987) Influence of pressure on permeability of normal and diseased muscular arteries to horseradish peroxidase. *Atherosclerosis*, **65**, 215–25.
43. Nabel, E. G., Plautz, G. and Nabel, G. J. (1990) Site-specific gene expression *in vivo* by direct gene transfer into the arterial wall. *Science*, **294**, 1285–8.
44. Fram, D. B., Aretz, T., Azrin, M. A. *et al.* (1994) Localized intramural drug delivery during balloon angioplasty using hydrogel-coated balloons and pressure-augmented diffusion. *J. Am. Coll. Cardiol.*, **23**, 1570–7.
45. Riessen, R., Rahimizadeh, H., Blessing, E. *et al.* (1993) Arterial gene transfer using pure DNA applied directly to a hydrogel coated angioplasty balloon. *Hum. Gene Ther.*, **4**, 749–58.
46. Fernandez-Ortiz, A., Meyer, B. J., Mailhac, A. *et al.* (1994) A new approach for local intravascular drug delivery. *Circulation*, **89**, 1518–22.
47. Riessen, R. and Isner, J. M. (1994) Prospects for site-specific delivery of pharmacologic and molecular therapies. *J. Am. Coll. Cardiol.*, **23**, 1234–44.
48. Hong, M. K., Bhatti, T., Matthews, B. J. *et al.* (1993) The effect of porous infusion balloon-delivered angiopeptin on myointimal hyperplasia after balloon injury in the rabbit. *Circulation*, **88**, 638–48.
49. Franklin, S. M., Kalan, J. M., Currier, J. W. *et al.* (1992) Effects of local delivery of doxorubicin or saline on restenosis following angioplasty in atherosclerotic rabbits. *Circulation*, **86**, I-52.
50. Wilensky, R. L., Gradus-Pizlo, I., March, K. L. *et al.* (1992) Efficacy of local intramural injection of colchicine in reducing restenosis following angioplasty in the atherosclerotic rabbit model. *Circulation*, **86**, I-52.
51. Lambert, C. R., Leone, J. E. and Rowland, S. M. (1993) Local drug delivery catheters: functional comparison of porous and microporous designs. *Cor. Art. Dis.*, **4**, 469–75.
52. Wilensky, R. L., March, K. L., Gradus-Pizlo, I. *et al.* (1993) Enhanced localization and retention of microparticles following intramural delivery into atherosclerotic arteries using a new delivery catheter. *J. Am. Coll. Cardiol.*, **21**, 185A.
53. Nunes, G. L., King, S. B., Hanson, S. R. *et al.* (1992) Hydrogel-coated PTCA balloon catheter delivery of an antithrombin inhibits platelet dependent thrombosis. *Circulation*, **86**, I-380.
54. Sheriff, M. U., Khetpal, V. and Spears, J. R. (1993) Method of application of local high dose heparin during balloon angioplasty. *J. Am. Coll. Cardiol.*, **21**, 188A.
55. Levine, M. J., Leonard, B. M., Burke, J. A. *et al.* (1990) Clinical and angiographic results of balloon-expandable intracoronary stents in right coronary arteries. *J. Am. Coll. Cardiol.*, **16**, 332–9.

56. Schatz, R. A., Palmaz, J. C., Tio, F. O. *et al.* (1987) Balloon-expandable intracoronary stents in the adult dog. *Circulation*, **76**, 450–7.
57. Schatz, R. A., Baim, D. S., Leon, M. *et al.* (1991) Clinical experience with the Palmaz–Schatz coronary stent: initial results of a multicenter study. *Circulation*, **83**, 148–61.
58. Sigwart, U., Puel, J., Mirkovitch, V. *et al.* (1987) Intravascular stents to prevent occlusion and restenosis after transluminal angioplasty. *N. Engl. J. Med.*, **316**, 701–6.
59. Serruys, P. W., Strauss, B. H., Beatt, K. J. *et al.* (1991) Angiographic follow-up of a self-expanding coronary-artery stent. *N. Engl. J. Med.*, **324**, 13–17.
60. Sigwart, U., Urban, P., Golf, S. *et al.* (1988) Emergency stenting for acute occlusion after coronary balloon angioplasty. *Circulation*, **78**, 1121–7.
61. Urban, P., Sigwart, U., Golf, S. *et al.* (1989) Intravascular stenting for stenosis of aortocoronary venous bypass grafts. *J. Am. Coll. Cardiol.*, **13**, 1085–91.
62. Puel, J., Rousseau, H., Joffre, F. *et al.* (1987) Intravascular stents to prevent restenosis after transluminal coronary angioplasty. *Circulation*, **76**, IV-27 (Abstract).
63. Sheth, S., Park, K. D., Dev, V. *et al.* (1994) Prevention of stent subacute thrombosis by segmented polyurethaneurea–polyethylene oxide–heparin coating in the rabbit carotid. *J. Am. Coll. Cardiol.*, **23**, 187A.
64. Cox, D. A., Anderson, P. G., Roubin, G. S. *et al.* (1991) Local delivery of heparin and methotrexate fails to inhibit *in vivo* smooth muscle cell proliferation. *Circulation*, **84**, II-71 (Abstract).
65. Cox, D. A., Anderson, P. G., Roubin, G. S. *et al.* (1992) Effect of local delivery of heparin and methotrexate on neointimal proliferation in stented porcine coronary arteries. *Cor. Art. Dis.*, **3**, 237–48.
66. Langer, R., Brown, L., Leong, K. *et al.* (1985) Controlled release and magnetically modulated systems for macromolecular drugs. *Ann. NY Acad. Sci.*, **446**, 1–13.
67. Langer, R., Brown, L. and Edelman, E. (1985) Controlled release and magnetically modulated release systems for macromolecules. *Methods Enzymol.*, **112**, 399–422.
68. Langer, R. (1990) New methods of drug delivery. *Science*, **249**, 1527–33.
69. Brown, L., Munoz, C., Seimer, L. *et al.* (1986) Controlled release of insulin from polymer matrices: control of diabetes in rats. *Diabetes*, **35**, 692–7.
70. Murray, J., Brown, L., Klagsbrun, M. and Langer, R. (1983) A micro sustained release system for epidermal growth factor. *In Vitro*, **19**, 743–8.
71. Edelman, E. R., Mathiowitz, E., Langer, R. and Klagsbrun, M. (1991) Controlled and modulated release of basic fibroblast growth factor. *Biomaterials*, **12**, 619–26.
72. Langer, R., Brem, H., Falterman, K. *et al.* (1976) Isolation of a cartilage factor that inhibits tumor neovascularization. *Science*, **192**, 70–2.
73. Langer, R. and Murray, J. B. (1983) Angiogenesis inhibitors and their delivery systems. *Appl. Biochem. Biotech.*, **8**, 9–24.
74. Levy, R. J., Wolfrum, J., Schoen, F. J. *et al.* (1985) Inhibition of calcification of bioprosthetic heart valves by local controlled-release diphosphonate. *Science*, **228**, 190–2.
75. Preis, I. and Langer, R. (1979) A single step immunization by sustained antigen release. *J. Immunol. Meth.*, **28**, 193–7.
76. Hanke, H., Hassenstein, S., Kamenz, J. *et al.* (1992) Prolonged proliferative response of smooth muscle cells after experimental intravascular stenting: a stent wire related phenomenon. *Circulation*, **86**, I-186 (Abstract).
77. Cavender, J. B., Anderson, P. and Roubin, G. S. (1990) The effects of heparin bonded tantalum stents on thrombosis and neointimal proliferation. *Circulation*, **82**, III-541 (Abstract).
78. Baird, A. and Ling, N. (1987) Fibroblast growth factors are present in the extracellular matrix produced by endothelial cells *in vitro*: implications for a role of heparinase-like enzymes in the neovascular response. *Biochem. Biophys. Res. Commun.*, **142**, 428–35.
79. Vlodavsky, I., Folkman, J., Sullivan, R. *et al.* (1987) Endothelial cell-derived basic fibroblast growth factor: synthesis and deposition into the subendothelial extracellular matrix. *Proc. Natl Acad. Sci. USA*, **84**, 2292–6.

80. Folkman, J., Klagsbrun, M., Sasse, J. *et al.* (1988) A heparin-binding angiogenic protein – basic fibroblast growth factor – is stored within basement membrane. *Am. J. Pathol.*, **130**, 393–400.
81. Bashkin, P., Doctrow, S., Klagsbrun, M. *et al.* (1989) Basic fibroblast growth factor binds to subendothelial extracellular matrix and is released by heparitinase and heparin-like molecules. *Biochemistry*, **28**, 1737–43.
82. Nugent, M. A. and Edelman, E. R. (1992) Kinetics of basic fibroblast growth factor binding to its receptor and heparan sulfate proteoglycan: a mechanism for cooperativity. *Biochemistry*, **31**, 8876–83.
83. Edelman, E. R., Nugent, M. A. and Karnovsky, M. J. (1993) Perivascular and intravenous bFGF administration: vascular and solid organ deposition. *Proc. Natl Acad. Sci. USA*, **30**, 1513–17.
84. Edelman, E. R., Nugent, M. A., Smith, L. T. and Karnovsky, M. J. (1992) Basic fibroblast growth factor enhances the coupling of intimal hyperplasia and proliferation of vasa vasorum in injured rat arteries. *J. Clin. Invest.*, **89**, 465–71.
85. Hayek, A., Culler, F. L., Beattie, G. M. *et al.* (1987) An *in vivo* model for study of the angiogenic effects of basic fibroblast growth factor. *Biochem. Biophys. Res. Commun.*, **147**, 876–80.
86. Thompson, J. A., Anderson, K. D., DiPietro, J. M. *et al.* (1988) Site-directed neovessel formation *in vivo*. *Science*, **241**, 1349–52.
87. Cordeiro, P. G., Seckel, B. R., Lipton, S. A. *et al.* (1989) Acidic fibroblast growth factor enhances peripheral nerve regeneration *in vivo*. *Plast. Reconstr. Surg.*, **83**, 1013–19.
88. Greisler, H., Cziplerele, D., Kim, D. *et al.* (1992) Enhanced endothelialization of expanded polytetrafluoroethylene grafts by fibroblast growth factor type I pretreatment. *Surgery*, **112**, 244–55.
89. Greisler, H., Klosak, J., Dennis, J. *et al.* (1987) Biomaterial pretreatment with ECGF to augment endothelial cell proliferation. *J. Vasc. Surg.*, **5**, 393–402.
90. Gospodarowicz, D. and Cheng, J. (1986) Heparin protects basic and acidic FGF from inactivation. *J. Cell. Physiol.*, **128**, 475–84.
91. Gospodarowicz, D., Neufeld, G. and Schweigerer, L. (1987) Fibroblast growth factor: structural and biological properties. *J. Cell. Physiol.* (Supp.), **5**, 15–26.
92. Thomas, K. A. and Gimenez-Gallego, G. (1986) Fibroblast growth factors: broad spectrum mitogens with potent angiogenic activity. *Trends Biochem. Sci.*, **11**, 81.
93. Presta, M., Moscatelli, D., Silverstein, J. J. and Rifkin, D. B. (1986) Purification from a human hepatoma cell line of a basic FGF like molecule that stimulates capillary endothelial cell plasminogen activator production DNA synthesis and migration. *Mol. Cell. Biol.*, **6**, 4060.
94. Vu, C. D., Edelman, E. R., Nugent, M. A. *et al.* (1993) The continuous release of bFGF to enhance the delay phenomenon in skin flaps: an experimental study. 38th meeting Plastic Surgery Research Council. *J. Plastic Surg.*, 85–7 (Abstract).
95. Harada, K., Grossman, W., Friedman, M. *et al.* (1994) Basic fibroblast growth factor improves myocardial function in chronically ischemic porcine hearts. *J. Clin. Invest.*, **94**, 623–30.
96. Selke, F. W., Yang, S. Y., Harada, K. *et al.* (1994) Basic-fibroblast growth factor enhances endothelial-dependent relaxation of the collateral-perfused porcine coronary microcirculation. *Am. J. Physiol.*, **267** (*Heart Circ., Physiol.*, **36**) H1303–11.
97. Simons, M., Edelman, E. R., Langer, R. *et al.* (1992) Antisense c-*myb* oligonucleotides inhibit intimal arterial smooth muscle accumulation *in vivo*. *Nature*, **359**, 69–73.
98. Edelman, E. R. and Karnovsky, M. J. (1994) Contrasting effects of the intermittent and continuous administration of heparin in experimental restenosis. *Circulation*, **89**, 770–6.
99. Rogers, C. and Edelman, E. R. (1992) Controlled release of heparin reduces neointimal hyperplasia in stented rabbit arteries: ramifications for local therapy. *J. Interven. Cardiol*, **5**, 195–202.
100. Baserga, R., Reiss, K., Alder, H. *et al.* (1992) Inhibition of cell cycle progression by antisense oligodeoxynucleotides. *Ann. NY Acad. Sci.*, **660**, 64–9.

101. Bennett, M. R., Anglin, S., McEwan, J. R. *et al.* (1994) Inhibition of vascular smooth muscle cell proliferation *in vitro* and *in vivo* by c-*myc* antisense oligodeoxynucleotides. *J. Clin. Invest.*, **93**, 820–8.
102. Morishita, R., Gibbons, G., Ellison, K. E. *et al.* (1994) Intimal hyperplasia after vascular injury is inhibited by antisense cdk2 kinase oligonucleotides. *J. Clin. Invest.*, **93**, 1458–64.
103. Bolling, S. F., Lin, H., Annesley, T. M. *et al.* (1991) Local cyclosporine immunotherapy of heart transplants in rats enhances survival. *J. Heart Lung Transplant.*, **10**, 577–83.
104. Villa, A. E., Guzman, L. A., Chen, W. *et al.* (1994) Local delivery of dexamethasone for prevention of neointimal proliferation in a rat model of balloon angioplasty. *J. Clin. Invest.*, **93**, 1243–9.
105. Muller, D. W. M., Golomb, G., Gordon, D. *et al.* (1992) Local adventitial hirulog delivery for the prevention of stent thrombosis and neointimal thickening. *Circulation*, **86**, I-381 (Abstract).
106. Slepian, M. J. and Massia, S. P. (1993) Local delivery of a cyclic RGD peptide inhibits neointimal hyperplasia following balloon injury. *Circulation*, **88**, I-372 (Abstract).
107. Ortu, P., LaMuraglia, G. M., Roberts, W. G. *et al.* (1992) Photodynamic therapy of arteries: a novel approach for treatment of experimental intimal hyperplasia. *Circulation*, **85**, 1189–96.
108. March, K. L., Patton, B. L., Wilensky, R. L. and Hathaway, D. R. (1993) 8-Methoxypsoralen and longwave ultraviolet irradiation are a novel antiproliferative combination for vascular smooth muscle. *Circulation*, **87**, 184–91.
109. Edelman, E. R., Simons, M., Sirois, M. G. and Rosenberg, R. D. (1995) The role of c-*myc* in vascular injury. *Circ. Res.*, **76**, 176–182.
110. Oberhoff, M., Herdeg, C., Shamet, K. *et al.* (1993) Delivery of low molecular weight heparin via porous balloon catheter for the prevention of smooth muscle cell proliferation. *Circulation*, I-661 (Abstract).
111. Wilensky, R. L., March, K. L. and Hathaway, D. R. (1991) Restenosis in an atherosclerotic rabbit model is reduced by a thiol protease inhibitor. *J. Am. Coll. Cardiol.*, **17**, 268A.
112. Soria, I., Hassinger, N. L., Owen, W. G. and Chesebro, J. H. (1993) Local delivery of hirudin into rabbit carotid arteries with an iontophoretic balloon catheter. *Circulation*, **88**, I-660.
113. Gradus-Pizlo, I., Wilensky, R. L., March, K. L. *et al.* (1993) Local delivery of biodegradable microparticles containing colchicine or colchicine analog does not block restenosis in atherosclerotic rabbit femoral arteries. *Circulation*, **88**, I-372.
114. Avitall, B., Hare, J. and Zander, G. (1992) Iontophoretic transmyocardial drug delivery. A novel approach to antiarrhythmic drug delivery. *Circulation*, **85**, 1582–93.
115. Singh, J. and Roberts, M. S. (1989) Transdermal delivery of drugs by iontophoresis. *Drug Des. Deliv.*, **4**, 1–12.

3

Targeted Therapies for Accelerated Arteriopathies

A. Daniel Johnson
S. Ward Casscells

Introduction

One factor uniting accelerated arteriopathies such as carotid endarterectomy or post-PTCA restenosis, transplantation atherosclerosis, and coronary or peripheral venous graft occlusion is their dependence upon an initial injury to the vessel wall to induce vascular remodeling and subsequent narrowing or occlusion. Most commonly, the injury occurs during interventions to treat pre-existing cardiovascular disease. As a result, a significant percentage of primary interventions fail within 3–6 months, requiring additional treatment. While there are unique facets to each of the arteriopathies, they also share several of the following characteristics: moderate-to-severe endothelial injury, minor-to-severe endothelial denudation, activation of the smooth-muscle cells to proliferate/migrate to form a neointima, invasion of leukocytes (especially T-lymphocytes and macrophages) into the site of injury, and expansion of the neointima by extracellular matrix deposition. Because of this relatively uniform etiology, treatment modalities developed for one pathology (such as restenosis) may be applicable to the other conditions. This chapter will outline some of the basic principles underlying targeted therapies for accelerated arteriopathies. It will then briefly review recent work by our laboratory and others on inhibiting smooth-muscle cell proliferation after percutaneous transluminal angioplasty, as a means to prevent restenosis. Other potential treatments which are at various stages of testing will also be discussed briefly. Where appropriate, unique features and experimental data demonstrating applicability to the other accelerated arteriopathies will also be noted.

Goals and problems of targeted vascular therapies

The current concept of direct, selective targeting and inhibition of specific subclasses of cells initially arose from studies in cancer biology. Antibodies were developed against tumor cell-specific surface markers, which were then used to locally deliver and concentrate cytotoxins such as ricin, *Pseudomonas* exotoxin A, and diphtheria toxin, causing tumor cell death.[1-3] This technique has been modified to direct biologically active molecules to sites of vascular injury, which can then modify the progression of the repair process. Ideally, a single targeted compound could promote re-endothelialization, inhibit smooth-muscle growth, and limit both leukocytic involvement as well as matrix deposition; these effects would occur only at the site(s) of vascular injury, without affecting distal tissues. However, given the complexity of vascular reparative responses (as reviewed in Ref. 4), experimental models to date have focused on altering single components of the process.

The limiting step in localization of therapeutic compounds has been identification of surface markers that are unique to injured vasculature. While targeting specificity has proven to be increasingly important as investigations continue, there is unfortunately a paucity of such markers. This is especially true for the arterial smooth-muscle cells (aSMCs), which along with their extracellular matrix comprise the structural bulk of hyperplastic occlusions.[5,6] Autoantibodies to smooth muscle have been described in patients with biliary cirrhosis, chronic active hepatitis, migraines, and malaria; however, the specificity of these antibodies and the identity of their antigens are not known and as yet have not been cloned.[7-9] Commonly used identification markers for aSMCs such as α-actin, various cytoskeletal protein isoform variants such as high-molecular-weight caldesmin, smooth-muscle myosins, calponin, etc.,[10-15] are intracellular components which cannot be utilized for targeting intact cells (though their promoter regions could be used to achieve cell-specific expression of a foreign gene). Recent work on the role of cell-adhesion molecules (CAMs) in coordinating vascular inflammatory responses, as well as data on aSMC migration and interactions with extracellular matrix, have suggested there may be a specific profile of several proteins which are coordinately expressed only by aSMCs (as will be discussed later). Furthermore, analyses of RNA expression in neural crest-derived versus mesenchyme-derived aSMCs have suggested there are also isoforms of cadherins (a subclass of adhesion molecules[16-19]) which may differ between the two cell types (M. Majesky, pers. comm.). However, all of the aSMC surface proteins which have been well characterized to date have subsequently been found to be expressed at significant levels or have critical roles elsewhere in the body. Therefore, targeting of proliferating aSMCs has focused on disrupting the signaling pathways of the various peptide growth factors controlling aSMC growth, as will be discussed in more detail later. Modulation of extracellular matrix expression by aSMCs is a still newer area of effort, which will also be discussed.

Endothelial cells (ECs) present different problems than do aSMCs. Several surface markers are well characterized in ECs, the most notable being Factor VIII-related antigen (also called von Willebrand's factor, a component of the instrinsic coagulation pathway[20-24]), *Ulex* lectin binding of fucose-conjugated surface glycoproteins,[25-28] and the presence of vascular endothelial growth factor (VEGF) receptors.[29,30] However, regulation of re-endothelialization appears to be more complex than for smooth-muscle cell proliferation. Therapeutic rejuvenation of an intact endothelial lining within an injured vessel requires specific activation of both EC proliferation and migration, without induction of occlusive smooth-muscle growth; this is especially difficult since there are few mitogens for ECs (except for VEGF, and possibly platelet-derived endothelial cell growth factor (PD-ECGF)[31–33]) which do not also stimulate aSMCs. Moreover, endothelial cells must migrate back into denuded areas across extracellular matrices which may not support such movement, as will be discussed in the section on vascular matrix. In light of this greater complexity, it is not surprising that few studies have attempted to stimulate endothelial regeneration as a means for limiting arteriopathies. Conversely though, studies of transplant atherosclerosis have begun to define the stages of the initial injury to the endothelium, in hopes of preventing EC loss. A brief overview of the current data regarding mechanisms for leukocyte-induced endothelial damage will be discussed later in the context of CAMs in early inflammation.

Targeted compounds that prevent vascular occlusion are further constrained by two additional factors. The first problem is the utilization of targeted vascular signaling pathways by other body systems. Non-specific side effects are common with many current drugs, but frequently these effects are minimal or tolerable. However, the present generation of targeted therapeutics utilize endogenous or semi-endogenous agonists which have the potential for both random activation of cells, as well as for inhibition of vital cellular pathways in other body systems.[34,35] The second difficulty which must be overcome is an apparent redundancy in repair signals within the vasculature. As an example, current evidence supports basic fibroblast growth factor as the primary inducer of smooth-muscle proliferation postinjury; yet inhibition of bFGF alone has proven insufficient to prevent neointimal formation in some *in vivo* models, but not others.[34,36–41] It is quite possible that with additional studies, other components which signal for repair will be determined, which also must be addressed in order to completely block aSMC hyperplasia. Therefore, the compounds which will be described here should be considered as 'proof of concept' models, and not the final agents of choice. Further work is needed in order to develop more accurate targeting systems, based on our evolving understanding of the basic biology of vascular injury.

Chemical atherectomy: selective ablation of proliferating smooth-muscle cells

The goal of selectively ablating proliferating aSMCs to prevent restenosis has been greatly aided by recent experimental studies of the vascular response to injury. Data from numerous laboratories have demonstrated that mechanical or chemical injury induces a tremendous variety of mitogenic molecules by a subset of aSMCs; these mitogens subsequently initiate autocrine and paracrine loops which stimulate reparative growth.[37,39,40,42] Currently, the most important mitogens for vascular targeting are peptide growth factors and their receptors, which include acidic and basic fibroblast growth factors (a- and bFGF), platelet-derived growth factor (PDGF), epidermal growth factor (EGF), transforming growth factor beta-1 (TGF-β_1), insulin-like growth factor-1 (IGF-1), and others (see Refs 36 and 42 for a review). The receptors for these mitogens are internalized by receptor-mediated endocytosis upon ligand binding, carrying the ligand along. In theory, conjugation of a ligand with a toxin which cannot normally cross into cells both targets the toxin to cells expressing a particular receptor, and allows the toxin access to the intracellular spaces. Once internalized, the toxin then kills receptor-bearing cells. In the case of angioplasty, the toxin would destroy proliferating smooth-muscle cells only, presumably leaving the nonactivated aSMCs, which express fewer receptors for mitogens, relatively intact.

One mitogen–toxin combination which has been tested against proliferating smooth muscle is TGFα–PE40, a recombinant chimera of transforming growth factor alpha (TGFα) with a 40-kDa fragment of *Pseudomonas* exotoxin A (PE40).[43] TGFα–PE40 retains the native toxin's ADP-ribosyltransferase, which terminates protein synthesis by inactivating elongation factor 2. However, PE40 toxin fragment lacks the normal binding site for cell-surface receptors; instead, TGFα–PE40 targets and binds specifically to EGF receptor-bearing cells. Studies of rabbit aSMCs in culture showed significant dose-dependent decreases in both cell number and cellular protein synthesis upon treatment with TGFα–PE40 ($ID_{50} = 4.0 \pm 1.7$ ng ml^{-1}).[43] Furthermore, proliferating smooth-muscle cells were 30-fold more sensitive than quiescent cells to TGFα–PE40, and TGFα–PE40 toxicity could be competitively inhibited by excess EGF.

The utility of TGFα–PE40 was limited *in vivo*, due to hepatotoxicity resulting from high constitutive levels of EGF receptors in the liver.[35] Therefore, additional modifications were made of the subunit proteins to further increase specificity. First, the N-terminal DNA sequence corresponding to the heparin-binding domain of a second mitogen, heparin-binding epidermal growth factor (HB-EGF), was transferred to the TGFα–toxin prokaryotic expression construct. The rationale was to increase smooth-muscle delivery of toxin by causing its accumulation within vascular extracellular matrices which are rich in heparin sulfate proteoglycans. Domain analysis of wild-type exotoxin A also determined that the C-terminal amino acid sequence, REDLK, is required for translocation of the toxin to a cytosolic compartment after internalization. A second change was made in the C-terminal sequence of the expression construct, which exchanged the native translocation signal sequence for the residues KDEL. Addition of this conserved endoplasmic reticulum retention sequence[44] further increased the toxicity of the chimera.[45,46] The combined HB–TGFα–KDEL protein demonstrated a six-fold increase in toxicity against rat aSMCs compared to the original chimera, without a concomitant increase in high-affinity binding to the EGF receptor. This suggests that hepatotoxicity via EGF receptor uptake in the liver could be less using this construct, but no *in vivo* data have been published.

Targeting of the EGF receptor is the strategy behind another chimera, DAB$_{389}$EGF, which is a fusion of EGF with the diphtheria toxin A fragment.[47] Again, diphtheria toxin A fragment lacks its native receptor-binding domain, using EGF instead for targeting. For human arterial smooth-muscle cells in culture, DAB$_{389}$EGF caused a dose-dependent decrease in protein synthesis, with an ID_{50} of 40 pM. Similar to TGFα–PE40, cytotoxicity was inhibited by excess EGF or a neutralizing monoclonal antibody to the EGF receptor. Especially interesting was the ability of DAB$_{389}$EGF to inhibit smooth-muscle cell outgrowth from human atherosclerotic plaques, as assessed using explant cultures. However, no *in vivo* data are available.

Other groups, including ours, have focused on different growth factors and toxins. Current evidence from balloon-injured artery models indicates that release of basic FGF is a major signal for smooth-muscle proliferation postinjury.[37,40] Moreover, there is significant upregulation of the FGF receptors within the arterial wall, both in animal models and in human tissues at various times postangioplasty[34,37,39,40] (and our unpublished results). Additionally, other mitogens for smooth muscle, notably thrombin, interleukin-1β, and PDGF, can upregulate local paracrine or autocrine loops involving bFGF and its receptor.[48–51] Therefore, blockade or ablation of the cells which respond to bFGF could significantly limit restenosis by depressing aSMC replication. We have used a conjugate of bFGF with saporin, a plant toxin originally derived from *Saponaria officinalis* to attack proliferating smooth-muscle cells. Saporin is a highly thermostable, proteolytically resistant enzyme that cleaves ribose from adenine in the 28S RNA of the 60S ribosomal subunit, thereby blocking protein synthesis.[52] Saporin alone is nearly impermeable to cell membranes, and minimally affects cell viability; in contrast, FGF–saporin has a potent effect upon cell proliferation, both *in vitro* and *in vivo*.[53] While the data outlined below are specific to FGF–saporin, they are a model for effects generally seen for mitogen–toxin conjugates.

For rat arterial smooth-muscle cells grown in 10% serum, 10 nM bFGF–saporin significantly inhibits protein synthesis by 14 hours, and DNA synthesis by 24 hours. Cell death begins by 24–48 hours, and continues for 3–6 days.[34] This process is essentially irreversible with as little as 1 hour of exposure to toxin. These effects are not seen in the presence of 400-fold excess bFGF, and pure saporin alone inhibited cell growth only at 500-fold higher concentrations than the toxin conjugate. By 72 hours after toxin addition to subconfluent human smooth-muscle cells grown in different serum levels, a variable number of viable cells remain (Figure 3.1). Percentage survival depends upon a number of factors, but can range from <10% to as high as 80% (A. D. Johnson, unpublished results). Among the critical factors determining toxicity appears to be time within cell cycle, with the most actively proliferating cells being the most sensitive; in contrast, our data indicate that postconfluent, quiescent smooth-muscle cells, which express few FGF receptors, are resistant to toxicity.[34] However, in human aSMCs there appears to be additional heterogeneity in toxic responsiveness, which cannot be explained by differences in mean cell population doubling time (Figure 3.1). The survival of some aSMCs when exposed to bFGF–saporin may be due to failure of the toxin to bind or enter those cells, or resistance to the saporin once internalized. Indeed, we and others have developed both smooth-muscle and non-muscle cell lines which exhibit partial resistance to bFGF–saporin (A. Baird, pers. comm.). Additionally, there are interspecies differences in toxicity; a comparision of porcine and human aSMCs showed human cells were less sensitive, possibly because their higher endogenous bFGF production competed with toxin for high-affinity receptors (B. Sosnowski, in review).

We have also found that the initial response to low (0.1–1 nM) concentrations of bFGF–saporin was an increase in protein and DNA synthesis, and in some cases, a mild proliferative effect.[34] Presumably, the bFGF component of the chimera exerted its effects prior to those seen with saporin. Another similar finding is that endothelial

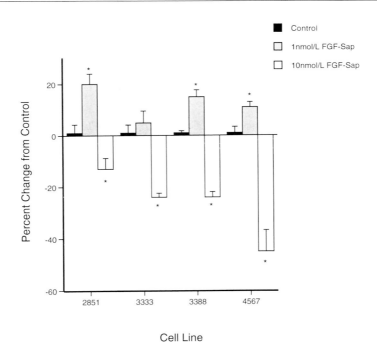

Figure 3.1 Differences in cytotoxicity of bFGF/saporin–C96S to human aSMCs. Human aSMCs derived by explant culture were plated at subconfluence, then 24 hours later treated with 0–10 nmol L^{-1} bFGF–saporin/C96S for 72 hours. Cell survival was then determined by crystal violet staining and expressed as a percentage of non-toxin treated controls. Data shown are for cells treated with toxin in 1% fetal calf serum; values are expressed as the percentage change in cell number for each treatment after 72 hours, relative to 1% serum only controls, ±SEM, n = three replicates. An asterisk indicates a significant ($P < 0.05$) difference from controls for that cell line. Significant heterogeneity ($P < 0.0001$ overall) existed between the four human aSMC lines shown, and similar differences in proliferation in response to bFGF (not shown) were also seen. Similar variations in toxicity were also observed for cells treated in the presence of 15% serum. At the lower dose of toxin in 1% serum, some stimulation of growth was observed, in agreement with other studies; no such stimulation was observed in 15% FCS.

cells are relatively resistant to bFGF–saporin. Indeed, we have repeatedly found that aortic endothelium was stimulated by toxin at the doses where smooth-muscle cell killing was observed, and EC death required nearly 50-fold higher levels than for smooth-muscle cell ablation. The resistance of ECs to the bFGF–saporin may be explained by the four-fold lower density of FGF receptors than on smooth-muscle cells. Endothelial cells may not take up enough toxin to terminally disrupt protein synthesis, while sufficient bFGF-mediated signaling occurs to induce proliferation. Use of differential drug sensitivities between two or more target tissues have been a strategy employed with classical pharmaceutical drugs for a number of years. Therefore, designing 'therapeutic dosage windows' for targeted chimeric compounds is unlikely to present insurmountable difficulties, compared to their initial identification and synthesis.

In vivo studies in the rat carotid artery balloon injury model have also demonstrated potential efficacy of bFGF–saporin for prevention of smooth hyperplasia (Figure 3.2). Basic FGF–saporin given intravenously at $100\,\mu g\,kg^{-1}$, 24–72 hours

(A)

(B)

(C)

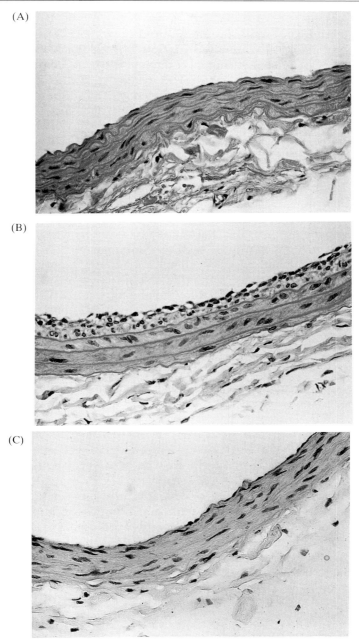

Figure 3.2   Rat carotid arteries pre- and postballoon injury, with versus without bFGF–saporin inhibition of smooth-muscle cell proliferation. After overinflation injury using a 2F Fogarty balloon catheter, vessels were formalin fixed at various times, embedded in paraffin, then sectioned and stained with hematoxylin and eosin. Final magnification shown is 40×. A. Normal, uninjured control vessel. B. Carotid artery 14 days postinjury; animal injected with saline vehicle alone. C. Carotid artery 14 days postinjury, with intravenous injection of 100 μg kg^{-1} body weight of bFGF–saporin 24 hours after initial ballooning. bFGF–saporin reduced neointimal mass to near non-injured levels at 14 days, but by 28 days postinjury, neointimal size was the same for mitotoxin-treated and vehicle only-treated animals.

after balloon denudation injury in rats reduced neointimal formation 83% compared to saline-treated, balloon-injured controls 14 days postsurgery.[34] However, these results were not persistent; animals examined 28 days after injury and bFGF–saporin treatment showed no benefit. This could be due to proliferation of a subpopulation of aSMCs with aberrant or reduced FGF receptors (A. D. Johnson, in review), which would be unable to bind bFGF–saporin. Evidence that bFGF initially induces proliferation postinjury, while PDGF promotes aSMC migration into the intima from the media,[24,41] supports the possibility that additional components of the restenotic cascade must also be blocked to completely inhibit neointimal formation.

Like TFGα–PE40,[35] bFGF–saporin at $100\,\mu g\,kg^{-1}$ intravenously causes cachexia and hepatotoxicity *in vivo*,[34] suggesting a lack of specificity. The earliest studies on bFGF–saporin used a heterogeneous mixture containing several conjugate isoforms, each with potentially different toxicities due to different molar ratios of saporin to bFGF. This prompted the synthesis of single, homogeneous isoforms of bFGF–saporin by two different methods.[54] For chemical synthesis, saporin was derivatized then purified to yield molecules containing a single reactive sulfhydryl site. This moiety was then chemically conjugated to recombinant bFGF which had undergone site-directed mutagenesis to delete one of the two potential cysteine residues available for sulfhydryl addition. The result was formation of a homogeneous species of chimera with a molar toxin/ligand ratio of 1:1, which demonstrated equal toxicity as the original compound in a number of fibroblastoid cell lines. This compound, or a recombinant bFGF–saporin which has been recently synthesized (A. Baird, pers. comm.), may prove to have less nonspecific toxicity than the original compound used in our studies.

In addition to bFGF–saporin, recent work has also described a recombinantly expressed chimera of either acidic or basic FGF linked to the same *Pseudomonas* exotoxin A fragments, PE40 or PE4E-KDEL, as used for HB–TGFα described above.[55] Human aortic smooth-muscle cells in culture were sensitive to both aFGF and bFGF conjugates, while endothelial cells were sensitive to bFGF conjugates only. Furthermore, the time for maximal toxicity varied significantly between aFGF– and bFGF–PE40, which suggests that differences in mitogen affinities for different isoforms of receptors or differences in ligand–receptor complex processing may be exploited to improve selectivity of chimeric toxins. However, both the interactions of growth factors with their surface receptors, and the processing of the receptor–ligand complexes, must be better understood before rational design of conjugates can fully take advantage of unique attributes within targeted cells.

Cell-adhesion molecules: breaking the ties that bind

The rapidity with which arteriopathies develop is not due solely to autocrine/paracrine mitogens derived from aSMCs. Recent observations have shown vascular occlusion is additionally accelerated by recruitment of activated T-lymphocytes and monocyte-macrophages from the circulation into the vascular wall, particularly after vascular grafting or cardiac transplantation.[56–59] There is also mounting evidence

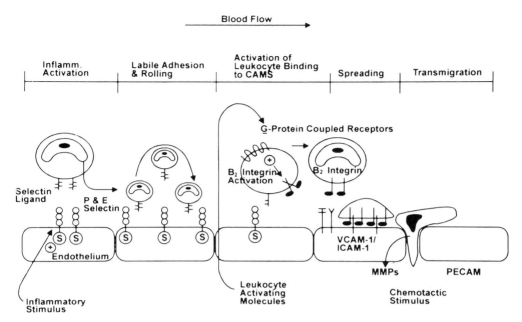

Figure 3.3 Schematic diagram of leukocytic adhesion to endothelial cells during inflammation. For a detailed description, see text. Briefly, transient binding of leukocyte glycoproteins to selectins expressed at the endothelial luminal surface slows blood-borne cells sufficiently to contact the endothelium. Leukocytes become activated, gain firm attachment via integrin/cell adhesion molecule interactions, then undergo extravasation and move towards chemotactic and inflammatory stimuli. S, selectin; MMPs, matrix metalloproteinases; VCAM/ICAM, vascular and intercellular adhesion molecules; PECAM, platelet–endothelial cell adhesion molecule; inflamm., inflammatory.

that leukocytes play a significant role in postangioplasty restenosis.[60–62] Considerable advances have been made in our understanding of the molecular interactions required for leukocyte and platelet adhesion to vessels and their therapeutic potential. A complete survey of the myriad cell-adhesion molecules and their behavior is not possible here; several recent reviews cover current concepts in detail.[63] What is important to this discussion is that leukocyte recruitment is a multistep cascade, in which each step must occur in sequential order. Data from several studies will be briefly reviewed that demonstrate how disruption of this cascade may significantly reduce vascular hyperresponsive repair stimuli, preventing vascular occlusion.

Intravital microscopy and *in vitro* reconstitution models[63–65] of generalized leukocytic recruitment to the vascular wall (as occurs during an inflammatory response) have shown that six essential steps occur: EC activation, labile adhesion, rolling, leukocyte activation, high-affinity adhesion and transmigration to the subendothelial spaces (Figure 3.3). ECs are activated initially by inflammatory stimuli such as thrombin, histamine, interleukin-1 (IL-1), lipopolysaccharide, interferon-gamma (IFN-γ) or tumor necrosis factor (TNF).[56,60] The ECs respond by surface presentation of P- and E-selectins, two members of a class of Ca^{2+}-dependent carbohydrate binding cell-adhesion molecules.[66–68] The selectins bind to specific glycoprotein ligands on blood-borne leukocytes with high affinity, but also with high lability; thus, initial selectin binding slows circulating cells and brings them in proximity of the EC monolayer. Rolling of leukocytes subsequently occurs as selectin binding is broken transiently by the flow of blood, then re-established. Rolling stops when leukocyte activating molecules from ECs (such as platelet activating factor (PAF) or chemokines such as IL-8 and macrophage chemotactic protein-1 (MCP-1)) bind to G-protein dependent, seven membrane-spanning receptors on leukocytes, causing activation of the cytoplasmic domains of $\beta2$ (CD11/CD18+) class integrins.[57,63] The activated integrins bind with high affinity to vascular or intercellular adhesion molecule-1 (VCAM-1 or ICAM-1, respectively) on the surface of the ECs; at this point, the leukocytes no longer roll, and exhibit a spread morphology. Postspreading transmigration between ECs requires a chemotactic gradient to direct migration towards the inflammatory stimulus, and both adhesion molecules such as platelet–endothelial cell adhesion molecule-1 (PECAM-1),[65] as well as matrix metalloproteinases such as stromelysin and 72 kDa gelatinase.[69,70]

It appears that much if not all of the fibroproliferative occlusion during chronic rejection, as well as a significant portion of occlusion after angioplasty, requires a fully active leukocyte recruitment pathway in order to occur. Early studies of balloon injury-induced neointimal formation in normal rats noted little effect of corticosteroids or cyclosporine, at least at the dosages used. Similarly, athymic nude rats lacking T-lymphocytes developed a neointima equivalent to normal rats, suggesting that T-lymphocytes are not involved in the response to balloon injury.[71] However, in rat, murine, rabbit and canine transplantation models the number of T-lymphocytes correlated with both progression and severity of vascular occlusion.[58,72–74] In transplanted vessels, ECs bind to circulating T-lymphocytes via surface class I and II HLA antigens.[56] The endothelium is activated, with subsequent recruitment of additional T-lymphocytes and monocyte/macrophages via an E-selectin/ICAM-1 dependent pathway. Initially, accumulating T-lymphocytes probably inhibit smooth-muscle proliferation by releasing IFN-γ,[72] so may not directly induce intimal thickening. However, T-lymphocytes also recruit macrophages that secrete copious smooth-muscle mitogens and chemotactic proteins (particularly IL-1, PDGF, bFGF, IGF-1, and TGF-β) that induce aSMC proliferation and migration.[5,36,39,42,75,76] In addition to stimulation of aSMCs, recruited cytotoxic (CD8$^+$) T-lymphocytes and macrophages attack the foreign endothelium directly,[56] while antibody-induced localization of complement proteins causes EC lysis.[77,78] The exposed subendothelial collagen binds platelets via $\alpha2\beta1$ integrins,[79] activating a thrombotic cascade. The underlying aSMCs, if stimulated by cytokine release, also express adhesion molecules and mediate further binding of leukocytes;[57,73] likewise, in inflammation due to mechanical injury, T-lymphocytes and monocytes are directly recruited by the exposed aSMCs, via ICAM-1.[80]

Murine and rabbit cardiac transplantation studies have confirmed that ICAM-1 is a major requirement for T-lymphocyte recruitment, and that ICAM-1 is upregulated in ECs of both epicardial and small arteries during early rejection.[58,63,73] More recently, the percentage of vessels expressing ICAM-1 in human cardiac allografts undergoing rejection has also been reported.[81,82] Endothelial expression in vessels at baseline is 50–60% prior to initiation of rejection, but reaches up to 92% in cases of moderate-to-severe rejection. Additionally, aSMCs were observed to begin expressing ICAM-1 concurrently with initial T-lymphocyte infiltration. Interestingly, aSMCs in primary atherosclerotic plaques also express both VCAM-1 and ICAM-1, and in culture upon stimulation by pro-inflammatory cytokines.[83–88] Adhesion molecule expression is especially intense in sites of activated aSMC growth *in vivo*,[73,83] while in relatively quiescent fibrotic plaques, expression of adhesion molecules by aSMCs is minimal.[85]

Given the requirement for sequential action by adhesion molecules in leukocyte recruitment as well as their prominent expression prior to occlusion, therapeutic antagonists which block cell adhesion are under active development. While several show significant initial promise, few clinical trials are currently underway. The early steps in the cascade, endothelial activation and labile adhesion via selectins, have been exploited only to a limited extent. Imaging of endothelium during joint inflammation has been demonstrated in pig models using ^{111}In-labeled monoclonal antibodies to E-selectin,[89] but has not been used in the context of predicting early stages of rejection. Studies have shown that E-selectin is generally upregulated after endothelial trauma, and that in animal models,[90,91] antagonists of E-selectin inhibit monocytic influx at sites of inflammation, as well as improve transplant survival. However, there are equivocal data as to whether E-selectin is consistently induced in human hearts by transplantation (reviewed in Ref. 59), bringing into question whether E-selectin is the primary mediator for rejection in humans. This suggests that other, as-yet-undefined cascades may exist in man which additionally mediate rejection. There are some data showing that P-selectin is upregulated over primary atherosclerotic plaques,[92] but no evidence to date that P-selectin is involved with vascular occlusion. However, the role of neutrophils (which are preferentially recruited by P-selectin[63]) has not been clearly established in either primary athero-sclerosis or in accelerated arteriopatheis. Likewise, the effect of increased display of P-selectin by aggregated platelets upon the cells underlying the platelet mass is still unknown. Therefore, P-selectin remains a factor to consider in future studies.

Inhibition of ICAM-1 and VCAM-1 interactions have proven to have significant protective effects against transplant rejection as well as associated diffuse arterio-sclerosis.[72,74,93,94] Monoclonal antibodies against either ICAM-1 or the leukocyte CD11a/CD18 to which ICAM-1 binds inhibited approximately 30% of the binding of activated T-lymphocytes to aSMCs *in vitro*, while an additional 30% inhibition was possible using antibodies that blocked VCAM-1 adhesion.[57] However, there appeared to be T-lymphocyte binding which could not be inhibited by either VCAM-1 or ICAM-1 inhibition, suggesting there are additional recruitment paths which are currently undescribed. Rejection and vascular occlusion have also been inhibited in mouse and rabbit *in vivo* models using a pair of monoclonal antibodies to simul-taneously neutralize both ICAM-1 and its ligand LFA-1,[95] as well as by adminis-tration of antibodies against VCAM-1.[72] In the rabbit model, it was found that blockade of the VCAM-1 receptor molecule (VLA-4) reduced vascular rejection more than did inhibition of ICAM-1 receptor (CD18) binding.[74] In contrast, renal allograft rejection (which is essentially equivalent to massive vascular rejection) has been successfully inhibited by anti-ICAM-1 antibodies in the monkey.[96] ICAM-1 inhi-bition is especially attractive, since both MHC molecules and ICAM-1 are required for antigen presentation to T-lymphocytes;[97] ICAM-1 blockade may therefore inhibit two critical steps in vascular graft injury rather than one. More recently, a distinct class of anti-inflammatory compounds, termed leumedins, have been developed which specifically inhibit upregulation of the ICAM-1 receptor molecule. The leumedin NPC15669 has been used to block recruitment of neutrophils at inflammatory foci,[98–101] and the hyperacute phase of xenograft rejection in guinea pig to Lewis rat transplants has been efficiently inhibited by use of NPC15669 to block neutrophils.[102] To date though, no studies have examined the effects of leumedins upon vascular occlusion during chronic rejection.

The final transmigration step in T-lymphocyte recruitment, as well as other components of chronic rejection, have also been exploited to inhibit vascular occlusion. Monoclonal antibodies to PECAM-1 have been used to prevent intraperitoneal thioglycollate induced leukocyte emigration for up to 48 hours in a mouse model,[103] suggesting that PECAM-1 inhibition would also prevent rejection. One of the integrins, $\alpha V\beta 3$, required for aSMC migration in response to mitogens from macrophages has been blocked using both monoclonal antibodies and soluble RGD-type competitive binding peptides;[61] $\alpha V\beta 3$ blockade has been shown in rabbit carotid injury models to significantly reduce aSMC migration into the site of injury. Similar to $\alpha V\beta 3$ blockade, a neutralizing monoclonal antibody against platelet IIb/IIIa integrin (which mediates the final common pathway for platelet aggregation[104]) has been found to cross-react with intimal smooth-muscle integrins, blocking migration.[105] As stated previously, there is also evidence suggesting IFN-γ has an endogenous antiproliferative effect upon aSMCs, and administration of IFN-γ has successfully prevented immune-mediated aSMC proliferation in animal models.[106] Exogenous IFN-γ administered to balloon-injured rats daily for seven days resulted in 50% reduction of neointimal area two weeks postinjury, with the effects persisting up to 10 weeks postsurgery. Finally, soluble complement receptor 1 (sCR1) has also significantly improved graft heart survival in a guinea pig to Lewis rat cardiac xenograft model,[102] presumably by inhibiting the complement cascade which causes de-endothelialization.

Although recent advances are cause for optimism, it has been a recurring problem that animal models do not accurately reflect clinical reality, particularly in controlled trials to prevent restenosis. Unfortunately, there are minimal data on cell-adhesion blockade in human subjects on which to base areas of future emphasis, so considerably more data are needed before efficient inhibition of adhesion molecules becomes a clinical reality. An additional problem is the reliance upon monoclonal antibodies to inhibit adhesion cascades. Widespread use of neutralizing antibodies increases the potential for development of 'anti-antibody antibodies'; this has been observed previously with generation of antimurine antibodies during monoclonal therapies (i.e. the HAMA response[107]). However, there are new approaches to monoclonal antibody generation which may circumvent these important issues; these will be discussed in the next section. Drugs similar to the leumedins eliminate some of the problems associated with the use of neutralizing antibodies or inhibitory peptides, but a potentially better scenario would be rational drug design based on understanding and modeling adhesive protein–protein interactions at the molecular level. Selective inhibitors would then be chemically synthesized like any other pharmaceutical drug. Finally, there again is the problem seen with the first generation of mitogen–toxin conjugates: non-specificity. Inflammatory-cell recruitment is essential to normal immune monitoring, and more important for transplantation arteriosclerosis, it appears from animal studies that at least some T-lymphocyte infiltration is essential if recipients are to develop long-term acceptance of donated tissues.[57,63] Since general adhesion blockade may raise immunosuppression issues, additional specificity for particular vascular sites only continues to be a principal concern.

Monoclonal antibodies: seek and subdue

Data for a variety of monoclonal antibodies that inhibit cell-adhesion molecule cascades were described in the preceding section. However, other neutralizing antibodies have also been tested for treatment of accelerated arteriopathies. The earliest monoclonal antibody specifically targeted to transplant rejection, OKT3,[108,109] was approved in the mid-1980s. Yet the most promising clinical data to date are for Centocor's 7E3 mouse/human chimeric monoclonal antibody which neutralizes platelet integrin IIb/IIIa, the receptor mediating the final common pathway for platelet aggregation.[104] Endothelial damage of venous and arterial grafts, as well as during transplantation is well documented; such damage frequently leads to thrombotic occlusion.[57,60,110,111] As was discussed previously, the aggregated platelets can also express selectins that potentiate the immune response, in addition to releasing mitogens and chemotactic compounds for aSMCs. Animal trials (Refs 112–114, and numerous others) have tested monoclonal antibody 7E3 for efficacy in prevention of platelet aggregation. 7E3 significantly reduces both platelet adhesion and thrombosis, and has subsequently proven beneficial in human clinical studies such as the EPIC trials.[115,116] However, 7E3 has demonstrated some potential problems, such as an increased risk for bleeding;[116] therefore more selective targeting, as discussed previously, may eventually be preferable.

Emerging clinical evidence suggests that antibodies to cardiac myosin can assist in diagnosing myocardial infarction, myocarditis, and most important for this discussion, transplant rejection.[117] There is also increasing evidence that imaging of the thrombus can have clinical utility.[110] Other cellular molecules required for the rejection reaction and subsequent neointimal formation offer additional targets for monoclonal antibody diagnosis or therapies. IL-2 appears to play a significant role in development of chronic rejection and hence transplant arteriosclerosis;[118] therefore, monoclonal antibodies against the IL-2 receptor have been tested both in animal studies[119] and a small human trial.[120] In three human subjects with multiple advanced rejection episodes, anti-IL-2 receptor antibody administration for 12 days resulted in 90% inhibition of mixed lymphocyte reactions and reduced rejection (determined by biopsy) from an average of Grade 3A to Grade 0–1A. Studies *in vitro* and in animal models have also used neutralizing antibodies against the mitogenic growth factors to attain similar results as mitogen–toxin chimeras in blocking neointimal formation.[121–123] Administration of a goat anti-PDGF polyclonal antibody to athymic rats after carotid artery balloon de-endothelialization resulted in nearly 100% blockade of aSMC migration into a neointima 8 days postinjury, thus successfully inhibiting PDGF signaling;[123] approximately 80% blockade of early proliferation was observed using rabbit anti-bFGF antibodies both in culture and in rat carotid injury models.[36,38,122]

The principal problem with monoclonal antibody therapies as a whole has been recognition of therapeutic antibodies as foreign proteins. However, if such difficulties can be resolved, antibody-mediated neutralization or detection of paths specific to accelerated arteriopathies will remain clinically viable alternatives. Several groups have developed alternatives to classical murine monoclonal antibodies that may eliminate or reduce the HAMA reaction. Some groups have made 'humanized' murine antibodies by recombinant expression of modified murine antibody variable regions linked to human Fc (constant) regions.[124] Additional novel approaches include phage-directed display of human Fab fragments in an *E. coli* expression system,[125] allowing completely human antibody protein sequences to be isolated and purified in quantity. Other promising innovations include purification of human antibodies from long-term cultures of human B-lymphocytes[126] as well as selection of B-lymphocytes specific for particular antigens by a method termed subtractive immunization.[127] There has also been recent success in creating transgenic mice which express human immunoglobulin genes.[128] These new approaches may allow for an even greater variety of monoclonal antibodies to become available for clinical trials.

Extracellular matrix: it's what is outside that counts

Restenosis is not comprised solely of cellular elements; extracellular matrix is an essential component of vascular repair as well. Recent evidence suggests that smooth muscle and matrix elastic recoil, as well as matrix expansion and remodeling, may be as important as smooth-muscle hyperplasia in formation of occlusions.[83,129] There has been a particular emphasis on matrix changes which alter the ability of aSMCs and ECs to proliferate and migrate in response to the various extracellular mitogens, including provisional matrix components which activate smooth-muscle proliferation and migration.[130,131] Unfortunately, these areas have not yet come to clinical fruition; what follows should be considered a very superficial preview of an emerging area in our understanding of accelerated arteriopathies, which may be applicable to targeted therapies in the future, or an adjunct to increase specificity of therapies already mentioned.

Reconstruction of damaged vascular wall requires two distinct phases of aSMC activity. First, aSMCs must 'loosen' their pericellular matrix to permit migration into sites of repair; this step depends upon proteases, including urokinase, metalloproteinases and others.[132–136] Second, once aSMCs have migrated to the site of repair, new matrix must be produced. The initial matrix which is synthesized is provisional and counteradhesive, allowing aSMCs to remain motile; later, this matrix is degraded, and replaced by a strongly adhesive matrix similar to that in normal adult vasculature.[129] There is little information available on how aSMCs regulate the total size of the final matrix, which would provide an ideal cellular pathway for intervention. More data are available concerning the composition of provisional matrix, which helps direct aSMC migration.

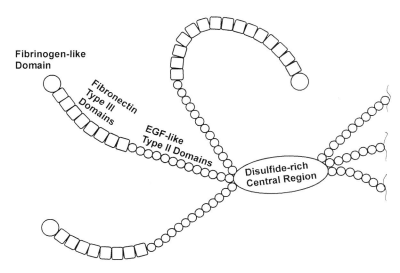

Figure 3.4 Schematic structure of tenascin. Tenascin is a hexameric oligomer, joined centrally by multiple disulfide linkages at the C-termini, with each N-terminal arm extending radially. Each monomeric arm in turn has protein domains with distinct biochemical features and interactions. These repeating domains are active in cell–cell or cell–matrix binding, calcium sequestration and interactions between multiple extracellular matrix molecules.

Two molecules, tenascin (TN) and thrombospondin (TSP) (Figures 3.4 and 3.5, respectively), appear to be the major counteradhesive proteins within the early provisional matrix.[131,137] TSP is a multi-subunit trimer, that is a predominant protein within platelet-alpha granules; yet the source for arterial wall deposition after balloon injury appears to be synthesis by aSMCs and ECs.[138,139] TN, which is a hexamer, is like TSP in that it is comprised of multiple subunit domains, each with distinctive biochemical properties.[140–142] TN has been detected as a significant mRNA species in actively proliferating, neointimal smooth-muscle cells in the balloon injured rat model, so the large quantities within early matrix are probably of aSMC origin.[143–145] Both TSP and TN act as counteradhesive molecules because they have subunit domains that can disrupt the assembly of focal adhesion proteins expressed by aSMCs or ECs, which normally form the cellular binding sites to fibronectin in the extracellular matrix.[146,147] In ECs, this appears to inhibit migration into injured areas,[139,146,148] but for aSMCs it allows cell migration within what is normally a highly adhesive milieu.[131] TSP also appears to inhibit re-endothelialization of injured sites by directly blocking EC proliferation, while acting as a significant mitogen for aSMCs.[131,149] There is further evidence that some of the progression and migratory effects of soluble mitogens on aSMCs during vascular injury are a result of increased TSP synthesis and deposition.[150–152] Given the negative clinical effects which TSP and TN deposition may have upon injured sites, they would seem strong candidates for therapeutic inhibition; unfortunately, no *in vivo* data are available to date.

Extant matrix and matrix-derived molecules not only regulate migration of aSMCs and ECs, but also organization and synthesis of additional extracellular components

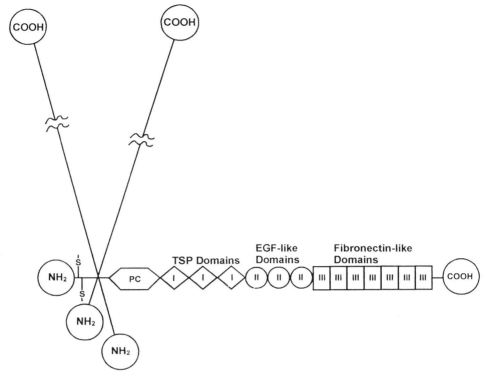

Figure 3.5 Similar to tenascin, thrombospondin comprises multiple repeating molecular domains; however, thrombospondin is a homotrimer, linked by disulfide bridges near the amino terminus. The linking arms and globular C-terminal domains spread in three directions, allowing considerable flexibility and thereby increasing potential interactions with other matrix components. Note especially that two of the subunit domain types (Type II or EGF-like, and Type III or fibronectin-like) are highly similar between thrombospondin and tenascin (Figure 3.4). The TSP domain is unique to thrombospondin and is not present in tenascin.

(Figure 3.6). For example, an important feature of maturation of new vascular matrix appears to be contraction of the collagen fibrils, which contributes to the late vascular narrowing after balloon injury.[153–156] This process is beginning to be understood in terms of the actin and myosin isoforms involved,[157] but being intracellular proteins, they remain poor targets. Matrix contraction could be interrupted by drugs that inhibit anchoring of collagen fibrils to the cellular Ib and IIb/IIIa integrin receptors that transmit the force of the acto-myosin complex to the wall as a whole.[158–160] As a second example, heparin administration in balloon injured rats decreases both elastin and collagen content of the new matrix, suggesting that heparin may prevent late elastic recoil in the rat model, in addition to its antimitogenic effects.[161] Therefore, inhibition of elastogenesis or collagen synthesis/deposition may be plausible alternatives for prevention of occlusion due to matrix contraction. Similarly, a more complete understanding of the effects of TGF-β_1 and PDGF[162] upon matrix synthesis and degradation may offer new strategies for targeted therapy.

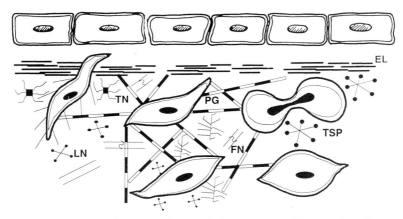

Figure 3.6 Schematic diagram of the arterial extracellular matrix. In addition to thrombospondin (TSP) and tenascin (TN), proteoglycans (PG), laminin (LN), fibronectin (FN), and elastin (EL) form a complex interactive milieu, underlying the endothelium and surrounding the smooth-muscle cells. The ability of different extracellular matrix molecules to determine functional characteristics of smooth-muscle cells *in vitro* has been observed for decades. More recently, we have begun to understand how the composition of matrix is actively controlled by cells after injury, in order to change cellular migration rates, contractility and proliferation capacity. For additional details on the interactions of matrix molecules that regulate smooth muscle and endothelial functions, see Refs 104, 105 and 129–142.

Summary

Recent advances in our understanding of vascular injury have made it increasingly possible to develop therapeutic strategies that uniquely target and prevent accelerated arteriopathies. Knowing the specific signaling roles played by mitogenic growth factors has allowed the proliferative cascade itself to be disrupted. Some therapies have emphasized blockage of the initial signal, while others 'hijack' the effector molecules to inhibit cell proliferation. In contrast, DNA-based therapies have targeted the postreceptor cascades that are activated prior to smooth-muscle proliferation associated with intimal hyperplasia, as well as the final common pathways used by all proliferating cells. Using a complementary combination of both these approaches may ultimately yield a better clinical outcome than will any single system alone. It still remains to be demonstrated whether any of the targeted therapies described will be more efficacious in routine use than any of the therapies which have resulted in disappointing clinical trials so far. However, we remain cautiously optimistic that accelerated arteriopathies are a controllable clinical problem.

References

1. Vitetta, E. S., Fulton, R. J., May, R. D. *et al.* (1987) *Science*, **238**, 1098–104.
2. FitzGerald, D. and Pastan, I. (1989) Targeted toxin therapy for the treatment of cancer. *J. Natl Cancer Inst.*, **81**, 1455–63.
3. Pai, L. H. and Pastan, I. (1993) The use of immunotoxins for cancer therapy. *Eur. J. Cancer*, **29A**, 1606–9.

4. Ip, J. H., Fuster, V., Badimon, L. *et al.* (1990) Syndromes of accelerated atherosclerosis: role of vascular injury and smooth muscle cell proliferation. *J. Am. Coll. Cardiol.*, **15**, 1667–87.

5. Clowes, A. W. and Reidy, M. A. (1991) Prevention of stenosis after vascular reconstruction: pharmacologic control of intimal hyperplasia – a review. *J. Vasc. Surg.*, **13**, 885–91.

6. Anderson, H. V., Vignale, S. J., Benedict, C. R. and Willerson, J. T. (1993) Restenosis after coronary angioplasty. *J. Intervent. Cardiol.*, **6**, 187–202.

7. Ludwig, C. L., Stiller, J. W., Burns, P. J. and Phillips, T. M. (1988) Migraine headaches, migraine equivalents, and anti-smooth muscle antibodies. *Headache*, **28**, 332–6.

8. Dighiero, G., Lymberi, P., Monot, C. and Abuaf, N. (1990) Sera with high levels of anti-smooth muscle and anti-mitochondrial antibodies frequently bind to cytoskeleton proteins. *Clin. Exptl Immunol.*, **82**, 52–6.

9. Daniel-Ribeiro, C., Slama, L. B. and Gentilini, M. (1991) Anti-nuclear and anti-smooth muscle antibodies in Caucasians, Africans, and Asians with acute malaria. *J. Clin. Lab. Immunol.*, **35**, 109–12.

10. Gadeau, A-P., Campan, M., Millet, D. *et al.* (1993) Osteopontin overexpression is associated with arterial smooth muscle cell proliferation *in vitro*. *Arterioscler. Thromb.*, **13**, 120–5.

11. Birukov, K. G., Frid, M. G., Rogers, J. D. *et al.* (1993) Synthesis and expression of smooth muscle phenotype markers in primary culture of rabbit aortic smooth muscle cells: influence of seeding density and media and relation to cell contractility. *Exptl Cell Res.*, **204**, 46–53.

12. Fatigati, V. and Murphy, R. A. (1984) Actin and tropomyosin variants in smooth muscles: dependence on tissue type. *J. Biol. Chem.*, **259**, 14383–8.

13. Rovner, A. S., Murphy, R. A. and Owens, G. K. (1994) Expression of smooth muscle and nonmuscle myosin heavy chains in cultured vascular smooth muscle cells. *J. Biol. Chem.*, **261**, 14740–5.

14. Nikkari, S. T., Koistinaho, J. and Jaakkola, O. (1990) Changes in the composition of cytoskeletal and cytocontractile proteins of rat aortic smooth muscle cells during aging. *Differentiation*, **44**, 216–21.

15. Shirinsky, V. P., Birukov, K. G., Koteliansky, V. E. *et al.* (1991) Density-related expression of caldesmin and vinculin in cultured rabbit aortic smooth muscle cells. *Exptl Cell Res.*, **194**, 186–9.

16. Birchmeier, W. and Behrens, J. (1994) Cadherin expression in carcinomas: role in the formation of cell junctions and the prevention of invasiveness. *Biochim. Biophys. Acta (Mol. Cell Res.)*, **1198**, 11–26.

17. Pavalko, F. M. and Otey, C. A. (1994) Role of adhesion molecule cytoplasmic domains in mediating interactions with the cytoskeleton. *Proc. Soc. Exptl Biol. Med.*, **205**, 282–93.

18. Gilbertson-Beadling, S. K. and Fisher, C. (1993) A potential role for *N*-cadherin in mediating endothelial cell-smooth muscle cell interactions in the rat vasculature. *Lab. Invest.*, **69**, 203–9.

19. Lazard, D., Sastre, X., Frid, M. G. *et al.* (1993) Expression of smooth muscle-specific proteins in myoepithelium and stromal myofibroblasts of normal and malignant human breast tissue. *Proc. Natl Acad. Sci. USA*, **90**, 999–1003.

20. Wagner, D. D. and Bonfanti, R. (1991) von Willebrand factor and the endothelium. *Mayo Clin. Proc.*, **66**, 621–7.

21. Ruggeri, Z. M. and Ware, J (1993) von Willebrand factor. *FASEB J.*, **7**, 308–16.

22. Nurden, A. T. and Nurden, P. (1993) A review of the role of platelet membrane glycoproteins in the platelet–vessel wall interaction. *Baillière's Clin. Haematol.*, **6**, 653–90.

23. Pearson, J. D. (1993) The control of production and release of haemostatic factors in the endothelial cell. *Baillière's Clin. Haematol.*, **6**, 629–51.

24. Liaw, L. and Schwartz, S. M. (1993) Comparison of gene expression in bovine aortic endothelium *in vivo* versus *in vitro*: differences in growth regulatory molecules. *Arterioscler. Thromb.*, **13**, 985–93.

25. Rafii, S., Shapiro, F., Rimarachin, J. *et al.* (1994) Isolation and characterization of human bone marrow microvascular endothelial cells: hematopoietic progenitor cell adhesion. *Blood*, **84**, 10–19.
26. Grafe, M., Graf, K., Auch-Schwelk, W. *et al.* (1993) Cultivation and characterization of micro- and macrovascular endothelial cells from the human heart. *Eur. Heart J.*, **14** (Supp. 1), 74–81.
27. Whyte, A., Garratt, L., James, P. S. and Binns, R. M. (1993) Distribution of saccharides in pig lymph-node high-endothelial venules and associated lymphocytes visualized using fluorescent lectins and confocal microscopy. *Histochem. J.*, **25**, 726–34.
28. Siflinger-Birnboim, A., Schnitzer, J., Lum, H. *et al.* (1991) Lectin binding to gp60 decreases specific albumin binding and transport in pulmonary artery endothelial monolayers [published erratum appears in *J. Cell. Physiol.*, June 1992, **151**(3), 642]. *J. Cell. Physiol.*, **149**, 575–84.
29. Millauer, B., Wizigmann-Voos, S., Schnurch, H. *et al.* (1993) High affinity VEGF binding and developmental expression suggest flk-1 as a major regulator of vasculogenesis and angiogenesis. *Cell*, **72**, 835–46.
30. Kim, K. J., Li, B., Winer, J. *et al.* (1993) Inhibition of vascular endothelial growth factor-induced angiogenesis suppresses tumour growth *in vivo*. *Nature*, **362**, 841–44.
31. Waltenberger, J., Usuki, K., Fellstrom, B. *et al.* (1992) Platelet-derived endothelial cell growth factor. Pharmacokinetics, organ distribution and degradation after intravenous administration in rats. *FEBS Lett.*, **313**, 129–32.
32. Heldin, C. H., Usuki, K. and Miyazono, K. (1991) Platelet-derived endothelial cell growth factor. *J. Cell. Biochem.*, **47**, 208–10.
33. Miyazono, K., Usuki, K. and Heldin, C. H. (1991) Platelet-derived endothelial cell growth factor. *Progr. Growth Factor Res.*, **3**, 207–17.
34. Casscells, S. W., Lappi, D. A., Olwin, B. B. *et al.* (1992) Elimination of smooth muscle cells in experimental restenosis: targeting of fibroblast growth factor receptors. *Proc. Natl Acad. Sci. USA*, **89**, 7159–63.
35. Mesri, E. A., Kreitman, R. J., Fu, Y. M. *et al.* (1993) Heparin-binding transforming growth factor a–*Pseudomonas* exotoxin A. A heparin sulfate-modulated recombinant toxin cytotoxic to cancer cells and proliferating smooth muscle cells. *J. Biol. Chem.*, **268**, 4853–62.
36. Reidy, M. A., Fingerle, J. and Lindner, V. (1992) Factors controlling the development of arterial lesions after injury. *Circulation*, **86** (Supp. III), III-43–III-46.
37. Lindner, V., Lappi, D. A., Baird, A. *et al.* (1991) Role of basic fibroblast growth factor in vascular lesion formation. *Circ. Res.*, **68**, 106–13.
38. Olson, N. E., Chao, S., Lindner, V. and Reidy, M. A. (1992) Intimal smooth muscle cell proliferation after balloon catheter injury: the role of basic fibroblast growth factor. *Am. J. Pathol.*, **140**, 1017–23.
39. Lindner, V. and Reidy, M. A. (1993) Expression of basic fibroblast growth factor and its receptor by smooth muscle cells and endothelium in injured rat arteries: an *en face* study. *Circ. Res.*, **73**, 589–95.
40. Jackson, C. L. and Reidy, M. A. (1993) Basic fibroblast growth factor: its role in the control of smooth muscle cell migration. *Am. J. Pathol.*, **143**, 1024–31.
41. Casscells, S. W. (1992) Migration of smooth muscle and endothelial cells: critical events in restenosis. *Circulation*, **86**, 723–9.
42. Libby, P., Schwartz, D., Brogi, E. *et al.* (1992) A cascade model for restenosis: a special case of atherosclerosis progression. *Circulation*, **86** (Supp. III), III-47–III-52.
43. Epstein, S. E., Siegall, C. B., Biro, S. *et al.* (1991) Cytotoxic effects of a recombinant chimeric toxin on rapidly proliferating vascular smooth muscle cells. *Circulation*, **84**, 778–87.
44. Pelham, H. R. B. (1989) Heat shock and the sorting of luminal ER proteins. *EMBO J.*, **8**, 3171–6.
45. Chaudhary, V. K., Jinno, Y., FitzGerald, D. and Pastan, I. (1990) *Pseudomonas* exotoxin contains a specific sequence at the carboxyl terminus that is required for cytotoxicity. *Proc. Natl Acad. Sci. USA*, **87**, 308–12.

46. Seetharam, S., Chaudhary, V. K., FitzGerald, D. and Pastan, I. (1991) Increased cytotoxic activity of *Pseudomonas* exotoxin and two chimeric toxins in KDEL. *J. Biol. Chem.*, **266**, 17376–81.
47. Pickering, J. G., Bacha, P. A., Weir, L. *et al.* (1993) Prevention of smooth muscle cell outgrowth from human atherosclerotic plaque by a recombinant cytotoxin specific for the epidermal growth factor receptor. *J. Clin. Invest.*, **91**, 724–9.
48. Ali, S., Davis, M. G., Becker, M. W. and Dorn, G. W. II (1993) Thromboxane A$_2$ stimulates vascular smooth muscle hypertrophy by up-regulating the synthesis and release of endogenous basic fibroblast growth factor. *J. Biol. Chem.*, **268**, 17397–403.
49. Weiss, R. H. and Maduri, M. (1992) The mitogenic effect of thrombin in vascular smooth muscle cells is largely due to basic fibroblast growth factor. *J. Biol. Chem.*, **268**, 5724–7.
50. Winkles, J. A. and Gay, C. G. (1991) Serum, phorbol ester, and polypeptide mitogens increase class 1 and 2 heparin-binding (acid and basic fibroblast) growth factor gene expression in human vascular smooth muscle cells. *Cell Growth Differentiation*, **2**, 531–40.
51. Sato, Y., Hamanaka, R., Ono, J. *et al.* (1991) The stimulatory effect of PDGF on vascular smooth muscle cell migration is mediated by the induction of endogenous basic FGF. *Biochem. Biophys. Res. Commun.*, **174**, 1260–6.
52. Lappi, D. A., Ying, W., Barthelemy, I. *et al.* (1994) Expression and activities of a recombinant basic fibroblast growth factor–saporin fusion protein. *J. Biol. Chem.*, **269**, 12552–8.
53. Lappi, D. A., Matsunami, R., Martineau, D. and Baird, A. (1993) Reducing the heterogeneity of chemically conjugated targeted toxins: homogeneous basic FGF–saporin. *Anal. Biochem.*, **212**, 446–51.
54. Mifflin, L. C. and Cohen, R. E. (1994) hsc70 moderates the heat shock (stress) response in *Xenopus laevis* oocytes and binds to denatured protein inducers. *J. Biol. Chem.*, **269**, 15718–23.
55. Gawlak, S. L., Pastan, I. and Siegall, C. B. (1993) Basic fibroblast growth factor–*Pseudomonas* exotoxin chimeric proteins: comparison with acidic fibroblast growth factor–*Pseudomonas* exotoxin. *Bioconj. Chem.*, **4**, 483–9.
56. Colvin, R. B. (1991) The pathogenhesis of vascular rejection. *Transplant. Proc.*, **23**, 2052–5.
57. Hansson, G. K., Geng, Y. J., Holm, J. and Stemme, S. (1993) Lymphocyte adhesion and cellular immune reactions in chronic rejection and graft arteriosclerosis. *Transplant. Proc.*, **25**, 2050–1.
58. Russell, P. S., Chase, C. M., Winn, H. J. and Colvin, R. B. (1994) Coronary atherosclerosis in transplanted mouse hearts. I. Time course and immunogenetic and immunopathological considerations. *Am. J. Pathol.*, **144**, 260–74.
59. Tanio, J. W., Basau, C. B., Albelda, S. M. and Eisen, H. J. (1994) Differential expression of the cell adhesion molecules ICAM-1, VCAM-1, and E-selectin in normal and posttransplantation myocardium: cell adhesion molecule expression in human cardiac allografts. *Circulation*, **89**, 1760–8.
60. Hansson, G. K. (1993) Immune and inflammatory mechanisms in the development of atherosclerosis. *Br. Heart J.*, **69** (Supp.), S38–S41.
61. Choi, E. T., Engel, L., Callow, A. D. *et al.* (1994) Inhibition of neointimal hyperplasia by blocking alpha-V beta-3 integrin with a small peptide antagonist GpenGRGDSPCA. *J. Vasc. Surg.*, **19**, 125–34.
62. Sluiter, W., Pietersma, A., Lamers, J. M. and Koster, J. F. (1993) Leukocyte adhesion molecules of the vascular endothelium: their role in the pathogenesis of cardiovascular disease and the mechanisms underlying their expression. *J. Cardiovasc. Pharmacol.*, **22**, S37–S44.
63. Springer, T. A. (1994) Traffic signals for lymphocyte recirculation and leukocyte emigration: the multistep paradigm. *Cell*, **76**, 301–14.
64. Lawrence, M. B. and Springer, T. A. (1991) Leukocytes roll on a selectin at physiologic flow rates: distinction from and prerequisite for adhesion through integrins. *Cell*, **65**, 859–73.

65. Albelda, S. M., Smith, C. W. and Ward, P. A. (1994) Adhesion molecules and inflammatory injury. *FASEB J.*, **8**, 504–12.
66. Luscinskas, F. W. and Lawler, J. (1994) Integrins as dynamic regulators of vascular function. *FASEB J.*, **8**, 929–38.
67. Weis, W. I. (1994) Lectins on a roll: the structure of E-selectin. *Structure*, **2**, 147–50.
68. Varki, A. (1994) Selectin ligands. *Proc. Natl Acad. Sci. USA*, **91**, 7390–7.
69. DiCorleto, P. E. (1993) Cellular mechanisms of atherogenesis. *Am. J. Hypertens.*, **6**, 314S–318S.
70. Henney, A. M., Wakeley, P. R., Davies, M. J. *et al.* (1991) Localization of stromelysin gene expression in atherosclerotic plaques by *in situ* hybridization. *Proc. Natl Acad. Sci. USA*, **88**, 8154–8.
71. Ferns, G. A. A., Reidy, M. A. and Ross, R. (1991) Balloon catheter de-endothelialization of the nude rat carotid: response to injury in the absense of functional T lymphocytes. *Am. J. Pathol.*, **138**, 1045–57.
72. Pelletier, R., Ohye, R., Kincade, P. *et al.* (1993) Monoclonal antibody to anti-VCAM-1 interferes with murine cardiac allograft rejection. *Transplant. Proc.*, **25**, 839–41.
73. Tanaka, H., Sukhova, G. K., Swanson, S. J. *et al.* (1994) Endothelial and smooth muscle cells express leukocyte adhesion molecules heterogeneously during acute rejection of rabbit cardiac allografts. *Am. J. Pathol.*, **144**, 938–51.
74. Sadahiro, M., McDonald, T. O. and Allen, M. D. (1993) Reduction in cellular and vascular rejection by blocking leukocyte adhesion molecule receptors. *Am. J. Pathol.*, **142**, 675–83.
75. Thyberg, J., Hedin, U., Sjolund, M. *et al.* (1990) Regulation of differentiated properties and proliferation of arterial smooth muscle cells. *Arteriosclerosis*, **10**, 966–90.
76. Munro, J. M. and Cotran, R. S. (1988) The pathogenesis of atherosclerosis: atherogenesis and inflammation. *Lab. Invest.*, **58**, 249–61.
77. Jooste, S. V., Colvin, R. B. and Winn, H. J. (1981) The vascular bed as the primary target in the destruction of skin grafts by antiserum. II. Loss of sensitivity to antiserum in long-term xenografts of skin. *J. Exptl Med.*, **154**, 1332.
78. Winn, H. J. (1992) Antibody-mediated rejection. In: Williams, G. M., Burdick, J. F. and Solez, K. (eds) *Kidney Transplant Rejection: Diagnosis and Treatment*, pp. 318–32. New York: Marcel Dekker.
79. Polanowska-Grabowska, R., Geanacopoulos, M. and Gear, A. R. (1993) Platelet adhesion to collagen via the alpha-2 beta-1 integrin under arterial flow conditions causes rapid tyrosine phosphorylation of pp125FAK. *Biochem. J.*, **296**, 543–7.
80. Ikeda, U., Ikeda, M., Seino, Y. *et al.* (1993) Expression of intercellular adhesion molecule-1 on rat vascular smooth muscle cells by pro-inflammatory cytokines. *Atherosclerosis*, **104**, 61–8.
81. Cybulsky, M. I. and Gimbrone, M. A., Jr (1991) Endothelial expression of a mononuclear leukocyte adhesion molecule during atherogenesis. *Science*, **251**, 788–91.
82. Carlos, T., Gordon, D., Fishbein, D. *et al.* (1992) Vascular cell adhesion molecule-1 is induced on endothelium during acute rejection in human cardiac allografts. *J. Heart Lung Transpl.*, **11**, 1103–9.
83. O'Brien, E. R., Alpers, C. E., Stewart, D. K. *et al.* (1993) Proliferation in primary and restenotic coronary atherectomy tissue: implications for antiproliferative therapy. *Circ. Res.*, **73**, 223–31.
84. Li, H., Cybulsky, M. I., Gimbrone, M. A., Jr and Libby, P. (1993) Inducible expression of vascular cell adhesion molecule-1 by vascular smooth muscle cells *in vitro* and within rabbit atheroma. *Am. J. Pathol.*, **143**, 1551–9.
85. Poston, R. N., Haskard, D. O., Coucher, J. R. *et al.* (1992) Expression of intercellular adhesion molecule-1 in atherosclerotic plaques. *Am. J. Pathol.*, **140**, 665–73.
86. Couffinhal, T., Duplaa, C., Moreau, C. *et al.* (1994) Regulation of vascular cell adhesion molecule-1 and intercellular adhesion molecule-1 in human vascular smooth muscle cells. *Circ. Res.*, **74**, 225–34.
87. Wood, K. M., Cadogan, M. D., Ramshaw, A. L. and Parums, D. V. (1993) The distribution of adhesion molecules in human atherosclerosis. *Histopathology*, **22**, 437–44.

88. van der Wal, A. C., Das, P. K., Tigges, A. J. and Becker, A. E. (1992) Adhesion molecules on the endothelium and mononuclear cells in human atherosclerotic lesions. *Am. J. Pathol.*, **141**, 1427–433.

89. Keelan, E. T. M., Harrison, A. A., Chapman, P. T. *et al.* (1994) Imaging vascular endothelial activation: an approach using radiolabeled monoclonal antibodies against the endothelial cell adhesion molecule E-selectin. *J. Nucl. Med.*, **35**, 276–81.

90. Picker, L. J. and Butcher, E. C. (1992) Physiological and molecular mechanisms of lymphocyte homing. *Annu. Rev. Immunol.*, **10**, 561–91.

91. Mulligan, M. S., Varani, J., Dame, M. K. *et al.* (1991) Role of endothelial–leukocyte adhesion molecule 1 (ELAM-1) in neutrophil-mediated lung injury in rats. *J. Clin. Invest.*, **88**, 1396–406.

92. Johnson-Tidey, R. R., McGregor, J. L., Taylor, P. R. and Poston, R. N. (1994) Increase in the adhesion molecule P-selectin in endothelium overlying atherosclerotic plaques: coexpression with intercellular adhesion molecule-1. *Am. J. Pathol.*, **144**, 952–61.

93. Orosz, C. G., Ohye, R. G., Pelletier, R. P. *et al.* (1993) Treatment with anti-vascular cell adhesion molecule 1 monoclonal antibody induces long-term murine cardiac allograft acceptance. *Transplantation*, **56**, 453–60.

94. Pelletier, R. P., Ohye, R. G., Vanbuskirk, A. *et al.* (1992) Importance of endothelial VCAM-1 for inflammatory leukocytic infiltration *in vivo*. *J. Immunol.*, **149**, 2473–81.

95. Isobe, M., Yagita, H., Okumura, K. and Ihara, A. (1992) Specific acceptance of cardiac allograft after treatment with antibodies to ICAM-1 and LFA-1. *Science*, **255**, 1125–7.

96. Cosimi, A. B., Conti, D. and Delmonico, F. L. (1990) *In vivo* effects of monoclonal antibody to ICAM-1 (CD54) in nonhuman primates with renal allografts. *J. Immunol.*, **144**, 4604–12.

97. Altmann, D. M., Hogg, N. and Trowsdale, J. (1989) Cotransfection of ICAM-1 and HLA-DR reconstitutes human antigen presenting function in mouse L cells. *Nature*, **338**, 512.

98. Naccache, P. H., Jean, N., Liao, N. W. *et al.* (1994) Regulation of stimulated integrin surface expression in human neutrophils by tyrosine phosphorylation. *Blood*, **84**, 616–24.

99. Otterbein, L., Lowe, V. C., Kyle, D. J. and Noronha-Blob, L. (1993) Additive effects of a bradykinin antagonist, NPC 17761, and a leumedin, NPC 15669, on survival in animal models of sepsis. *Agents Actions*, **39** (Spec. Issue), C125–C127.

100. Sekine, S., Hayashi, Y., Ando, T. *et al.* (1993) [An outbreak of gastroenteritis due to group C rotavirus in Tokyo]. *Kansenshogaku Zasshi*, **67**, 110–15.

101. Navab, M., Hama, S. Y., Van Lenten, B. J. *et al.* (1993) A new antiinflammatory compound, leumedin, inhibits modification of low density lipoprotein and the resulting monocyte transmigration into the subendothelial space of cocultures of human aortic wall cells. *J. Clin. Invest.*, **91**, 1225–30.

102. Zehr, K. J., Herskowitz, A., Lee, P. C. *et al.* (1994) Neutrophil adhesion and complement inhibition prolongs survival of cardiac xenografts in discordant species. *Transplantation*, **57**, 900–6.

103. Bogen, S., Pak, J., Garifallou, M. *et al.* (1994) Monoclonal antibody to murine PECAM-1 (CD31) blocks acute inflammation *in vivo*. *J. Exptl Med.*, **179**, 1059–64.

104. Kaplan, A. V., Leung, L. L., Leung, W. H. *et al.* (1991) Roles of thrombin and platelet membrane glycoprotein IIb/IIIa in platelet-subendothelial deposition after angioplasty in an *ex vivo* whole artery model. *Circulation*, **84**, 1279–88.

105. Otey, C. A., Pavalko, F. M. and Burridge, K. (1990) An interaction between alpha-actinin and the beta-1 integrin subunit *in vitro*. *J. Cell Biol.*, **111**, 721–9.

106. Hansson, G. K. and Holm, J. (1991) Interferon-gamma inhibits arterial stenosis after injury. *Circulation*, **84**, 1266–72.

107. McAfee, J. G. (1994) Imaging vascular endothelial activation [editorial]. *J. Nucl. Med.*, **35**, 281.

108. Kimball, J. A., Norman, D. J., Shield, C. F. *et al.* (1993) OKT3 antibody response study (OARS): a multicenter comparative study. *Transplant. Proc.*, **25**, 558–60.

109. Light, J. A., Khawand, N., Ali, A. *et al.* (1989) Comparison of Minnesota antilymphocyte globulin and OKT3 for induction of immunosuppression in renal transplant patients. *Transplant. Proc.*, **21**, 1738–40.

110. Cerqueira, M. D., Stratton, J. R., Vracko, R. *et al.* (1992) Noninvasive arterial thrombus imaging with ^{99m}Tc monoclonal antifibrin antibody. *Circulation*, **85**, 298–304.
111. Underwood, M. J., Pringle, S. and de Bono, D. P. (1992) Reduction of thrombus formation *in vivo* using a thrombolytic agent targeted at damaged endothelial cells. *Br. J. Surg.*, **79**, 915–17.
112. Rote, W. E., Nedelman, M. A., Mu, D. X. *et al.* (1994) Chimeric 7E3 prevents carotid artery thrombosis in cynomolgus monkeys. *Stroke*, **25**, 1223–32.
113. Rote, W. E., Mu, D. X., Bates, E. R. *et al.* (1994) Prevention of rethrombosis after coronary thrombolysis in a chronic canine model. I. Adjunctive therapy with monoclonal antibody 7E3 F(ab')2 fragment. *J. Cardiovasc. Pharmacol.*, **23**, 194–202.
114. Bates, E. R., McGillem, M. J., Mickelson, J. K. *et al.* (1991) A monoclonal antibody against the platelet glycoprotein IIb/IIIa receptor complex prevents platelet aggregation and thrombosis in a canine model of coronary angioplasty. *Circulation*, **84**, 2463–9.
115. Topol, E. J., Califf, R. M., Weisman, H. F. *et al.* (1994) Randomized trial of coronary intervention with antibody against platelet IIb/IIIa integrin for reduction of clinical restenosis: results at six months. *Lancet*, **343**, 881–6.
116. Anonymous (1994) Use of a monoclonal antibody directed against the platelet glyco-protein IIb/IIIa receptor in high-risk coronary angioplasty. *N. Engl. J. Med.*, **330**, 956–61.
117. Ballester, M., Obrador, D., Carrio, I. *et al.* (1992) Early postoperative reduction of monoclonal antimyosin antibody uptake is associated with absent rejection-related complications after heart transplantation. *Circulation*, **85**, 61–8.
118. Kupiec-Weglinski, J. W., Diamantstein, R. and Tilney, N. (1988) Interleukin-2 receptor targeted therapy: rationale and applications in organ transplantation. *Transplantation*, **46**, 785–92.
119. Kupiec-Weglinski, J. W., Diamantstein, T., Tilney, N. L. and Strom, T. B. (1986) Therapy with monoclonal antibody to interleukin-2 receptor spares suppressor T cells and prevents or reverses acute allograft rejection in rats. *Proc. Natl Acad. Sci. USA*, **83**, 2624–7.
120. van Gelder, T., Balk, A. H. M. M., Mochtar, B. and Weimar, W. (1992) Reversal of graft rejection with monoclonal anti-interleukin-2 receptor. *Lancet*, **339**, 873.
121. Russell, W. E., van Wyk, J. J. and Pledger, W. J. (1984) Inhibition of the mitogenic effects of plasma by a monoclonal antibody to somatomedin C. *Proc. Natl Acad. Sci. USA*, **81**, 2389–92.
122. Lindner, V. and Reidy, M. A. (1991) Proliferation of smooth muscle cells after vascular injury is inhibited by an antibody against basic fibroblast growth factor. *Proc. Natl Acad. Sci. USA*, **88**, 3739–43.
123. Ferns, G. A. A., Raines, E. W., Sprugel, K. H. *et al.* (1991) Inhibition of neointimal smooth muscle accumulation after angioplasty by an antibody to PDGF. *Science*, **233**, 1129–32.
124. Lockwood, C. M., Thiru, S., Isaacs, J. D. *et al.* (1993) Long-term remission of intractable systemic vasculitis with monoclonal antibody therapy. *Lancet*, **341**, 1620–2.
125. Barbas, C. F., III, Crowe, J. E., Jr, Cababa, D. *et al.* (1992) Human monoclonal Fab fragments derived from a combinatorial library bind to respiratory syncitial virus F glycoprotein and neutralize infectivity. *Proc. Natl Acad. Sci. USA*, **89**, 10164–8.
126. Williamson, R. A., Burioni, R., Sanna, P. P. *et al.* (1993) Human monoclonal antibodies against a plethora of viral pathogens from single combinatorial libraries. *Proc. Natl Acad. Sci. USA*, **90**, 4141–5.
127. Brooks, P. C., Lynn, J. M., French, D. L. and Quigly, J. P. (1993) Subtractive immunization yields monoclonal antibodies that specifically inhibit metastasis. *J. Cell Biol.*, **122**, 1351–9.
128. Morrison, S. L. (1994) Success in specification. *Nature*, **368**, 812–13.
129. Majesky, M. (1994) Neointimal formation after acute vascular injury: role of counterad-hesive extracellular matrix proteins. *Texas Heart Inst. J.*, **21**, 78–85.
130. Schwartz, S. M., Heimark, R. L. and Majesky, M. W. (1990) Developmental mechanisms underlying pathology of arteries. *Physiol. Rev.*, **70**, 1177–209.
131. Majesky, M. W., Giachelli, C. M., Reidy, M. A. and Ross, R. (1992) Rat carotid neointimal smooth muscle cells reexpress a developmentally regulated mRNA phenotype during repair of arterial injury. *Circ. Res.*, **71**, 759–68.

132. Bendeck, M. P., Zempo, N., Clowes, A. W. *et al*. (1994) Smooth muscle cell migration and matrix metalloproteinase expression after arterial injury in the rat. *Circ. Res.*, **75**, 539–45.

133. Zempo, N., Kenargy, R. D., Au, Y. P. *et al*. (1994) Matrix metalloproteinases of vascular wall cells are increased in balloon-injured rat carotid artery. *J. Vasc. Surg.*, **20**, 209–17.

134. Pauly, R. R., Passaniti, A., Bilato, C. *et al*. (1994) Migration of cultured vascular smooth muscle cells through a basement membrane barrier requires type IV collagenase activity and is inhibited by cellular differentiation. *Circ. Res.*, **75**, 41–54.

135. Kenagy, R. D., Nikkari, S. T., Welgus, H. G. and Clowes, A. W. (1994) Heparin inhibits the induction of three matrix metalloproteinases (stromelysin, 92-kD gelatinase, and collagenase) in primate arterial smooth muscle cells. *J. Clin. Invest.*, **93**, 1987–93.

136. Yanagi, H., Sasaguri, Y., Sugama, K. *et al*. (1991) Production of tissue collagenase (matrix metalloproteinase 1) by human aortic smooth muscle cells in response to platelet-derived growth factor. *Atherosclerosis*, **91**, 207–16.

137. Scott-Burden, T. (1994) Extracellular matrix: the cellular environment. *News Physiol. Sci.*, **9**, 110–15.

138. Raugi, G. J., Mullen, J. S., Bark, D. H. *et al*. (1990) Thrombospondin deposition in rat carotid artery injury. *Am. J. Pathol.*, **137**, 179–85.

139. DiPietro, L. A., Nebgen, D. R. and Polverini, P. J. (1994) Downregulation of endothelial cell thrombospondin 1 enhances *in vitro* angiogenesis. *J. Vasc. Res.*, **31**, 178–85.

140. Bornstein, P. (1992) Thrombospondins: structure and regulation of expression [published erratum appears in *FASEB J.*, January 1993, **7**(1), 237]. *FASEB J.*, **6**, 3290–9.

141. Vrucinic-Filipi, N. and Chiquet-Ehrismann, R. (1993) Tenascin function and regulation of expression. *Symp. Soc. Exptl Biol.*, **47**, 155–62.

142. Venstrom, K. A. and Reichardt, L. F. (1993) Extracellular matrix. 2: Role of extracellular matrix molecules and their receptors in the nervous system. *FASEB J.*, **7**, 996–1003.

143. Majesky, M. W., Giachelli, C. M., Reidy, M. A. and Schwartz, S. M. (1992) Rat carotid neointimal smooth muscle cells reexpress a developmentally regulated mRNA phenotype during repair of arterial injury. *Circ. Res.*, **71**, 759–68.

144. Giachelli, C., Bae, N., Lombardi, D. *et al*. (1991) Molecular cloning and characterization of 2B7, a rat mRNA which distinguishes smooth muscle cell phenotypes *in vitro* and is identical to osteopontin (secreted phosphoprotein I, 2aR). *Biochem. Biophys. Res. Commun.*, **177**, 867–73.

145. Mackie, E. J., Scott-Burden, T., Hahn, A. W. *et al*. (1992) Expression of tenascin by vascular smooth muscle cells. Alterations in hypertensive rats and stimulation by angiotensin II [see comments]. *Am. J. Pathol.*, **141**, 377–88.

146. RayChaudhury, A., Frazier, W. A. and D'Amore, P. A. (1994) Comparison of normal and tumorigenic endothelial cells: differences in thrombospondin production and responses to transforming growth factor-beta. *J. Cell Sci.*, **107**, 39–46.

147. Sriramarao, P., Mendler, M. and Bourdon, M. A. (1993) Endothelial cell attachment and spreading on human tenascin is mediated by alpha-2 beta-1 and alpha v beta-3 integrins. *J. Cell Sci.*, **105**, 1001–12.

148. Tolsma, S. S., Volpert, O. V., Good, D. J. *et al*. (1993) Peptides derived from two separate domains of the matrix protein thrombospondin-1 have anti-angiogenic activity. *J. Cell Biol.*, **122**, 497–511.

149. Tschoepe, D., Schultheiss, H. P., Kolarov, P. *et al*. (1993) Platelet membrane activation markers are predictive for increased risk of acute ischemic events after PTCA. *Circulation*, **88**, 37–42.

150. Frazier, W. A. (1987) Thrombospondin: a modular adhesive glycoprotein of platelets and nucleated cells. *J. Cell Biol.*, **105**, 625–32.

151. Thie, M., Harrach, B., Schonherr, E. *et al*. (1993) Responsiveness of aortic smooth muscle cells to soluble growth mediators is influenced by cell–matrix contact. *Arterioscler. Thromb.*, **13**, 994–1004.

152. Sharifi, B. G., LaFleur, D. W., Pirola, C. J. *et al*. (1992) Angiotensin II regulates tenascin gene expression in vascular smooth muscle cells. *J. Biol. Chem.*, **267**, 23910–15.

153. Heistad, D. D. and Armstrong, M. L. (1994) Sick vessel syndrome: can atherosclerotic arteries recover? *Circulation*, **89**, 2447–50.
154. Kakuta, T., Currier, J. W., Haudenschild, C. C. *et al.* (1994) Differences in compensatory vessel enlargement, not intimal formation, account for restenosis after angioplasty in the hypercholesterolemic rabbit model. *Circulation*, **89**, 2809–15.
155. Post, M. J., Borst, C. and Kuntz, R. E. (1994) The relative importance of arterial remodeling compared with intimal hyperplasia in lumen renarrowing after balloon angioplasty: a study in the normal rabbit and the hypercholesterolemic Yucatan micropig. *Circulation*, **89**, 2816–21.
156. Gibbons, G. H. and Dzau, V. J. (1994) The emerging concept of vascular remodeling. *N. Engl. J. Med.*, **330**, 1431–8.
157. Aikawa, M., Sivam, P. N., Kuro-o, M. *et al.* (1993) Human smooth muscle myosin heavy chain isoforms as molecular markers for vascular development and atherosclerosis. *Circ. Res.*, **73**, 1000–12.
158. Glass, W. F., Jr and Kreisberg, J. I. (1993) Regulation of integrin-mediated adhesion at focal contacts by cyclic AMP. *J. Cell. Physiol.*, **157**, 296–306.
159. Fujio, Y., Yamada, F., Takahashi, K. and Shibita, N. (1993) Altered fibronectin-dependent cell adhesion by PDGF accompanies phenotypic modulation of vascular smooth muscle cells. *Biochem. Biophys. Res. Commun.*, **196**, 997–1002.
160. Bauer, J. S., Varner, J., Schreiner, C. *et al.* (1993) Functional role of the cytoplasmic domain of the integrin alpha 5 subunit. *J. Cell Biol.*, **122**, 209–21.
161. Snow, A. D., Bolender, R. P., Wight, T. N. and Clowes, A. W. (1990) Heparin modulates the composition of the extracellular matrix domain surrounding arterial smooth muscle cells. *Am. J. Pathol.*, **137**, 313–30.
162. Majesky, M. W., Lindner, V., Twardzik, D. R. *et al.* (1991) Production of transforming growth factor B1 during repair of arterial injury. *J. Clin. Invest.*, **88**, 904–10.

4

Accelerated Arteriopathies: Molecular Approach

Michael Simons

Introduction

Rapid advances in molecular biology over the past decade have led to a new understanding of the etiology and pathogenesis of a number of cardiovascular diseases. In this chapter we will review molecular events involved in development of postangioplasty restenosis and will discuss new therapeutic approaches evolving from the knowledge of these processes. Although we will primarily be concerned with molecular biology of restenosis as a prototypical accelerated arteriopathy, the discussion will be relevant to a number of closely related syndromes such as arteriopathies seen in cardiac transplant recipient's coronary arteries, postcoronary bypass vein grafts and accelerated hypertension syndromes. We will first briefly discuss molecular pathology of vascular lesions seen in accelerated arteriopathy, then describe current understanding of pathophysiology of this process and finally will concentrate on emerging novel molecular therapies.

Molecular pathology of vascular lesions

The predominant feature of vascular lesions seen in postangioplasty restenosis is abundant proliferation of smooth-muscle cells (SMCs) accompanied by extensive production of extracellular matrix.[1] In addition, a variety of other cell types, including macrophages and T-lymphocytes are present as well. The source of SMCs seen in these lesions remains a matter of some debate. Although in animals devoid of SMCs in the intima (such as rat carotid artery) neointimal lesions clearly consist of SMCs having migrated from the media, in larger animals (such as pigs) possessing SMCs in the intima, the situation is less clear with both intimal and medial SMCs probably contributing to the final lesion. This source of neointimal SMCs is not purely of theoretical interest since agents capable of blocking SMC migration may not be effective in treatment of this process if migration is not a major event. In particular, this putative difference between the origin of neointimal SMCs in small and large animals may be partially responsible for the failure of angiotensin converting-enzyme inhibitors to prevent postangioplasty restenosis in patients[2] and large animals,[3] while being very effective in rats.[4]

The SMCs found in neointimal lesions seen in these syndromes appear phenotypically different from their medial counterparts (Table 4.1). In particular they possess abundant rough endoplasmic reticulum, suggesting active protein synthesis, are capable of cell division (proliferation) and exhibit a number of changes in cytoskeletal protein composition demonstrating decrease in expression of contractile proteins (such as smooth-muscle actin and myosin) and a corresponding increase in nonmuscle isoforms. In addition, neointimal cells express large amounts of growth factor receptors as well as secrete growth factors (such as PDGF and IGF-1) themselves. These and other changes in neointimal SMC phenotype including expression of osteopontin, tropoelastin and procollagen resemble the phenotype seen in immature (developing) SMCs,[5] leading some authors to suggest that remnant immature SMCs are responsible for the formation of lesions seen in accelerated arteriopathies.[6] This point of view considers neointimal cells to be the result of expansion of dormant precursor cells rather than a consequence of 'phenotypic modulation' of normal medial SMCs.

While a lot of the information described above was gleaned from experimental studies in animal models, advent of coronary and peripheral atherectomy has provided a unique opportunity to study atherosclerotic and restenotic plaques in

Table 4.1 Smooth-muscle cell phenotypes

	Contractile	Synthetic
Functional		
Contractility	+	−
Proliferation	−	+
Matrix synthesis	−	++++
Rough endoplasmic reticulum	+	++++
Thick filaments	+	−
*Contractile proteins**		
α-Actin	80%	45%
β, γ-Actin	20%	55%
SMMHC	90%	15%
NMMHC	10%	85%
Growth factors		
PDGF-A	+	+++
PDGF-α receptor	±	+++
PDGF-B	++	+
PDGF-β receptor	++	+
IGF-1	+	+++
TGF-β	−	+++
Other proteins		
Osteopontin	−	+++
Matrix GIa protein	−	+++
Tropoelastin	+++	+
Phospholamban	+++	±

*SMMHC, smooth-muscle myosin heavy chain; NMMHC, nonmuscle myosin heavy chain. The plus signs indicate the extent of gene expression.

live patients and correlate their molecular phenotypes with subsequent clinical course. Molecular analysis of atherectomy tissue demonstrated that many features associated with proliferating SMCs and endothelial cells *in vitro* and in animal models are present in restenotic human coronary lesions (Table 4.2). However, some of the SMCs in primary (i.e. previously uninstrumented) atherosclerotic lesions also appear to have undergone phenotypic transformation displaying morphological appearance and molecular markers typical of cells in restenotic lesions (Figure 4.1). Thus, there is a continuous spectrum of phenotypic variations between SMCs observed in primary atherosclerotic lesions and lesions seen in accelerated arteriopathies with the latter condition being perhaps a more aggressive variant of the former.

Given the observation that SMCs in accelerated arteriopathy lesions demonstrate phenotypes typical of proliferating SMCs in culture, it is interesting to consider the rate of cell proliferation in these lesions. Several investigators have examined atherectomy specimens from a number of lesions looking for expression of proliferating cell nuclear antigen (PCNA), protein expressed predominantly during S-phase of the cell cycle and thus associated with cell division and proliferation. While some studies reported high proliferative indices in restenotic but not in primary lesions,[7] others have found minimal PCNA expression in all types of lesions examined with an exception of arteriovenous dialysis shunts.[8–10] It should be noted that interpretation of these experiments is complicated by differences in fixation protocols, composition, variability, and age of the lesions analyzed, and criteria used for determining positive staining. However, it appears that in most cases, only a modest level of cell proliferation is present in mature lesions associated with a number of accelerated arteriopathy syndromes. These observations gave rise to a notion suggesting that cell proliferation does not play an important role in pathogenesis of these lesions and that therapy should not be targeted toward control of cell proliferation, but rather, toward other aspects of lesion formation such as inflammation or matrix production.[8] However, studies in a variety of animal models

Table 4.2 Gene expression in accelerated arteriopathy lesions

Gene	Smooth muscle cells	Endothelial cells
PDGF-A	+++	+
PDGF-B	−	++
aFGF	+	+
bFGF	+	+
TGF-β	++	No data
IGF-1	+++	No data
MCSF	+	+
ICAM-1	+	+
VCAM-1	+	+
IL-1	+	+
IL-6	+++	+
IL-8	No data	+
TNF	+	−
MHC-DR	+	+

The plus signs indicate the extent of gene expression. Modified from ref. 18.

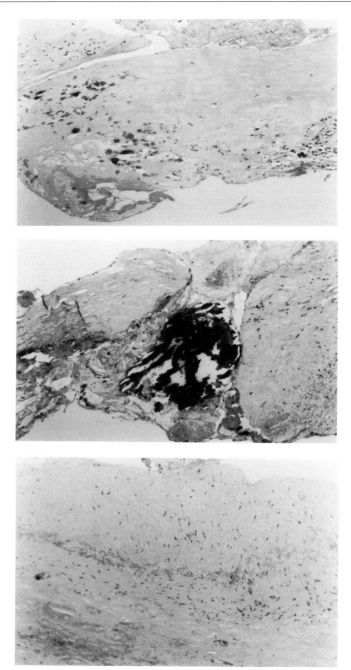

Figure 4.1   Histologic appearance of primary and restenotic coronary lesions. Low-power views of primary atherectomy specimen showing no areas of intimal hyperplasia (top), primary atherectomy specimen with extensive intimal hyperplasia (middle) and secondary (restenotic) atherectomy specimen demonstrating sheets of proliferating smooth muscle cells (bottom). (Courtesy of Dr S. Schnitt, Beth Israel Hospital, Boston.)

contradict this conclusion. In a rat model of carotid artery injury, SMC proliferation in the media reaches a peak 72 hours after injury while SMC proliferation in the forming neointima reaches a maximum 7 days after injury.[11] Markers of cell proliferation (such as BudR uptake or PCNA staining) are down to low levels 14 days after injury. Similar kinetics have been observed in rabbit iliac artery[12] and baboon vascular grafts[13] suggesting that a short burst of proliferation is sufficient to fully account for neointimal development in all of these models. Since most of the human specimens examined are obtained at later time points, it is not particularly surprising to see low level of proliferation in these lesions. Furthermore, since proliferative burst is relatively time-limited, it presents a better target for a short-term intervention than relatively chronic processes of inflammation and matrix deposition.

However, despite findings of low proliferative indices in most restenotic lesions, 'synthetic' SMCs derived from restenotic tissues display faster growth rate than their normal arterial wall counterparts cultured *in vitro,* suggesting higher potential for formation of proliferative lesions. The appearance of such cells is not limited to restenotic tissues. Primary atherosclerotic plaques frequently contain sheets of SMCs morphologically similar to cells seen in secondary (restenotic) lesions[14] and displaying similar molecular markers and proliferative potential (Figure 4.2). Indeed, subsequent occurrence of angiographic restenosis has been correlated with the number of 'activated' (i.e. potentially proliferative) cells in primary and secondary lesions undergoing atherectomy.[15]

Whereas cellular proliferation has received most attention in analysis of accelerated arteriopathic lesions, recently attention has turned to other features of this syndrome including extracellular matrix proteins and the involvement of immune/inflammatory cells. A number of immune mediators are present in these lesions including macrophages, monocytes and T and B lymphocytes thus suggesting that the immune system is involved in lesion development. This may be especially true in the case of accelerated arteriopathy seen in cardiac transplant recipients. In addition to normal expression of class I major histocompatibility complex (MHC) antigens (HLA-A, B and C), endothelial cells and SMCs in these lesions frequently express class II MHC antigens (MHC-DR) thus suggesting direct interaction with T cells. Furthermore, cells in accelerated arteriopathy lesions show expression of a number of receptors such as ICAM-1 and VCAM-1[16,17] involved in mediating adhesion of lymphocytes and macrophages. While the exact role played by these cells is uncertain, they are capable of producing a number of cytokines including M-CSF and the interleukins IL-1, IL-6 and IL-8[18] all capable of stimulation of cellular proliferation.

The extracellular matrix is another important component of these lesions frequently accounting for most of the lesion volume. However, little is known regarding its composition or formation. Initiation of smooth-muscle proliferation has been shown to be associated with production of a number of extracellular matrix proteins including tenascin,[19] type I and type IV collagen,[20–22] fibronectin[23] and proteoglycans.[24,25] The increased production of the latter may be especially important since proteoglycan components of extracellular matrix are capable of binding and sequestering herapin-binding growth factors such as FGFs and VEGF.[26–30] Therefore, it is easy to see how modulation in this component of extracellular matrix

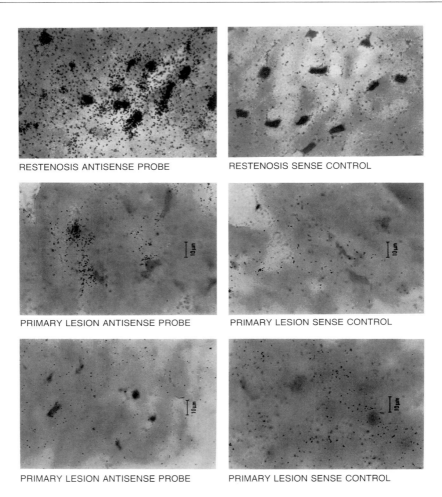

RESTENOSIS ANTISENSE PROBE   RESTENOSIS SENSE CONTROL

PRIMARY LESION ANTISENSE PROBE   PRIMARY LESION SENSE CONTROL

PRIMARY LESION ANTISENSE PROBE   PRIMARY LESION SENSE CONTROL

Figure 4.2 Molecular markers in atherosclerotic plaques. Material retrieved from atherectomy specimens was fixed in paraformaldehyde and hybridized with antisense and sense probes for nonmuscle
myosin heavy-chain B (myosin isoform found mostly in proliferative smooth-muscle cells). Left panels
show hybridization with antisense and right panels sense (control) probe. Top. Restenotic lesion showing
intense hybridization in all cells. Middle. Primary atheroma showing hybridization in some cells. Bottom.
Primary atheroma showing no hybridization in any cells. (From Simons *et al.* (1993) *N. Engl. J. Med.*, **328**,
608–13, with permission.)

composition might result in alteration in a number of cellular processes including
migration, proliferation and secretion of extracellular material mediated by these
growth factors.

Molecular pathogenesis of accelerated arteriopathies

Studies discussed in the previous section suggest that alterations in the vessel-wall
milieu result in the development of lesions characterized by the presence of sheets of
phenotypically   modulated   SMCs,   newly   secreted   extracellular   matrix   and

inflammatory/immune cells. In this section we will briefly discuss what factors are involved in generation of these lesions. Once again in our discussion we will use postangioplasty restenosis as a prototypical accelerated arteriopathy.

A number of factors come into play after an angioplasty of an arterial lesion. These include vessel-wall stretch, loss of endothelial surface, rupture of atherosclerotic plaque, and, frequently, rupture of internal elastic lamina. These events are followed by platelet deposition on exposed wall surface and formation of mural thrombus. Each of these factors by itself is capable of stimulating smooth-muscle proliferation. Thus, vessel-wall stretch, in the absence of endothelial denudation or injury to the wall itself, has been shown to stimulate medial smooth-muscle proliferation[31] presumably via a putative 'stretch receptor'. Loss of endothelial surface with attendant deposition and degranulation of platelets exposes underlying SMCs to a number of growth factors including PDGF, EGF and TGF-β. Formation of mural thrombus leads to generation of high local concentration of thrombin, another potent SMC mitogen. In addition, SMCs themselves, once stimulated begin producing a number of mitogens including PDGF, EGF and IGF-1. Furthermore, cell death and destruction following angioplasty release bFGF and, potentially, other heparin-binding growth factors (Table 4.2).

The importance of individual elements of this mitogen soup has been critically analyzed in a number of animal models. All isoforms of PDGF (PDGF-AA, AB and BB) are capable of stimulating SMC proliferation and migration *in vitro*. *In vivo*, platelets are a predominant source of PDGF-BB while SMCs in restenotic and atherosclerotic lesions have been shown to produce PDGF-AA. At the same time, vascular SMCs predominantly express PDGF-α receptor that can be stimulated by PDGF-AA and AB but not BB isoforms. Following arterial injury, SMCs in the vessel wall upregulate expression of PDGF-A gene and downregulate expression of PDGF-β receptor.[32,33] The importance of platelet-derived PDGF is suggested by observations that neointimal lesion formation is reduced in thrombocytopenic rats.[34] Furthermore, mice subjected to arterial injury treated with anti-PDGF antibody also show decreased neointimal formation.[35] In both of these models, PDGF effects appear primarily related to inhibition of SMC migration, since the first wave of proliferation seen after injury in the arterial wall is preserved.

Basic FGF is another potent SMC mitogen both under *in vitro* and *in vivo* conditions. Exposure of vessel wall to the growth factor either via gene transfer[36] or continuous administration,[37,38] leads to abundant neointimal proliferation. Further demonstration of bFGF's role in mediating initial SMC proliferation seen in the media after arterial injury comes from observations of reduced proliferation in mice treated with anti-bFGF antibody.[39] Interestingly, this treatment did not affect eventual neointimal lesion formation suggesting that other growth factors are capable of stimulating the process in the absence of bFGF.

EGF, IGF-1 and thrombin are also mitogenic for SMCs *in vitro*, especially in combination with other growth factors such as PDGF and may well play a similar role *in vivo*. IGF-1 production is increased by stimulation of quiescent SMCs in culture[40,41] and in the arterial wall[42] and clinical observations suggest higher frequency of restenosis in patients with type II diabetes mellitus,[43] a disease characterized by elevated plasma insulin and IGF-1 levels.[44] Furthermore, several animal studies suggested that treatment with angiopeptin, a somatostatin analog (IGF-1 inhibitor), may lead to reduced lesion formation after arterial injury.[45,46] In addition, angiopeptin administration has been suggested to reduce the extent of coronary arteriopathy in an animal transplant model.[47] However, evidence of angiopeptin's efficacy has been less clear in clinical trials.[48,49] Although capable of stimulating cell growth *in vitro*, perhaps via interaction with other growth factors[33] thrombin's role in regulation of smooth muscle proliferation *in vivo* has not been clearly defined. A number of anticoagulants have not been shown to be effective in reducing restenosis in either animal or clinical trials.[50] More specific thrombin antagonists, such as hirudin and hirulog, are currently being evaluated for their antiproliferative activity.

TGF-β also has an important role in vascular lesion development. Although present in normal vascular SMCs, growth factor expression increases after injury[51] and elevated factor levels have been observed in restenotic coronary specimens.[52] The mitogen is capable of stimulating cell proliferation in low concentrations (while suppressing in high concentrations). However, most importantly, TGF-β stimulates matrix production both *in vivo* and *in vitro*[53,54] and thus may contribute importantly to overall lesion formation. It is uncertain whether important changes in matrix production *per se* occur in the absence of cellular proliferation since evaluation of a number of therapies that have demonstrated antiproliferative effectiveness in animal models also lead to reduced extracellular matrix production as well (see below).

Finally, angiotensin II is also capable of stimulating SMC migration and proliferation *in vivo*. Thus, its infusion into rats following balloon injury potentiates neointimal formation.[55] However, given in the absence of other mitogens, angiotensin II induces SMC hypertrophy but not proliferation.[56] Angiotensin II-stimulated SMCs in culture can synthesize both PDGF-AA and TGF-β. Since PDGF-AA stimulates SMC proliferation and TGF-β inhibits it, a net result might be hypertrophy of the cell and the balance between TGF-β and PDGF-AA production may determine the extent of proliferation versus hypertrophy in any given setting.[56] If the supposition that angiotensin II induces SMC proliferation *in vivo* via stimulation of PDGF-AA synthesis is correct, it is not surprising that it is not mitogenic *in vitro*, since cultured SMCs do not express the PDGF-α receptor. The potential role of angiotensin II in accelerated arteriopathies *in vivo* is further emphasized by the success of angiotensin converting-enzyme inhibitor blockade in preventing neointimal formation after balloon injury in a rat carotid artery,[4] a model fully dependent on migration and replication of medial SMCs.

Molecular therapeutics and antisense technology

Identification of a number of genes and molecular pathways involved in pathogenesis of accelerated arteriopathic lesions allowed development of novel therapeutic strategies to control these processes. The principal approach discussed in this chapter is aimed at inhibition of expression of proteins important for lesion development using antisense technology. An alternative strategy (see Chapter 3) aims to prevent lesion formation by selective targeting of cells involved in its

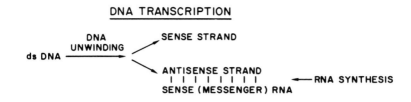

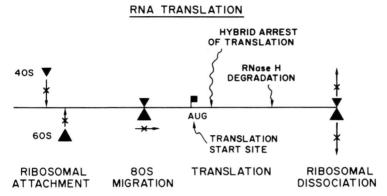

Figure 4.3 The process of protein synthesis and sites of action of antisense oligonucleotides. Sites of potential action of antisense oligonucleotides are indicated with X.

development. Yet another evolving approach utilizes gene therapy by expressing proteins capable of inhibiting the process of SMC proliferation and deposition of extracellular matrix.

Nature of antisense sequences

Antisense technology refers to the use of synthetic oligonucleotides or RNA transcripts designed to interrupt synthesis of specific proteins. In the course of protein synthesis, genetic information encoded in a double-stranded DNA molecule is transcribed into a single-stranded (sense) messenger RNA chain (mRNA) that is then translated into a protein (Figure 4.3). Numerous steps during this process can thus be targeted in order to disrupt the final outcome. One group of approaches targets specific RNA molecules (anti-RNA strategy) by introducing oligonucleotides that can specifically bind to coding (sense) RNA (hence, 'antisense' oligonucleotides). Such oligonucleotides can then interfere with a number of processes during RNA translation including mRNA transport from the nucleus to the cytoplasm, intracellular sequestration of the molecule and ribosome assembly. In addition, such oligonucleotides can cause hybrid arrest of translation by introducing non-readable double-stranded areas in the molecule or can mark the mRNA for destruction by creating double-stranded regions that can be cleaved by RNAase H, a naturally occurring enzyme.

Alternative approaches (anti-DNA strategy) aims to disrupt DNA transcription by designing oligonucleotides capable of binding to specific DNA elements. Such oligonucleotides can then impede DNA unwinding, interfere with binding of specific transcription factors or inhibit function of RNA polymerase (Figure 4.3). While anti-DNA strategy presents a very interesting and potentially highly viable approach to control of gene expression, there is relatively little experience to date in the use of this technology. In the following pages we will concentrate exclusively on the use of anti-RNA strategy and the reader is referred to several recent reviews for consideration of the anti-DNA approach.[57,58]

Oligonucleotides employed in antisense studies are typically 15–25 nucleotide long molecules that can be rapidly synthesized in any desired sequence. The sequence of the oligonucleotide is dictated by the sequence of a specific target mRNA molecule thus allowing, at least in theory, considerable precision in suppressing selected genes. Any part of the mRNA molecule can be targeted with antisense oligonucleotides and published studies have reported usage of antisense sequences aimed at 5'-untranslated region, ATG codon (site of initiation of protein synthesis), exon/intron boundaries, 3'-untranslated region as well as other parts of the message. Unfortunately, there is no accurate way to predict what oligonucleotide will be most successful in achieving the desired effect. Indeed, even a three-nucleotide difference in position of antisense sequence has been reported to produce major differences in terms of biological potency.[59] Thus, a number of antisense sequences must be synthesized and tested for each desired target sequence. The length of the antisense oligonucleotide is dictated by thermodynamic considerations of stability of the RNA–oligonucleotide hybrid (determined by 'melting temperature' that is dependent on base composition of the oligonucleotide) and specificity of binding (determined by the number of basepair matches required for binding to a unique nucleotide sequence). Although both of these considerations would favor longer oligonucleotide sequences, in practice shorter (15–18 bp) sequences appear to be most efficient. Finally, the choice of antisense sequence is also dictated by the *specificity of effect*, a major problem in the antisense field.

Standard ('unmodified' or phosphodiester oligonucleotides) have a rather short half-life (<2–3 hours) in cells and tissue due to nuclease degradation. However, a number of chemical modifications in the oligonucleotide backbone have been introduced in order to prolong survivial of these molecules (Figure 4.4). Of these, phosphorothioates (with sulfur replacing oxygen) and methylphosphonates (methyl group instead of oxygen) have been used most frequently. Both modifications provide markedly increased *in vitro* and *in vivo* survival (half-life >24 hours) combined with low toxicity and ease of synthesis, although a variety of other modifications have been tested as well.[60] In addition to chemical modifications introduced to increase oligonucleotide survival in cells, a number of modifications to the structure of the molecules have been introduced in order to increase its binding specificity thus reducing nonspecific effects.[61,62]

Evaluation of antisense effect

Administration of an ideal antisense oligonucleotide would result in a sequence-specific suppression of target gene function thus leading to production of a desired

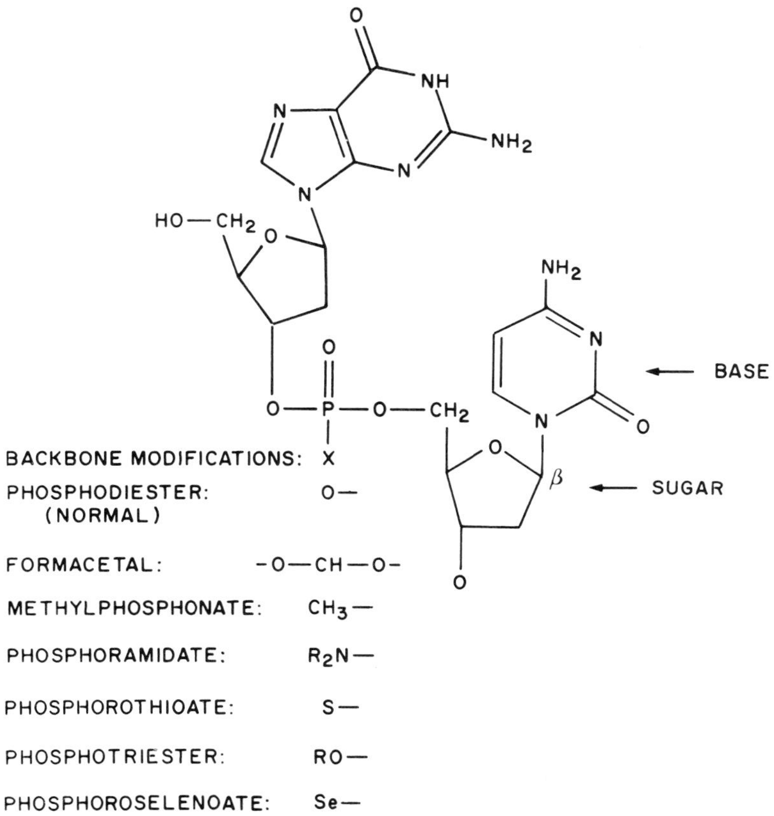

Figure 4.4 Chemical modifications of oligonucleotide backbone.

phenotype. Furthermore, it would not affect other mRNAs and proteins and would not be cytotoxic. However, oligonucleotide administration can result in disruption of synthesis of unwanted mRNAs due to the existence of partial sequence matches between oligonucleotides and other mRNA. Thus, although a 13 nucleotide-long sequence would be expected to be unique in a human genome (the probability of more than one such sequence occurring, 4^{13}, approaches zero given the size of the genome), there could be multiple shorter nucleotide matches with other sequences, that, under certain conditions, could interfere with processing of these sequences. Such occurrence of nonspecific degradation of mRNA sequences has been demonstrated to occur under *in vitro* conditions[63] as well as in *Xenopous* oocytes.[64,65] The other source of nonspecificity may result from oligonucleotides binding to intercellular proteins[66] thus interfering with their function. Finally, production of double-stranded RNA molecules (RNA–oligonucleotide hybrids) may potentially result in activation of enzymes such as p68 kinase[67] that can affect synthesis of a number of molecules.

Thus, an apparent phenotype resulting from oligonucleotide administration can be due to unintended suppression of different genes and proteins rather than that of the targeted sequence. Therefore, extensive controls are needed in order to demonstrate sequence specificity of effect and the lack of nonspecific toxicity (Table 4.3). These should include the use of multiple nonoverlapping antisense sequences with the same phenotype resulting from administration of each antisense sequence. Such a control minimizes the chance of an observed biological effect being due to nonspecific interactions since it is unlikely that two or more overlapping sequences would interact with the same unintended mRNAs or proteins producing identical effect. In addition, 'scrambled' sequences (oligonucleotide of the same base composition as an antisense sequence but synthesized in a different order) and 'missense' sequences (sequences with two-to-three nucleotide mismatches) should demonstrate no biological effect in terms of desired phenotype (such as, for example, cell proliferation) and should not affect the targeted gene's mRNA and protein levels. This control assures that the observed phenotype is not due to nonspecific chemical toxicity of the oligonucleotide. Furthermore, suppression of an unrelated gene not expected to alter cell phenotype should be used to demonstrate that formation of RNA–oligonucleotide structures *per se* does not lead to nonspecific degradation of multiple messages. Finally, overexpression of the targeted gene should be used to show that the observed antisense effect is indeed a function of suppressed gene function.

While any gene may, in principle, be selected for antisense suppression, inhibition of certain genes may be more biologically effective. Important considerations in this regard include message abundance, protein half-life, and the existence of isozymes or other closely related proteins capable of carrying out similar function. Message abundance is important since relatively small amounts of oligonucleotides can be delivered intracellularly given current technologies. In this regard it should be noted that most successful antisense studies have targeted low abundance messages (see Tables 4.4 and 4.5). The half-life of the target protein is another important consideration since even complete shut off of transcription and destruction of the entire message pool of a particular gene will achieve no biological effect if the long-lived protein itself already exists in the cell. Fortunately, half-lives of most proteins involved in cell proliferation are rather short. This is not the case, however, for most

Table 4.3   Controls in antisense experiments

Target gene's suppression
mRNA level
Protein level
Phenotype

Sequence-specific effect
Two or more nonoverlapping antisense sequences producing the same phenotype
Two missense (>two nucleotide mismatch) oligonucleotides show no effect
Target gene's overexpression increases antisense oligonucleotide requirements

Oligonucleotide toxicity
Scrambled sequence shows no effect

Activation of p68 system
Antisense oligonucleotides against biologically unrelated gene decrease the level of specific mRNA/
   protein but do not produce the same phenotype

---

structural proteins including extracellular matrix proteins. One potential for dealing with long-lived proteins is to begin antisense oligonucleotide administration prior to initiation of protein synthesis. Finally, the selected target should be unique in its biological function.

Antisense treatment of restenosis

Having discussed general principles of antisense technology, we will now turn to specific applications of antisense to treatment of accelerated arteriopathies. Advances in understanding of molecular mechanisms involved in the development of these lesions have lead to the description of a large number of mitogens capable of stimulating SMC proliferation that in turn generate a variety of second messenger pathways that can all lead to initiation of DNA synthesis (Figure 4.5). The multitude of mitogens and intracellular messenger pathways involved in, and capable of, stimulation of cell growth makes it unlikely that inhibition of function of any of these genes would be sufficient to stop the process. However, regardless of the mode of activation and nature of the proliferative signal, the cell must go through the cell cycle in order to proliferate. The genes involved in this final common pathway thus represent an appealing target for the antisense approach. Two other features make these genes attractive. First, cell-cycle proteins tend to be expressed only during their respective parts of the cycle. Second, the level of expression of these genes

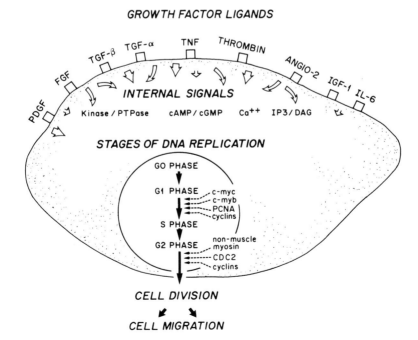

Figure 4.5   Molecular events involved in activation of smooth-muscle cell proliferation.

tends to be low (as low as 10 molecules per cell) especially compared to expression levels of growth factors and growth factor receptors (often in the 10^5 molecules per cell range). Thus, antisense therapy can be initiated prior to appearance of a low-abundance protein frequently possessing a very short half-life. Given these considerations, it is not surprising that practically all attempts at antisense control of SMC proliferation dealt with cell cycle-specific genes.

A number of genes are involved in regulation of cell-cycle progression. The cycle begins with a G_1-phase (defined as the time from application of proliferative stimulus to the onset of DNA synthesis) during which events necessary for subsequent DNA replication take place. This phase is followed by the S-phase (time of DNA synthesis) during which the process of DNA replication occurs. Once DNA replication has been completed, the cell enters the G_2-phase (defined as the time from the end of DNA synthesis to initiation of mitosis) during which preparation for mitosis takes place and finally the cell enters the M- (mitosis) phase. A number of genes critical to each of these stages have been identified. These include such G_1

Table 4.4 *In vitro* antisense studies

Gene†	SMC species	Growth suppression (%)	Reference
c-*myb*	Rat	48	Simons and Rosenberg[72]
	Bovine	70*	Brown *et al.*[73]
c-*myc*	Human	78	Ebbecke *et al.*[76]
	Rat	50	Biro *et al.*[75]
	Rat	75	Bennett *et al.*[77]
	Human	65	Shi *et al.*[74]
NMMHC	Rat	65	Simons and Rosenberg[72]
PCNA	Rat	50	Speir and Epstein[59]
	Human	57	Pickering *et al.*[78]

*Percentage cells in DNA synthesis.
†NMMHC, non-muscle myosin heavy chain; PCNA, proliferating cell nuclear antigen.

Table 4.5 *In vivo* antisense studies

Gene	Species	Delivery mode	Intimal suppression (%)	Reference
c-*myb*	Rat	Pluronics®	84	Simons *et al.*[79]
	Rat	EVAc	80	Edelman *et al.*[83]
	Pig	Hydrogel catheter	20†	Azrin *et al.*[85]
	Pig	Transport catheter	65	Gunn *et al.*[113]
c-*myc*	Rat	Pluronics®	53	Bennett *et al.*[77]
	Rat	EVAc**	90	Edelman *et al.*[83]
	Pig	Perfusion balloon	70	Shi *et al.*[86]
cdc2/PCNA	Rat	HVJ virus	68	Morishita *et al.*[84]
cdc2	Rat	Pluronics®	47	Abe *et al.*[82]
cdk2	Rat	Pluronics®	55	Abe *et al.*[82]
cdk2	Rat	HVJ virus	40	Morishita *et al.*[114]
*PCNA**	Rat	Pluronics®	80	Simons *et al.*[81]

*PCNA, proliferating cell nuclear antigen.
**EVAc, ethylene vinylacetate copolymer.
†Decrease in PCNA expression.

proteins as protooncogenes c-*myc* and c-*myb* (both involved in regulation of the S-phase entry), G_1/S and G_2/S cyclins such as cdc2 and cdk2 kinases, proliferating cell nuclear antigen (PCNA, a subunit of DNA polymerase, an S-phase protein), and nonmuscle myosin (a protein involved in mitosis). Prior *in vitro* studies have demonstrated that antisense suppression of these molecules affects proliferation of a number of cell types including fibroblasts, myeloid cells and numerous cancer cell lines.[68–71]

First, the feasibility of this approach to control of SMC growth has been tested *in vitro* (Table 4.4). These experiments not only defined targets suitable for *in vivo* experiments but also were used to investigate the specificity of antisense effect in SMCs. Thus, addition of antisense but not sense nonmuscle myosin heavy-chain oligonucleotides results in decreased cell proliferation in response to serum stimulation in a dose-dependent manner (Figure 4.6). This downregulation of proliferation is accompanied by a drop in mRNA (Figure 4.7) and protein levels.[72] Similar results have been obtained with antisense but not sense or missense c-*myb* oligonucleotides.[72,73] At the same time, suppression of thrombomodulin expression, a protein not involved in SMC proliferation, does not affect proliferation suggesting that formation of double-stranded RNA complex *per se* does not lead to non-specific effects in this system. Similar results have been obtained in other *in vitro* studies.[59,74–78] As a further control, Bennett *et al.* overexpressed c-myc protein in their SMCs and demonstrated lack of effectiveness of antisense c-*myc* suppression in cell expression high amounts of c-*myc* but not in untransfected controls.[77]

Given the success of these experiments, a number of investigators initiated studies of antisense in *in vivo* models of arterial injury (Table 4.5). However, while there is a considerable body of knowledge regarding the *in vitro* application of antisense oligonucleotides, there is little information regarding their usage *in vivo*. Oligonucleotides can be delivered to the desired arterial-wall segment in a variety of ways (Figure 4.8). A local *extravascular delivery* can be carried out by placing oligonucleotide-containing polymer in close proximity with the vessel wall, insuring a high local concentration of oligonucleotides and minimizing blood flow washout. Alternatively, local *intravascular delivery* may be attempted by direct injection of oligonucleotides into the arterial wall using a perfusion balloon catheter, or double balloon catheters that allow creation of a central chamber that can be used to 'bathe' an isolated arterial-wall segment with an oligonucleotide-containing solution either in the 'naked' form or in the presence of liposome particles that would facilitate cell absorption. Further, balloon catheters or stents coated with oligonucleotide-containing polymers have been tried as well.

In addition to mechanical devices, antisense therapy can be accomplished using local viral-mediated delivery. This approach allows potentially higher efficiency of delivery but introduces potential for infectious and immunogenic complications. Finally, systemic intravenous administration of antisense oligonucleotides has been tried as well. This has the obvious drawback of high cost due to substantial oligonucleotide dose requirement as well as a potential for systemic toxicity.

The first reported *in vivo* antisense study was carried out in a rat carotid injury model using a polaxamer (Pluronic® F 127) gel to extravascularly deliver antisense c-*myb* oligonucleotides immediately after a balloon injury.[79] The gel compound used

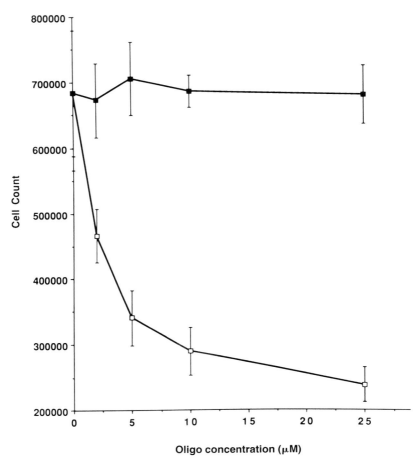

Figure 4.6 Effects of antisense nonmuscle myosin heavy-chain oligonucleotides on smooth-muscle cell proliferation. The antisense (□) and sense (■) nonmuscle myosin heavy-chain phosphorothioate oligonucleotides have been added at varying concentrations (μM) to growth-arrested SV40LT SMCs prior to serum stimulation and cell counts were obtained 72 hours later. The data are displayed as mean ± SD. (From Simons and Rosenberg (1992), *Circ. Res.*, **70**, 835–43, with permission.)

in the study has a unique temperature-inversion property existing as a liquid at 4°C and in a gel form at body temperature. Once applied to the artery *in vivo*, the gel is rapidly resorbed providing relatively short bolus delivery of oligonucleotides. However, even this short (<2 hours) arterial-wall exposure to antisense oligonucleotide results in a prolonged (two weeks) biologic effect with antisense-treated arteries demonstrating little neointimal formation (Figure 4.9). Morphometric analysis of the arteries treated with antisense and sense oligonucleotides, as well as arteries exposed to the gel alone or completely untreated arteries, demonstrated that antisense c-*myb* oligonucleotides suppressed neointimal formation while not affecting arterial media (Figure 4.10). This observation is consistent with known c-*myb* expression in proliferating but not quiescent cells.[80] As in the case of *in vitro* studies,

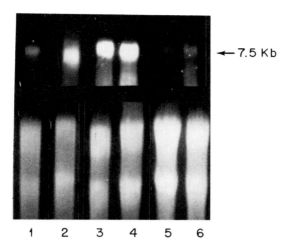

Figure 4.7 Effect of antisense oligonucleotide administration on target mRNA levels. Total RNA from SV40LT SMCs was examined with a probe for nonmuscle myosin heavy chain. Upper panels. Autoradiography analysis. Lower panels. Ethidium bromide-stained gel. Lanes: 1, growth arrest cells; 2, proliferating cells; 3 and 4, cells treated with sense oligonucleotides; 5 and 6, cells treated with antisense oligonucleotides. (From Simons and Rosenberg (1992) *Circ. Res.*, **70**, 835–43, with permission.)

specificity of effect was demonstrated by the lack of suppression of neointimal growth with missense oligonucleotides. An interesting feature of the study was a remarkably local effect of antisense delivery (Figure 4.11). While the entire length of carotid artery is ballooned during the study, the gel containing oligonucleotides is applied only to the cervical part of the artery and it is only this arterial segment that shows suppression of neointimal proliferation.

Subsequently, the same local extravascular polaxamer gel delivery was used to deliver antisense c-*myc*,[77] PCNA[81] as well as cdc2 and cdk2[82] oligonucleotides achieving similar results. Specificity of the anti-c-*myc* effect was demonstrated using mismatched sequences and the effect of oligonucleotides on target gene function was shown by decrease in mRNA expression.[77] As previously demonstrated in the c-*myb* study, the antiproliferative effect of antisense c-*myc* oligonucleotides was also localized to the site of gel application. In the case of the cdc2/cdk2 study, the specificity of the antisense effect was shown by demonstration of the decrease in specific kinase function in antisense- but not in sense oligonucleotide-treated arteries.[82] Proliferative cell nuclear antigen is thought to be one of the critical proteins involved in DNA replication. Its role in formation of postballoon injury neointima *in vivo* was confirmed by demonstrating a close correlation between PCNA protein expression and the 'first wave' of medial SMC proliferation (Figure 4.12; see Ref. 81). A different polymer (ethylene vinylacetate) capable of providing sustained zero-order release kinetics of packaged oligonucleotides was also shown to be an effective means of extravascular delivery of antisense c-*myc* and c-*myb* oligonucleotides.[83] Given its prolonged time course of delivery, the use of this polymer might be particularly suitable to inhibition of expression of long-lived proteins or genes whose expression is likely to persist for a prolonged period of time.

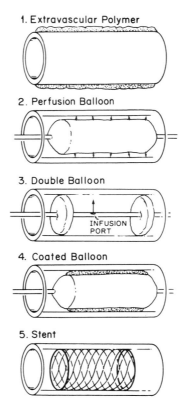

Figure 4.8 Oligonucleotide delivery strategies.

Using a different delivery strategy, Morishita et al.[84] demonstrated that a single intraluminal administration of antisense cdc2 kinase and PCNA oligonucleotides in the presence of inactivated viral particles used as delivery vehicles also resulted in suppression of neointimal formation when given immediately after angioplasty in a rat carotid artery. This study further extended the range of 'single bolus' antisense therapy by demonstrating the persistence of effect for up to six weeks after treatment (Figure 4.13). Furthermore, the study suggests that a combination of antisense oligonucleotides against different genes may be more effective in suppressing proliferation than a single antisense target. The evaluation of antisense therapy of postangioplasty restenosis has now been extended to large animals. Preliminary studies, now underway in a number of laboratories, suggest that intravascular balloon-mediated delivery of antisense c-myc[85] and c-myb[86,113] oligonucleotides is capable of inhibition of neointimal proliferation in porcine coronary and carotid arteries.

Although most of the application of antisense technologies so far has centered on treatment of restenosis, the technique is now being applied to other forms of accelerated arteriopathies. Thus, antisense oligonucleotides have been shown to suppress expression of a cell-adhesion molecule ICAM-1,[87] expression of bFGF[88]

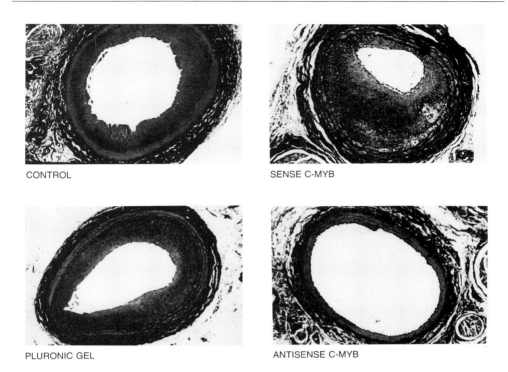

Figure 4.9 Effect of antisense and sense c-*myb* oligonucleotides on neointimal formation in rat carotid arteries subjected to balloon angioplasty. Representative cross-sections from the carotid artery of an untreated rat (control), a rat treated with Pluronic® gel containing 200 μg of sense oligonucleotide, a rat treated with Pluronic® gel and a rat treated with Pluronic® gel containing 200 μg of antisense oligonucleotide (Masson trichrome, magnification ×80). (From Simons *et al.* (1992) *Nature*, **359**, 67–70, with permission.)

and IL-1[89] receptors as well as a number of other targets that may well prove useful for clinical management. Preliminary studies demonstrate that intravenous infusion of anti-ICAM-1 antisense oligonucleotides is capable of delaying cardiac transplant rejection in a mouse transplant model.[90] However, encouraging as these studies are at the moment, the eventual acceptance of the antisense approach to treatment will depend on successful demonstration of effectiveness in a variety of large animal models and, eventually, in clinical trials.

Problems of antisense technology and future directions

Although antisense treatment of accelerated arteriopathies shows a lot of promise, a number of very important problems remain. Foremost among them are the frequency of nonspecific effects, toxicity associated with the use of oligonucleotides and effective delivery of these molecules to the target site. A number of approaches are being developed to increase the specificity of hybridization to the target sequence and to avoid binding to unintended sequences via partial matches. Reducing the length of oligonucleotide to the 10–12 nucleotide range is one such

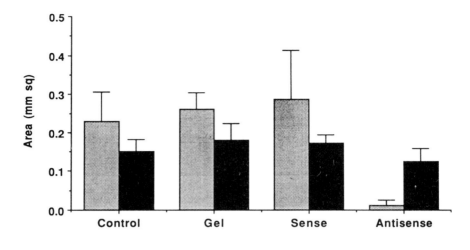

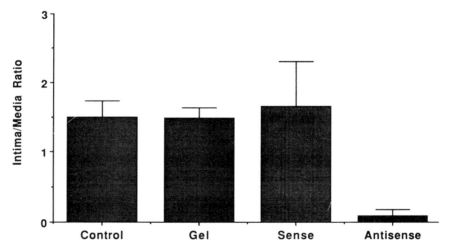

Figure 4.10   Intimal and medial cross-sectional areas, as well as intimal:medial ratios of untreated and treated rat carotid arteries. The upper panel shows mean cross-sectional areas of the intimal (light stippled bars) and medial (dark stippled bars) regions of rat carotid arteries which were untreated, treated with Pluronic® gel, treated with Pluronic® gel containing 200 μg of sense oligonucleotide and Pluronic® gel containing 200 μg of antisense oligonucleotide. The lower panel depicts the ratio of intimal to medial areas (stippled bars) for the same four groups of animals. The data are provided as mean ± SD. (From Simons *et al.* (1992) *Nature*, **359**, 67–70, with permission.)

approach. Synthesis of chimeric backbones (a combination of methylphosphomono-diester and phosphodiester structures) has been shown to result in increased binding specificity and enhanced RNase H cleavage.[61] A number of other modifications said to result in improved specificity including the introduction of pyrano-syl,[91] (2′–5′)oligoadenylate[92] or 5′-cholesteryl[93] groups have recently been introduced.

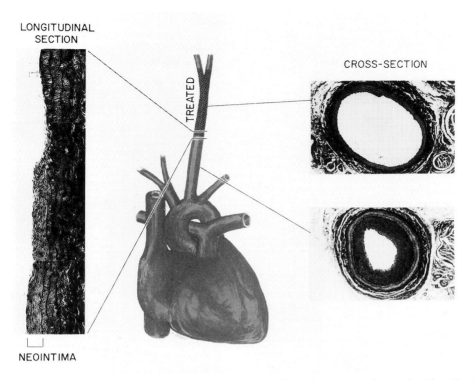

Figure 4.11 Spatial distribution of the antiproliferative effect of antisense oligonucleotides. Typical cross-sections (Masson trichrome, ×80) from treated and untreated segments of the left carotid artery of a rat are shown on the right side of the panel and a longitudinal section of the transitional area between these zones (Masson trichrome, ×200) is depicted on the left side of the panel. The shaded area represents the extent of application of Pluronic® gel. (From Simons *et al.* (1992) *Nature*, **359**, 67–70, with permission.)

Additional avenues being pursued by a variety of investigators include use of oligonucleotides to block translation via specific binding to RNA hairpin structures,[94] synthesis of RNA enzymes (ribozymes) capable of digesting specific RNA sequences,[95] and the use of oligonucleotides directed at inhibition of DNA transcription.[96] Furthermore, recent investigations have suggested that the presence of four consecutive G (guanine) nucleotides in the oligonucleotide sequence may have a nonspecific antiproliferative effect[96a] by preventing bFbF or other growth factor binding to their receptors.[96b]

Another major issue facing antisense therapy is effective delivery of oligonucleotides to the target tissue and cells. None of the existing delivery systems provides effective means of local delivery and systemic administration at the moment appears prohibitively expensive as well as potentially toxic. The problem is compounded by our rudimentary knowledge of oligonucleotide transport into cells even under *in vitro* conditions. Two groups of investigators have reported oligonucleotide uptake via active membrane transport and postulated the existence of oligonucleotide receptor.[97,98] However, in tissue culture, the majority of oligonucleotides appear to be taken up via endocytosis as suggested by punctate distribution of fluorescent

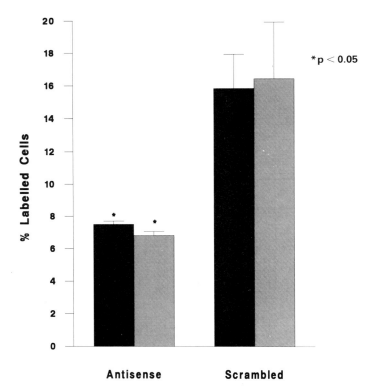

Figure 4.12 Immunocytochemical analysis of BudR and PCNA expression in medial smooth-muscle cells. Rats were subjected to balloon injury, sacrificed at 72 hours, left carotid arteries were perfusion fixed and representative sections were stained for BudR and PCNA. The fraction of labeled cells was determined as a ratio of cells stained with anti-BudR or anti-PCNA antibody to the total number of cells in each section. The bar graph shows the percentage of cells expressing PCNA (dark bars) or labeled with BudR (stippled bars) in rats treated with antisense 1 (left) or sense 1 oligonucleotides (right). The data are displayed as mean ± SD.

labeled oligonucleotides in the cells characteristic of endosomal vesicles. Oligonucleotide can escape from the endosomal compartment during fusion with other intracellular vesicles (such as lysosomes) thus ending up free inside the cytoplasm. The subsequent fate of oligonucleotides is not clear with some being retained in the cytoplasm while intranuclear localization is noted for some sequences.[99] Chemical modifications have been used to overcome these problems as well. Thus, the use of lipoprotein[100] or neoglycoprotein[101] conjugates improves tissue survival as well as increases in oligonucleotide uptake by cells. Other techniques being tested to facilitate molecule transport include the use of liposomes,[102,103] lipofectin[104] and cationic lipids.[105] Interestingly, once inside tissues, oligonucleotide stability appears to be quite high with significant concentrations of intact molecules being present 3–7 days after administration.[106–108] Finally, administration of synthetic molecules carries a potential for significant toxicity. To date, however, surprisingly little systemic side effects have been noted from administration of large doses of phosphorothioate oligonucleotides.

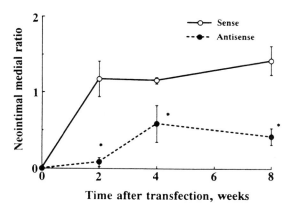

Figure 4.13 Long-term efficiency of antisense oligonucleotides. Long-term efficiency of cdc2 kinase/ PCNA antisense and sense administration on intima:media ratio in a rat model of arterial injury. (From Morishita *et al.* (1993) *Proc. Natl Acad. Sci. USA*, **90**, 8474–8, with permission.)

Despite these problems, the use of antisense oligonucleotides has been increasing. Local delivery has been found effective to modulate gene expression in the brain[109–111] and systemic intravenous administration has been used to successfully treat leukemia in mice.[112] It is hoped that continuous advances in our understanding and development of this exciting technique may one day provide us with a new tool for treatment of some of the more recalcitrant clinical problems.

References

1. Liu, M. W., Roubin, G. S. and King, S. B. III (1989) Restenosis after coronary angioplasty. Potential biological determinants and the role of intimal hyperplasia. *Circulation*, **79**, 1374–87.
2. Anonymous (1992) Does the new angiotensin converting enzyme inhibitor cilazapril prevent restenosis after percutaneous transluminal coronary angioplasty? Results of the MERCATOR study: a muilticenter, randomized, double-blind placebo-controlled trial. *Circulation*, **86**, 100–10.
3. Lam, J. Y., Lacoste, L. and Bourassa, M. G. (1992) Cilazapril and early atherosclerotic changes after balloon injury of porcine carotid arteries. *Circulation*, **85**, 1542–7.
4. Powell, J. S., Clozel, J-P., Muller, R. K. M. *et al.* (1989) Inhibitors of angiotensin-converting enzyme prevent myointimal proliferation after vascular injury. *Science*, **245**, 186–8.
5. Majesky, M. W., Giachelli, C. M., Reidy, M. A. and Schwartz, S. M. (1992) Rat carotid neointimal smooth muscle cells reexpress a developmentally regulated mRNA phenotype during repair of arterial injury. *Circ. Res.*, **71**, 759–68.
6. Weissberg, P. L., Grainger, D. J., Shanahan, C. M. and Metcalfe, J. C. (1993) Approaches to the development of selective inhibitors of vascular smooth muscle cell proliferation. *Cardiovasc. Res.*, **27**, 1191–8.
7. Pickering, J. G., Weir, L., Jekanowski, J. *et al.* (1993) Proliferative activity in peripheral and coronary atherosclerotic plaques among patients undergoing percutaneous revascularization. *J. Clin. Invest.*, **91**, 1469–80.
8. Stewart, D. K., Ferguson, M., Tran, N. *et al.* (1993) Proliferation in primary and restenotic coronary atherectomy tissue. Implications for antiproliferative therapy. *Circ. Res.*, **73**, 223–31.
9. Gordon, D., Reidy, M. A., Benditt, E. P. and Schwartz, S. M. (1990) Cell proliferation in human coronary arteries. *Proc. Natl Acad. Sci. USA*, **87**, 4600–4.

10. Gordon, D. (1992) Cell proliferation in human arteries. *Cardiovasc. Pathol.*, **1**, 259–62.
11. Clowes, A. W., Reidy, M. A. and Clowes, M. M. (1983) Kinetics of cellular proliferation after arterial injury. I. Smooth muscle growth in the absence of endothelium. *Lab. Invest.*, **49**, 327–33.
12. Hanke, H., Strohschneider, T., Oberhoff, M. *et al.* (1990) Time course of smooth muscle cell proliferation in the intima and media of arteries following experimental angioplasty. *Circ. Res.*, **67**, 651–9.
13. Geary, R. L., Kohler, T. R., Vergel, S. *et al.* (1993) Time course of flow-induced smooth muscle cell proliferation and intimal thickening in endothelialized baboon vascular grafts. *Circ. Res.*, **74**, 14–23.
14. Safian, R. D., Gelbfish, J. S., Erny, R. E. *et al.* (1990) Coronary atherectomy: clinical, angiographic, and histological findings and observations regarding potential mechanisms. *Circulation*, **82**, 69–79.
15. Simons, M., Leclerc, G., Safian, R. D. *et al.* (1993) Activated smooth muscle cells in coronary lesions. *N. Engl. J. Med.*, **328**, 608–13.
16. O'Brien, K. D., Allen, M. D., McDonald, T. O. (1993) Vascular cell adhesion molecule-1 is expressed in human atherosclerotic plaques. *J. Clin. Invest.*, **92**, 945–51.
17. Poston, R. N., Haskard, D. O., Coucher, J. R. *et al.* (1992) Expression of intercellular adhesion molecule 1 in atherosclerotic plaques. *Am. J. Pathol.*, **140**, 665–73.
18. Libby, P., Schwartz, D., Brogi, E. *et al.* (1992) A cascade model for restenosis. *Circulation*, **86** (Supp. III), III-47–52.
19. Hedin, U., Holm, J. and Hansson, G. K. (1991) Induction of tenascin in rat arterial injury. Relationship to altered smooth muscle cell phenotype. *Am. J. Pathol.*, **139**, 649–56.
20. Okada, Y., Katsuda, S., Matsui, Y. *et al.* (1990) Collagen synthesis by cultured arterial smooth muscle cells during spontaneous phenotypic modulation. *Acta Pathol. Jpn.*, **40**, 157–64.
21. Katsuda, S., Okada, Y., Minamoto, T. *et al.* (1992) Collagens in human atherosclerosis. Immunohistochemical analysis using collagen type-specific antibodies. *Arterioscler. Thromb.*, **12**, 494–502.
22. Ang, A. H., Tachas, G., Campbell, J. H. *et al.* (1990) Collagen synthesis by cultured rabbit aortic smooth-muscle cells. Alteration with phenotype. *Biochem. J.*, **265**, 461–9.
23. Clausell, N., Molossi, S. and Rabinovitch, M. (1993) Increased interleukin-1β and fibronectin expression are early features of the development of the postcardiac transplant coronary arteriopathy in piglets. *Am. J. Pathol.*, **142**, 1772–86.
24. Asundi, V., Cowan, K., Matzura, D. *et al.* (1990) Characterization of extracellular matrix proteoglycan transcripts expressed by vascular smooth muscle cells. *Eur. J. Cell Biol.*, **52**, 98–104.
25. Carey, D. J. (1992) Vascular smooth muscle extracellular matrix. *J. Vasc. Surg.*, **15**, 917–19.
26. Bernfield, M. and Sanderson, R. D. (1990) Syndecan, a developmentally regulated cell surface proteoglycan that binds extracellular matrix and growth factors. *Phil. Trans. R. Soc. Lond. (Biol.)*, **327**, 171–86.
27. Mali, M., Elenius, K., Miettinen, H. M. and Jalkanen, M. (1993) Inhibition of basic fibroblast growth factor-induced growth promotion by overexpression of syndecan-1. *J. Biol. Chem.*, **32**, 24215–22.
28. Salmivirta, M., Heino, J. and Jalkanen, M. (1992) Basic fibroblast growth factor–syndecan complex at cell surface or immobilized to matrix promotes cell growth. *J. Biol. Chem.*, **267**, 17606–10.
29. Jalkanen, M., Elenius, K. and Salmivirta, M. (1992) Syndecan – a cell surface proteoglycan that selectively binds extracellular effector molecules. *Adv. Exp. Med. Biol.*, **313**, 79–85.
30. Gitay-Goren, H., Soker, S., Vlodavsky, I. and Neufeld, G. (1992) The binding of vascular endothelial growth factor to its receptors is dependent on cell surface-associated heparin-like molecules. *J. Biol. Chem.*, **267**, 6093–8.
31. Clowes, A. W., Clowes, M. M., Fingerle, J. and Reidy, M. A. (1989) Kinetics of cellular proliferation after arterial injury. V. Role of acute distension in the induction of smooth muscle proliferation. *Lab. Invest.*, **60**, 360–4.

32. Miano, J. M., Vlasic, N., Tota, R. R. and Stemerman, M. B. (1993) Smooth muscle cell immediate–early gene and growth factor activation follows vascular injury. *Arterioscler. Thromb.*, **13**, 211–19.

33. Okazaki, H., Majessky, M. W., Harker, L. A. and Schwartz, S. M. (1992) Regulation of platelet-derived growth factor ligand and receptor gene expression by α-thrombin in vascular smooth muscle cells. *Circ. Res.*, **71**, 1285–93.

34. Fingerle, J., Johnson, R., Clowes, A. W. *et al.* (1989) Role of platelets in smooth muscle cell proliferation and migration after vascular injury in rat carotid artery. *Proc. Natl Acad. Sci. USA*, **86**, 8412–16.

35. Ferns, G. A., Raines, E. W., Sprugel, K. H. *et al.* (1991) Inhibition of neointimal smooth muscle accumulation after angioplasty by an antibody to PDGF. *Science*, **253**, 1129–32.

36. Nabel, E. G., Yang, Z. Y., Plautz, G. *et al.* (1993) Recombinant fibroblast growth factor-1 promotes intimal hyperplasia and angiogenesis in arteries *in vivo*. *Nature*, **362**, 844–6.

37. Edelman, E. R., Nugent, M. A., Smith, L. T. and Karnovsky, M. J. (1992) Basic fibroblast growth factor enhances the coupling of intimal hyperplasia and proliferation of vasa vasorum in injured rat arteries. *J. Clin. Invest.*, **89**, 465–73.

38. Cuevas, P., Gonzales, A. M., Carceller, F. and Baird, A. (1991) Vascular response to basic fibroblast growth factor when infused onto the normal adventitia or into the injured media of the rat carotid artery. *Circ. Res.*, **69**, 360–9.

39. Lindner, V. and Reidy, M. A. (1991) Proliferation of smooth muscle cells after vascular injury is inhibited by an antibody against basic fibroblast growth factor. *Proc. Natl Acad. Sci. USA*, **88**, 3739–43.

40. Delafontaine, P., Bernstein, K. E. and Alexander, R. W. (1991) Insulin-like growth factor I gene expression in vascular cells. *Hypertension*, **17**, 693–9.

41. Delafontaine, P., Lou, H. and Alexander, R. W. (1991) Regulation of insulin-like growth factor I messenger RNA levels in vascular smooth muscle cells. *Hypertension*, **18**, 742–7.

42. Fath, K. A., Alexander, R. W. and Delafontaine, P. (1993) Abdominal coarctation increases insulin-like growth factor I mRNA levels in rat aorta. *Circ. Res.*, **72**, 271–7.

43. Carrozza, J. P. Jr, Kuntz, R. E., Fishman, R. F. and Baim, D. S. (1993) Restenosis after arterial injury caused by coronary stenting in patients with diabetes mellitus. *Ann. Intern. Med.*, **118**, 344–9.

44. Bornfeldt, K. E., Arnqvist, H. J. and Capron, L. (1992) *In vivo* proliferation of rat vascular smooth muscle in relation to diabetes mellitus insulin-like growth factor I and insulin. *Diabetalogica*, **35**, 104–8.

45. Lundergan, C., Foegh, M. L., Vargas, R. *et al.* (1989) Inhibition of myointimal proliferation of the rat carotid artery by the peptides, angiopeptin and BIM 23034. *Atherosclerosis*, **80**, 49–55.

46. Santoian, E. D., Schneider, J. E., Gravanis, M. B. *et al.* (1993) Angiopeptin inhibits intimal hyperplasia after angioplasty in porcine coronary arteries. *Circulation*, **88**, 11–14.

47. Foegh, M. L., Khirabadi, B. S., Chambers, E. *et al.* (1989) Inhibition of coronary artery transplant atherosclerosis in rabbits with angiopeptin, an octapeptide. *Atherosclerosis*, **78**, 229–36.

48. Eriksen, U. H., Amtorp, O., Bagger, J. P. *et al.* (1993) Continuous angiopeptin infusion reduces coronary restenosis following balloon angioplasty. *Circulation*, **88** (Supp. I), 3198 (Abstract).

49. Emanuelsson, H., Bagger, J-P., Balcon, R. *et al.* (1994) Long-term effects of angiopeptin treatment in coronary angioplasty – reduction of clinical events but not of angiographic restenosis. *J. Am. Coll. Cardiol.*, **23**, 714 (Abstract).

50. Herrman, J-P. R., Hermans, W. R. M., Vos, J. and Serruys, P. W. (1993) Pharmacological approaches to the prevention of restenosis following angioplasty. *Drugs*, **46**, 18–52, 249–62.

51. Majesky, M. M., Lindner, V., Twardzik, D. R. *et al.* (1991) Production of transforming factor β1 during repair of arterial injury. *J. Clin. Invest.*, **88**, 904–10.

52. Nikol, S., Isner, J. M., Pickering, J. G. *et al.* (1992) Expression of transforming growth factor-β1 is increased in human vascular restenotic lesions. *J. Clin. Invest.*, **90**, 1582–92.

53. Chen, J-K., Hoshi, H. and McKeehan, W. L. (1987) Transforming growth factor type β specifically stimulates synthesis of proteoglycan in human adult arterial smooth muscle cells. *Proc. Natl Acad. Sci. USA*, **84**, 5287–91.

54. Nabel, E. G., Shum, L., Pompili, V. J. *et al.* (1993) Direct transfer of transforming growth factor beta 1 gene into arteries stimulates fibrocellular hyperplasia. *Proc. Natl Acad. Sci. USA*, **92**, 10759–63.

55. Daemen, M. J. A. P., Lombardi, D. M., Bosman, F. T. and Schwartz, S. M. (1991) Angiotensin II induces smooth muscle cell proliferation in the normal and injured rat arterial wall. *Circ. Res.*, **68**, 450–6.

56. Owens, G. K. (1989) Control of hypertrophic versus hyperplastic growth of vascular smooth muscle cells. *Am. J. Physiol.*, **257**, H1755–65.

57. Helene, C. (1992) Control of gene expression by antisense and antigene oligonucleotide-intercalator conjugates. In: Erickson, R. P. and Izant, J. G. (eds) *Gene Regulation: Biology of Antisense RNA and DNA*, pp. 109–118. New York: Raven Press.

58. Helene, C., Thuong, N. T. and Harel-Bellan, A. (1992) Control of gene expression by triple helix-forming oligonucleotides. The antigene strategy. *Ann. NY Acad. Sci.*, **660**, 27–36.

59. Speir, E. and Epstein, S. E. (1992) Inhibition of smooth muscle cell proliferation by an antisense oligodeoxynucleotide targeting the messenger RNA encoding proliferating cell nuclear antigen. *Circulation*, **86**, 538–47.

60. Wickstrom, E. (1992) Antisense DNA therapeutics: neutral analogs and their stereo-chemistry. In: Erickson, R. P. and Izant, J. G. (eds) *Gene Regulation: Biology of Antisense RNA and DNA*, pp. 261–72. New York: Raven Press.

61. Giles, R. V. and Tidd, D. M. (1992) Increased specificity for antisense oligodeoxynucleo-tide targeting of RNA cleavage by RNase H using chimeric methylphosphonodiester/phosphodiester structures. *Nucl. Acids Res.*, **20**, 763–70.

62. Hoke, G. D., Draper, K., Freier, S. *et al.* (1991) Effects of phosphorothioate capping on antisense oligonucleotide stability, hybridization and antiviral efficacy versus herpes simplex infection. *Nucl. Acids Res.*, **19**, 5743–8.

63. Mirabelli, C. K., Bennett, C. F., Anderson, K. and Crooke, S. T. (1991) *In vitro* and *in vivo* pharmacologic activities of antisense oligonucleotides. *Anti-Cancer Drug Design*, **6**, 647–61.

64. Woolf, T. M., Jennings, C. G., Rebagliati, M. and Melton, D. A. (1990) The stability, toxicity and effectiveness of unmodified and phosphorothioate antisense oligodeoxy-nucleotides in *Xenopus* oocytes and embryos. *Nucl. Acids Res.*, **18**, 1763–9.

65. Woolf, T. M., Melton, D. A. and Jennings, C. G. (1992) Specificity of antisense oligonu-cleotides *in vivo*. *Proc. Natl Acad. Sci. USA*, **89**, 7305–9.

66. Block, L. C., Griffin, L. C., Latham, J. A. *et al.* (1992) Selection of single-stranded DNA molecules that bind and inhibit human thrombin. *Nature*, **355**, 564–6.

67. Offerman, M. K. and Medford, R. M. (1993) Induction of VCAM-1 gene expression by double-stranded RNA occurs by a p68 kinase-dependent pathway in endothelial cells. *Clin. Res.*, **41**, 262a (Abstract).

68. Degols, G., Leonetti, J. P., Mechti, N. and Lebleu, B. (1991) Antiproliferative effects of antisense oligonucleotides directed to the RNA of c-*myc* oncogene. *Nucl. Acids Res.*, **19**, 945–8.

69. Citro, G., Perrotti, D., Cucco, C. *et al.* (1992) Inhibition of leukemia cell proliferation by receptor-mediated uptake of c-*myb* antisense oligodeoxynucleotides. *Proc. Natl Acad. Sci. USA*, **89**, 7031–5.

70. Melani, C., Rivoltini, L., Parmiani, G. *et al.* (1991) Inhibition of proliferation by c-*myb* antisense oligodeoxynucleotides in colon adenocarcinoma cell lines that express c-*myb*. *Cancer. Res.*, **51**, 2897–901.

71. Neckers, L., Whitesell, L., Rosolen, A. and Geselowitz, D. A. (1992) Antisense inhibition of oncogene expression. *Crit. Rev. Oncog.*, **3**, 175–231.

72. Simons, M. and Rosenberg, R. D. (1992) Antisense nonmuscle myosin heavy chain and c-*myb* oligonucleotides suppress smooth muscle cell proliferation *in vitro*. *Circ. Res.*, **70**, 835–43.

73. Brown, K. E., Kindy, M. S. and Sonenshein, G. E. (1992) Expression of the c-*myb* proto-oncogene in bovine vascular smooth muscle cells. *J. Biol. Chem.*, **267**, 4625–30.

74. Shi, Y., Hutchinson, H. G., Hall, D. J. and Zalewski, A. (1993) Downregulation of c-*myc* expression by antisense oligonucleotides inhibits proliferation of human smooth muscle cells. *Circulation*, **88**, 1190–5.
75. Biro, S., Fu, Y. M., Yu, Z. X. and Epstein, S. E. (1993) Inhibitory effects of antisense oligodeoxynucleotides targeting c-*myc* mRNA on smooth muscle cell proliferation and migration. *Proc. Natl Acad. Sci. USA*, **90**, 654–8.
76. Ebbecke, M., Unterberg, C., Buchwald, A. *et al.* (1992) Antiproliferative effects of a c-*myc* antisense oligonucleotide on human arterial smooth muscle cells. *Basic. Res. Cardiol.*, **87**, 585–91.
77. Bennett, M. R., Anglin, S., McEwan, J. R. *et al.* (1994) Inhibition of vascular smooth muscle cell proliferation *in vitro* and *in vivo* by c-*myc* antisense oligodeoxynucleotides. *J. Clin. Invest.*, **93**, 820–8.
78. Pickering, G., Weir, L., Jekanowski, J. and Isner, J. M. (1992) Inhibition of proliferation of human vascular smooth muscle cells using antisense oligonucleotides to PCNA. *J. Am. Coll. Cardiol.*, **19**, 165A.
79. Simons, M., Edelman, E. R., DeKeyser, J. L. *et al.* (1992) Antisense c-*myb* oligonucleotides inhibit intimal arterial smooth muscle cell accumulation *in vivo*. *Nature*, **359**, 67–70.
80. Thompson, C. B., Challoner, P. B., Neiman, P. E. and Groudine, M. (1986) Expression of the c-*myb* proto-oncogene during cellular proliferation. *Nature*, **319**, 374–80.
81. Simons, M., Edelman, E. R. and Rosenberg, R. D. (1994) Antisense PCNA oligonucleotides inhibit intimal hyperplasia in a rat carotid injury model. *J. Clin. Invest.*, **93**, 2351–6.
82. Abe, J., Zhou, W., Taguchi, J. *et al.* (1994) Suppression of neointimal smooth muscle cell accumulation *in vivo* by antisense cdc2 and cdk2 oligonucleotides in rat carotid artery. *Biochem. Biophys. Res. Commun.*, **198**, 16–24.
83. Edelman, E. R., Simons, M. and Rosenberg, R. D. (1995) c-Myc in vasculoproliferative disease. *Circ. Res.*, **76**, 176–82.
84. Morishita, R., Gibbons, G. H., Ellison, K. E. *et al.* (1993) Single intraluminal delivery of antisense cdc2 kinase and proliferating-cell nuclear antigen oligonucleotides results in chronic inhibition of neointimal hyperplasia. *Proc. Natl Acad. Sci. USA*, **90**, 8474–8.
85. Azrin, M. A., Mitchel, J. F., Pedersen, C. *et al.* (1994) Inhibition of smooth muscle cell proliferation *in vivo* following local delivery of antisense c-*myb* oligonucleotides during angioplasty. *J. Am. Coll. Cardiol.*, **23**, 396A.
86. Shi, Y., Fard, A., Vermani, P. and Zalewski, A. (1994) c-*myc* antisense oligomers reduce neointimal formation in porcine coronary arteries. *J. Am. Coll. Cardiol.*, **23**, 395A.
87. Chiang, M. Y., Chan, H., Zounes, M. A. *et al.* (1991) Antisense oligonucleotides inhibit intercellular adhesion molecule 1 expression by two distinct mechanisms. *J. Biol. Chem.*, **266**, 18162–71.
88. Morrison, R. S. (1991) Suppression of basic fibroblast growth factor expression by antisense oligodeoxynucleotides inhibits the growth of transformed human astrocytes. *J. Biol. Chem.*, **266**, 728–34.
89. Burch, R. M. and Mahan, L. C. (1991) Oligonucleotides antisense to the interleukin 1 receptor mRNA block the effects of interleukin 1 in cultured murine and human fibroblasts and in mice. *J. Clin. Invest.*, **88**, 1190–6.
90. Bennett, E. F. (1994) Regulation of leukocyte-endothelial cell adhesion molecule expression with synthetic oligonucleotides. *J. Cell. Biochem.*, (Supp. 18A), E021 (Abstract).
91. Augustyns, K., Godard, G., Hendrix, C. *et al.* (1993) Hybridization specificity, enzymatic activity and biological (Ha-*ras*) activity of oligonucleotides containing 2,4-dideoxy-beta-D-erythro-hexopyranosyl nucleosides. *Nucl. Acids Res.*, **21**, 4670–6.
92. Torrence, P. F., Maitra, R. K., Lesiak, K. *et al.* (1993) Targeting RNA for degradation with a (2′–5′)oligoadenylate-antisense chimera. *Proc. Natl Acad. Sci. USA*, **90**, 1300–4.
93. Krieg, A. M., Tonkinson, J., Matson, S. *et al.* (1993) Modification of antisense phosphodiester oligodeoxynucleotides by a 5′ cholesteryl moiety increases cellular association and improves efficacy. *Proc. Natl Acad. Sci. USA*, **90**, 1048–52.
94. Brossalina, E., Pascolo, E. and Toulme, J. J. (1993) The binding of an antisense oligonucleotide to a hairpin structure via triplex formation inhibits chemical and biological reactions. *Nucl. Acids Res.*, **21**, 5616–22.

95. Parker, R., Muhlrad, D., Deshler, J. O. *et al.* (1992) Ribozymes: principles and designs for their use as antisense and therapeutic agents. In: Erickson, R. P. and Izant, J. G. (eds) *Gene Regulation: Biology of Antisense RNA and DNA*, pp. 55–70. New York: Raven Press.

96. Nagai, K. and Hecht, S. M. (1991) Site-specific DNA cleavage by antisense oligonucleotides covalently linked to phenazine di-N-oxide. *J. Biol. Chem.*, **266**, 23994–4002.

96a. Burgess, T. L., Fisher, E. F., Ross, S. L. *et al.* (1995) The antiproliferative activity of c-myb and c-myc antisense oligonucleotides in smooth muscle cells is caused by a nonantisense mechanism. *Proc. Natl Acad. Sci. USA*, **92**, 4051–55.

96b. Guvakova, M. A., Yakubov, L. A., Vlodavsky, I. *et al.* (1995) Phosphorothioate oligodeoxynucleotides bind to basic fibroblast growth factor, inhibit its binding to cell surface receptors, and remove it from low affinity binding sites on extracellular matrix. *J. Biol. Chem.*, **270**, 2620–7.

97. Yakubov, L. A., Deeva, E. A., Zarytova, V. F. *et al.* (1989) Mechanism of oligonucleotide uptake by cells: involvement of specific receptors? *Proc. Natl Acad. Sci. USA*, **86**, 6454–8.

98. Loke, S. L., Stein, C. A., Zhang, X. H. *et al.* (1989) Characterization of oligonucleotide transport into living cells. *Proc. Natl Acad. Sci. USA*, **86**, 3474–8.

99. Leonetti, J. P., Mechti, N., Degols, G. *et al.* (1991) Intracellular distribution of microinjected antisense oligonucleotides. *Proc. Natl Acad. Sci. USA*, **88**, 2702–6.

100. de Smidt, P. C., Le Doan, T., de Falco, S. and van Berkel, T. J. (1991) Association of antisense oligonucleotides with lipoproteins prolongs the plasma half-life and modifies the tissue distribution. *Nucl. Acids Res.*, **19**, 4695–700.

101. Bonfils, E., Depierreux, C., Midoux, P. *et al.* (1992) Drug targeting: synthesis and endocytosis of oligonucleotide–neoglycoprotein conjugates. *Nucl. Acids Res.*, **20**, 4621–9.

102. Thierry, A. R. and Dritschilo, A. (1992) Liposomal delivery of antisense oligodeoxynucleotides. Application to the inhibition of the multidrug resistance in cancer cells. *Ann. NY Acad. Sci.*, **660**, 300–2.

103. Juliano, R. L. and Akhtar, L. (1992) Liposomes as a drug delivery system for antisense oligonucleotides. *Antisense Res.*, **2**, 165–76.

104. Yeoman, L. C., Danels, Y. J. and Lynch, M. J. (1992) Lipofectin enhances cellular uptake of antisense DNA while inhibiting tumor cell growth. *Antisense Res.*, **2**, 51–9.

105. Capaccioli, S., Di Pasquale, G., Mini, E. *et al.* (1993) Cationic lipids improve antisense oligonucleotide uptake and prevent degradation in cultured cells and in human serum. *Biochem. Biophys. Res. Commun.*, **197**, 818–25.

106. Agrawal, S., Temsamani, J. and Tang, J. Y. (1991) Pharmacokinetics, biodistribution, and stability of oligodeoxynucleotide phosphorothioates in mice. *Proc. Natl Acad. Sci. USA*, **88**, 7595–9.

107. Temsamani, J., Tang, J. Y. and Agrawal, S. (1992) Capped oligodeoxynucleotide phosphorothioates. Pharmacokinetics and stability in mice. *Ann. NY Acad. Sci.*, **660**, 318–20.

108. Goodarzi, G., Watabe, M. and Watabe, K. (1992) Organ distribution and stability of phosphorothioated oligodeoxyribonucleotides in mice. *Biopharm. Drug Dispos.*, **13**, 221–7.

109. Wahlestedt, C., Golanov, E., Yamamoto, S. *et al.* (1993) Antisense oligodeoxynucleotides to NMDA-R1 receptor channel protect cortical neurons from excitotoxicity and reduce focal ischaemic infarctions. *Nature*, **363**, 260–3.

110. Gyurko, R., Wielbo, D. and Phillip, M. I. (1993) Antisense inhibition of AT1 receptor mRNA and angiotensinogen mRNA in the brain of spontaneously hypertensive rats reduces hypertension of neurogenic origin. *Regul. Peptides*, **49**, 167–74.

111. Harrison, P. (1993) Antisense: into the brain. *Lancet*, **342**, 254–5.

112. Ratajczak, M. Z., Kant, J. A., Luger, S. M. *et al.* (1992) *In vivo* treatment of human leukemia in a SCID mouse model with c-*myb* antisense oligodeoxynucleotides. *Proc. Natl Acad. Sci. USA*, **89**, 11823–7.

113. Gunn, J., Holt, C. M., Shepherd, L. *et al.* (1995) Local delivery of c-myb antisense attenuates neo-intimal thickening in porcine model of coronary angioplasty. *J. Am. Coll. Cardiol.*, **25**, 201A (abstract).

114. Morishita, R., Gibbons, G. H., Ellison, K. E. *et al.* (1994) Intimal hyperplasia after vascular injury is inhibited by antisense cdk-2 oligonucleotides. *J. Clin. Invest.*, **93**, 1458–64.

5

Thrombotic Heart Disease and Myocardial Infarction: Introduction and Contemporary Therapies

Daniel I. Simon
Clyde R. Meckel

Introduction

The contemporary treatment of acute myocardial infarction (MI) exemplifies the notion that an understanding of the pathophysiologic mechanisms of disease can be translated into successful therapeutic approaches that save lives. These interventions are responsible for an appriximately 80% reduction in average inhospital mortality from MI since the 1960s (Figure 5.1).[1] This chapter will discuss the pathology, pathophysiology, and state-of-the-art management of MI and related acute ischemic syndromes. In addition, this review provides a background and

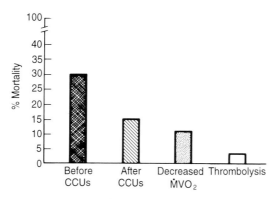

Figure 5.1   Decrease in the mortality rate of patients with acute MI correlating with three milestones in the management of MI: widespread use of coronary care units (CCUs), interventions to decrease myocardial oxygen consumption (MVO₂) and thrombolytic therapy. (From Sobel, B. E. (1989) Coronary thrombolysis and the new biology. *J. Am. Coll. Cardiol.*, **14**, 850–60, with permission.)

rationale for future therapeutic strategies that employ principles of molecular biology and local drug delivery that will be discussed below.

Pathophysiology

Pathologic, angiographic and angioscopic studies indicate that myocardial infarction results from the acute occlusion of a coronary artery secondary to atherosclerotic plaque disruption and thrombus formation. The central role of thrombosis in acute myocardial infarction was initially proposed by Herrick[2] in 1912, but remained controversial in the prethrombolytic decades due to autopsy findings contradicting the frequency and pathophysiologic significance of coronary artery thrombi.[3] In 1980, DeWood and coworkers resolved this controversy by performing coronary angiography early in the course of myocardial infarction and demonstrating an 87% incidence of total coronary occlusion in the infarct-related vessel.[4]

Thrombus formation is the result of the complex and dynamic interplay between the following: coronary atherosclerosis and plaque rupture; platelet adhesion/aggregation; endothelial products including prostacyclin, endothelium-derived relaxing factor, heparan sulfate, and tissue-type plasminogen activator; plasma clotting factors; and local shear forces. Coronary atherosclerosis and specific plaque morphology are key determinants of thrombotic occlusion. The extent and severity of atherosclerosis in autopsied patients with a history of myocardial infarction has been quantified by Roberts[5] and colleagues: severe narrowing (76–100%) of the cross-sectional area was present in 20–45% of all coronary segments, moderate narrowing (51–75%) in up to 66% of coronary segments, and mild narrowing (26–50%) in approximately 33% of coronary segments. Recently, there have been important observations from angiographic studies performed in patients before and after infarction regarding the severity of the atherosclerotic lesions responsible for myocardial infarction. Mild and moderate stenoses are often the site of subsequent myocardial infarctions. Stenoses in the infarct-related artery of <50% on initial angiograms were observed in 48% of patients prior to infarction by Ambrose and coworkers[6] and in 66% by Little and colleagues.[7] It has been hypothesized that mild and moderate stenoses are more likely to destabilize and undergo plaque disruption and thrombosis than more severe stenoses, which may progress to asymptomatic, chronic occlusion.[8]

Plaque activation or disruption probably occurs via two distinct mechanisms: (1) plaque fissuring[9–11] and (2) intraplaque hemorrhage originating from extensive *vasa vasorum*.[12,13] Histologic features associated with a propensity for plaque disruption include soft plaques with a higher lipid content, increased numbers of macrophages and foam cells, and eccentricity.[14] Shear forces fron intraluminal blood flow and other physical forces imparted by, for example, artery curvature and bending with systole, may play an important role in promoting plaque disruption.[8,15] Specific angiographic features are also associated with atherosclerotic plaques responsible for infarction. Angiography in patients with a recent myocardial infarction and a patent infarct-related artery demonstrates eccentric stenoses with irregular borders and intraluminal lucencies suggestive of residual throm-bus.[16,17]

Q Wave versus non-Q wave infarction

Myocardial infarction can be classified electrocardiographically as Q wave MI or non-Q wave MI (NQWMI). MI has also been classified using the pathologic designations transmural or nontransmural (subendocardial). While Q wave MI is generally associated with transmural infarction and NQWMI with nontransmural infarction, electrocardiographic designation remains more clinically relevant than pathologic designation in terms of natural history and prognosis. In general, Q wave infarcts are larger as assessed by peak creatine kinase,[18] associated with a higher inhospital mortality, and are usually caused by acute coronary occlusion;[19] in contrast, NQWMIs are smaller, associated with a lower inhospital mortality, and are more often caused by incomplete occlusion of the infarct-related artery.[20] Thus, the early and late risks for the two types of MI are very different. While Q wave MI is associated with a higher inhospital mortality, NQWMI patients are at significant risk for recurrent ischemia and infarction, leading to an overall long-term mortality that is equivalent.[21] Importantly, from a management standpoint, certain interventions that have resulted in significant mortality reductions in MI, such as thrombolysis and beta-blockade, are associated with Q wave rather than NQWMI.

Management of myocardial infarction

The primary rationale for intervening in MI is to prolong survival by limiting infarct size, reinfarction and mechanical complications (e.g. cardiac rupture, ventricular septal defect) that lead to pump failure and by preventing sudden death secondary to arrhythmias. It is therefore useful to broadly categorize interventions into those that increase myocardial blood flow (thrombolytic agents, primary revasculariza-tion, antithrombotic agents), decrease myocardial oxygen consumption (beta-blockers, nitrates, calcium-channel blockers), or prevent sudden, arrhythmic death (lidocaine, beta-blockers) (see Table 5.1). Some interventions – magnesium and angiotensin converting enzyme (ACE) inhibitors – have multiple effects that may in concert positively impact on MI therapy.

Risk stratification

Before considering specific therapeutic strategies, risk stratification of MI patients is important because MI is heterogeneous with mortality ranging from 1.5% in 'low risk' subgroups to over 80% in 'high risk' subgroups with cardiogenic shock. In the prethrombolytic era, patients with MI were classified clinically into four groups with variable prognosis depending on the presence of signs of congestive heart failure or cardiogenic shock (Table 5.2). In the thrombolytic era, risk stratification according to clinical variables has also been elucidated by the Thrombolysis in Myocardial Infarction (TIMI) investigators (Table 5.3).

In evaluating the randomized, prospective trials and meta-analyses presented below that provide the rationale for current MI management, it is prudent to consider the patient populations studied in light of these disparate prognostic categories. Randomized trials tend to exclude the sickest patients. For example, in the landmark Gruppo Italiano per lo Studio della Streptochinasi nell'Infarto Miocardico (GISSI-1) trial, overall mortality averaged <13% in those randomized to placebo.[22] Nonetheless, current MI therapy, guided by trials in well over 200 000

Table 5.1 Management of myocardial infarction

Increase myocardial oxygen supply
Reperfusion therapy – thrombolysis, primary angioplasty or bypass grafting
Antiplatelet agents – aspirin
Anticoagulation – heparin

Decrease myocardial oxygen consumption
Beta-blockers
Nitrates
Calcium-channel blockers

Antiarrhythmic therapy
Beta-blockers
Liodocaine

Multifactorial
ACE inhibitors
Magnesium

Table 5.2 Risk stratification: Killip classification*

Class	Examination	MI patients (%)	Mortality (%)
I	No rales and no S_3	33	6
II	Rales or S_3 present	38	30
III	Rales > 50%	10	38
IV	Shock	19	81

*Adapted from Killip, T. and Kimball, J. T. (1967) Treatment of myocardial infarction in a coronary care unit: a two year experience with 250 patients. *Am. J. Cardiol.*, **20**, 457–64.

Table 5.3 Risk stratification: TIMI classification*

Risk factors (n)†	Patients (%)	Mortality (%)
0	26	1.5
1	42	2.3
2	21	7.0
3	7	13.0
≥4	3	17.2

*Adapted from Hillis, L. D., Forman, S., Braunwald, E. (1990) and the Thrombolysis in Myocardial Infarction Investigators. Risk stratification before thrombolytic therapy in patients with acute myocardial infarction. *J. Am. Coll. Cardiol.*, **16**, 313–15.
†Risk factors: anterior MI, prior MI, age >70 years, female, diabetes, atrial fibrillation, rales >1/3, hypotension and sinus tachycardia.

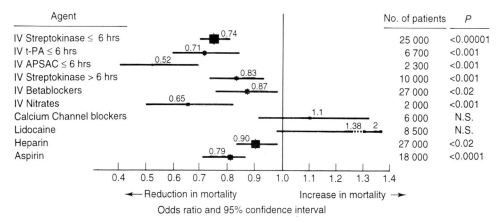

Figure 5.2 Summary of various treatments on mortality in acute MI. Odds ratios and their 95% confidence intervals are plotted. The size of the square is related to the variance of the data. Larger squares reflect more data, and narrower confidence intervals indicate more precise estimates of treatment effect. IV, intravenous; t-PA, tissue plasminogen activator; APSAC, anisoylated plasminogen–streptokinase activator complex; NS, not significant. (From Yusef, S., Sleight, P., Held, P. and McMahon, S. (1990) Routine medical management of acute myocardial infarction. Lessons from overviews of recent randomized controlled trials. *Circulation,* **82** (Supp. II), 117–34, with permission.)

patients worldwide, has resulted in mortality reductions ranging from 15 to 25% for individual drug treatments (Figure 5.2).[23,24]

Reperfusion therapy

Thrombolysis

Prolonged thrombotic occlusion of the infarct-related artery results in myocardial necrosis. The rationale of reperfusion therapy is based on the concept that irreversible ischemic myocardial cell injury develops in an increasing number of cells as the duration of coronary occlusion is prolonged and, therefore, ischemic but viable myocardium is available for pharmacologic or percutaneous transluminal coronary angioplasty (PTCA)/surgical salvage. This 'wavefront phenomenon' or ischemic cell death was advanced by the seminal observations of Reimer and coworkers[25,26] demonstrating that irreversible injury develops at variable times with a wave of cell death beginning in the subendocardium and progressing toward the subepicardium (Figure 5.3a). Circumflex occlusion in the dog for 15 minutes was completely reversible in that reperfusion completely prevented necrosis. However, after 40 minutes of occlusion, subendocardial necrosis developed that extended with focal involvement of the mid- and subepicardial myocardium if occlusion is allowed to persist for 3 hours. By 6 hours, necrosis was nearly transmural and the proportion of ischemic muscle which was viable and potentially salvageable beyond this point was limited (Figure 5.3b). Importantly, Reimer and coworkers demonstrated that reperfusion preserved viable myocytes and resulted in smaller average transmural infarcts if reperfusion occurred at 3 hours; in contrast, no change in infarct size was

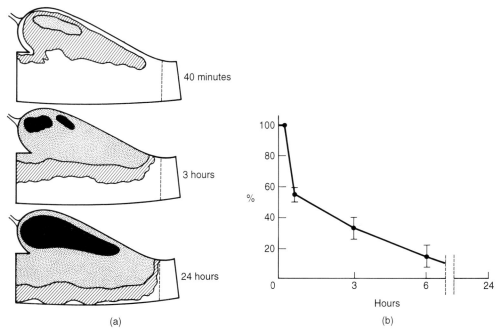

(a)   (b)

Figure 5.3 (a) Diagram summarizing the wavefront of ischemic cell death with respect to duration of coronary occlusion. Necrosis (all shaded areas) proceeds from the subendocardium toward the subepicardium with progressive transmural extension of the ischemic zone as occlusion time increases. The vertical dashed line indicates the anatomic boundary of the ischemic coronary bed. Microvascular injury, evidenced by interstitial hemorrhage (horizontal cross-hatching), progresses at a lower pace. Complete cessation of microvascular perfusion may occur and results in a central core (dotted areas) of necrotic muscle devoid of either hemorrhage or inflammatory response. Up to 3 hours after occlusion there is typically a significant amount of subepicardial myocardium which is viable and salvageable by reperfusion. (b) Proportion of ischemic muscle which is viable and potentially salvageable as a function of time after coronary occlusion. Data are plotted as a percentage of 24-hour infarct size. (From Reimer, K. A., Lowe, J. E., Rasmussen, M. M. and Jennings, R. B. (1977) The wavefront phenomenon of ischemic cell death. I. Myocardial infarct size vs duration of coronary occlusion in dogs. *Circulation*, **56**, 786–94, with permission.)

seen if reperfusion was performed at 6 hours. In addition to reperfusion, myocardial oxygen consumption at the time of experimental coronary artery occlusion, and for up to 3 hours thereafter, was found to be an important determinant of infarct size.[27] These experimental studies form the basis for current reperfusion therapy (thrombolysis or primary revascularization with PTCA/coronary artery bypass grafting (CABG)) in MI. While the size and number of collateral vessels differs in dog and man, Reimer and coworkers accurately predicted the applicability of their observations in man by emphasizing that 'since the amount of potentially salvageable myocardium progressively decreases as the period of ischemia is prolonged, time is the most critical variable involved in delaying or preventing ischemic myocardial cell death'.

The landmark angiographic trial of DeWood[4] ushered in the thrombolytic era by unequivocally demonstrating that acute MI is caused by thrombotic occlusion of the infarct-related artery and that cardiac catheterization/angiography could be performed safely in the setting of MI. The Western Washington trial of intracoronary streptokinase (SK) in acute MI was the first thrombolytic study to document a reduction in mortality[28] and establish that infarct artery-related patency at the time of hospital discharge was associated with improved 12-month survival compared to an occluded infarct-related artery.[29]

Limitations of intracoronary administration led to the extensive intravenous thrombolytic trials that have now definitively shown in prospective, randomized studies, as recently evaluated by the Fibrinolytic Therapy Trialists' (FTT) Collaborative Group,[30] to reduce MI mortality by 18% (95% CI 13–23%; $2P < 0.00001$) (Figure 5.4). Current Food and Drug Administration-approved thrombolytic agents for MI include SK, tissue-type plasminogen activator (t-PA) and anistreplase (anisoylated plasminogen streptokinase activator complex, APSAC). SK is a nonfibrin specific fibrinolytic agent that forms a 1:1 stoichiometric complex with plasminogen, which in turn converts uncomplexed plasminogen to plasmin, the major fibrinolytic protease.[31] APSAC, a modified form of SK that requires deacylation for plasmin generation resulting in a longer plasma half-life conducive for bolus administration, is also a non-fibrin specific activator and thus leads to significant hypofibrinogenemia. t-PA, an endogenous plasminogen activator, binds fibrin, leading to an enhancement in plasmin generation due to the formation of a kinetically favorable ternary complex between fibrin, plasminogen and t-PA.[32] This tends to limit t-PA activity to the fibrin clot as reflected by a less marked reduction in plasma fibrinogen compared to nonfibrin specific agents. Fibrin specificity is generally associated with an increased rate of clot lysis (Figure 5.5), but also an increased reocclusion rate (13.5% (95% confidence interval 11–16%)) for t-PA versus 8% (3–10%) for the non-fibrin specific agents SK, APSAC or urokinase[33] secondary to the lack of fibrinogenolysis and production of antithrombotic fibrinogen degradation products. The intravenous administration of SK (1.5 million units over 1 hour) resulted in 43–55% patency (defined as TIMI 2 or 3 flow) at 90 minutes;[34,35] administration of nonfront-loaded t-PA (100 mg over 3 hours) achieved 70% and front-loaded or accelerated t-PA (100 mg over 90 minutes) 81% patency,[36] respectively. It is important to note, however, that 'catch-up' in patency occurs with no significant differences at 180 minutes.

As demonstrated by GISSI-1 and ISIS-2 (Second International Study of Infarct Survival),[36] intravenous SK reduced mortality by 18% and 25%, respectively. The Anglo-Scandinavian Study of Early Thrombolysis (ASSET)[38] trial reported a 26% reduction in mortality for t-PA, APSAC Intervention Mortality Study (AIMS)[39] a 50% reduction in mortality for APSAC. Despite the consistent benefit of thrombolysis, only a minority (<25%) of MI patients actually receive thrombolytic therapy (Figure 5.6).[40] Broader use of thrombolytic therapy is now further supported by recent data from the EMERAS[41] and LATE[42] trials demonstrating significant mortality reduction (15%) when treatment is initiated up to 12 hours. The recent report by the FTT Collaborative Group has provided a thorough examination of the benefits of thrombolysis within a wide range of clinically relevant subgroups and demographic parameters, including age, hour from presentation, gender and ECG and hemodynamics at presentation (Figure 5.4).

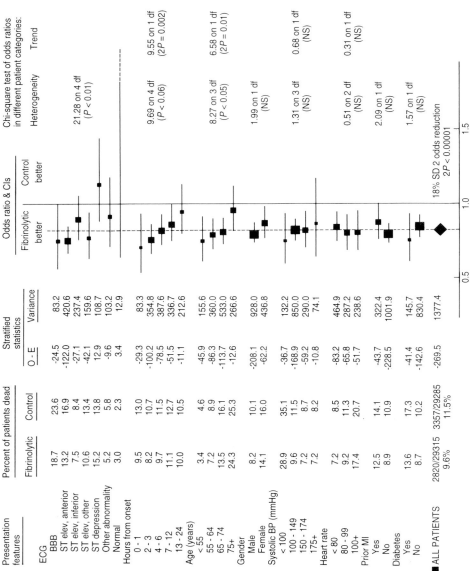

Presentation features	Percent of patients dead		Stratified statistics		Odds ratio & CIs	Chi-square test of odds ratios in different patient categories:	
	Fibrinolytic	Control	O – E	Variance	Fibrinolytic better / Control better	Heterogeneity	Trend
ECG						21.28 on 4 df ($P < 0.01$)	
BBB	18.7	23.6	-24.5	83.2			
ST elev, anterior	13.2	16.9	-122.0	420.6			
ST elev, inferior	7.5	8.4	-27.1	237.4			
ST elev, other	10.6	13.4	-42.1	159.6			
ST depression	15.2	13.8	12.9	108.7			
Other abnormality	5.2	5.8	-9.6	103.2			
Normal	3.0	2.3	3.4	12.9			
Hours from onset						9.69 on 4 df ($P < 0.06$)	9.55 on 1 df ($2P = 0.002$)
0 - 1	9.5	13.0	-29.3	83.3			
2 - 3	8.2	10.7	-100.2	354.8			
4 - 6	9.7	11.5	-78.5	387.6			
7 - 12	11.1	12.7	-51.5	336.7			
13 - 24	10.0	10.5	-11.1	212.6			
Age (years)						8.27 on 3 df ($P < 0.05$)	6.58 on 1 df ($2P = 0.01$)
<55	3.4	4.6	-45.9	155.6			
55 - 64	7.2	8.9	-86.3	360.0			
65 - 74	13.5	16.1	-113.7	533.0			
75+	24.3	25.3	-12.6	266.6			
Gender						1.99 on 1 df (NS)	
Male	8.2	10.1	-208.1	928.0			
Female	14.1	16.0	-62.2	436.8			
Systolic BP (mmHg)						1.31 on 3 df (NS)	0.68 on 1 df (NS)
<100	28.9	35.1	-36.7	132.2			
100 - 149	9.6	11.5	-168.9	850.0			
150 - 174	7.2	8.7	-59.2	290.0			
175+	7.2	8.2	-10.8	74.1			
Heart rate						0.51 on 2 df (NS)	0.31 on 1 df (NS)
<80	7.2	8.5	-83.2	464.9			
80 - 99	9.2	11.3	-65.8	287.2			
100+	17.4	20.7	-51.7	238.6			
Prior MI						2.09 on 1 df (NS)	
Yes	12.5	14.1	-43.7	322.4			
No	8.9	10.9	-228.5	1001.9			
Diabetes						1.57 on 1 df (NS)	
Yes	13.6	17.3	-41.4	145.7			
No	8.7	10.2	-142.6	830.4			
■ **ALL PATIENTS**	2820/29315 9.6%	3357/29285 11.5%	-269.5	1377.4	18% SD 2 odds reduction $2P < 0.00001$		

Figure 5.4

Figure 5.4 (Opposite) Proportional effects of fibrinolytic therapy on mortality during days 0–35 according to subgroup analysis. 'Observed minus expected' (O − E) number of events among fibrinolytic-allocated patients (and its variance) is given for respective clinical subgroup at MI presentation. This is used to calculate odds ratios (ORs) of death among patients allocated to fibrinolytic therapy to that among those allocated to control. ORs (black squares with areas proportional to amount of 'statistical information' contributed by the trials) are plotted with their 99% CIs (horizontal lines). Squares to the left of the solid vertical line indicate benefit (significant at $2P < 0.01$ only where entire CI is to the left of the vertical line). Overall result and 95% CI represented by diamond, with overall proportional reduction in the odds of death and statistical significance given alongside. Chi-square tests for evidence of heterogeneity of, or trends in, size of ORs in subdivisions of each presentation feature are also given. (From Fibrinolytic Therapy Trialists Collaborative Group (1994) Indications for fibrinolytic therapy in suspected acute myocardical infarction: collaborative overview of early mortality and major morbidity results from all randomized trials of more than 1000 patients. *Lancet*, **343**, 311–22, with permission.)

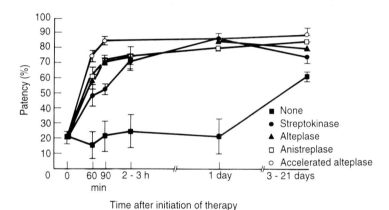

Time after initiation of therapy

Figure 5.5 Pooled analysis of angiographic patency rates over time for various thrombolytic agents: patency rates are highest following t-PA, early rates with conventional or non-accelerated t-PA and anistreplase (APSAC) are strikingly similar. The patency rate following SK has 'caught up' to conventional t-PA and APSAC within 2–3 hours. Includes 13 728 angiographic observations. (From Granger, C. B., Califf, R. M. and Topol, E. J. (1992) Thrombolytic therapy for acute myocardial infarction. A review. *Drugs*, **44**, 293–325, with permission.)

Considerable controversy surrounds the thrombolytic trials directly comparing SK and t-PA.[43–46] GISSI-2, which compared 1.5 million units of SK and non-accelerated t-PA, with or without subcutaneous heparin, demonstrated no mortality difference between tPA and SK (8.9% vs 8.5%).[47] ISIS-3, which compared 1.5 million units of SK, 30 units of APSAC and 0.6 million units kg^{-1} of two-chain t-PA, also revealed no mortality advantages (10.5%, 10.6% and 10.3%, respectively).[48] In both trials, SK was associated with the lowest stroke rates. Both trials have been criticized for the lack of adequate intravenous heparin therapy with the fibrin-specific plasminogen activator, t-PA, which may be particularly dependent on conjunctive heparin use for maintaining infarct-artery patency as suggested by the Heparin Aspirin Reperfusion (HART)[49] and European Cooperative Study Group-6 (ECSG-6)[50] trials. The Global Utilization Streptokinase Tissue-Plasminogen Activator for

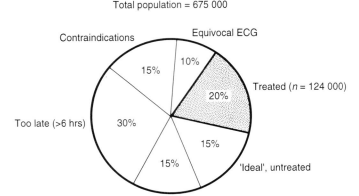

Figure 5.6   The approximate proportions of patients eligible and ineligible for thrombolysis according to current recommendations and therapeutic practices. (From Muller, D. W. M. and Topel, E. J. (1990) Selection of patients with acute myocardial infarction for thrombolytic therapy. *Ann. Intern. Med.*, **113**, 949–60, with permission.)

Occlusive Coronary Arteries (GUSTO) trial attempted to investigate optimal thrombolytic strategies and therefore compared four different regimens: accelerated t-PA with intravenous heparin, SK with subcutaneous heparin, SK with intravenous heparin and combination SK and t-PA with intravenous heparin.[51] This accelerated t-PA regimen resulted in a 14% mortality reduction (6.3% t-PA vs 7.3% pooled SK), corresponding to nine net lives saved per 1000 patients treated. While some investigators have questioned the outcome of this trial,[43–46] the angiographic subtrial of GUSTO has dramatically demonstrated that early artery patency with normal flow (grade TIMI 3) is a powerful predictor of mortality with 8.9%, 7.4% and 4.4% mortality rates for TIMI 0/1, TIMI 2 or TIMI 3 flow, respectively (Figure 5.7). Because accelerated t-PA achieves TIMI 3 flow at 90 minutes in only 54% of patients,

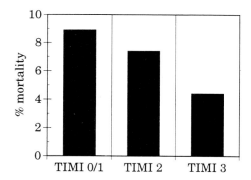

Figure 5.7   Relation of mortality from acute MI to TIMI flow seen 90 minutes after thrombolytic therapy. (Adapted from the GUSTO angiographic investigators (1993) The effects of tissue plasminogen activator, streptokinase, or both on coronary artery patency, ventricular function, and survival after acute myocardial infarction. *N. Engl. J. Med.*, **329**, 1615–22, with permission.)

even further modification of present dosing regimens (e.g. double bolus t-PA) and/or new agents will be required to optimize mortality reduction.

Primary revascularization

Despite the consistent benefit of thrombolysis, only a minority of MI patients are eligible (approximately 33%) or actually receive (approximately 20%) thrombolytic therapy due to multiple factors including presenting 'too late', borderline ECG, age and absolute/relative contraindications.[40] As illustrated in Figure 5.8, it is precisely these patients who are at greatest mortality risk in the setting of acute MI. Reperfusion with primary or direct revascularization by coronary angioplasty or bypass grafting offers an alternative to salvage ischemic but viable myocardium. There is now accumulating and compelling evidence that such a strategy is not only feasible, but worthy of head-to-head comparison with thrombolysis. Primary PTCA results in early and rapid infarct-related artery patency with >90% technical success and inhospital mortality of 7.2–8.3%.[52,53] The Primary Angioplasty in Myocardial Infarction (PAMI)[54] trial demonstrated significantly decreased death or nonfatal reinfarction at six months with immediate angioplasty (9%) compared to thrombolysis with t-PA (17%). In addition, PTCA was accompanied by a 0% stroke rate and shorter mean time to resolution of chest pain (290 vs 354 minutes). Additional randomized primary angioplasty trials[55,56] support the notion that mechanical revascularization is at least equivalent to thrombolysis with respect to infarct size and may result in improvement in ejection fraction. In patients who have coronary anatomy not conducive to angioplasty, emergency coronary artery bypass surgery may be offered to provide immediate reperfusion with acceptable mortality.[57,58] The results of GUSTO showing that mortality is directly related to early and rapid artery patency provides a compelling basis for further evaluating the role of primary revascularization versus thrombolysis in the treatment of MI.

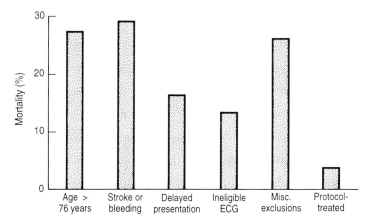

Figure 5.8 Mortality rates for patients excluded from thrombolytic therapy by exclusion subgroup (including patients with multiple exclusions) and for patients treated with thrombolytic therapy. (From Cragg, D. R., Friedman, H. Z., Bonema, J. D. *et al.* (1991) Outcome of patients with acute myocardial infarction who are ineligible for thrombolytic therapy. *Ann. Intern. Med.*, **115**, 173–7, with permission.)

Aspirin

Platelet adhesion and aggregation contribute significantly to occlusive thrombus formation at the site of plaque rupture.[8] The occlusive thrombus is platelet-rich on pathologic[59] and angioscopic[60] examinations which demonstrate a white (platelet/fibrin-rich) 'head' with a red (erythrocyte/fibrin-rich) 'tail'; platelet microemboli have also been found in the territory distal to thrombotic occlusions.[61] The importance of platelet activation in acute ischemic syndromes *in vivo* has also been demonstrated by the association of increased platelet thromboxane (TXA$_2$) production with symptomatic ischemia/infarction.[62] Aspirin possesses antiplatelet properties by virtue of its ability to irreversibly acetylate cyclooxygenase and inhibit TXA$_2$ synthesis.[63,64] ISIS-2 showed that the administration of aspirin (160 mg daily) up to 24 hours after the onset of symptoms of acute suspected MI reduced five-week mortality by 23% (Figure 5.9), nonfatal MI by 49%, and nonfatal stroke by 46% compared with the placebo control group.[65] Importantly, the effect of aspirin on mortality was additive to that of SK: SK alone resulted in a 25% reduction and the combination of SK and ASA in a 42% reduction in mortality compared with the double placebo control group. Aspirin is also effective in secondary prevention after MI. The Antiplatelet Trialists Collaborative Group has performed a meta-analysis on 10 post-MI trials showing that antiplatelet treatment, with aspirin being just as effective as aspirin plus either dipyridamole or sulfinpyrazone, reduced the risk of vascular death by 13%, nonfatal reinfarction by 31% and nonfatal stroke by 42%.[66]

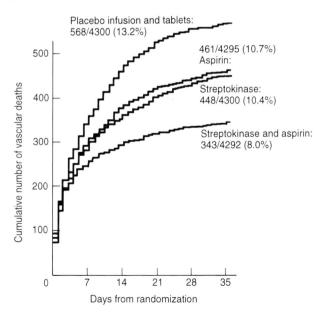

Figure 5.9 Cumulative vascular mortality at five weeks in the ISIS-2 trial: aspirin results in nearly the same benefit as streptokinase, and the effects of aspirin and streptokinase are additive. See text for explanation of trial name abbreviation. (From Yusef, S., Sleight, P., Held, P. and McMahon, S. (1990) Routine medical management of acute myocardial infarction. Lessons from overviews of recent randomized controlled trials. *Circulation*, **82** (Supp. II), 117–34, with permission.)

Anticoagulation

Despite its widespread use, evidence demonstrating a survival advantage for anticoagulation in the setting of MI is limited. In the prethrombolytic era, meta-analysis of 32 studies, including nonrandomized and randomized trials, has demonstrated approximately a 22% reduction in mortality ($P < 0.001$) that is still significant if only the three large randomized trials (Medical Research Council, Bronx Municipal Hospital and Veterans Administration Cooperative Studies) are considered ($P < 0.01$).[67–69] Anticoagulation was also associated with a significant reduction in systemic embolization and a trend toward decreased reinfarction rates.

Thrombin has emerged as the central focus of adjuvant therapy for acute MI in the thrombolytic era. It is not only responsible for converting fibrinogen to fibrin, but is a potent platelet agonist that induces aggregation. Thrombolytic therapy and the resultant increase in plasmin activity leads directly to enhanced thrombin generation as shown independently by Eisenberg,[70] Owen[71] and Rapold.[72] Thrombin level, as reflected by thrombin–antithrombin III complex formation, is an early predictor of reocclusion after successful thrombolysis.[73]

Mortality reductions with the antithrombin agent, heparin, as adjunct to thrombolytic therapy for acute MI, remain controversial due to the lack of appropriately designed trials.[74] The ISIS-2 trial, although not designed to assess the effect of heparin, revealed that mortality was the lowest in patients who received SK and aspirin without heparin (8.0%) compared to patients who received SK and aspirin with intravenous heparin (8.3%) or subcutaneous heparin (9.0%). Data pooled from GISSI-2 and ISIS-3 also demonstrate no survival benefit from the additon of aspirin plus heparin (death at 35 days 10.0%) or aspirin alone (10.2%, $P = 0.37$) to thrombolysis. In contrast, the SCATI trial investigated the use of subcutaneous heparin in acute myocardial infarction with and without concomitant SK and found that mortality was significantly lower in heparin-treated patients both overall (5.8% vs 10%) and in the SK group (4.6% vs 8.8%).[75]

There is evidence from patency trials (HART and ECSG-6) suggesting that the addition of heparin to aspirin and t-PA may lead to enhanced patency rates. GUSTO investigated the strategy of intravenous heparin and accelerated t-PA in comparison to SK with intravenous or subcutaneous heparin, but did not directly compare t-PA with and without heparin, which therefore raises further questions. Subanalysis of the recent LATE trial suggests that survival is improved with the use of t-PA and adjunctive heparin compared to t-PA alone (mortality 6.6% vs 10.3%, respectively); however, the use of heparin was not randomized. This issue is important because several studies have demonstrated an increased risk of serious bleeding with the use of adjunctive heparin (major hemorrhage pooled GISSI-2 and ISIS-3: aspirin plus heparin 1.0% vs aspirin alone 0.7%, $P < 0.001$).

Beta-blockers

Salvaging ischemic but viable myocardium also requires medical intervention on the 'demand' side. Beta-blockers reduce myocardial oxygen consumption by lowering heart rate, contractility and wall stress, which has been shown to decrease infarct size in experimental models. In a meta-analysis of 27 trials, intravenous beta-blockers reduced inhospital mortality by 13%, reinfarction by 19% and cardiac arrest/ventricular fibrillation by 16%.[76] The long-term use of oral beta-blockers is also associated with an impressive 22% reduction in mortality and 27% reduction in reinfarction. The mechanism of mortality reduction with beta-blockers is multifactorial. Immediate beta-blockade has been reported to prevent cardiac rupture and ventricular fibrillation,[77] chronic beta-blockade primarily sudden death. A strategy of immediate, intravenous beta-blockade has been found to significantly reduce reinfarction and recurrent angina compared to 'deferred' or delayed oral beta-blockers and should be employed unless specific contraindications, such as congestive heart failure and heart block, at MI presentation dictate otherwise.[78]

Nitrates

Nitrates reduce preload and afterload, thereby decreasing wall stress and myocardial oxygen consumption. Additional benefit may also be derived from their ability to increase coronary blood flow. Intravenous nitroglycerin was found to lower mortality by 49% when the results of six trials were pooled.[79] In one of these trials reported by Judgutt and Warnica, intravenous nitroglycerin limited infarct size and expansion, increased left-ventricular ejection fraction, and was associated with fewer infarct-related complications, such as left-ventricular thrombus, cardiogenic shock and infarct extension.[80] However, this impressive impact on survival has not been confirmed in two recent, randomized trials, ISIS-4 (oral mononitrate)[81] and GISSI-3 (intravenous for the first 24 hours followed by transdermal).[82] In GISSI-3, nitrate use was associated with no difference in death rate, clinical heart failure or proportion of patients with ejection fraction <35% or extent of akinesis/dyskinesis. There were slightly lower rates of postinfarction angina and cardiogenic shock among nitrate-allocated patients.

Angiotensin converting-enzyme (ACE) inhibitors

Incontrovertible evidence supports the use of ACE inhibitors to improve survival in patients with symptomatic congestive heart failure[83–85] and in asymptomatic patients with left-ventricular dysfunction starting days after myocardial infarction.[86,87] The mechanism(s) of benefit is based upon the ability of ACE inhibition to reduce angiotensin II-mediated vasoconstriction and sodium retention and to increase the level of bradykinin and vasodilator prostaglandins that also contribute to an overall improved hemodynamic and neurohormonal profile. Interestingly, ACE inhibition decreased both progressive heart failure and sudden death in these studies.

The use of ACE inhibitors in the acute MI setting is based upon the remodeling hypothesis of Pfeffer and coworkers that ACE inhibitors interrupt the pathophysiologic sequence of excessive work load and increased wall stress, which begets dilatation/hypertrophy leading to progressive left-ventricular enlargement and dysfunction.[88] Also emerging from this hypothesis is the importance of patency of the infarct-related artery, which is an independent determinant of left ventricular enlargement in their studies.[89] The results of ACE inhibitor trials in acute MI are somewhat inconclusive. The Cooperative North Scandinavian Enalapril Survival Study (CONSENSUS) II trial, which randomized patients to enalapril or placebo on the first day of MI, was terminated after interim analysis revealed no significant change in survival at three months.[90] However, ISIS-4 (captopril versus placebo)[91] and GISSI-3 (lisinopril versus placebo)[82] demonstrated significant survival benefit when administered on the first day of MI: 6.9% vs 7.3% and 6.3% vs 7.1%, respectively, corresponding to approximately 5 lives saved per 1000 patients treated. In GISSI-3, lisinopril treatment resulted in a smaller percentage of patients with ejection fraction <35% (4.8% vs 5.3%), but had no effect on akinetic/dyskinetic score or clinical heart failure rates. The overall beneficial effect of ACE inhibition may be related not only to infarct remodeling, but perhaps to emerging evidence that ACE inhibition may favorably enhance endogenous fibrinolytic mechanisms by inhibiting plasminogen activator-1 production.[92] Such an effect may be partially responsible for the finding that ACE inhibition has been found to decrease recurrent MI by up to 25%.[86]

Calcium-channel blockers

Calcium-channel blockers are able to decrease myocardial oxygen consumption and possibly increase coronary blood flow that together could act favorably to reduce mortality after MI. In either short-term studies in the setting of acute MI or long-term studies after MI, no benefit on survival is seen with the administration of calcium-channel blockers (verapamil, nifedipine, diltiazem or lidoflazine).[93] The data surrounding diltiazem and NQWMI are particularly illustrative of the difficulty in demonstrating a significant impact on survival. While diltiazem has been associated with a reduction in recurrent angina and reinfarction in patients with NQWMI,[94] the subsequent mortality trial showed no benefit for diltiazem over placebo unless subgroup analysis was performed.

Magnesium

The Second Leicester Intravenous Magnesium Intervention trial (LIMIT-2)[95] and meta-analysis of seven smaller trials catapulted the use of magnesium into the forefront of acute MI interventions. LIMIT-2 reported 25% reductions in both mortality and clinical heart failure in patients randomized to intravenous magnesium for 24 hours compared to placebo; the meta-analysis suggested an even more impressive 35% (95% CI 17–49%) mortality reduction.[95] The mechanism(s) of magnesium's benefit in MI has been attributed to the reduction of calcium influx into myocardial cells thereby limiting reperfusion injury,[96] antiplatelet effects,[97] afterload reduction[98] and antiarrhythmic properties.[99] However, ISIS-4, which randomized over 50 000 patients, was unable to detect any benefit of magnesium whatsoever.[100] In fact, magnesium was associated with a nonsignificant *excess* of mortality (4 per 1000 patients treated), cardiogenic shock (5 per 1000 patients treated) and heart failure (5 per 1000 patients treated). Therefore, the routine use of magnesium can no longer be recommended in acute MI.

Lidocaine

While beta-blockers have been shown to reduce the incidence of peri-infarct ventricular fibrillation/cardiac arrest, the prophylactic use of lidocaine is not associated with improved survival.[101] Lidocaine is effective in reducing the incidence of ventricular fibrillation by approximately 36%, but is associated with significant bradycardia and asystole, which may contribute to excess mortality.

Unstable angina

The development of unstable angina is precipitated by activation of the atherosclerotic plaque and, generally, nonocclusive thrombus formation. Angioscopy performed at the time of bypass surgery has revealed intracoronary thrombus in up to 90% of patients with unstable angina.[102] A primary pathophysiologic role for platelets in unstable angina has been elucidated by experimental evidence demonstrating elevated urinary metabolites of TXA_2 in patients with unstable angina[103] as well as from the Folts model, which has shown that cyclic coronary flows are secondary to platelet aggregate formation.[104]

Patients who present unstable angina have a significantly increased risk of nonfatal infarction (2–20%) and inhospital mortality (2–21%), as reported in several series.[105–108] Aspirin significantly reduces the risk of nonfatal MI and death in the setting of unstable angina.[109,110] In the Veterans Administration study, in which patients were randomized to aspirin (324 mg day^{-1}) or placebo and followed for three months, aspirin reduced mortality by 51% and MI by 55%.[91] Anticoagulation with heparin is also highly efficacious in unstable angina. The Montreal Heart Study showed that heparin reduced the risk of refractory angina by 57%, fatal and nonfatal MI by 85% and the total event rate by 57%.[94] It has been recently demonstrated that the discontinuation of heparin after completing a short course in the setting of unstable angina led to a 2.8-fold reactivation rate of clinically significant ischemia compared to patients treated with aspirin alone or aspirin plus heparin.[111] These results suggest that antiplatelet therapy is required to prevent reactivation of a presumably persistently thrombogenic culprit lesion. While unstable angina is associated with nonocclusive thrombus, thrombolytic therapy has not had a beneficial impact on infarction or mortality rates as demonstrated by the Thrombolysis in Myocardial Infarction (TIMI) IIIb study: death, MI or failure (54.2% t-PA vs 55.5% placebo; P = NS); fatal/nonfatal MI (7.4% t-PA vs 4.9% placebo.).[112] Coronary angioplasty has a role in both initially stabilized and refractory unstable angina in terms of reducing the incidence of recurrent chest pain, MI and death compared to historic control populations.[113]

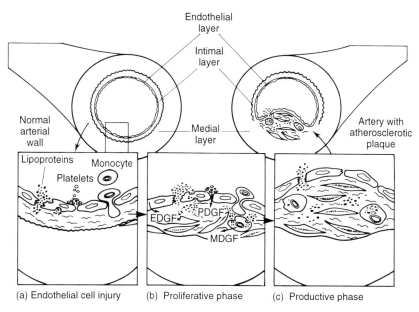

Figure 5.10 In the genesis of an atherosclerotic plaque, endothelial cell injury (a) leads to excessive influx of lipoproteins, invasion of monocytes/macrophages and adherence of platelets. This leads to a proliferative phase (b) in which a macrophage reaction and release of growth factors (EDGF, MDGF, PDGF) set in motion a process of smooth-muscle proliferation, eventually resulting in a productive phase (c) in which connective-tissue elements are formed leading to distinct plaque formation. (From Hurst, J. W., Becker, A. E. and Wilcox, B. R. (1988) Coronary heart disease. In: Hurst, J. W., Anderson, R. E., Becker, A. E. and Wilcox, B. R. (eds) *Atlas of the Heart*, pp. 6.1–6.44. New York: Gower Medical.)

Future directions

Reimer's hypothesis that '. . . time is the most critical variable involved in delaying or preventing ischemic myocardial cell death' and the results of GUSTO demonstrating that mortality is directly related to early and rapid artery patency have focused present research efforts on developing improved reperfusion strategies. These include modifying the dosing regimens of existing thrombolytic agents (i.e. 'double bolus' t-PA that increased the proportion of patients with TIMI 3 flow[114]), designing new agents (e.g. 'second-generation' t-PA that is fibrin-specific, plasminogen activator inhibitor-1 resistant and designed for increased half-life allowing bolus administration[115]), and investigating new antithrombotic agents (novel thrombin and factor Xa inhibitors and the new class of platelet GPIIb/IIIa integrin inhibitors). Exciting preliminary data from trials using hirudin and hirulog suggest that direct thrombin inhibitors, which unlike heparin do not require antithrombin-III complex formation and are thus capable of inhibiting clot-bound fibrin, may be more efficacious than existing anticoagulant regimens.[116,117]

Basic research and developing therapeutics for the treatment of MI are directed at the earliest stages of atherogenesis and plaque development to the much later events of post-MI myocardial salvage with, for example, free-radical scavenging agents to limit reperfusion injury,[118] or potentially even myocardial 'regeneration' facilitated by gene transfer to induce replication of myocardial cells.[119] The 'response-to-injury' hypothesis[120] formulated by Ross and modified by others (Figure 5.10) provides a framework to introduce the key 'players' that will be the subject of other chapters. In this hypothesis, injury to the endothelium leads to a critical sequence of cellular interactions involving monocytes, platelets, lymphocytes, and their secreted growth factors and cytokines that culminates in the formation of atherosclerotic plaques. Interventions along this path may provide a therapeutic mechanism to interrupt this progression and prevent MI.

References

1. Sobel, B. E. (1989) Coronary thrombolysis and the new biology. *J. Am. Coll. Cardiol.*, **14**, 850–60.
2. Herrick, J. B. (1912) Certain clinical features of sudden obstruction of coronary arteries. *JAMA*, **59**, 2015–20.
3. Roberts, W. C. and Buja, L. M. (1972) The frequency and significance of coronary arterial thrombi and other observations in fatal acute myocardial infarction. *Am. J. Med.*, **52**, 425–43.
4. DeWood, M., Spores, J., Notske, R. *et al.* (1980) Prevalence of total coronary occlusion during the early hours of transmural myocardial infarction. *N. Engl. J. Med.*, **303**, 897–902.
5. Roberts, W. C. (1989) Qualitative and quantitative comparison of amounts of narrowing by atherosclerotic plaques in the major epicardial coronary arteries at necropsy in sudden death, transmural acute myocardial infarction, transmural healed myocardial infarction, and unstable angina pectoris. *Am. J. Cardiol.*, **64**, 324–8.
6. Ambrose, J. A., Tannenbaum, M. A., Alexopoulos, D. *et al.* (1988) Angiographic progression of coronary artery disease and the development of myocardial infarction. *J. Am. Coll. Cardiol.*, **12**, 56–62.
7. Little, W. C., Constantinescu, M., Applegate, R. J. *et al.* (1988) Can coronary angiography predict the site of a subsequent myocardial infarction in patients with mild to moderate coronary artery disease? *Circulation*, **78**, 1157–66.
8. Fuster, V., Badimon, L., Badimon, J. J. and Cheseboro, J. (1992) The pathogenesis of coronary artery disease and the acute ischemic syndromes. *N. Engl. J. Med.*, **326**, 242–50.
9. Constantinides, P. (1996) Plaque fissure in human coronary thrombosis. *J. Atheroscl. Res.*, **1**, 1–17.
10. Davies, M. J. and Thomas, A. (1984) Thrombosis and acute coronary lesions in sudden cardiac ischemic death. *N. Engl. J. Med.*, **310**, 1137–40.
11. Davies, M. J. and Thomas, A. C. (1985) Plaque fissuring – the cause of acute myocardial infarction, sudden ischemic death, and crescendo angina. *Br. Heart J.*, **53**, 363–73.
12. Barger, A. C., Beeuwkes, R., Lainey, L. L. and Silverman, K. J. (1984) Hypothesis: vasa vasorum and neovascularization of human coronary arteries. *N. Engl. J. Med.*, **310**, 175–77.
13. Barger, C. A., Beeuwkes, R., Lainey, L. L. and Silverman, K. J. (1984) Hypothesis: vasa vasorum and neovascularization of human coronary arteries – a possible role in the pathophysiology of atherosclerosis. *N. Engl. J. Med.*, **310**, 175–7.
14. Richardson, P. D., Davies, M. J. and Born, G. V. R. (1989) Influence of plaque configuration and stress distribution on fissuring of coronary atherosclerotic plaques. *Lancet*, **ii**, 941–4.
15. Falk, E. (1989) Morphologic features of unstable atherothrombotic plaques underlying acute coronary syndromes. *Am. J. Cardiol.*, **63**, 114E–120E.
16. Ambrose, J. A., Winters, S. L., Arora, R. R. *et al.* (1985) Coronary angiographic morphology in myocardial infarction: a link between the pathogenesis of unstable angina and myocardial infarction. *J. Am. Coll. Cardiol.*, **6**, 1233–8.

17. Levin, D. C. and Fallon, J. T. (1982) Significance of the angiographic morphology of localized coronary stenoses: histopathologic correlations. *Circulation*, **66**, 316–20.
18. Hackel, D. B., Reimer, K. A., Ideker, R. E. *et al.* (1984) Comparison of enzymatic and anatomic estimates of myocardial infarct size in man. *Circulation*, **70**, 824–35.
19. Lavie, C. L. and Gersh, B. J. (1990) Acute myocardial infarction: initial manifestations, management, prognosis. *Mayo Clin. Proc.*, **65**, 531–48.
20. O'Brien, T. X. and Ross, J. (1989) Non-Q wave myocardial infarction. Incidence, pathophysiology, and clinical course compared with Q wave infarction. *Clin. Cardiol.*, **12** (Supp. III), 3.
21. Nicod, P., Gilpin, E., Dittrich, H. *et al.* (1989) Short- and long-term clinical outcome after Q-wave and non-Q-wave myocardial infarction in a large patient population. *Circulation*, **79**, 528–36.
22. Gruppo Italiano per lo Studio della Streptochinasi nell'Infarto Miocardico (GISSI) (1986) Effectiveness of intravenous thrombolytic treatment in acute myocardial infarction. *Lancet*, **i**, 397–402.
23. Yusuf, S., Wittes, J. and Friedman, L. (1988) Overview of results of randomized clinical trials in heart disease. I. Treatments following myocardial infarction. *JAMA*, **260**, 2088–93.
24. Yusuf, S., Sleight, P., Held, P. and McMahon, S. (1990) Routine medical management of acute myocardial infarction. Lessons from overviews of recent randomized controlled trials. *Circulation*, **82** (Supp. II), 117–34.
25. Reimer, K. A., Lowe, J. E., Rasmussen, M. M. and Jennings, R. B. (1977) The wavefront phenomenon of ischemic cell death. I. Myocardial infarct size vs duration of coronary occlusion in dogs. *Circulation*, **56**, 786–94.
26. Reimer, K. A. and Jennings, R. B. (1979) The 'wavefront phenomenon' of myocardial ischemic cell death: II. Transmural progression of necrosis within the framework of ischemic bed size (myocardium at risk) and collateral flow. *Lab. Invest.*, **40**, 633–44.
27. Maroko, P. R., Kjeshus, J. K., Sobel, B. E. *et al.* (1971) Factors influencing infarct size following experimental coronary artery occlusions. *Circulation*, **43**, 67–82.
28. Kennedy, J. W., Ritchie, J. L., Davis, K. B. and Fritz, J. K. (1983) Western Washington trial of intracoronary streptokinase in acute myocardial infarction. *N. Engl. J. Med.*, **309**, 1477–82.
29. Kennedy, J. W., Ritchie, J. L., Davis, K. B. *et al.* (1985) The Western Washington randomized trial of intracoronary streptokinase in acute myocardial infarction. *N. Engl. J. Med.*, **312**, 1073–8.
30. Fibrinolytic Therapy Trialists' Collaborative Group (1994) Indications for fibrinolytic therapy in suspected acute myocardial infarction: collaborative overview of early mortality and major morbidity results from all randomised trials of more than 1000 patients. *Lancet*, **343**, 311–22.
31. Keaney, J. F., Jr and Loscalzo, J. (1994) Pharmacology of thrombolytic agents. In: Loscalzo, J. and Schafer, A. I. (eds) *Thrombosis and Hemorrhage*, pp. 1173–206. Boston: Blackwell Scientific Publications.
32. Hoylaerts, M., Rijken, D. C., Lijnen, H. R. and Collen, D. (1982) Kinetics of the activation of plasminogen by human tissue plasminogen activator. Role of fibrin. *J. Biol. Chem.*, **257**, 2912–19.
33. Granger, C. B., Califf, R. M. and Topol, E. J. (1992) Thrombolytic therapy for acute myocardial infarction. *Drugs*, **44**, 293–325.
34. Chesboro, J. H., Knautterud, G., Roberts, R. *et al.* (1987) Thrombolysis in Myocardial Infarction (TIMI) trial, phase I: A comparison between intravenous tissue-type plasminogen activator and intravenous streptokinase. *Circulation*, **76**, 142–54.
35. Verstraete, M., Bory, M., Collen, D. *et al.* (1985) Randomized trial of intravenous recombinant tissue-type plasminogen activator versus intravenous streptokinase in acute myocardial infarction (ECSG-2). *Lancet*, **i**, 842–7.

36. The GUSTO angiograhic investigators (1993) The effects of tissue plasminogen activator, streptokinase, or both on coronary artery patency, ventricular function, and survival after acute myocardial infarction. *N. Engl. J. Med.*, **329**, 1615–22.
37. ISIS-2 Collaborative Group (1988) Randomized trial of intravenous streptokinase, oral aspirin, both, or neither among 17 187 cases of suspected myocardial infarction. *Lancet*, **ii**, 349–60.
38. Wilcox, R. G., von der Lippe, G., Olsson, C. G. *et al.* (1988) Trial of tissue plasminogen activator for mortality reduction in acute myocardial infarction. *Lancet*, **ii**, 349–60.
39. AIMS Trial Study Group (1988) Effect of intravenous APSAC on mortality after acute myocardial infarction: preliminary report of placebo-controlled trial. *Lancet*, **i**, 842–7.
40. Muller, D. W. and Topol, E. J. (1990) Selection of patients with acute myocardial infarction for thrombolytic therapy. *Ann. Intern. Med.*, **113**, 949–60.
41. EMERAS (Estudio Multicentrico Estreptoquinsa Republicas de America del Sur) Collaborative Group (1993) Randomised trial of late thrombolysis in patients with suspected acute myocardial infarction. *Lancet*, **342**, 767–72.
42. LATE Study Group (1993) Late assessment of thrombolytic efficacy (LATE) study with alteplase 6–24 hours after onset of acute myocardial infarction. *Lancet*, **342**, 759–66.
43. Fuster, V. (1993) Coronary thrombolysis – A perspective for the practicing physician [Editorial]. *N. Engl. J. Med.*, **329**, 723–5.
44. Sleight, P. (1993) Thrombolysis after GUSTO: A European perspective. *J. Myocard. Ischemia*, **5**, 25–30.
45. Ridker, P. M., O'Donnell, C., Marder, V. J. and Hennekens, C. H. (1993) Large-scale trials of thrombolytic therapy for acute myocardial infarction: GISI-2, ISIS-3, and GUSTO-1 [Editorial]. *Ann. Intern. Med.*, **119**, 530–2.
46. Lee, K. L., Califf, R. M., Simes, J. *et al.* (1994) Holding GUSTO up to the light. *Ann. Intern. Med.*, **120**, 876–81.
47. Gruppo Italiano per lo Studio della Sopravvivenza nell'Infarto Miocardico: GISSI-2 (1990) A factorial randomized trial of alteplase versus streptokinase and heparin versus no heparin among 14 490 patients with acute myocardial infarction. *Lancet*, **336**, 65–71.
48. The International Study Group (1990) In-hospital mortality and clinical course of 20 891 patients with suspected acute myocardial infarction randomized between alteplase and streptokinase with or without heparin. *Lancet*, **336**, 71–5.
49. Hsia, J., Kleinman, N., Aguirre, F. *et al.* for the HART Investigators (1992) Heparin-induced prolongation of partial thromboplastin time after thrombolysis; relation to coronary artery patency. *J. Am. Coll. Cardiol.*, **20**, 31–5.
50. de Bono, D. P., Simoons, J. L., Tijssen, J. *et al.* for the European Cooperative Study Group (1992) Effect of early intravenous heparin on coronary patency, infarct size, and bleeding complications after alteplase thrombolysis: results of a randomized double blind European Cooperative Study Group trial (ECSG 6). *Br. Heart J.*, **67**, 122–8.
51. The GUSTO Investigators (1993) An international randomized trial comparing four thrombolytic strategies for acute myocardial infarction. *N. Engl. J. Med.*, **329**, 673–82.
52. Eckman, M. H., Wong, J. B., Salem, D. N. and Pauker, S. G. (1992) Direct angioplasty for acute myocardial infarction. *Ann. Intern. Med.*, **117**, 667–76.
53. O'Keefe, J. H., Rutherford, B. D., McConahay, D. R. *et al.* (1989) Early and late results of coronary angioplasty with and without antecedent thrombolytic therapy for acute myocardial infarction. *Am. J. Cardiol.*, **64**, 1221–30.
54. Grines, C. L., Browne, K. F., Marco, J. *et al.* for the Primary Angioplasty in Myocardial Infarction Study Group (1993) A comparison of immediate angioplasty with thrombolytic therapy for acute myocardial infarction. *N. Engl. J. Med.*, **328**, 673–9.
55. Gibbons, R. J., Holmes, D. R., Reeder, G. S. *et al.* (1993) Immediate angioplasty compared with the administration of a thrombolytic agent followed by conservative treatment for myocardial infarction. *N. Engl. J. Med.*, **328**, 685–91.
56. Zijlstra, F., deBoer, M. J., Hoorntje, J. C. A. *et al.* (1993) A comparison of immediate coronary angioplasty with intravenous streptokinase in acute myocardial infarction. *N. Engl. J. Med.*, **328**, 680–4.

57. DeWood, M. A., Spores, J., Notske, R. N. *et al.* (1979) Medical and surgical management of myocardial infarction. *Am. J. Cardiol.*, **44**, 1356–64.
58. Phillips, S. J., Kongtahworn, C., Zeff, R. H. *et al.* (1979) Emergency coronary revascularization: a possible therapy for acute myocardial infarction. *Circulation*, **60**, 241–6.
59. Friedman, M. and Van den Bovenkamp, G. J. (1966) The pathogenesis of a coronary thrombus. *Am. J. Pathol.*, **48**, 19–44.
60. Mizuno, K., Satomura, K., Miyamoto, A. *et al.* (1992) Angioscopic evaluation of coronary-artery thrombi in acute coronary syndrome. *N. Engl. J. Med.*, **326**, 287–91.
61. Davies, M. J. and Thomas, A. (1984) Thrombosis and acute coronary-artery lesions in sudden cardiac ischemic death. *N. Engl. J. Med.*, **310**, 1137–40.
62. Fitzgerald, D. J., Roy, L., Catella, F. *et al.* (1986) Platelet activation in unstable coronary disease. *N. Engl. J. Med.*, **315**, 983–9.
63. Vane, J. R. (1971) Inhibition of prostaglandin synthesis as a mechanism of action for aspirin-like drugs. *Nature*, **231**, 232–5.
64. Roth, G. J. and Majerus, P. W. (1975) The mechanism of the effect of aspirin on human platelets. I. Acetylation of a particulate fraction protein. *J. Clin. Invest.*, **56**, 624–32.
65. ISIS-2 Collaborative Group (1988) Randomized trial of i.v. streptokinase, oral aspirin, both, or neither among 17 187 cases of suspected acute myocardial infarction. *Lancet*, **ii**, 349–60.
66. Antiplatelet Trialists' Collaborative (1988) Secondary prevention of vascular disease by prolonged antiplatelet treatment. *BMJ*, **296**, 320–31.
67. Peto, R. (1978) Clinical trial methodology. *Biomed. Pharmacother.*, **28**, 24–36.
68. Mitchell, J. R. A. (1981) Anticoagulants in coronary heart disease: retrospect and prospect. *Lancet*, **i**, 257–62.
69. Drapkin, A. and Merskey, L. (1972) Anticoagulation therapy after acute myocardial infarction: relation of therapeutic benefit to patient's age, sex and severity of infarction. *JAMA*, **222**, 541–8.
70. Eisenberg, P. R., Sherman, L. A. and Jaffe, A. S. (1987) Paradoxic elevation of fibrinopeptide A after streptokinase: evidence for continued thrombosis despite intense fibrinolysis. *J. Am. Coll. Cardiol.*, **10**, 527–9.
71. Owen, J., Friedman, K. D., Grossman, B. A. *et al.* (1988) Thrombolytic therapy with tissue plasminogen activator or streptokinase induces transient thrombin activity. *Blood*, **72**, 616–20.
72. Rapold, H. J. (1990) Promotion of thrombin activity by thrombolytic therapy without simultaneous anticoagulation. *Lancet*, **i**, 481–2.
73. Gulba, D. C., Barthels, M., Reil, G. H. and Lichten, P. R. (1988) Thrombin/antithrombin-III complex level as early predictor of reocclusion after successful thrombolysis. *Lancet*, **ii**, 97.
74. Ridker, P. M., Hebert, P. R., Fuster, V. and Hennekens, C. H. (1993) Are both aspirin and heparin justified as adjuncts to thrombolytic theraphy for acute myocardial infarction? *Lancet*, **341**, 1574–7.
75. The SCATI (Studio sulla Calciparina nell'Angina e nella Trombosi Ventricolare nell'Infarto) Group (1989) Randomised controlled trial of subcutaneous heparin in acute myocardial infarction. *Lancet*, **ii**, 182–6.
76. Yusuf, S., Peto, R., Lewis, J. *et al.* (1985) Beta blockade during and after myocardial infarction: an overview of the randomized trials. *Prog. Cardiovasc. Dis.*, **27**, 335–71.
77. ISIS-1 (First International Study of Infarct Survival) Collaborative Group (1988) Possible mechanisms for the early mortality reduction produced by beta-blockade started early in acute myocardial infarction. *Lancet*, **i**, 921–3.
78. Roberts, R., Rogers, W. J., Mueller, H. S. *et al.* (1991) Immediate versus deferred β-blockade following thrombolytic therapy in patients with acute myocardial infarction. Results of the Thrombolysis in Myocardial Infarction (TIMI) II-B study. *Circulation*, **83**, 422–37.
79. Yusuf, S., Collins, R., MacMahon, S. and Peto, R. (1988) Effect of i.v. nitrates on mortality in acute myocardial infarction: an overview of the randomised trials. *Lancet*, **i**, 1088–92.

80. Judgutt, B. I. and Warnica, J. W. (1988) Intravenous nitroglycerin therapy to limit myocardial infarct size, expansion, and complications. Effect of timing, dosage, and infarct location. *Circulation*, **78**, 906–19.
81. ISIS Collaborative Group (1993) ISIS-4: randomised study of oral isosorbide mononitrate in over 50 000 patients with suspected acute myocardial infarction. *Circulation*, **88**, I-394.
82. GISSI-3 (1994) Effects of lisinopril and transdermal glyceryl trinitrate singly and together on 6-week mortality and ventricular function after acute myocardial infarction. *Lancet*, **343**, 1115–22.
83. CONSENSUS Trial Study Group (1987) Effects of enalapril on mortality in severe congestive heart failure. *N. Engl. J. Med.*, **316**, 1429–35.
84. The SOLVD Investigators (1991) Effect of enalapril on survival in patients with reduced left ventricular ejection fractions and congestive heart failure. *N. Engl. J. Med.*, **325**, 293–302.
85. Cohn, J. N., Archibald, D. G., Ziesche, S. *et al.* (1986) Effect of vasodilator therapy on mortality in chronic congestive heart failure. Results of a Veterans Administration Cooperative Study. *N. Engl. J. Med.*, **314**, 1547–52.
86. Pfeffer, M. A., Braunwald, E., Moye, L. A. *et al.* (1992) Effect of captopril on mortality and morbidity in patients with left ventricular dysfunction after myocardial infarction. Results of the Survival and Ventricular Enlargement Trial. *N. Engl. J. Med.*, **327**, 669–77.
87. The SOLVD Investigators (1992) Effect of enalapril on mortality and the development of heart failure in asymptomatic patients with reduced left ventricular ejection fractions. *N. Engl. J. Med.*, **327**, 685–91.
88. Pfeffer, M. A. and Braunwald, E. (1990) Ventricular remodelling after myocardial infarction. *Circulation*, **81**, 1161–72.
89. Pfeffer, M. A., Lamas, G. A., Vaughan, D. E. *et al.* (1988) Effect of captopril on progressive ventricular dilatation after anterior myocardial infarction. *N. Engl. J. Med.*, **319**, 80–6.
90. Swedberg, K., Held, P., Kjekshus, J. *et al.* (1992) Effects of the early administration of enalapril on mortality in patients with acute myocardial infarction. Results of the Cooperative New Scandanavian Enalapril Survival Study II (CONSENSUS II). *N. Engl. J. Med.*, **327**, 678–84.
91. ISIS Collaborative Group (1993) ISIS-4: randomised study of oral captopril in over 50 000 patients with suspected acute myocardial infarction. *Circulation*, **88**, I-394.
92. Ridker, P. M., Gadboury, C. L., Seely, E. W. *et al.* (1993) Stimulation of plasminogen activator inhibitor-1 *in vivo* by infusion of angiotensin II. Evidence of a potential interaction between the renin–angiotensin system and fibrinolytic function. *Circulation*, **87**, 1969–73.
93. Yusuf, S. and Furberg, C. D. (1987) Effects of calcium channel blockers on survival after myocardial infarction. *Cardiovasc. Drugs Ther.*, **1**, 343–4.
94. Gibson, R. S., Boden, W. E., Theroux, P. *et al.* (1986) Diltiazem and reinfarction in patients with non Q wave MI. *N. Engl. J. Med.*, **315**, 423–9.
95. Woods, K. L., Fletcher, S., Roffe, C. H. and Haider, Y. (1992) Intravenous magnesium sulphate in suspected acute myocardial infarction: results of the second Leicester Intravenous Magnesium Intervention Trial (LIMIT-2). *Lancet*, **339**, 1553–8.
96. Shine, K. I. (1979) Myocardial effects of magnesium. *Am. J. Physiol.*, **237**, H413–23.
97. Adams, J. H. and Mitchell, J. R. (1979) The effects of agents which modify platelet behaviour and of magnesium ions on thrombus formation *in vivo*. *Thromb. Haemost.*, **42**, 603–10.
98. Turplaty, P. D. and Altura, B. M. (1978) Extracellular magnesium ions control calcium exchange and content of vascular smooth muscle. *Eur. J. Pharmacol.*, **52**, 421–3.
99. Perticone, F., Adinolfi, I. and Bonaduce, D. (1986) Efficiency of magnesium sulfate in the treatment of torsade de pointes. *Am. Heart J.*, **112**, 847–9.
100. ISIS-4 Collaborative Group (1993) ISIS-4: randomised study of intravenous magnesium in over 50 000 patients with suspected acute myocardial infarction. *Circulation*, **88**, I-292.

101. McMahon, S. and Yusuf, S. (1987) Effects of lidocaine on ventricular fibrillation, asystole, and early death in patients with suspected acute myocardial infarction. In: Califf, R. M. and Wagner, G. S. (eds) *Acute Coronary Care*, pp. 51–60. Boston: Martinus Nijhoff.

102. Sherman, C. T., Litvack, F., Grundfest, W. *et al.* (1986) Coronary angioscopy in patients with unstable angina pectoris. *N. Engl. J. Med.*, **315**, 913–19.

103. Grande, P., Grauholt, A. M. and Madsen, J. K. (1990) Unstable angina pectoris. Platelet behavior and prognosis in progressive angina and intermediate coronary syndrome. *Circulation*, **I** (Supp.), 16–19.

104. Folts, J. D., Crowell, E. B. and Rowe, G. G. (1976) Platelet aggregation in partially obstructed vessels and its elimination with aspirin. *Circulation*, **54**, 365–70.

105. Bertolasi, C. A., Tronge, J. E., Ricitelli, M. A. *et al.* (1976) Natural history of unstable angina with medical or surgical therapy. *Chest*, **70**, 596–605.

106. Hultgren, H. N., Shettigar, U. R. and Miller, D. C. (1982) Medical versus surgical treatment of unstable angina. *Am. J. Cardiol.*, **50**, 663–70.

107. Lewis, D. H., Davis, J. W., Archibald, D. G. *et al.* (1983) Protective effects of aspirin against acute myocardial infarction and death in men with unstable angina. *N. Engl. J. Med.*, **309**, 396–403.

108. Olson, H. G., Lyons, K. P., Aronow, W. S. *et al.* (1981) The high risk angina patient. *Circulation*, **64**, 674–84.

109. Cairns, J. A., Gent, M., Snger, J. *et al.* (1985) Aspirin, sulfinpyrazone, or both in unstable angina. *N. Engl. J. Med.*, **313**, 1369–75.

110. Theroux, P., Ourelette, H., McCans, J. *et al.* (1988) Aspirin and heparin or both to treat acute unstable angina. *N. Engl. J. Med.*, **319**, 1105–11.

111. Theroux, P., Waters, D., Lam, J. *et al.* (1992) Reactivation of unstable angina following discontinuation of heparin. *N. Engl. J. Med.*, **327**, 141–5.

112. TIMI IIIb Trial (1994) Effects of t-PA and a comparison of early and invasive strategies in unstable angina and non Q wave myocardial infarction. Results of TIMI IIIb trial. *Circulation*, **89**, 1545–56.

113. de Feyter, P. J. and Serruys, P. W. (1994) Percutaneous transluminal coronary angioplasty for unstable angina. In: Topol, E. J. (ed.) *Textbook of Interventional Cardiology*, pp. 274–91. Philadelphia: W. B. Saunders.

114. Purvis, J. A., McNeill, A. J., Siddiqui, R. A. *et al.* (1994) Efficacy of 100 mg of double-bolus alteplase in achieving complete perfusion in the treatment of acute myocardial infarction. *J. Am. Coll. Cardiol.*, **23**, 6–10.

115. Refino, C. J., Paoni, N. F., Keyt, B. A. *et al.* (1993) A variant of t-PA (T103N, KHRR 296-299 AAAA) that, by bolus, has increased potency and decreased systemic activation of plasminogen. *Thromb. Haemost.*, **70**, 313–19.

116. Cannon, C. P., McCabe, C. H., Henry, T. D. *et al.* (1994) A pilot trial of recombinant desulfatohirudin compared with heparin in conjunction with tissue-type plasminogen activator and aspirin for acute myocardial infarction: results of the Thrombolysis in Myocardial Infarction (TIMI-5). *J. Am. Coll. Cardiol.*, **23**, 993–1003.

117. Lindon, R. M., Theroux, P., Juneau, M. *et al.* (1993) Initial experience with a direct antithrombin, hirulog, in unstable angina. Anticoagulant, antithrombotic, and clinical effects. *Circulation*, **88**, 1495–501.

118. Forman, M. B. and Virmani, R. (1991) Pathogenesis and modification of myocardial reperfusion injury. In: Gersh, B. J. and Rahimtoola, S. H. (eds) *Current Topics in Cardiology: Acute Myocardial Infarction*, pp. 349–70. New York: Elsevier.

119. von Harsdorf, R., Schott, R. J., Shen, Y. T. *et al.* (1993) Gene injection into canine myocardium as a useful model for studying gene expression in the heart of large mammals. *Circ. Res.*, **72**, 688–95.

120. Ross, R. (1986) The pathogenesis of atherosclerosis – an update. *N. Engl. J. Med.*, **314**, 488–500.

6

Thrombotic Heart Disease and Myocardial Infarction: Local Therapy

Campbell Rogers

Introduction

Atherosclerosis causes chronic tissue ischemia because of fixed arterial narrowings and acute tissue necrosis after sudden vascular occlusion. Sudden occlusion by intraluminal arterial thrombosis causes nearly all acute transmural myocardial infarctions and thrombotic occlusion of noncoronary arteries can result in limb loss, stroke or visceral infarction. The mechanism underlying acute thrombosis is increasingly recognized as rupture of pre-existing atherosclerotic plaques into the lumen, exposure of thrombogenic vessel-wall elements to the bloodstream, stimulation of platelet adhesion and aggregation, and fibrin generation.[1,2]

The acute treatment of such arterial occlusions has focused on relieving obstruction by removing the offending intraluminal thrombus. Methods for accomplishing this include mechanical removal via surgical or catheter-based techniques, or pharmacologic removal via agents which dissolve thrombus and/or prevent its extension or recurrence. Because the site of thrombotic occlusion is only a very small fraction of the arterial tree, and systemic treatments are prone to hemorrhagic complications, attempts have been made to design techniques for treating only the thrombosed arterial segment using local delivery of antithrombotic or thrombolytic agents.

As will be outlined in this chapter, local treatment for arterial thrombotic diseases encompasses two discrete concepts: (1) *anatomic targeting*, i.e. methods designed to deliver highest drug concentrations to thrombosed arterial segments; and (2) *biochemical targeting*, i.e. drugs designed to be systemically delivered but to act primarily at sites of thrombosis. Each of these approaches has been applied to the treatment of acute coronary ischemic syndromes, and in experimental models of arterial thrombosis, novel techniques of antithrombotic drug delivery continue to show promising results.

Acute myocardial infarction

Thrombolytic agents

DeWood *et al.* in 1980 defined angiographically the pathophysiology of acute myocardial infarction, demonstrating thrombotic coronary occlusion in 87% of patients within four hours of transmural infarction.[3] This discovery spurred the development of drugs for dissolving thrombus and ushered in an era in which thrombolytic therapy has reduced mortality from myocardial infarction over 30%. In 1958, the first use of intravenous streptokinase to treat myocardial infarction was reported[4] followed soon after by attempts at local delivery via coronary sinus retroperfusion.[5] Based on only marginal clinical benefits and high complication rates reported in early trials of prolonged intravenous infusions of streptokinase,[6–8] in the early 1980s trials of thrombolytic agents were undertaken employing anatomic targeting to achieve local effects while theoretically minimizing systemic toxicities. In these trials, streptokinase was injected as originally described by Rentrop *et al.*[9] directly into occluded coronary arteries through catheters placed percutaneously and guided into the coronary ostia. Kennedy *et al.* in the Western Washington Intracoronary Streptokinase Trial enrolled 250 patients under 76 years old, presenting with less than 12 hours of chest pain and ST-segment elevations on electrocardiogram, and treated them with either nitroglycerine or streptokinase, 250 000–350 000 u via intracoronary infusion. Patients receiving streptokinase had lower mortality after 30 days[10] and after 12 months,[11] with 12-month follow-up demonstrating the primacy of a patent infarct-related artery above and beyond treatment group.[11] Similar studies from Khaja *et al.*[12] and Anderson *et al.*[13] supported the angiographic and clinical benefit from intracoronary streptokinase, although another angiographic study[14] demonstrated that after 10–14 days spontaneous recanalization had occurred in 67% of untreated patients, not significantly different from the recanalization rate of 73% in those receiving streptokinase.

These small studies had as a cornerstone local delivery of thrombolytic agents to sites of coronary thrombosis, anticipating that this might enhance efficacy while limiting systemic toxicity. On the other hand, such local delivery required access to emergency cardiac catheterization facilities, delayed administration of streptokinase until after angiography, and heightened potential bleeding risks from vascular access sites. The balance of these advantages and disadvantages was tested in several randomized trials comparing intracoronary and intravenous streptokinase for acute myocardial infarction. Two trials of patients randomized *after* coronary arteriography reported systemic hypofibrinogenemia after either route of administration, and marginally more frequent although no faster recanalization with intracoronary than intravenous delivery.[15–16] Conversely, in a study of 50 patients randomized on presentation,[17] those assigned to immediate intravenous treatment had more rapid treatment and were left with better left-ventricular function after 10 days than those randomized to coronary arteriography first, followed by intracoronary streptokinase treatment. There was no significant difference in bleeding complications between the two groups.

Despite the hope that systemic exposure to thrombolytic agents would be lessened by regional infusion, systemic overflow out of, or through, occluded arteries clearly produces a systemic lytic state,[15,18-23] and successful reperfusion after regional infusion was in fact *dependent on* systemic depletion of fibrinogen:[23] those patients who acquired a systemic lytic state were much more likely to have reperfusion (12 of 12) than those who did not (none of 7).

These observations led to virtual abandonment of intracoronary thrombolytic administration as a first-line treatment for acute myocardial infarction, and attention was turned to the design of systemically administered, but *biochemically local* therapy with agents whose fibrinolytic activity would be most pronounced at sites of intra-arterial thrombosis. In the early 1980s, the human serine protease tissue-type plasminogen activator (t-PA) was isolated and purified, and produced in large quantities by recombinant-DNA techniques.[24-26] Tissue-type plasminogen activator has a marked affinity for the binary complex of plasminogen bound to fibrin, giving it a theoretical advantage over streptokinase as a selective fibrinolytic agent.

As might be anticipated from the outcomes of trials with intracoronary or intravenous streptokinase, such fibrin selectivity has advantages and disadvantages compared to nonselective agents. On the one hand, clinical angiographic trials have conclusively shown that clot lysis in patients with acute myocardial infarction is significantly more rapid with t-PA than with streptokinase.[27,28] In the Thrombolysis in Myocardial Infarction (TIMI) Phase I trial, patency after 90 min was 60% in patients treated with t-PA and 40% in those treated with streptokinase.[27] Similarly, in the Global Utilization of Streptokinase and Tissue Plasminogen Activator for Occluded Coronary Arteries (GUSTO) trial, a large difference in arterial patency was seen after 90 min, with 81% of patients receiving accelerated t-PA but only 54–60% of patients receiving streptokinase having patent arteries.[28] A recent meta-analysis of studies with either or both thrombolytic agents[29] found that after 90 min, patency in t-PA-treated patients was 68–72% with conventional dosing and 82–87% with an accelerated dosing regimen, while in streptokinase-treated patients patency after 90 min was seen in 48–55%.

On the other hand, although systemic plasminogen activation does occur after systemic t-PA infusion,[30] more frequent reocclusion after fibrin-selective thrombo-lysis has been attributed to the failure of t-PA to produce as profound systemic hypofibrinogenemia as streptokinase.[30-32] In the GUSTO trial, patency after 180 min was not significantly different between groups receiving t-PA or streptokinase,[28] and in Granger's overview, patency rates after 2–3 hours were no different (65–80% with t-PA and 65–75% with streptokinase).[29] The explanation for the failure of t-PA to maintain angiographic benefit over time compared to streptokinase may reflect precisely the local targeting for which it was developed, with rapid local clot lysis but less systemic inhibition of recurrent clot formation.

Fibrin specificity has also led to slightly more frequent serious bleeding compli-cations in patients treated with t-PA compared to streptokinase,[33-35] probably because of direct targeting by t-PA of hemostatic plugs present within other vessels at sites of minor vascular disruption. In the GUSTO trial, for example, an excess incidence of two strokes per 1000 patients treated was reported with t-PA compared with streptokinase.[35]

The clinical implications of the additional risks and benefits derived from bio-chemically local thrombolytic therapy using a fibrin-selective agent are not clear.[36,37] Two large trials in Europe comparing streptokinase and t-PA in a randomized fashion showed no difference in survival or left-ventricular function,[33,34] while the GUSTO trial showed significantly better survival after 30 days in those patients randomized to t-PA.[35]

Antithrombin agents

In addition to thrombolytic therapy, antithrombotic compounds, principally heparin, have become central elements of treatment regimens for acute myocardial infarction. The lesser degree of systemic hypofibrinogenemia induced by t-PA than by streptokinase has placed even greater emphasis on concomitant antithrombotic treatment in order to reduce the risk of rethrombosis after t-PA-mediated clot lysis. As with thrombolytic agents, local targeting of antithrombotic drugs has also been proposed as a means of enhancing their efficacy while reducing systemic drug-related morbidity. Local delivery of these agents in clinical settings has centered on biochemical rather than anatomic targeting, using systemic delivery of direct antithrombin agents most active at sites of ongoing thrombus formation. The theoretical benefit of these agents is greater inhibition of thrombin activity and of fibrin generation than that achieved by heparin, which does not bind directly to thrombin but requires the cofactor antithrombin III and is less able to penetrate established thrombi.[38]

The targeted agents used most widely to date have been recombinant hirudin and related specific thrombin inhibitors such as hirulog (Biogen, Cambridge, MA). Hirudin is a 65-amino acid polypeptide derived from the medicinal leech *Hirudo medicinalis*. In animal studies, more effective enhancement of thrombolysis has been observed with these agents than with heparin.[39–46] Two pilot clinical trials of direct thrombin inhibitors as adjunctive therapy with thrombolysis have been reported. Lidon *et al.* used hirulog with streptokinase[47] and showed enhancement of early patency (77% of hirulog-treated arteries with TIMI grade 2 or 3 flow after 90 min compared to 47% of heparin-treated arteries). Cannon *et al.* used desulfatohirudin with t-PA[48] and found only slightly better early patency (83% vs 79% at 90 min in hirudin- and heparin-treated patients, respectively) but significantly better later patency (99% vs 93%, respectively, after 18–36 hours) and less frequent reocclusion (1% vs 7%, respectively). Adverse events such as bleeding were not significantly different in either study between groups receiving heparin or the direct thrombin inhibitor. Ongoing large studies will provide more complete information about the relative clinical benefits and risks of such biochemically localized antithrombotic drugs used in conjunction with thrombolytic agents to treat acute myocardial infarction.

Unstable angina pectoris

Unstable coronary ischemic syndromes, without frank transmural infarction, are also considered to originate with athersclerotic plaque disruption and thrombus formation, although most often without persistent complete luminal occlusion.[2,49–53] As with myocardial infarction, therapy for unstable angina has been directed at removing thrombus burden from the culprit artery, and local treatments have been proposed to minimize toxicity while maximizing effectiveness.

Thrombolytic therapy using systemic administration of fibrin-selective or non-selective agents has been compared with routine antithrombotic therapy in several observational and randomized trials. Small studies using streptokinase,[54] urokinase[55,56] or t-PA[57,58] have shown effective resolution of thrombus, but clinical benefit beyond that achieved with heparin and/or aspirin has not been demonstrated.[59–61] In fact the risk of complications, including more frequent myocardial infarctions and intracranial hemorrhages, was higher with thrombolytic treatment, even with a fibrin-selective agent, in these trials.

In contrast to the results of targeted thrombolytic treatment, targeted antithrombotic therapy for unstable angina has shown more promise in early pilot studies. Testing the hypothesis that hirudin would be more effective than heparin at preventing the accumulation of intracoronary thrombus, because of its potent and specific effect on thrombin, Topol *et al.* treated 146 patients with either heparin or increasing doses of hirudin.[62] Angiographic outcomes after 3–5 days favored those patients treated with hirudin, who showed less luminal obstruction than those treated with heparin. As in the trials of thrombolytic therapy for unstable angina, there was no difference in clinical outcomes between groups, but in contrast to those same thrombolytic trials, there were no intracranial hemorrhagic events reported in either treatment group.

Coronary angioplasty

Percutaneous transluminal coronary angioplasty using balloons or other devices (e.g. atherectomy cutters, lasers, and stents) fails in 5–10% of cases because of luminal thrombus present at the outset, or because of acute vessel closure including thrombosis and mural dissection provoked by arterial injury from the angioplasty itself. Furthermore, thrombus present before angioplasty heightens the risk of procedural complications including myocardial infarction.[63–65] Local pharmacologic treatment for each of these indications has included intracoronary thrombolytic agent infusion and/or biochemically antithrombotic compounds.

Zeiher *et al.* studied the use of intracoronary urokinase in all patients undergoing angioplasty.[66] They enrolled 251 patients in a double-blind comparison with heparin. Angiographic signs of intraluminal thrombus were present in only 9% of the urokinase group and 17% of the heparin group, and angiographic success, incidence of infarction and acute closure was not different between groups. In settings where extensive thrombosis is evident at the outset, intracoronary infusion of thrombolytic agents has shown somewhat more promising results. Grill *et al.* administered intracoronary streptokinase or t-PA to patients with intravascular thrombus and showed marked angiographic resolution. Kiesz *et al.* delivered an intracoronary bolus of urokinase to 29 patients with acute infarction, unstable angina or postinfarction angina. Eighty-three percent of patients showed complete resolution of angiographically demonstrable thrombus. In a case-control retrospective study, Pavlides *et al.* compared the outcomes after angioplasty in 80 patients with unstable angina who received intracoronary urokinase with the outcomes of 167 matched controls, finding that those with intraluminal thrombosis had a lower incidence of ischemic complications (3% vs 18%), while those with evidence for mural dissection fared worse with thrombolytic therapy. Finally, in the Thrombolysis and Angioplasty in Unstable Angina pilot study, Ambrose *et al.* randomized patients with unstable angina to intracoronary urokinase or placebo immediately before angioplasty.[67] They found that, in this small study, the presence of thrombus after angioplasty was lower in those patients receiving urokinase, but the incidence of acute closure no different.

Regionally localized thrombolytic therapy has also been used in specific high-risk angioplasty subgroups. Chronic total occlusions of aortocoronary saphenous vein bypass grafts have poor long-term patency rates after angioplasty, and the local infusion of thrombolytic agents has been proposed as a means of improving outcomes[68] although large series of patients treated with this approach have not been reported. Acute closure after angioplasty has also been treated with local infusion of thrombolytic agents, although prospective randomized data are lacking. A large series including 48 patients with impending or established vessel closure during angioplasty was reported to have 94% incidence of vessel patency after intracoronary administration of urokinase and further balloon inflations.[69] In contrast, in two other series, no benefit was observed with streptokinase[70] or with t-PA or urokinase.[71] In this circumstance, where local administration has a concomitant risk of causing hemorrhage into a postangioplasty arterial dissection and promoting a mural hematoma,[72] the drawbacks of the method may outweigh its benefits, and prospective controlled trials are needed.

Biochemically localized antithrombotic therapy has also been used as a routine adjunctive treatment to angioplasty. The importance of adequate anticoagulation during routine angioplasty has been demonstrated using heparin, with lower clotting parameters and heparin levels correlating with higher rates of procedural complications such as acute closure.[73,74] The high therapeutic:toxic ratio of heparin, and its attendant bleeding risks and other toxicities, including thrombocytopenia,[75] osteoporosis,[76] skin necrosis[77] and hypersensitivity reactions,[78] spread over the large numbers of patients undergoing angioplasty, have prompted the evaluation of direct thrombin inhibitors as alternative adjunctive antithrombotic therapy for angioplasty. Two dose ranging pilot studies[79,80] have demonstrated a trend toward fewer episodes of acute vessel closure in patients treated with direct thrombin inhibitors than in those treated with heparin, although in one of these series, a higher rate of vascular access site hemorrhage was observed with hirudin than with heparin.[79] Larger trials examining the relative risks and benefits of these agents as adjunctive treatment for angioplasty are underway.

Novel approaches

All of the clinical therapeutic regimens discussed so far have attempted to use fairly large doses of antithrombotic or thrombolytic agents, either infused regionally, or

Table 6.1 Attributes of local antithrombotic drug delivery systems

Delivery of adequate dose for sufficient period of time
Deposition of drug into necessary sites
Low systemic drug levels
Feasibility for catheter- or surgical-based delivery
Vascular injury attendant to delivery does not offset therapeutic benefit of drug

infused systemically but targeted regionally. As an alternative to these approaches, several experimental systems have been designed which are intended to provide more truly local drug delivery to the vascular wall, at much lower doses, with much less systemic exposure. Such systems, in order to be clinically applicable, must have the attributes outlined in Table 6.1.

Transluminal methods

The first experimental method described for delivering antithrombotic drugs was a perforated balloon catheter used by Wolinsky and Thung.[81] This modified angioplasty balloon included 300 pores (25 μm) in its outer surface, through which fluid instilled into the lumen of the balloon was expelled outward in a radial direction. Wolinsky delivered fluorescein-labeled heparin or the tracer molecule horseradish peroxidase to canine brachial arteries via this technique, demonstrating the position of each throughout the arterial media, with depth and quantity of penetration determined by instillation pressure. After 24–72 hours, little heparin was detectable in the vessel wall, and histologic study at these time points showed that extensive necrosis of medial smooth-muscle cells had occurred, related to the pressure of infusion.

Other balloon-based techniques have used modifications in which smaller pores or lower instillation pressures are used,[82,83] in order to lessen vascular injury from the drug delivery, although preliminary studies with heparin,[84,85] Phe-Pro-Arg-CH_2Cl (PPACK)[86] and hirudin[85] have been unable to demonstrate either prolonged deposition of drug within the vessel wall or biologic responses in *in vivo* models of arterial thrombosis.

More recently, hoping to further minimize vascular disruption caused by the delivery of drug itself, two other balloon-based techniques have been reported. One, iontopheresis, uses electric current to force charged molecules into the arterial wall from the lumen. A recent report described the delivery of hirudin by iontopheresis to porcine carotid arteries.[87] Hirudin was detectable in the vessel wall, but fell to control levels after three hours. Systemic effects were not found, and biologic endpoints not measured in this preliminary study. The second recently reported balloon-based method is coating of a balloon with an inert hydrogel, which in turn absorbs an active agent. After balloon inflation, the absorbed drug diffuses passively out of the hydrogel and into the arterial wall. Preliminary studies using horseradish peroxidase and heparin have shown deposition into arterial walls, but rapid washout left minimal amounts of either agent in the arterial wall after 60–90 min.[88]

Using a similar system, Nunes *et al.* delivered PPACK to prosthetic vascular grafts in a porcine model, and demonstrated a reduction in platelet deposition, although no measurement was made of drug deposition in this nonarterial model. Further studies in systems allowing longer-term measurements of biologic outcomes are necessary in order to define better whether these acute treatment systems will reduce arterial thrombosis.

Stents

Endovascular stents are another potential route for the transluminal delivery of antithrombotic drugs. Stents are metal or polymeric mesh, collapsed onto deflated angioplasty balloons, and expanded inside arteries by balloon inflation. After expansion, the balloon is deflated and withdrawn, leaving the stent behind. Clinical use of stents has centered on their providing a scaffolding for repairing angioplasty-induced arterial dissections, preventing acute closure.[89-94] Stents provoke thrombosis[95] because of vascular injury they impose[96] compounded by their thrombogenic material within the bloodstream. They also, however, have the potential for providing prolonged local drug administration. The balance between these attributes depends on specifics of drug, stent material and artery.

We, and others, have used metal stents coated with ionically bound heparin in animal models.[97,98] Heparin is released from these stents in extremely small amounts over several days[98] and produces no detectable deposition within the vessel wall. However, in a model using balloon denudation followed by stent placement in rabbit iliac arteries, designed to provide a high rate of spontaneous thrombosis similar to that reported in early trials of stents in human coronary arteries, we found that this small amount of heparin delivered at the arterial lumen was nearly as effective as continuous systemic heparin infusion at preventing thrombosis[98] (Figure 6.1). Bailey *et al.* found similar inhibition after 24 hours,[97] while in another system using stents in swine carotid arteries thrombosis was much less frequent and no effect of heparin was demonstrable (1 of 9 uncoated stents and none of 9 heparin-bound stents had thrombosis; $P = $ NS).[99]

An alternative to binding of small amounts of drugs to metal stents is the application of a polymer coating to metal stent struts, or fabrication of stents entirely from polymer compounds. This would allow incorporation of greater amounts of drug into the polymer material and might provide release over more prolonged periods of time after deployment. Furthermore, if the stent material were bioerodible, a device might be constructed which provided local drug release and then was gradually reabsorbed within the artery. Several polymer materials have been used for stent construction, and the thrombotic, inflammatory and vascular proliferative responses to the materials have been prohibitive to long-term use.[100] The feasibility of drug incorporation into, and release from, these stents has only been reported in preliminary *in vitro* models.[101]

The design of composite stents, i.e. coating metal struts with polymer materials, has also been proposed. Some inert polymers on metal stents have been shown to reduce platelet deposition, thrombosis and vascular spasm,[102-104] while others have

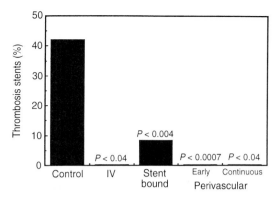

Figure 6.1 Bar graph shows the incidence of complete thrombosis in rabbit iliac arteries 14 days after endovascular stent implantation. Heparin was delivered systemically (IV), or locally from within the artery (stent bound) or adjacent to the artery (perivascular). *P* values reflect comparison with untreated controls. Differences between heparin-treated groups were not significant. (Adapted with permission from Rogers, C., Karnovsky, M. J. and Edelman, E. R. (1993). Inhibition of experimental neointimal hyperplasia and thrombosis depends on the type of vascular injury and the site of drug administration. *Circulation,* **88**, 1215–21. Copyright 1993 American Heart Association.)

produced inflammatory responses akin to those seen with polymeric stents. The incorporation of drugs into these polymers has not yet been reported.

Temporary metal stents also have been proposed as drug-release and scaffolding devices. Eigler *et al.* reported the implantation and removal of temporary metallic stents from canine coronary arteries.[105] These stents are constructed from nitinol, which undergoes shape changes at different temperatures. As late as one week after implantation, Eigler and coworkers instilled warm (75°C) lactated Ringer's solution into stented arteries, causing the stents to collapse and allowing removal via balloon. The feasibility of this technique clinically, the long-term effects of the arterial injuries caused by the stent or the warm solution, and the biologic efficacy of drugs delivered from this route all are unknown.

The proposed use of stents for delivering antithrombotic or antiproliferative drugs to arterial walls must consider the attributes listed in Table 6.1. Perhaps most important of these is the delivery of enough drug for sufficient time to provide biologic efficacy. We have compared the biologic efficacies of three routes of heparin administration as well as their efficiencies at accomplishing drug deposition.[98,106] In a model using metal stent placement in denuded rabbit iliac arteries, we delivered heparin locally via perivascular administration from ethylene vinylacetate copolymer (EVAc) slabs impregnated with heparin placed adjacent to the outside of stented arteries, or via intra-arterial administration from the stent surface itself. We found that inhibition of stent thrombosis after 14 days was equivalent from each route and no different from that seen with intravenous infusion (Figure 6.1).

The deposition of ^{125}I-heparin into these arteries, however, differed markedly depending on how, where, and to which artery the drug was delivered. Heparin released from the stent was not detectable within the arterial wall after two hours. Heparin released into the perivascular space was detectable after two hours of drug release, but within 15 minutes of removal of the polymeric slab, no heparin remained

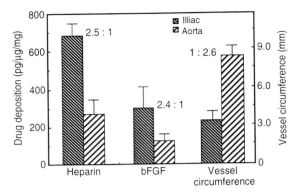

Figure 6.2 Bar graph shows deposition of heparin or the heparin-binding growth factor basic fibroblast growth factor (bFGF) in rabbit iliac arteries or aortae, and the artery sizes. Deposition of each compound from a unilateral perivascular source depended upon the artery's circumference.

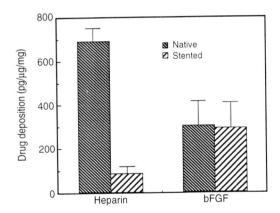

Figure 6.3 Bar graph shows the effect of stent placement within an artery on the deposition of heparin or basic fibroblast growth factor (bFGF) into the same artery after perivascular delivery. Stenting caused an eightfold reduction in the deposition of highly charged and soluble heparin, but caused no change in less-soluble, more avidly bound bFGF.

in the artery. Delivery to the relatively large aortae was less efficient than delivery to smaller iliac arteries (Figure 6.2). Finally, although perivascular delivery was sufficient to eliminate stent-induced thrombosis,[98] heparin deposition after perivascular delivery was reduced over eight-fold by stent placement (Figure 6.3). This effect may reflect alterations in geometry of the vessel imposed by the stent, such as increased circumference for perivascular drug to traverse, heightened charge concentration impeding diffusion of heparin into the vessel, or depletion of tissue water and therefore the volume of distribution for heparin because of radial compressive forces applied to the vessel by the stent.

Looking for a generalizable pattern of stent-based drug release, we compared these results with those for a heparin-binding growth factor, basic fibroblast growth

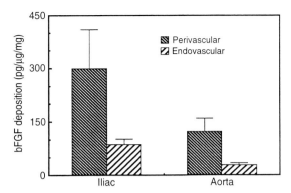

Figure 6.4   Bar graph shows the efficiencies of deposition of basic fibroblast growth factor into arteries of different sizes, after endovascular stent-based delivery or perivascular polymer-based delivery. Stent-based delivery was threefold less efficient in each case. Stent-based delivery of heparin produced no measurable levels within arteries.

factor (bFGF). Heparin-avid bFGF was bound to heparin-coated stents and delivered to rabbit iliac arteries or aortae *in vivo*. Basic FGF was also delivered into the perivascular space from polymeric devices prepared as described by Edelman *et al*.[107] We found that bFGF was deposited in significant amounts into arterial walls after *stent-based* release, in contrast to heparin which was undetectable. Basic FGF was even more efficiently deposited into arteries after perivascular release (Figure 6.4). Geometric parameters of vessel circumference determined deposition of either heparin or bFGF after perivascular release, likely reflecting circumferential distribution to equilibrium from a unilateral source. Altering the arterial state by balloon denudation reduced heparin deposition threefold and expansion of an endovascular stent reduced deposition eightfold. For bFGF delivered to identical arteries via the same routes, growth factor deposition did not change with denudation or stent placement, possibly reflecting its adhesiveness and the solubility of heparin (Figure 6.3). These studies demonstrated that antithrombotic arterial drug deposition after local release cannot be precisely predicted from simple tracer molecules alone, but rather that it depends on properties of the drug, the state of the artery and the mode of delivery.

Conclusion

Sudden thrombosis of a small atherosclerotic segment causes the vast majority of acute manifestations of arterial disease. Local treatment of such thrombosis is appealing because of heightened local effects and minimized systemic toxicities. Since the first attempts at local instillation of antithrombotic and thrombolytic drugs in the early 1960s, clinicians and basic scientists have sought safe and effective means for accomplishing local antithrombotic interventions. The common finding throughout all of these investigations has been the importance of addressing the precise agent under consideration, the particular vascular syndrome targeted and the arterial state into which the agent is delivered. With further examination of these parameters, anatomically or biochemically local management of acute myocardial infarction, unstable angina and abrupt arterial occlusion after angioplasty may become standard elements of vascular therapeutics.

References

1. Davies, M. J. and Thomas, A. C. (1985) Plaque fissuring – the cause of acute myocardial infarction, sudden ischaemic death, and crescendo angina. *Br. Heart. J.*, **53**, 363–73.
2. Fuster, V., Badimon, L., Badimon, J. J. and Chesebro, J. H. (1992) The pathogenesis of coronary artery disease and the acute coronary syndromes. *N. Engl. J. Med.*, **326**, 242–50, 310–18.
3. DeWood, M. A., Spores, J., Notske, R. *et al.* (1980) Prevalence of total coronary occlusion during the early hours of transmural myocardial infarction. *N. Engl. J. Med.*, **303**, 897–902.
4. Fletcher, A. P., Sherry, S., Alkjaersig, N. *et al.* (1959) The maintenance of a sustained thrombolytic state in man. II. Clinical observations on patients with myocardial infarction and other thromboembolic disorders. *J. Clin. Invest.*, **381**, 1111–19.
5. Boucek, R. J., Murphy, W. P. J., Sommer, L. S. and Voudoukis, I. J. (1960) Segmental perfusion of the coronary arteries with fibrinolysin in man following myocardial infarction. *Am. J. Cardiol.*, **6**, 525–33.
6. Simon, T. L., Ware, J. H. and Stengle, J. M. (1973) Clinical trials of thrombolytic agents in myocardial infarction. *Ann. Intern. Med.*, **79**, 712–19.
7. Duckert, F. (1979) Thrombolytic therapy in myocardial infarction. *Cardiovasc. Dis.*, **21**, 342–50.
8. European Cooperative Study Group (1979) Streptokinase in acute myocardial infarction. *N. Engl. J. Med.*, **301**, 797–802.
9. Rentrop, K. P., Blanke, H. and Karsch, K. R. (1979) Acute myocardial infarction: intracoronary application of nitroglycerine and streptokinase in combination with transluminal recanalization. *Clin. Cardiol.*, **2**, 354–63.
10. Kennedy, J. W., Ritchie, J. L., Davis, K. B. and Fritz, J. K. (1983) Western Washington randomized trial of intracoronary streptokinase in acute myocardial infarction. *N. Engl. J. Med.*, **309**, 1477–82.
11. Kennedy, J. W., Ritchie, J. L., Davis, K. B. *et al.* (1985) The western Washington randomized trial of intracoronary streptokinase in acute myocardial infarction: a 12-month follow-up report. *N. Engl. J. Med.*, **312**, 1073–8.
12. Khaja, F., Walton, J. A., Brymer, J. F. *et al.* (1983) Intracoronary fibrinolytic therapy in acute myocardial infarction: report of a prospective randomized trial. *N. Engl. J. Med.*, **308**, 1305–11.
13. Anderson, J. L., Marshall, H. W., Bray, B. E. *et al.* (1983) A randomized trial of intravenous and intracoronary streptokinase in the treatment of acute myocardial infarction. *N. Engl. J. Med.*, **308**, 1312–18.
14. Rentrop, K. P., Feit, F., Blanke, H. *et al.* (1984) Effects of intracoronary streptokinase and intracoronary nitroglycerine infusion on coronary angiographic patterns and mortality in patients with acute myocardial infarction. *N. Engl. J. Med.*, **311**, 1457–63.
15. Rogers, W. J., Mantle, J. A., Hood, W. P. *et al.* (1983) Prospective randomized trial of intravenous and intracoronary streptokinase in acute myocardial infarction. *Circulation*, **68**, 1051–61.
16. Alderman, E. L., Jutsky, K. R., Berte, L. E. *et al.* (1984) Randomized comparison of intravenous versus intracoronary streptokinase for myocardial infarction. *Am. J. Cardiol.*, **54**, 14–19.
17. Anderson, J. L., Marshall, H. W., Askins, J. C. *et al.* (1984) A randomized trial of intravenous and intracoronary streptokinase in patients with acute myocardial infarction. *Circulation*, **70**, 606–18.

18. Ganz, W., Buchbinder, N., Marcus, H. *et al.* (1981) Intracoronary thrombolysis in evolving myocardial infarction. *Am. Heart J.,* **101**, 4–13.
19. Rentrop, P., Blanke, H., Karsch, K. R. *et al.* (1981) Selective intracoronary thrombolysis in acute myocardial infarction and unstable angina pectoris. *Circulation,* **63**, 307–17.
20. Ganz, W., Geft, I. and Maddahi, J. (1983) Non-surgical reperfusion in evolving myocardial infarction. *J. Am. Coll. Cardiol.,* **1**, 1247–53.
21. Marder, V. J. (1983) Pharmacology of thrombolytic agents: implications for therapy of coronary artery thrombosis. *Circulation,* **68**, I-2–I-5.
22. Burket, M. W., Smith, M. R., Walsh, T. E. *et al.* (1985) Relation of effectiveness of intracoronary thrombolysis in acute myocardial infarction to systemic thrombolytic state. *Am. J. Cardiol.,* **56**, 441–4.
23. Rothbard, R. L., Fitzpatrick, P. G., Francis, C. W. *et al.,* (1985) Relationship of the lytic state to successful reperfusion with standard- and low-dose intracoronary streptokinase. *Circulation,* **71**, 562–70.
24. Matsuo, O., Rijken, D. C. and Collen, D. (1981) Thrombolysis by human tissue plasminogen activator and urokinase in rabbits with experimental pulmonary embolus. *Nature,* **291**, 590–1.
25. Hoylaerts, M., Rijken, D. C. and Collen, D. (1982) Kinetics of the activation of plasminogen by human tissue plasminogen activator: role of fibrin. *J. Biol. Chem.,* **257**, 2912–19.
26. Collen, D., Rijken, D. C., Van Damme, J. and Billiau, A. (1982) Purification of human tissue-type plasminogen activator in centigram quantities from human melanoma cell culture fluid and its conditioning for use *in vivo. Thromb. Haemost.,* **48**, 294–6.
27. Chesebro, J. H., Knatterud, G., Roberts, R. *et al.* (1987) Thrombolysis in Myocardial Infarction Trial, Phase I: a comparison between intravenous tissue plasminogen activator and intravenous streptokinase. *Circulation,* **76**, 142–54.
28. The GUSTO investigators (1993) The effects of tissue plasminogen activator, streptokinase, or both on coronary-artery patency, ventricular function, and survival after acute myocardial infarction. *N. Engl. J. Med.* **329**, 1615–22.
29. Granger, C. B., Califf, R. M. and Topol, E. J., (1992) Thrombolytic therapy for acute myocardial infarction. *Drugs,* **44**, 293–325.
30. Topol, E. J., Bell, W. R. and Weisfeldt, M. L. (1985) Coronary thrombolysis with recombinant tissue-type plasminogen activator: a hemtatologic and pharmacologic study. *Ann. Intern. Med.,* **103**, 837–43.
31. Rao, A. K., Pratt, C., Berks, A. *et al.* (1988) Thrombolysis in Myocardial Infarction Trial–Phase 1: Hemorrhagic manifestations and changes in plasma fibrinogen and the fibrinolytic system in patients treated with recombinant tissue plasminogen activator and streptokinase. *J. Am. Coll. Cardiol.,* **11**, 1–11.
32. Stump, D. C., Califf, R. M., Topol, E. J. *et al.* (1989) Pharmacodynamics of thrombolysis with recombinant tissue-type plasminogen activator: correlation with characteristics and clinical outcomes in patients with acute myocardial infarction. *Circulation,* **80**, 1222–30.
33. Gruppo Italiano per lo Studio della Sopravvivenza nell'Infarto Miocardio. GISSI-2 (1990) A factorial randomized trial of alteplase versus streptokinase and heparin versus no heparin among 14 490 patients with acute myocardial infarction. *Lancet,* **336**, 65–71.
34. ISIS-3 (Third International Study of Infarct Survival) Collaborative Group (1992) ISIS-3A. A randomized comparison of streptokinase vs tissue plasminogen activator vs anistreplase and of aspirin plus heparin vs aspirin alone among 41 299 cases of suspected acute myocardial infarction. *Lancet,* **339**, 753–70.
35. The GUSTO investigators (1993) An international randomized trial comparing four thrombolytic strategies for acute myocardial infarction. *N. Engl. J. Med.,* **329**, 673–82.
36. Lee, K. L., Califf, R. M., Simes, J. *et al.* (1994) Holding GUSTO up to the light. *Ann. Intern. Med.,* **120**, 876–81.
37. Ridker, P. M., O'Donnell, C. J., Marder, V. J. and Hennekens, C. H. (1994) A response to 'Holding GUSTO up to the light'. *Ann. Intern. Med.,* **120**, 882–5.

38. Weitz, J. I., Hudoba, M., Massel, D. *et al.* (1990) Clot-bound thrombin is protected from inhibition by heparin–antithrombin III but is susceptible to inactivation by antithrombin III-independent inhibitors. *J. Clin. Invest.*, **86**, 385–91.

39. Agnelli, G., Pasciucci, C., Cosmi, B. and Nenci, G. G. (1990) The comparative effects of recombinant hirudin and standard heparin on thrombus growth in rabbits. *Thromb. Haemost.*, **63**, 204–7.

40. Kaiser, B., Simon, A. and Markwardt, F. (1990) Antithrombotic effects of recombinant hirudin in experimental angioplasty and intravascular thrombolysis. *Thromb. Haemost.*, **63**, 44–7.

41. Maraganore, J. M., Bourdon, P., Jablonski, J. *et al.* (1990) Design and characterization of hirulogs: a novel class of bivalent peptide inhibitors of thrombin. *Biochemistry*, **29**, 7095–101.

42. Haskel, E. J., Prager, N. A., Sobel, B. E. and Abendschein, D. R. (1991) Relative efficacy of antithrombin compared with antiplatelet agents in accelerating coronary thrombolysis and preventing early reocclusion. *Circulation*, **83**, 1048–56.

43. Klement, P., Borm, A., Hirsh, J. *et al.* (1992) The effects of thrombin inhibitors on tissue plasminogen activator induced thrombolysis in a rat model. *Thromb. Haemost.*, **68**, 64–8.

44. Sitko, G. R., Ramjit, D. R., Stabilito, I. I. *et al.* (1992) Conjunctive enhancement of enzymatic thrombolysis and prevention of thrombotic reocclusion with the selective factor Xa inhibitor, tick anticoagulant peptide: comparison to hirudin and heparin in a canine model of acute coronary artery thrombosis. *Circulation*, **85**, 805–15.

45. Yao, S. K., Ober, J. C., Ferguson, J. J. *et al.* (1992) Combination of inhibition of thrombin and blockade of thromboxane A_2 synthetase and receptors enhances thrombolysis and delays reocclusion in canine coronary arteries. *Circulation*, **86**, 1993–9.

46. Rigel, D. F., Olson, R. W. and Lappe, B. W. (1993) Comparison of hirudin and heparin as adjuncts to streptokinase thrombolysis in a canine model of coronary thrombolysis. *Circ. Res.*, **72**, 1091–102.

47. Lidon, R-M., Theroux, P., Lesperance, J. *et al.* (1994) A pilot, early angiographic patency study using a direct thrombin inhibitor as adjunctive therapy to streptokinase in acute myocardial infarction. *Circulation*, **89**, 1567–72.

48. Cannon, C. P., McCabe, C. H., Henry, T. D. *et al.* (1994) A pilot trial of recombinant desulphatohirudin compared with heparin in conjunction with tissue-type plasminogen activator and aspirin for acute myocardial infarction: results in the TIMI 5 trial. *J. Am. Coll. Cardiol.*, **23**, 993–1003.

49. Falk, E. (1985) Unstable angina with fatal outcome: dynamic coronary thrombosis leading to infarction and/or sudden death. *Circulation*, **71**, 699–708.

50. Sherman, C. T., Litvack, F., Grundfest, T. *et al.* (1986) Coronary angioscopy in patients with unstable angina pectoris. *N. Engl. J. Med.* **315**, 913–19.

51. Ambrose, J. A., Hjemdahl-Monsen, C. E., Borrico, S. *et al.* (1988) Angiographic demonstration of a common link between unstable angina pectoris and non-Q wave acute myocardial infarction. *Am. J. Cardiol.*, **61**, 244–7.

52. Williams, A. E., Freeman, M. R., Chisholm, R. J. *et al.* (1988) Angiographic morphology in patients with unstable angina pectoris. *Am. J. Cardiol.*, **62**, 1024–7.

53. Chesebro, J. and Fuster, V. (1992) Thrombosis in unstable angina. *N. Engl. J. Med.*, **327**, 192–4.

54. Mandelkorn, J. B., Wolf, N. M., Singh, S. *et al.* (1983) Intracoronary thrombus in nontransmural myocardial infarction and in unstable angina pectoris. *Am. J. Cardiol.*, **52**, 1–6.

55. Gotoh, K., Minamino, T., Katoh, O. *et al.* (1988) The role of intracoronary thrombus in unstable angina: angiographic assessment and thrombolytic therapy during ongoing anginal attacks. *Circulation*, **77**, 526–34.

56. Schreiber, T., Rizik, D., White, C. *et al.* (1992) Randomized trial of thrombolysis versus heparin in unstable angina. *Circulation*, **86**, 1407–14.

57. DeZwaan, C., Bar, F. W., Janssen, J. H. A. *et al.* (1988) Effects of thrombolytic therapy in unstable angina: clinical and angiographic results. *J. Am. Coll. Cardiol.*, **12**, 301–9.
58. Nicklas, J., Topol, E. J., Kander, N. *et al.* (1989) Randomized, double-blind, placebo-controlled trial of tissue plasminogen activator in unstable angina. *J. Am. Coll. Cardiol.*, **13**, 434–41.
59. Williams, D. O., Topol, E. J., Califf, R. M. *et al.* (1990) Intravenous recombinant tissue-type plasminogen activator in patients with unstable angina pectoris. *Circulation*, **92**, 376–83.
60. Freeman, M. R., Langer, A., Wilson, R. F. *et al.* (1992) Thrombolysis in unstable angina: randomized double-blind trial of t-PA and placebo. *Circulation*, **85**, 150–7.
61. The TIMI IIIB Investigators (1994) Effects of tissue plasminogen activator and a comparison of early invasive and conservative strategies in unstable angina and non-Q wave myocardial infarction: results of the TIMI IIIB trial. *Circulation*, **89**, 1545–56.
62. Topol, E. J., Fuster, V., Harrington, R. A. *et al.* (1994) Recombinant hirudin for unstable angina pectoris. *Circulation*, **89**, 1557–66.
63. Mabin, T. A., Holmes, D. R. J. and Smith, H. C. (1985) Intracoronary thrombus: role in coronary occlusion complicating percutaneous transluminal coronary angioplasty. *J. Am. Coll. Cardiol.*, **5**, 198–202.
64. Sugrue, D. D., Holmes, D. R. J. and Smith, H. C. (1986) Coronary artery thrombus as a risk factor for acute vessel occlusion during percutaneous transluminal coronary angioplasty: improving results. *Br. Heart J.*, **56**, 62–6.
65. Ellis, S. G., Roubin, G. S., King, S. B. *et al.* (1988) Angiographic and clinical predictors of acute closure after native vessel coronary angioplasty. *Circulation*, **77**, 372–9.
66. Zeiher, A. M., Kasper, W., Gaissmaier, G. and Wollschlager, H. (1990) Concomitant intracoronary treatment with urokinase during PTCA does not reduce acute complications during PTCA: a double blind randomized trial. *Circulation*, **82**, III-189.
67. Ambrose, J. A., Torre, S. R. and Sharma, S. K. (1992) Adjunctive thrombolytic therapy for angioplasty in ischemic rest angina: results of a double-blind randomized pilot study. *J. Am. Coll. Cardiol.*, **20**, 1197–204.
68. Hartmann, J. R., McKeever, L. S., Stamato, M. J. *et al.* (1991) Recanalization of chronically occluded aortocoronary saphenous vein bypass grafts by extended infusion of urokinase: Initial results and short term clinical follow-up. *J. Am. Coll. Cardiol.* **18**, 1517–23.
69. Schieman, G., Cohen, B. M. and Kozina, J. (1990) Intracoronary urokinase for intracoronary thrombus accumulation complicating percutaneous transluminal coronary angioplasty in acute ischemic syndromes. *Circulation*, **82**, 2052–60.
70. de Feyter, P. J., van den Brand, M., Jaarman, G. *et al.* (1991) Acute coronary occlusion during and after percutaneous transluminal coronary angioplasty: frequency, prediction, clinical course, management, and follow-up. *Circulation*, **93**, 927–31.
71. Lincoff, A. M., Popma, J. J., Ellis, S. C. *et al.* (1992) Abrupt vessel closure complicating coronary angioplasty: clinical, angiographic, and therapeutic profile. *J. Am. Coll. Cardiol.*, **19**, 926–30.
72. Pavlides, G. S., Schreiber, T. L., Gangadharan, V. *et al.* (1991) Safety and efficacy of urokinase during elective coronary angioplasty. *Am. Heart J.*, **121**, 731–77.
73. Ferguson, J. J., Dougherty, K. G., Gaos, C. M. *et al.* (1994) Relation between procedu. activated coagulation time and outcome after PTCA. *J. Am. Coll. Cardiol.*, **23**, 1061–5.
74. McGarry, T. F., Gottlieb, R. S. and Morganroth, J. (1992) The relationship of anticoagulation level and complications after successful percutaneous transluminal coronary angioplasty. *Am. Heart J.*, **123**, 1445–51.
75. King, D. J. and Kelton, J. G. (1984) Heparin-associated thrombocytopenia. *Ann. Intern. Med.*, **100**, 535–40.
76. Ginsberg, J. S., Kowalchuk, G., Hirsh, J. *et al.* (1990) Heparin effect on bone density. *Thromb Haemost.*, **64**, 286–9.
77. White, P. W., Sadd, J. R. and Nensel, R. E. (1979) Thrombotic complications of heparin therapy. *Ann. Surg.*, **190**, 595–608.
78. Chernof, A. I. (1950) Anaphylactic reactions following injection of heparin. *N. Engl. J. Med.*, **242**, 315–19.

79. van den Bos, A. A., Heyndrickx, G. R., Laarman, G. J. *et al.* (1992) PTCA with hirudin is associated with less acute cardiac complications than with heparin. *Eur. Heart J.*, **13**, 256.
80. Topol, E. J., Bonan, R. and Kakkar, V. V. (1993) Use of a direct antithrombin, hirulog, in place of heparin during coronary angioplasty. *Circulation*, **87**, 1622–9.
81. Wolinsky, H. and Thung, S. N. (1990) Use of a perforated balloon catheter to deliver concentrated heparin into the wall of the normal canine artery. *J. Am. Coll. Cardiol.*, **15**, 475–81.
82. Hong, M. K., Farb, A., Unger, E. F. *et al.* (1992) A new PTCA balloon catheter with intramural channels for local delivery of drugs at low pressure. *Circulation*, **86**, I-380.
83. Lambert, C. R., Leone, J. and Rowland, S. (1992) The microporous balloon: a minimal trauma local drug delivery catheter. *Circulation*, **86**, I-381.
84. Cox, D. A., Anderson, P. G., Roubin, G. S. *et al.* (1991) Local delivery of heparin and methotrexate fails to inhibit *in vivo* smooth muscle cell proliferation. *Circulation*, **84**, II-71.
85. Gimple, L. W., Gertz, S. D., Haber, H. L. *et al.* (1992) Effect of chronic subcutaneous or intramural administration of heparin on femoral artery restenosis after balloon angioplasty in hypercholesterolemic rabbits. *Circulation*, **86**, 1536–46.
86. Leung, W.-H., Kaplan, A. V., Grant, G. W. *et al.* (1990) Local delivery of antithrombin agent reduces platelet deposition at the site of balloon angioplasty. *Circulation*, **82**, III-428.
87. Fernandez-Ortiz, A., Meyer, B. J., Mailhac, A. *et al.* (1994) A new approach for local intravascular drug delivery: iontophoretic balloon. *Circulation*, **89**, 1518–22.
88. Fram, D. B., Aretz, T., Azrin, M. A. *et al.* (1994) Localized intramural drug delivery during balloon angioplasty using hydrogel-coated balloons and pressure-augmented diffusion. *J. Am. Coll. Cardiol.*, **23**, 1570–7.
89. Sigwart, U., Urban, P., Golf, S. *et al.* (1988) Emergency stenting for acute occlusion after coronary balloon angioplasty. *Circulation*, **78**, 1121–7.
90. Levine, M. J., Leonard, B. M., Burke, J. A. *et al.* (1990) Clinical and angiographic results of balloon-expandable intracoronary stents in right coronary arteries. *J. Am. Coll. Cardiol.*, **16**, 332–9.
91. Fischman, D. L., Savage, M. P., Leon, M. B. *et al.* (1991) Effect of intracoronary stenting in intimal dissection after balloon angioplasty: results of quantitative and qualitative coronary analysis. *J. Am. Coll. Cardiol.*, **18**, 1445–51.
92. Carrozza, J. P., Kuntz, R. E., Levine, M. J. *et al.* (1992) Angiographic and clinical outcome of intracoronary stenting: immediate and long-term results from a large single-center experience. *J. Am. Coll. Cardiol.*, **20**, 328–37.
93. Roubin, G. S., Cannon, A. D., Agrawal, S. K. *et al.* (1992) Intracoronary stenting for acute and threatened closure complicating percutaneous transluminal coronary angioplasty. *Circulation*, **85**, 916–27.
94. Sutton, J. M., Ellis, S. G., Roubin, G. S. *et al.* (1994) Major clinical events after coronary stenting: the multicenter registry of acute and elective Gianturco–Roubin stent placement. *Circulation*, **89**, 1126–37.
95. Nath, F. C., Muller, D. W. M., Ellis, S. G. *et al.* (1993) Thrombosis of a flexible coil coronary stent: frequency, predictors and clinical outcome. *J. Am. Coll. Cardiol.*, **21**, 622–7.
96. Schwartz, R. S., Huber, K. C., Murphy, J. G. *et al.* (1991) Restenosis and proportional neointimal response to coronary artery injury: results in a porcine model. *J. Am. Coll. Cardiol.*, **19**, 267–74.
97. Bailey, S. R., Paige, S., Lunn, A. and Palmaz, J. (1992) Heparin coating of endovascular stents decreases subacute thrombosis in a rabbit model. *Circulation*, **86**, I-186.
98. Rogers, C., Karnovsky, M. J. and Edelman, E. R. (1993) Inhibition of experimental neointimal hyperplasia and thrombosis depends on the type of vascular injury and the site of drug administration. *Circulation*, **88**, 1215–21.
99. Cavender, J. B., Anderson, P. A. and Roubin, G. S. (1990) The effects of heparin bonded tantalum stents on thrombosis and neointimal proliferation. *Circulation*, **82**, III-541 (Abstract).
100. Murphy, J. G., Schwarts, R. S., Edwards, W. D. *et al.* (1992) Percutaneous polymeric stents in porcine coronary arteries. *Circulation*, **86**, 1569–604.

101. Ebecje, M., Buchwald, A., Stricker, H. and Wiegand V. (1991) *In vitro* assessment of polyactides as slow release drug carriers. *Circulation,* **84**, II-72.
102. Bailey, S. R., Guy, D. M., Garcia, O. J. *et al.* (1990) Polymer coating of Palmaz–Schatz stent attenuates vascular spasm after stent placement. *Circulation,* **82**, III-541.
103. van der Giessen, W. J., Strauss, B. H., van Beusekom, H. M. M. *et al.* (1990) Self-expandable mesh stents: an experimental study comparing polymer coated and uncoated stents in the coronary circulation of pigs. *Circulation,* **82**, III-542.
104. Rogers, C. and Edelman, E. R. (1995) Endovascular stent design dictates experimental restenosis and thrombosis. *Circulation.* In press.
105. Eigler, N. L., Khorsandi, M. J., Forrester, J. S. *et al.* (1994) Implantation and recovery of temporary metallic stents in canine coronary arteries. *J. Am. Coll. Cardiol.,* **22**, 1207–13.
106. Rogers, C., Nugent, M. A., Lovich, M. A. and Edelman, E. R. (1994) Efficiencies of local vascular delivery of heparin and heparin binding growth factors differ depending on compound, artery, and site of administration. *Circulation,* **90**, I-508.
107. Edelman, E. R., Nugent, M. A., Smith, L. T. *et al.* (1992) Basic fibroblast growth factor enhances the coupling of intimal hyperplasia and proliferation of vasa vasorum in injured rat arteries. *J. Clin. Invest.,* **89**, 465–73.

7

Antibody-targeted Thrombolytic and Antithrombotic Agents

Edgar Haber

Introduction

In most patients with myocardial infarction, coronary occlusion is caused by a thrombus forming on a fissured atherosclerotic plaque. Early reperfusion with thrombolytic agents can limit infarct size and reduce left-ventricular dysfunction and congestive heart failure, and thereby diminish early and late mortality. Streptokinase, recombinant tissue-type plasminogen activator (rtPA), and anisoylated plasminogen streptokinase activator complex (APSAC) – the three widely available thrombolytic agents – have been the subjects of several large, multicenter clinical trials. Although the AIMS,[1] GISSI (Gruppo Italiano per lo Studio della Sopravvivenza nell'Infarto miocardico)[2] and ISIS (International Study of Infarct Survival)[3] trials showed no significant differences among these three agents, the recent GUSTO (Global Utilization of Streptokinase and Tissue Plasminogen Activator for Occluded Coronary Arteries)[4] trial, which was designed to meet some of the methodological objections to the older trials, has shown that patients treated with rtPA have a modest increase (1%) in survival after myocardial infarction in comparison with patients treated with streptokinase. Of far greater interest than the survival data was the demonstration that early reperfusion (the opening of an artery to blood flow) correlated directly with improved survival. While these findings indicate that rtPA may be only modestly more effective than streptokinase, they also show that the advantage of rtPA lies in its ability to lyze thrombi more quickly and more completely. To investigators engaged in developing plasminogen activators that are more potent and more specific than those presently on the market, the results of the GUSTO trial provide great encouragement.

The most significant limitations of plasminogen activator therapy in its present state include failure to lyze all thrombi (15–20% of patients do not experience early reperfusion), delayed reperfusion (45–60 minutes), and high rates (15–20%) of early reocclusion after thrombolysis. If these limitations could be overcome, thrombolytic therapy would certainly have a more beneficial effect on morbidity and mortality from myocardial infarction.

In planning the discovery and development of new thrombolytic agents, properties to be sought include increased potency and speed of thrombolysis combined with the ability to prevent rethrombosis without increasing hemorrhagic complications. Research in this field has been very active, with efforts ranging from the search for plasminogen activators in species as diverse as the *Staphylococcus*[5] and the vampire bat[6,7] to the application of genetic engineering techniques in both the selective alteration of existing plasminogen activators and the creation of fusion proteins from elements of different plasminogen activators. So far, none of these efforts have produced an agent generally accepted to be superior to those already approved for clinical use. This chapter describes novel approaches to the development of plasminogen activators that are based on the concept of antibody targeting to a specific component of the thrombus.

Because the ideal plasminogen activator is not available, supplemental agents have been used in an effort to prevent rethrombosis or enhance the lysis of resistant thrombi, which are generally thought to be rich in platelets. These drugs, known as adjunctive agents,[8-10] act either by inhibiting the aggregation of platelets or by blocking the action of thrombin. Aspirin has long been recognized as an effective inhibitor of platelet aggregation and its value has been confirmed in a multicenter clinical trial.[11] Also, an antibody specific for the platelet GPIIb/IIIa receptor has been shown to reduce thrombosis following angioplasty, though its value in myocardial infarction has not as yet been established.[12] Since inhibitors of either platelet aggregation or the action of thrombin are likely to increase bleeding risk, at the end of the chapter the potential for targeting plasminogen activators to platelets and for targeting thrombin inhibitors to fibrin is discussed.

Generating a fibrin-specific antibody

In targeting to any component of the thrombus, it is essential that the antibody-combining site be specific for a component of the clot and not cross-react with soluble serum proteins or antigens present on endothelial cells. Most of the present author's work on antibody–plasminogen activator molecules is based on monoclonal antibody 59D8,[13] which was established by fusing the spleen cells of immunized mice with an SP2/0 hybridoma line by standard methods. Antibody 59D8 was raised in response to immunization with a peptide of the sequence GHRPLDK(C), which represents the seven amino terminal residues of the β-chain of fibrin combined with a carboxyl terminal cysteine for cross-linking to keyhole limpet hemocyanin. The choice of targeting the β-chain amino terminus was because it is generated as a result of one of two thrombin cleavages that initiate the conversion of the soluble serum protein fibrinogen to the insoluble constituent of the clot, fibrin. The amino terminus of the β-chain appears to be conformationally protected in fibrinogen, as evidenced by the fact that there is essentially no cross-reactivity between fibrin and fibrinogen when tested with the 59D8 antibody.

Another important consideration in selecting a target on the thrombus is whether the epitope recognized by the antibody persists during the course of clot dissolution. Contrary to some reservations, it has been shown that the epitope recognized by

59D8 was lost from the clot (during *in vitro* fibrinolysis) at a rate identical to the rate of clot dissolution.[14] Thus, epitope availability is sufficient for antibody binding throughout the course of fibrinolysis.

With an antibody that binds fibrin but not fibrinogen, it has been possible to contemplate targeting a plasminogen activator to a component of the thrombus that is not present in circulating plasma. Realization of this concept would ultimately require synthesis of a recombinant fusion protein containing elements of both an antibody-combining site and a plasminogen activator catalytic site. To test the potential utility of this approach, however, fibrin-specific antibodies or antibody fragments have been chemically cross-linked to various plasminogen activators.

The use of chemically cross-linked conjugates as models for fusion proteins

Chemically cross-linking an antibody to another protein is the most rapid and straightforward method for determining whether the production of a fusion product by recombinant DNA technology would be worthwhile. The cross-linking procedure can be carried out quickly and with little difficulty if both proteins are available, and, in contrast with the production of fusion proteins, the cross-linking procedure does not require cloned genes for each of the two proteins or the working out of effective bacterial or eukaryotic expression systems. Although this is not always the case, the chemically cross-linked model conjugate also often predicts attributes of the fusion protein.

Significant disadvantages of chemically cross-linked proteins – which recombinant fusion proteins do not share – include chemical heterogeneity, low yield, lack of stability, and immunogenicity associated with the cross-linking reagent's presence in the product. Chemical cross-linking reagents are often indiscriminate about the amino acid side chains with which they interact. For example, any of the ε-amino groups on the protein surface can participate. Also, should a reactive group be near an active site (on the antibody or the enzyme), the functional properties of either molecule can be altered.

The commonly used two-stage cross-linking reactions, which are designed to produce heterodimeric complexes, are often subject to side reactions that result in multimers. These multimers make necessary size fractionation steps that often reduce the ultimate yield of the conjugate. For example, it has been difficult to obtain active heterodimers in yields in excess of 10% (by the methods summarized below). Disulfide conjugates also lack stability on storage and *in vivo*, although there has been progress in refining cross-linking reactions to produce more stable conjugates. Finally, even though there has been no clear demonstration that cross-linking reagents increase immunogenicity, one would expect these protein-linked organic groups to behave like classic haptenic antigenic determinants.

Monoclonal antibody 59D8,[13] discussed above, is the cornerstone of this author's work in this area. This antibody and another monoclonal antibody of similar specificity, 64C5, was used in studies in which we cross-linked antibodies or their Fabs to plasminogen activators.[13,15,16] In similar experiments with monoclonal antibodies that have little reactivity with fibrinogen but react with fragment D of non-cross-linked fibrin or fragment D-dimer of cross-linked fibrin, Holvoet et al.[17] have confirmed the utility of targeting fibrin.

We first showed that a conjugate of two-chain urokinase plasminogen activator (tcuPA) and anti-fibrin antibody 64C5 substantially enhanced *in vitro* fibrinolysis in comparison with tcuPA.[15] We then showed that tcuPA conjugated to the 64C5 Fab' was equally active[16] and that single-chain urokinase plasminogen activator (scuPA) could be used in a plasminogen activator–59D8 Fab' conjugate.[18] Because the antigen for 59D8 and 64C5 is a hapten, it was possible to demonstrate unequivocally that the enhancement of fibrinolytic potency was solely due to the antigen–antibody reaction: a sufficient concentration of peptide GHRPLDK reduced the fibrinolytic activity of the conjugate to that of its urokinase plasminogen activator (uPA) parent.[15]

Even the activity of tissue-type plasminogen activator (tPA), by itself fibrin-selective, could be enhanced by coupling it to a fibrin-specific antibody.[19] *In vivo* results for a tPA–59D8 conjugate in a rabbit venous thrombosis model were very encouraging.[20]

Bifunctional antibodies

Rather than simply chemically cross-linking an antibody to a plasminogen activator, with all the disadvantages listed above, we thought a more elegant approach might be to create a bifunctional antibody that was able to bind both fibrin and a plasminogen activator (without diminishing its enzymatic activity). Such a bifunc-tional antibody would serve to bring the plasminogen activator into proximity with fibrin, without the need to chemically manipulate the enzyme. We first tested the feasibility of this approach with antibodies to tPA or uPA chemically cross-linked to fibrin-specific antibody 59D8.[21,22] A significant enhancement in fibrinolytic activity was demonstrated both *in vitro* and *in vivo* with the 59D8–anti-tPA conjugate[21] and *in vitro* with the 59D8–anti-uPA conjugate.[22] A conjugate of the anti-tPA Fab' and the Fab' of 59D8 was also as effective as the intact antibody conjugate.[23] Sakharov et al.[24] have demonstrated a 10-fold enhancement in plasma clot lysis *in vitro* with cross-linked antibodies specific for fibrin and uPA.

A better method for producing bispecific antibodies, which avoids the disadvan-tages of chemical cross-linking, is to use somatic cell fusion to produce bivalent antibodies that possess two different antigen-combining sites. This method was first elaborated in 1983 by Milstein and Cuello[25] and has been applied more recently in the design of bifunctional antibodies that bind both tPA and fibrin.[26]

Immunoglobulin G is a symmetrical molecule possessing two antigen-combining sites of the same specificity. Since the component chains of the molecule are assembled after their individual biosyntheses, it is possible to obtain molecules of mixed specificity from cells that are synthesizing two different antibodies.[27] Somatic cell fusion between a hybridoma line secreting antifibrin antibody 59D8 and another hybridoma line secreting anti-tPA antibody TCL8 resulted in a cell line that produced a mixture of antibodies. In addition to the antibodies characteristic of the parental lines and inactive immunoglobulins, the line secreted an antibody that was able to bind both tPA and fibrin. This antibody was isolated from mixtures in culture medium or ascites by two steps of affinity chromatography, using tPA as immobilized antigen in the first and a peptide at the amino terminus of the fibrin β-chain (GHRPLDK(C)) in the second. This bispecific antibody bound simultaneously to tPA and fibrin in a solid-phase immunoassay.

It would be expected that an antibody specific for both fibrin and tPA would not only bind to the fibrin matrix of a thrombus but would also bind to tPA in plasma, thereby increasing the concentration of tPA at the surface of the thrombus. This expectation was confirmed by *in vitro* clot lysis experiments showing that the 59D8–TCL8 bispecific antibody enhanced the potency of tPA 14-fold when added to the assay system before tPA and 22-fold when mixed with tPA to form an immunoconjugate before addition to the assay system. When the 59D8–TCL8 bispecific antibody was tested *in vivo* in the rabbit jugular vein model, a 1.6-fold enhancement in fibrinolytic activity was observed.[26] Kurokawa *et al.*[28] have extended this work and produced by cell fusion bispecific antibodies that bind uPA and fibrin and tPA and fibrin. In a baboon venous thrombosis model, Imura *et al.*[29] tested an immunoconjugate of rscuPA and a bifunctional antibody with both scuPA and fibrin specificities. The immunoconjugate had a fivefold higher thrombolytic potency than unconjugated rscuPA, as a result of both slower clearance from the plasma and fibrin targeting by the specific idiotype of the antibody.

The production of bifunctional antibodies by somatic cell fusion is severely limited by product yield. Because the method depends on a stochastic assortment of immunoglobulin chains within the fused cell, no product is secreted in large amounts. In the future, it is likely that bifunctional antibodies will be produced as fusion proteins by recombinant DNA methods.

Fusion proteins

The most practical approach to antibody targeting is to create, by recombinant DNA methods, a single molecule that contains both an antibody-combining site and a plasminogen activator. Not only does this avoid the difficulties of chemical cross-linking but production of the molecule in quantity by fermentation methods can also be envisioned.

Antifibrin antibody–tPA protein

Building on the pioneering work of Neuberger *et al.*[30,31] and on our experience with cross-linked antibody–enzyme model proteins, we used recombinant technology to create a fusion protein with the activities of antifibrin antibody 59D8 and tPA.[32] Methods for generating the protein are detailed in Love *et al.*[33,34] and are summarized below.

Cloning the rearranged immunoglobulin gene

During the somatic development of the B cell, germline variable (V) and joining (J) regions are juxtaposed to produce a unique rearranged VJ sequence that codes for the antigen-combining site of the heavy or light chain of the immunoglobulin. Also, during this process the heavy chain incorporates a diversity (D) segment at the joining region.[35] These rearrangements result in a unique VDJ or VJ exon sequence that codes for the antigen the antibody recognizes. Unfortunately, expression of a particular immunoglobulin chain can only occur after the unique rearrangement has been cloned. For the expression plasmid coding for the 59D8–tPA fusion protein, the VDJ segment of the rearranged heavy chain of 59D8 was cloned and incorporated into a previously generated immunoglobulin expression plasmid, pSVgpt/26-10VH.[36] The antifibrin 59D8 VDJ was inserted into a unique *Eco*RI site 5' of the constant region, in place of the antidigoxin 26-10 VDJ, to create pSV2gpt (Figure 7.1A). It was unnecessary to clone or otherwise manipulate the light-chain gene because heavy-chain constructs were transfected into cell lines that had lost the ability to express normal heavy chains but retained the ability to produce light chains. It is possible to obtain heavy-chain VDJ sequence either by cloning complementary DNAs (cDNAs) constructed from the mRNA of the hybridoma or by cloning genomic sequences from high-molecular-weight DNA derived from the hybridoma; although genomic sequences were initially used, it became evident later that expression plasmids could be constructed with equal facility by using cDNAs.

Constructing the expression vector for the antifibrin–tPA protein

tPA is secreted as a single-chain, 70-kDa protein that is subsequently cleaved by plasmin to form A and B chains attached by a single disulfide bond.[37,38] Each chain contains multiple, intrachain disulfide bridges. Because only the catalytic function of the plasminogen activator was of interest, we used sequences coding for the B chain in constructing the 59D8–tPA expression vector. The tPA sequence – obtained from a cDNA clone (pPA34'F) that had been constructed from HeLa cell mRNA[39] – was provided by Sandra J.F. Degen (Children's Hospital Research Foundation, Cincinnati, Ohio). The γ2b constant region 3' of the *Xho*I site in the hinge region was removed and replaced with tPA B chain cDNA sequence, and an *Sfa*NI site in the tPA cDNA was converted to an *Xho*I site by the addition of a synthetic oligonucleotide adapter (which also added a glycine residue to the fusion product). The cDNA fragment was thus inserted in-frame into the *Xho*I site in the heavy-chain hinge region of pSV2gpt to create the vector pSVtPA(tPA) (Figure 7.1B). Initially, the 3' untranslated (UT) portion of the tPA cDNA, which contains a polyadenylation signal, was not modified in the vector (the descriptor in parentheses at the end of the plasmid name refers to the 3' UT region). The importance of this sequence to the level of gene expression became apparent in subsequent work. (Modifications to the 3' UT are discussed below.)

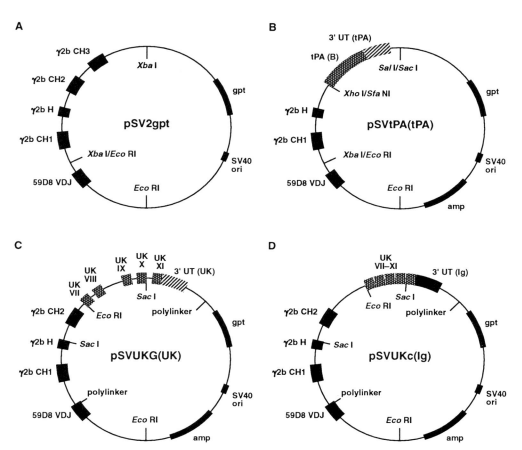

Figure 7.1 Construction of antibody–plasminogen activator plasmids. Coding sequences are indicated by labels outside the circles; restriction sites used in construction are indicated inside the circles.

A. The pSV2gpt vector was modified from that described by Near *et al.* (1990) *Mol. Immunol.*, **27**, 901, by substituting the genomic heavy chain variable region (VDJ) of antifibrin antibody 59D8 for the VDJ of antidigoxin antibody 26-10 at a unique *Eco*RI site. The pSV2gpt vector also contained an SV-40 promoter-driven *E. coli* guanine phosphoribosyltransferase (gpt) gene, serving as the selective marker in transfected hybridoma cells, and a partial pBR322 sequence for plasmid replication and clone selection in *E. coli*.

B. cDNA sequence coding for the tPA B chain and cDNA sequence coding for the tPA 3′ UT region were inserted into pSV2gpt to make pSVtPA(tPA), which codes for protein r59D8–tPA(B). (Modified from Schnee, J. M. *et al.* (1987) *Proc. Natl Acad. Sci. USA*, **84**, 6904.)

C. The genomic DNA encoding low-molecular-weight (32-kDa) scuPA, i.e. urokinase (UK) exons VII–XI, and the UK 3′ UT region were inserted in place of the tPA sequences in pSVtPA(tPA) to make pSVUKG(UK), which codes for r59D8–scuPA(32).

D. The genomic DNA encoding 32-kDa scuPA was replaced by cDNA encoding the same region (UK exons VII–XI) and the plasminogen activator 3′ UT region was replaced by the 59D8 (Ig) 3′ UT region to make pSVUKc(Ig), which also codes for r59D8–scuPA(32). (**C** and **D** modified from Runge, M. S. *et al.* (1991) *Proc. Natl Acad. Sci. USA*, **88**, 10337.)

Abbreviations: amp, pBR322 ampicillin resistance gene; CH1, 2 and 3, heavy-chain constant regions 1, 2, and 3; H, hinge; gpt, *E. coli* guanine phosphoribosyltransferase gene; SV40 ori, simian virus 40 origin of replication; tPA, tissue-type plasminogen activator; UK, urokinase; UT, untranslated region; VDJ, variable region.

Reprinted from Haber, E. (1994) Antibody–plasminogen activator conjugates and recombinant proteins. *Methods Mol. Genet.*, **5**, III–127.

Selecting loss variant cell lines

To select for heavy-chain loss variant hybridomas, we first grew the cells in soft agarose containing goat antimouse heavy-chain antiserum. Clusters secreting heavy chain developed halos. Cells without halos were picked and subcloned.

Transfecting the antifibrin–tPA expression plasmid

The pSVtPA(tPA) hybrid heavy-chain construct was transfected by electroporation into the heavy-chain loss variant hybridoma line. Selection occurred in medium containing xanthine, hypoxanthine and mycophenolic acid (see below).

Purifying and analyzing the antifibrin–tPA protein

The r59D8–tPA(B) protein was purified from cell supernatants and from ascites by sequential double-affinity chromatography.[40] One column consisted of the GHRPLDK(C) peptide (used to generate 59D8) linked to Sepharose, the other of an anti-(human) tPA monoclonal antibody (TCL8) linked to Sepharose.

Antifibrin antibody–scuPA protein

Although the r59D8–tPA(B) protein[32] described above retained both the fibrin antigen-binding and plasminogen activator activities of its parents, the fusion protein's ability to lyze plasma clots was suboptimal. It eventually became apparent that the tPA catalytic site had been an inappropriate choice – the loss in the construct of the amino terminal portion of the protein prevented the requisite enhancement of catalytic activity on fibrin binding.[41] With this experience in mind, we selected the catalytic site of urokinase, reasoning that it might function better in a fusion protein because its activity is independent of fibrin binding. The single-chain form, scuPA, was used because it has the additional advantage of being resistant to inactivation by plasminogen activator inhibitor-1 and α_2-antiplasmin. As it traveled through plasma, a fusion protein containing scuPA might resist circulating inhibitors and remain incapable of activating circulating plasminogen until it reached the plasmin-rich environment of the thrombus, where it would become active through cleavage of the plasmin-susceptible Lys-158–Ile-159 peptide bond.[42]

For the antifibrin–scuPA recombinant, like the antifibrin–tPA protein, we included only the Fab part of the antibody molecule to reduce the mass of the chimera to its essential components. In a similar vein, the urokinase kringle and growth factor regions were omitted and only the sequence corresponding to low-molecular-weight (32-kDa) scuPA, as described by Stump *et al.*,[43] was used. (This fragment is reported to be as active in fibrinolysis as the intact molecule.) Initially the CH2 domain of the antibody heavy chain and part of the CH3 domain had been included as a spacer between the antibody and the plasminogen activator; later experience (S.-Y. Shaw, unpublished observation) proved that this was not necessary. The r59D8–scuPA(32) protein contained antibody 59D8 heavy chain from residues 1 to

351 and, in contiguous peptide sequence, residues 144 to 411 of low-molecular-weight scuPA.[44]

Cloning and expressing the antifibrin–scuPA protein

Expression plasmid pSVUKG(UK) (Figure 7.1C) was constructed from a human urokinase (UK) gene. Exons coding for 32-kDa scuPA, from amino acid 144, were assembled in pGEM3 that had been modified to contain an *Xho*I site. Coding sequence upstream of the *Eco*RI site in exon VII was constructed from complementary synthetic oligonucleotides. An *Xho*I site was incorporated into the 5' end of this sequence. An internal *Eco*RI genomic fragment (1.3 kb) and a 3' *Eco*RI–*Sma*I fragment (3.4 kb) were assembled into the pGEM3 vector containing the 5' sequence. An *Xho*I–*Sal*I fragment containing the reconstructed UK genomic sequence was then inserted into pSVtPA(tPA) (Figure 7.1B),[32] replacing the tPA sequence to create pSVUKG(UK) (Figure 7.1C). (It is also possible to insert the cDNA sequence representing UK exons VII to XI instead of the genomic sequence, as shown by vector pSVUKc(Ig); Figure 7.1D.)

Transfecting and selecting the antifibrin–scuPA protein

The isolation of heavy-chain loss variants from the parental 59D8 cell line was as described above for the antifibrin–tPA protein. Expression constructs (Figure 7.2) were linearized by *Sal*I digestion and transfected by electroporation. A detailed description of the transfection and selection protocols has been published.[33] Essentially, loss variant cells were grown to half confluence, spun and resuspended in 1 ml of buffer containing 20–100 μg ml^{-1} plasmid DNA. The cells were exposed to a single pulse of 200 V (960 μF) and then transferred to growth medium in the absence of mycophenolic acid.

Selection for clones transfected with the *Escherichia coli* hypoxanthine guanine phosphoribosyltransferase gene was begun three days after electroporation by exposure to medium containing mycophenolic acid (0.5 μg ml^{-1}), xanthine (100 μg ml^{-1}) and hypoxanthine (15 μg ml^{-1}).

Recombinant protein expression levels

Although the structure and function of r59D8–scuPA(32) were as anticipated, the amount of protein secreted into the cell-culture supernatant was only 1% the amount secreted by the original hybridoma cell line. In later work, it became apparent that protein production could be greatly enhanced by modifying the 3' UT region of the mRNA (Figure 7.2). Love *et al.*[34] found that cell lines transfected with constructs in which the 3' UT region was coded by plasminogen activator genes – such as pSVtPA(tPA) and pSVUKG(UK) – produced very low levels of both mRNA and protein (0.008–0.06 μg ml^{-1}) in comparison with the parental 59D8 myeloma cell line (7.6–10 μg ml^{-1}). *In vitro* nuclear run-off analysis indicated that these low steady-state levels of mRNA did not result from a lower rate of transcription of the transfected gene (relative to the rate of transcription of the endogenous heavy-chain gene in the 59D8 parent cells). In contrast, cell lines tranfected with expression

r59D8–tPA(B) Constructs

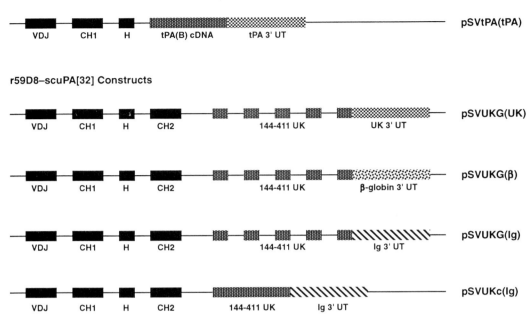

Figure 7.2   Genes transfected into 59D8 heavy chain loss variant cells. pSVtPA(tPA) contains a genomic variable (VDJ) region from fibrin-specific monoclonal antibody 59D8, cloned genomic constant region (CH1) and hinge (H) of a mouse γ2b antibody, and cDNA sequence coding for the B chain of tPA (amino acids 275 to 527) and the tPA 3' untranslated (UT) region. pSVUKG(UK) contains the 59D8 VDJ exon, γ2b constant regions, the coding regions from a genomic clone of scuPA containing urokinase (UK) exons VII to XI and a 3' UT sequence from the UK gene. Two modified plasmids were made by substituting the 3' UT region of either β-globin (pSVUKG(β)) or the mouse γ2b Ig gene (pSVUKG(Ig)). A third modified plasmid was made from pSVUKG(Ig) by substituting cDNA for the genomic DNA encoding UK exons VII to XI (pSVUKc(Ig)). All genes were assembled in the pSV2gpt vector to form their respective expression plasmids (see Figure 7.1).
Modified from Love, T. W. *et al.* (1993) *Thromb. Res.*, **69**, 221. Reprinted from Haber, E. (1994) Antibody–plasminogen activator conjugates and recombinant proteins. *Methods Mol. Genet.*, **5**, III–127.

plasmids in which the 3' UT region of the mouse γ2b heavy-chain gene (such as pSVUKG(Ig) and pSVUKc(Ig)) or the human β-globin gene (such as pSVUKG(β)) had been substituted for the 3' UT region of the plasminogen activator gene showed an increase in recombinant protein secretion of 68-fold.

Inserting the 3' UT region of the human β-globin or mouse γ2b heavy-chain gene

To generate pSVUKG(β) (Figure 7.2), we inserted a synthetic oligonucleotide containing *Eco*RI–*Xho*I–*Bam*HI–*Bgl*II–*Sal*I–*Hind*III sites into pUC19 to create pUC19M. The 5.0-kb *Xho*I to *Sal*I fragment from pSVUKG(UK), containing the scuPA gene, was inserted into the pUC19M vector to create pUKGXS. A synthetic oligo-nucleotide was made starting with the *Bam*HI site of urokinase exon XI and ending with *Bgl*II–*Sal*I sites immediately following the urokinase termination codon. This oligonucleotide was used to replace the *Bam*HI to *Sal*I fragment of pUKGXS to create pUKGXBS, eliminating the urokinase 3' UT region. The human β-globin 3' UT region and 3' flanking DNA was obtained by inserting the 217-bp *Alu*I fragment of pH(β)G1-D[45] into the *Sma*I site of the pLL10 vector[46] to create pH(β)UT. The human β-globin gene fragment was released from pH(β)UT by *Bam*HI digestion and ligated into the *Bgl*II site of pUC19M to create pUCH(β)UT. The β-globin sequence was then removed from pUCH(β)UT by *Bam*HI and *Sal*I digestion and ligated into the *Bam*HI and *Sal*I sites of pUKGXBS to create pUKG(β). Finally, the *Xho*I to *Sal*I fragment of pUKG(β) (containing the urokinase gene beginning at amino acid 144 of exon VII and a β-globin 3' UT element) was substituted for the *Xho*I to *Sal*I fragment in pSVUKG(UK) to generate pSVUKG(β).

pSVUKG(Ig) (Figure 7.2) was constructed by inserting the 3.3-kb *Sac*I to *Sal*I fragment of the γ2b heavy-chain gene (after the *Sac*I site had been blunted with T4 polymerase) into the *Sal*I and similarly blunted *Bgl*II sites of pUKGXBS (described above) to create pUKG(Ig). The *Xho*I to *Sal*I fragment of pUKG(Ig), containing the urokinase gene from amino acid 144 of exon VII and a γ2b 3' UT element, was then substituted for the *Xho*I to *Sal*I fragment of pSVUKG(UK) to generate pSVUKG(Ig). (All expression plasmids were then subjected to restriction-enzyme mapping and nucleotide-sequence analysis to confirm correct assembly.)

Producing r59D8–scuPA(32) in large quantity

Milligram quantities of r59D8–scuPA(32) were produced by growing cells to high density (total mass of approximately 4×10^{10} cells) in DMEM with 10% fetal calf serum in the extrafiber space of a CellMax (Type B) bioreactor (Cellco, Kensington, MD, USA) containing cellulose acetate hollow fibers with a sieving coefficient of approximately 4 kDa. Culture medium was harvested at 12-hour intervals and immediately frozen at $-70°C$. After the aliquots had been thawed and pooled, r59D8–scuPA(32) was purified from the medium (the initial concentration of recombinant protein varied between 0.05 and 0.3 mg ml^{-1}) by affinity chromatography on a resin containing Sepharose linked to the heptapeptide epitope for antibody 59D8.[19] The eluate contained a mixture of r59D8–scuPA(32) (15–35%) and enzymatically cleaved r59D8–scuPA(32) (85–65%). (Either thrombin or plasmin can cleave the scuPA portion of r59D8–scuPA(32) into low-molecular-weight two-chain urokinase.) r59D8–scuPA(32) was obtained by passing this mixture through a column of benzamidine–Sepharose.

Benzamidine–Sepharose chromatography was performed as described.[20] Rather than being used for affinity binding of the desired product (see Ref. 47 for a review), benzamidine–Sepharose was used to remove two-chain r59D8–scuPA(32) from the mixture of single- and two-chain forms. Purified r59D8–scuPA(32) (0.05–0.5 mg ml^{-1} in Tris-glycine buffer, pH 7.4) was used immediately in assays or frozen at $-70°C$, at which it remained stable for up to six weeks.

Properties of r59D8–scuPA(32)

To evaluate the functional properties of r59D8–scuPA(32), the specific amidolytic activity and kinetic parameters for activation of plasminogen by plasmin-cleaved

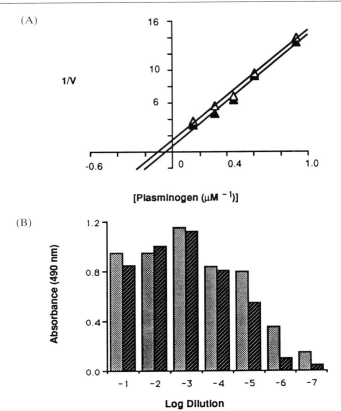

Figure 7.3 Kinetic and fibrin-binding properties of r59D8–scuPA(32). (A) Initial rates of reaction for two-chain urokinase (△) and the two-chain form of r59D8–scuPA(32) (▲). (B) Fibrin binding by native 59D8 (stippled bars) and r59D8–scuPA(32) (hatched bars). The means of duplicate determinations are shown. Reprinted from Runge, M. S. *et al.* (1991) *Proc. Natl Acad. Sci. USA*, **88**, 10337.

r59D8–scuPA(32) were compared with those of low-molecular-weight two-chain urokinase, and the fibrin-binding activity was compared with that of native 59D8. The specific amidolytic activity of tissue culture-derived scuPA was 85 000 u mg^{-1}. This material was >95% uncleaved (i.e. single-chain) when latent activity was compared with activity after cleavage to high-molecular-weight two-chain urokinase (scuPA and r59D8–scuPA(32) were converted to the two-chain form with plasmin–Sepharose).[20,48] Preparations of r59D8–scuPA(32) were 77.6% single chain, with a catalytic activity of 26 000 u mg^{-1} of protein after conversion to the two-chain form. Given the contribution, on a molar basis, of the 32-kDa scuPA portion of the 103-kDa r59D8–scuPA(32) molecule, the activity of the scuPA portion was 83 900 u mg^{-1} of scuPA. This is not significantly different from the activity of native scuPA. In addition, the K_m for activation of plasminogen by the plasmin-cleaved (two-chain) form of r59D8–scuPA(32) (16.6 μM) did not differ significantly from that of low-molecular-weight two-chain urokinase (9.1 μM) (Figure 7.3A). The fibrin-binding activity of r59D8–scuPA(32) (native 32-kDa scuPA does not bind fibrin directly) was compared with that of native 59D8 by measuring the binding of serial dilutions of either 59D8 or r59D8–scuPA(32) to fibrin monomer-coated, 96-well plates. The data shown in Figure 7.3B demonstrate that r59D8–scuPA(32) bound to fibrin in a manner similar to that of native 59D8. Although there was a trend toward diminished fibrin binding by r59D8–scuPA(32) (in comparison with fibrin binding by native 59D8) at dilutions of 10^{-5}, 10^{-6} and 10^{-7}, the observed differences were not statistically significant.

The preparations of r59D8–scuPA(32) used in the *in vitro* and *in vivo* assays that follow contained small amounts of two-chain material, probably resulting from thrombin cleavage of r59D8–scuPA(32). Thrombin-cleaved scuPA is considerably less active in fibrinolysis assays than is uncleaved scuPA. Thus, the effect of thrombin-generated two-chain r59D8–scuPA(32) would be to diminish any potential increase in thrombolytic potency due to increased fibrin binding by r59D8–scuPA(32).

In a human plasma clot lysis assay, r59D8–scuPA(32) was six times more potent than scuPA ($P < 0.0001$) (Figure 7.4A). At equivalent thrombolytic doses r59D8–scuPA(32) was more fibrin-specific, i.e. there was less consumption of fibrinogen and α_2-antiplasmin than with scuPA. In a typical plasma clot assay, at 3 hours with 800 u of scuPA, there was 66% ± 5% clot lysis. The fibrinogen level was 56% ± 5% that of control, and the α_2-antiplasmin level was 35% ± 9% that of control. With 200 u of r59D8–scuPA(32), clot lysis was 53% ± 4%, and fibrinogen and α_2-antiplasmin levels were 95% ± 1% and 85% ± 5%, respectively, those of controls. These data are comparable with those reported by Bode *et al.*,[18] who compared the fibrin specificity of scuPA with that of scuPA chemically coupled to antibody 59D8. The results were even more striking *in vivo*, when tested in the rabbit jugular vein model (the *in situ* formation of a human thrombus in the rabbit's vein). Compared with scuPA, r59D8–scuPA(32) displayed a remarkable 20-fold increase in thrombolytic potency *in vivo* over the entire dose–response range ($P < 0.0001$) (Figure 7.4B).[44] r59D8–scuPA(32) did not cause a decrease in fibrinogen concentration until 83% lysis was reached, at which point the fibrinogen concentration was 79% ± 4% that of the control. This represents a small but probably significant decrease in fibrinogen concentration.

The rabbit jugular vein model was selected for these studies because it allows quantitative comparisons of thrombolytic potency. Unfortunately, the model is not ideal for comparisons of fibrin specificity. For example, even very high doses of scuPA do not result in >40% thrombolysis in this model, precluding a comparison of specificity between scuPA and r59D8–scuPA(32) at a near maximal thrombolytic dose. Within the range where it was possible to compare plasma fibrinogen and α_2-antiplasmin concentrations between scuPA and r59D8–scuPA(32), the data resemble those previously published comparing tPA with tPA chemically conjugated to 59D8.[20]

M.S. Runge and coworkers (unpublished observations) have since studied the *in vitro* activities of r59D8–scuPA(32), scuPA and tPA in a baboon model that allows critical comparisons of thombolytic potency and inhibition of thrombus deposition in relation to both the dose and the plasma concentration of each plasminogen activator. r59D8–scuPA(32) was 8–10-fold more potent than rtPA and 15–20-fold more potent than rscuPA by dose administered and 2.8-fold more potent than rtPA

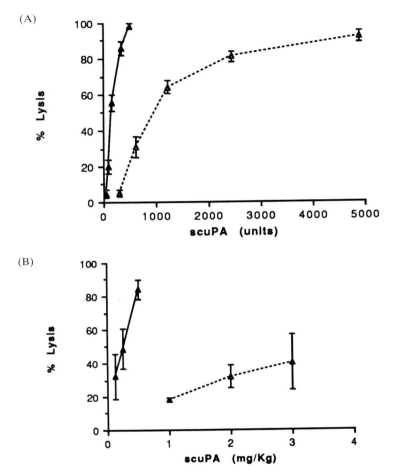

Figure 7.4 (A) Human plasma clot lysis assay. Clot lysis is shown at different concentrations (in units/ml) of scuPA (- - -Δ - - -) or r59D8–scuPA(32) (—▲—). Points represent clot lysis at 2 hours. The fold increase in potency was calculated by comparing the percent lysis curves in the plasma clot and rabbit jugular vein assays, which were fitted using a two-parameter exponential function (Runge, M. S. *et al.* (1988) *Biochemistry*, **27**, 1153). (B) Thrombolysis *in vivo*. Data represent the means of values from between 3 and 8 animals at each point. The 20-fold increase in potency for r59D8–scuPA(32) was derived as described in A. Reprinted from Runge, M. S. *et al.* (1991) *Proc. Natl Acad. Sci. USA*, **88**, 10337.

and 5.6-fold more potent than rscuPA by plasma concentration in the lysis of thrombi. This difference in potency, as calculated by the dose administered in comparison with plasma concentration, is explained by the observation that in the baboon the plasma half-life was 12 times longer for r59D8–scuPA(32) than for rscuPA. In an experiment in which pharmacokinetics does not play a role, r59D8–scuPA(32) was 11 times more potent than scuPA in the inhibition of thrombin deposition.

Of equally great interest is the observation that, at equipotent thrombolytic doses, template bleeding times in the baboon for r59D8–scuPA(32) were unchanged whereas those for tPA and scuPA were significantly prolonged. Since bleeding time prolongation apparently reflects the risk of clinical hemorrhage,[49] it would be of interest to determine whether r59D8–scuPA(32), in addition to being more potent, might also be safer.

Holvoet et al.[50] constructed an M_r 57 000 single-chain chimeric plasminogen activator consisting of a 33-kDa fragment of scuPA and an Fv derived from a fibrin-specific antibody directed at a cross-linked epitope of the D-dimer. This single-chain molecule was expressed by baculovirus-infected cells of the insect *Spodoptera frugiperda*. The recombinant molecule showed high affinity for binding the fibrin D-dimer fragment (essentially identical to that of the parent antibody molecule) and a very similar Michaelis–Menten constant for activating plasminogen. When tested in the lysis of a plasma clot *in vivo*, the recombinant single-chain molecule was 13-fold more potent than low-molecular-weight scuPA. In the hamster pulmonary embolism model, the thrombolytic potency of the antibody-targeted fusion protein was 23-fold greater than that of rscuPA. In rabbits with a jugular vein clot prepared from human plasma, the thrombolytic potency of the fusion protein was 11-fold higher than that of rscuPA. Further, in baboons with an autologous whole blood clot in the femoral vein, the chimera had a fivefold higher thrombolytic potency than scuPA.[51] Vandamme et al.[52] subsequently constructed a humanized version of the single-chain Fv contained in this fusion protein, which had very similar properties to the molecule containing the murine Fv, as described above.

Holvoet et al.[53] showed that the increase in fibrinolytic potency with the antifibrin Fv–scuPA fusion protein was due both to targeting of the activator to the clot through the single-chain Fv fragment (a sixfold increase) and to a more efficient conversion of the single-chain urokinase segment to its two-chain derivative (an eightfold increase). In a further examination of the relation between clearance rates and thrombolytic potency,[54,55] the Holvoet group studied the recombinant single chain molecule in a glycosylated and a nonglycosylated form (Glu was substituted for Asn-88 to abolish the glycosylation signal). The nonglycosylated form showed a fourfold slower clearance in the hamster but a less efficient targeting. Overall, the potency of the two forms was similar; however, the prolonged half-life of the nonglycosylated form compensated for its lower specific activity. Thus, the thrombolytic potency of a chimeric antibody-targeted plasminogen activator can be improved by increasing its specific thrombolytic activity or by reducing its rate of clearance, or both.

Yang et al.[56] described an interesting fusion protein that contains a fibrin-specific antibody-combining site and a modified scuPA catalytic domain. The design of this molecule was predicated on the observation that there is a high concentration of thrombin in the vicinity of an intravascular thrombus. Although thrombin is capable of cleaving and inactivating native scuPA, the urokinase-derived catalytic segment contained in the fusion protein was modified by site-directed mutagenesis so that the peptide bond normally cleaved by plasmin (to activate urokinase) would now be cleaved by thrombin. Thus, a selective thrombin cleavage site in a molecule targeted to fibrin would initiate clot lysis after thrombin activation. The specific change effected in the urokinase domain was the deletion of Phe-157 and Lys-158. According-ing to its design, r59D8–scuPA-T was activated by thrombin but not by plasmin, whereas the fusion protein discussed above, r59D8–scuPA(32), was activated by plasmin but not by thrombin. When activated by thrombin, r59D8–scuPA-T converted plasminogen to plasmin. *In vitro* plasma clot lysis assays showed that r59D8–scuPA-T lyzed clots that resulted from the action of thrombin and that heparin and hirudin could prevent clot lysis. When incorporated as part of a thrombin-induced clot, only r59D8–scuPA-T was able to lyze the clot, whereas r59D8–scuPA(32) and high-molecular-weight scuPA were ineffective. These results suggest that this thrombin-activatable form of r59D8–scuPA has the potential to selectively lyze fresh clots, which are thrombin rich, more effectively than older clots, which generally do not contain as much thrombin. A clinical event requiring thrombolysis – such as a coronary or cerebral artery occlusion – usually presents acutely and is the consequence of a very recent thrombus. The therapeutic aim is to dissolve that thrombus but not to disturb older thrombi that might be beneficially preventing undesirable hemorrhage, such as at the site of a peptic ulcer. Targetability engendered in fresh thrombi by a high local concentration of thrombin may well be the key to an important increase in specificity.

Targeting plasminogen activators to the platelet receptor

Arterial thrombi contain a high concentration of activated platelets, and it is likely that platelet-rich thrombi are particularly resistant to thrombolysis.[57] Highly platelet-rich thrombi may be a major reason for the failure to obtain reperfusion after thrombolytic therapy, and the accumulation of platelets at thrombi may lead to reocclusion.[57] Platelet aggregation is mediated by fibrinogen binding to the membrane-bound glycoprotein (GP)IIb/IIIa receptor.[57] An antibody specific for this receptor, 7E3, has been shown to enhance the speed of reperfusion and reduce the rate of reocclusion in animal models of arterial thrombosis.[58,59] It was of interest to determine whether the targeting of a plasminogen activator to the GPIIb/IIIa receptor through 7E3 would enhance the antibody's ability to accelerate clot lysis. We reasoned that a conjugate of 7E3 and uPA, in addition to blocking the GPIIb/IIIa receptor's access to fibrinogen by virtue of 7E3 binding to GPIIb/IIIa, would also produce a high local concentration of plasmin that could lyze the bound fibrin molecules responsible for aggregating the platelets.

Using chemical cross-linking, we conjugated high-molecular-weight two-chain urokinase (tcuPA) to 7E3 Fab' to produce, after fractionation, a 100-kDa molecule that was predominantly a 1:1 complex of Fab' and tcuPA.[60] The tcuPA–7E3 Fab' conjugate bound purified GPIIb/IIIa and intact platelets and exhibited plasminogen activator activity. At the concentrations tested, tcuPA showed very little activity against the clots, whereas the conjugate was 970-fold more active. An equimolar mixture of tcuPA and 7E3 was no more effective than uPA alone. The rate of lysis related to the concentration of platelets in the clot, and no enhancement in lysis by the conjugate over uPA was apparent in clots containing few platelets. Thus, uPA targeted to GPIIb/IIIa by conjugation to the antibody accounted for an improvement in fibrinolytic potency that was substantially greater than that achieved by uPA and the antibody alone.

Dewerchin *et al.*[61] have also studied several other antibodies to the ligand-induced binding sites on GPIIb/IIIa in conjugates with recombinant scuPA. They extended our observations by showing that the conjugates were more effective than scuPA in the lysis of platelet-rich thrombi *in vivo* in a hamster model of pulmonary embolism. There is little doubt that the next refinement to platelet targeting will require the construction of a recombinant molecule that contains both a binding site specific for activated platelets and a plasminogen activator catalytic site.

The disadvantage of using 7E3 as a targeting antibody is that it interacts with GPIIb/IIIa on both activated and resting platelets and thus does not target specifically to the thrombus.[57] Some of the antibodies described by Dewerchin *et al.*[61] may be more selective for activated platelets.

Targeting the thrombin inhibitor hirudin to fibrin

Recently Bode *et al.*[62] synthesized a bifunctional molecule that incorporates an antifibrin antibody and the thrombin inhibitor hirudin. The intent was to inhibit further fibrin deposition at sites of thrombosis while avoiding systemic anticoagulation. *In vitro* observations demonstrated an approximately tenfold reduction in fibrin deposition on a clot suspended in plasma in the presence of the antibody–hirudin conjugate in comparison with equimolar concentrations of hirudin. The construction of a fusion protein based on this principle is in progress.

Conclusion

In the decade since the first description of a fibrin-targeted plasminogen activator[15] there has been considerable progress. Simple chemical conjugates have evolved into elegant chimeric proteins, the smallest of which comprises only the minimal antibody-combining site, the Fv, and the catalytic site of urokinase.[50] These agents have been shown to be more effective than their parent plasminogen activators in a variety of animal models, including one resembling arterial thrombosis in the baboon. In addition to increased efficacy, early studies suggest that safety, as exemplified by diminished effects on hemostasis, may also be enhanced. An antibody specific for a platelet receptor has also been used to target a plasminogen activator. *In vitro* studies suggest that this approach may help dissolve platelet-rich thrombi, which are generally resistant to the presently available plasminogen activators. The thrombin inhibitor hirudin has also been targeted to fibrin, indicating that local, rather than systemic, anticoagulation may be possible. Confirmation of the utility of this approach awaits initiation of clinical studies.

There are many potential applications of antibody–enzyme chimeras beyond the field of thrombolytic agents. One example that has been widely exploited is the expression of a chimera that targets a cancer-associated cell-surface antigen – concentrating at the cell surface an enzyme that activates a cancer-chemotherapeutic prodrug and resulting in a high concentration of active drug in the vicinity of a tumor.[63] Another application, which has not yet been tested, is the use of appropriate antibody–enzyme chimeras to treat vascular occlusion without the need of mechanical or surgical intervention. Antigens specific for epitopes unique to arteriosclerotic plaques would be fused to enzymes such as collagenase that could degrade components of the plaque and thereby increase the diameter of the blood-vessel lumen.

References

1. AIMS Trial Study Group (1988) Effect of intravenous APSAC on mortality after acute myocardial infarction: preliminary report of a placebo-controlled clinical trial. *Lancet*, **i**, 545–9.
2. Gruppo Italiano per lo Studio della Sopravvivenza nell'Infarto miocardico (1990) GISSI-2: a factorial randomised trial of alteplase versus streptokinase and heparin versus no heparin among 12 490 patients with acute myocardial infarction. *Lancet*, **336**, 65–71.
3. ISIS-3 (Third International Study of Infarct Survival) Collaborative Group (1992) ISIS-3: a randomised comparison of streptokinase vs tissue plasminogen activator vs anistreplase and of aspirin plus heparin vs aspirin alone among 41 299 cases of suspected acute myocardial infarction. *Lancet*, **339**, 753–70.
4. Global Utilization of Streptokinase and Tissue Plasminogen Activator for Occluded Coronary Arteries (GUSTO) Investigators (1993) An international randomized trial comparing four thrombolytic strategies for acute myocardial infarction. *N. Engl. J. Med.*, **329**, 673–82.
5. Lijnen, H. R., Van, H. B., De Cock, F. *et al.* (1991) On the mechanism of fibrin-specific plasminogen activation by staphylokinase. *J. Biol. Chem.*, **266**, 11826–32.
6. Witt, W., Baldus, B., Bringmann, P. *et al.* (1992) Thrombolytic properties of *Desmodus rotundus* (vampire bat) salivary plasminogen activator in experimental pulmonary embolism in rats. *Blood*, **79**, 1213–17.
7. Gardell, S. J., Duong, L. T. Diehl, R. E. *et al.* (1989) Isolation, characterization, and cDNA cloning of a vampire bat salivary plasminogen activator. *J. Biol. Chem.*, **264**, 17947–52.
8. Popma, J. J. and Topol, E. J. (1991) Adjuncts to thrombolysis for myocardial reperfusion. *Ann. Intern. Med.*, **115**, 34–44.
9. Ellis, S. G., Bates, E. R., Schaible, T. *et al.* (1991) Prospects for the use of antagonists to the platelet glycoprotein IIb/IIIa receptor to prevent post-angioplasty restenosis and thrombosis. *J. Am. Coll. Cardiol.*, **17**, 89B–95B.
10. Imura, Y., Stassen, J. M., Bunting, S. *et al.* (1992) Antithrombotic properties of L-cysteine, N-(mercaptoacetyl)-D-Tyr-Arg-Gly-Asp-sulfoxide (G4120) in a hamster platelet-rich femoral vein thrombosis model. *Blood*, **80**, 1247–53.
11. ISIS-2 (Second International Study of Infarct Survival) Collaborative Group (1988) Randomised trial of intravenous streptokinase, oral aspirin, both, or neither among 17 187 cases of suspected acute myocardial infarction: ISIS-2. *Lancet*, **ii**, 349–60.
12. The EPIC Investigation (1994) Use of a monoclonal antibody directed against the platelet glycoprotein IIb/IIIa receptor in high-risk coronary angioplasty. *N. Engl. J. Med.*, **330**, 956–61.
13. Hui, K. Y., Haber, E. and Matsueda, G. R. (1983) Monoclonal antibodies to a synthetic fibrin-like peptide bind to human fibrin but not fibrinogen. *Science*, **222**, 1129–32.
14. Chen, F., Haber, E. and Matsueda, G. R. (1992) Availability of the B beta(15–21) epitope on cross-linked human fibrin and its plasmic degradation products. *Thromb. Haemost.*, **67**, 335–40.
15. Bode, C., Matsueda, G. R., Hui, K. Y. and Haber, E. (1985) Antibody-directed urokinase: a specific fibrinolytic agent. *Science*, **229**, 765–7.
16. Bode, C., Runge, M. S., Newell, J. B. *et al.* (1987) Thrombolysis by a fibrin-specific antibody Fab'–urokinase conjugate. *J. Mol. Cell. Cardiol.*, **19**, 335–41.

17. Holvoet, P., Stassen, J. M., Hashimoto, Y. *et al.* (1989) Binding properties of monoclonal antibodies against human fragment D-dimer of cross-linked fibrin to human plasma clots in an *in vivo* model in rabbits. *Thromb. Haemost.*, **61**, 307–13.

18. Bode, C., Runge, M. S., Schönermark, S. *et al.* (1990) Conjugation to antifibrin Fab' enhances fibrinolytic potency of single-chain urokinase plasminogen activator. *Circulation*, **81**, 1974–80.

19. Runge, M. S., Bode, C., Matsueda, G. R. and Haber, E. (1988) Conjugation to an antifibrin monoclonal antibody enhances the fibrinolytic potency of tissue plasminogen activator *in vitro*. *Biochemistry*, **27**, 1153–7.

20. Runge, M. S., Bode, C., Matsueda, G. R. and Haber, E. (1987) Antibody-enhanced thrombolysis: targeting of tissue plasminogen activator *in vivo*. *Proc. Natl Acad. Sci. USA.* **84**, 7659–62.

21. Bode, C., Runge, M. S., Branscomb, E. E. *et al.* (1989) Antibody-directed fibrinolysis. An antibody specific for both fibrin and tissue plasminogen activator. *J. Biol. Chem.*, **264**, 944–8.

22. Charpie, J. R., Runge, M. S., Matsueda, G. R. and Haber, E. (1990) A bispecific antibody enhances the fibrinolytic potency of single-chain urokinase. *Biochemistry*, **29**, 6374–8.

23. Runge, M. S., Bode, C., Savard, C. E. *et al.* (1990) Antibody-directed fibrinolysis: a bispecific (Fab')$_2$ that binds to fibrin and tissue plasminogen activator. *Bioconjug. Chem.*, **1**, 274–7.

24. Sakharov, D. V., Sinitsyn, V. V., Kratasjuk, G. A. *et al.* (1988) Two-step targeting of urokinase to plasma clot provides efficient fibrinolysis. *Thromb. Res.*, **49**, 481–8.

25. Milstein, C. and Cuello A. C. (1983) Hybrid hybridomas and their use in immunohistochemistry. *Nature*, **305**, 537–40.

26. Branscomb, E. E., Runge, M. S., Savard, C. E. *et al.* (1990) Bispecific monoclonal antibodies produced by somatic cell fusion increase the potency of tissue plasminogen activator. *Thromb. Haemost.*, **64**, 260–6.

27. Suresh, M. R., Cuello, A. C. and Milstein, C. (1986) Bispecific monoclonal antibodies from hybrid hybridomas. *Methods Enzymol.*, **121**, 210–28.

28. Kurokawa, T., Iwasa, S. and Kakinuma, A. (1990) Enhancement of fibrinolysis by bispecific monoclonal antibodies reactive to fibrin and plasminogen activators. *Thromb. Res. (Supp.)*, **10**, 83–9.

29. Imura, Y., Stassen, J. M., Kurokawa, T. *et al.* (1992) Thrombolytic and pharmacokinetic properties of an immunoconjugate of single-chain urokinase-type plasminogen activator (u-PA) and a bispecific monoclonal antibody against fibrin and against u-PA in baboons. *Blood*, **79**, 2322–9.

30. Neuberger, M. S., Williams, G. T. and Fox, R. O. (1984) Recombinant antibodies possessing novel effector functions. *Nature*, **312**, 604–8.

31. Williams, G. T. and Neuberger, M. S. (1986) Production of antibody-tagged enzymes by myeloma cells: application to DNA polymerase I Klenow fragment. *Gene*, **43**, 319–24.

32. Schnee, J. M., Runge, M. S., Matsueda, G. R. *et al.* (1987) Construction and expression of a recombinant antibody-targeted plasminogen activator. *Proc. Natl Acad. Sci. USA*, **84**, 6904–8.

33. Love, T. W., Runge, M. S., Haber, E., Quertermous, T. (1989) Recombinant antibodies possessing novel effector functions. *Methods Enzymol.*, **178**, 515–27.

34. Love, T. W., Quertermous, T., Zavodny, P. J. *et al.* (1993) High-level expression of antibody–plasminogen activator fusion proteins in hybridoma cells. *Thromb. Res.*, **69**, 221–9.

35. Tonegawa, S. (1983) Somatic generation of antibody diversity. *Nature*, **302**, 575–81.

36. Near, R. I., Ng, S. C., Mudgett-Hunter, M. *et al.* (1990) Heavy and light chain contributions to antigen binding in an anti-digoxin chain recombinant antibody produced by transfection of cloned anti-digoxin antibody genes. *Mol. Immunol.*, **27**, 901–9.

37. Gething, M. J., Adler, B., Boose, J. A. *et al.* (1988) Variants of human tissue-type plasminogen activator that lack specific structural domains of the heavy chain. *EMBO. J.*, **7**, 2731–40.

38. Harris, T. J. (1987) Second-generation plasminogen activators. *Protein Eng.*, **1**, 449–58.
39. Fisher, R., Waller, E. K., Grossi, G. *et al*. (1985) Isolation and characterization of the human tissue-type plasminogen activator structural gene including its 5' flanking region. *J. Biol. Chem.*, **260**, 11223–30.
40. Bode, C., Runge, M. S. and Haber, E. (1992) Purifying antibody–plasminogen activator conjugates. *Bioconjug. Chem.*, **3**, 269–72.
41. Love, T. W., Quertermous, T., Runge, M. S. *et al*. (1994) Attachment of an antifibrin antibody to the amino terminus of tissue-type plasminogen activator impairs stimulation by fibrin. *Fibrinolysis*, **8**, 326–32.
42. Declerck, P. J., Lijnen, H. R., Verstreken, M. *et al*. (1990) A monoclonal antibody specific for two-chain urokinase-type plasminogen activator. Application to the study of the mechanism of clot lysis with single-chain urokinase-type plasminogen activator in plasma. *Blood*, **75**, 1794–800.
43. Stump, D. C., Lijnen, H. R. and Collen, D. (1986) Purification and characterization of a novel low molecular weight form of single-chain urokinase-type plasminogen activator. *J. Biol. Chem.*, **261**, 17120–6.
44. Runge, M. S., Quertermous, T., Zavodny, P. J. *et al*. (1991) A recombinant chimeric plasminogen activator with high affinity for fibrin has increased thrombolytic potency *in vitro* and *in vivo*. *Proc. Natl Acad. Sci. USA*, **88**, 10337–41.
45. Lawn, R. M., Efstratiadis, A., O'Connell, C. and Maniatis, T. (1980) The nucleotide sequence of the human beta-globin gene. *Cell*, **21**, 647–51.
46. Rothstein, R. J., Lau, L. F., Bahl, C. P. *et al*. (1979) Synthetic adapters for cloning DNA. *Methods Enzymol.*, **86**, 98–109.
47. Haber, E., Quertermous, T., Matsueda, G. R. and Runge, M. S. (1989) Innovative approaches to plasminogen activator therapy. *Science*, **243**, 51–6.
48. Dewerchin, M., Lijnen, H. R., Van Hoef, B. *et al*. (1989) Biochemical properties of conjugates of urokinase-type plasminogen activator with a monoclonal antibody specific for cross-linked fibrin. *Eur. J. Biochem.*, **185**, 141–9.
49. Gimple, L. W., Gold, H. K., Leinbach, R. C. *et al*. (1989) Correlation between template bleeding times and spontaneous bleeding during treatment of acute myocardial infarction with recombinant tissue-type plasminogen activator. *Circulation*, **80**, 581–8.
50. Holvoet, P., Laroche, Y., Lijnen, H. R. *et al*. (1991) Characterization of a chimeric plasminogen activator consisting of a single-chain Fv fragment derived from a fibrin fragment D-dimer-specific antibody and a truncated single-chain urokinase. *J. Biol. Chem.*, **266**, 19717–24.
51. Dewerchin, M., Vandamme, A. M., Holvoet, P. *et al*. (1992) Thrombolytic and pharmacokinetic properties of a recombinant chimeric plasminogen activator consisting of a fibrin fragment D-dimer specific humanized monoclonal antibody and a truncated single-chain urokinase. *Thromb. Haemost.*, **68**, 170–9.
52. Vandamme, A. M., Dewerchin, M., Lijnen, H. R. *et al*. (1992) Characterization of a recombinant chimeric plasminogen activator composed of a fibrin fragment-D-dimer-specific humanized monoclonal antibody and a truncated single-chain urokinase. *Eur. J. Biochem.*, **205**, 139–46.
53. Holvoet, P., Laroche, Y., Lijnen, H. R. *et al*. (1992) Biochemical characterization of single-chain chimeric plasminogen activators consisting of a single-chain Fv fragment of a fibrin-specific antibody and single-chain urokinase. *Eur. J. Biochem.*, **210**, 945–52.
54. Holvoet, P., Laroche, Y., Stassen, J. M. *et al*. (1993) Pharmacokinetic and thrombolytic properties of chimeric plasminogen activators consisting of a single-chain Fv fragment of a fibrin-specific antibody fused to single-chain urokinase. *Blood*, **81**, 696–703.
55. Holvoet, P., Dewerchin, M., Stassen, J. M. *et al*. (1993) Thrombolytic profiles of clot-targeted plasminogen activators. Parameters determining potency and initial and maximal rates. *Circulation*, **87**, 1007–16.
56. Yang, W. P., Goldstein, J., Procyk, R. *et al*. (1994) Design and evaluation of a thrombin-activable plasminogen activator. *Biochemistry*, **33**, 606–12.
57. Coller, B. S. (1990) Platelets and thrombolytic therapy. *N. Engl. J. Med.*, **322**, 33–42.

58. Yasuda, T., Gold, H. K., Fallon, J. T. *et al.* (1988) Monoclonal antibody against the platelet glycoprotein (GP)IIb/IIIa receptor prevents coronary artery reocclusion after reperfusion with recombinant tissue-type plasminogen activator in dogs. *J. Clin. Invest.*, **81**, 1284–91.
59. Gold, H. K., Coller, B. S., Yasuda, T. *et al.* (1988) Rapid and sustained coronary artery recanalization with combined bolus injection of recombinant tissue-type plasminogen activator and monoclonal antiplatelet GPIIb/IIIa antibody in a canine preparation. *Circulation*, **77**, 670–7.
60. Bode, C., Meinhardt, G., Runge, M. S. *et al.* (1991) Platelet-targeted fibrinolysis enhances clot lysis and inhibits platelet aggregation. *Circulation*, **84**, 805–13.
61. Dewerchin, M., Lijnen, H. R., Stassen, J. M. *et al.* (1991) Effect of chemical conjugation of recombinant single-chain urokinase-type plasminogen activator with monoclonal antiplatelet antibodies on platelet aggregation and on plasma clot lysis *in vitro* and *in vivo*. *Blood*, **78**, 1005–18.
62. Bode, C., Hudelmayer, M., Mehwald, P. *et al.* (1994) Fibrin-targeted recombinant hirudin inhibits fibrin deposition on experimental clots more efficiently than recombinant hirudin. *Circulation*, **90**, 1956–63.
63. Senter, P. D., Wallace, P. M., Svensson, H. P. *et al.* (1991) Activation of prodrugs by antibody–enzyme conjugates. *Adv. Exp. Med. Biol.*, **303**, 97–105.

8

Molecular Approaches to the Therapy of Ischemic Heart Disease and Myocardial Infarction

Sung W. Lee
David A. Dichek

Introduction

Application of the techniques and concepts of molecular biology to the understanding and treatment of ischemic heart disease has led to numerous recent diagnostic and therapeutic advances. Among the molecular biologic techniques for which applications to the treatment of ischemic heart disease are now being pursued, perhaps none has received more attention and generated more hope than gene transfer. This chapter will review the status of gene transfer as a therapeutic approach to ischemic heart disease.

Gene transfer includes a variety of physical and biologic techniques by which foreign genetic material can be inserted into living cells, either *in vitro* or *in vivo*.[1] Gene transfer, when used to cure or ameliorate a human disease condition is known as 'gene therapy'.[2] The potential of gene-transfer techniques to become therapeutic tools for the treatment of human disease is most obvious in diseases caused by a genetic defect involving a single gene. Replacement of the defective gene is expected to lead in a very direct manner to amelioration or cure of the disease. Several human gene therapy trials are now being carried out in patients with diseases based on single-gene defects.[3–6]

In contrast to disease based on single-gene defects, the disease processes underlying ischemic and thrombotic heart disease (i.e. atherosclerosis and thrombosis) are complex with both polygenic and environmental factors. There is virtually never a specific genetic defect that can be targeted. Nevertheless, gene-therapy strategies for the treatment of ischemic heart disease are currently under widespread development, involving gene delivery to the vessel wall, liver and heart. Given the general absence of well-defined genetic defects in the pathogenesis of ischemic heart disease, the potential mechanisms by which gene transfer into these organs might affect the development of ischemic heart disease requires clarification.

The use of gene transfer into the vessel wall for the treatment of ischemic heart disease is based on current models of the pathogenesis of coronary atherosclerosis and thrombosis, models which invoke abnormal vascular gene expression in the etiology of both atherosclerosis and thrombosis. According to a widely held view[7] the pathway leading to coronary atherosclerosis may begin with a nondenuding injury to arterial endothelial cells. This injury initiates a program of pathologic gene expression in the endothelium, resulting in a series of complex vascular-cell responses, local inflammation, smooth-muscle cell and monocyte migration, and extracellular matrix and lipid deposition, leading ultimately to atherosclerosis.[7,8] Local gene transfer into the vessel wall might be undertaken in order to reprogram this pathologic gene expression in particular dysfunctional vascular cells, and thereby reverse or prevent the progression of atherosclerosis.

Focal thrombosis in an atherosclerotic coronary artery may also result from perturbations in vascular-cell gene expression, in the form of deficient endothelial expression of anticoagulant and fibrinolytic molecules such as tissue plasminogen activator[9] or nitric oxide.[10,11] Alternatively, thrombosis might result from local over-expression of procoagulant molecules such as plasminogen activator inhibitor-1[12,13] or tissue factor.[14] In both cases, thrombosis results from an imbalance in pro- and anticoagulant gene expression. Again, local gene transfer into the vessel wall might be used to correct this imbalance.

The above-cited model of atherosclerosis proposes that nondenuding arterial injury caused by stimuli such as hypercholesterolemia both initiate and exacerbate atherosclerosis and thrombosis. It is logical, therefore, to attempt to intervene therapeutically by reducing or eliminating these pathologic stimuli. As the genetic basis of hypercholesterolemia becomes more clearly defined, gene transfer is again becoming recognized as an extremely powerful tool for the treatment of hyper-cholesterolemia. In this case, the target for gene transfer is the liver, the key organ in lipid and lipoprotein metabolism. The therapeutic sequelae of gene transfer are more direct, resulting from direct manipulation of plasma lipid and lipoprotein levels with secondary effects on vessel-wall arteriosclerosis and thrombosis. In comparison to arterial gene transfer, hepatic gene transfer involves a more systemic approach with gene transfer affecting systemic parameters such as plasma cholesterol and specific circulating lipoprotein levels. This strategy, which potentially affects the whole organism rather than specific vascular sites, may be both more powerful and more feasible than widespread arterial gene transfer.

A third gene-transfer approach that may be taken to treat ischemic heart disease is gene transfer into the myocardium to promote the formation of collateral vessels. In this setting, genes that are capable of promoting angiogenesis would be introduced into ischemic areas of myocardium, leading to the formation of collateral vessels that provide these areas with an increased blood supply, effectively bypassing throm-bosed and stenotic epicardial vessels. To achieve this goal, gene transfer would be performed directly into the myocardium rather than into the arteries or liver.

We will discuss some of the advances made in developing gene transfer as a therapeutic approach to ischemic heart disease. Vascular, hepatic and myocardial strategies will be considered and compared as to their current status and future prospects.

Gene transfer into the vessel wall

The vessel wall is the principal site of the proliferative and occlusive lesions that lead to myocardial ischemia and infarction and is therefore a logical target of gene-transfer techniques aimed at the prevention and treatment of ischemic heart disease. Certain features in the development and progression of vascular lesions make gene transfer an attractive therapeutic approach, particularly when contrasted with other currently available therapies. First, atherosclerotic lesions are focal in nature, justifying an approach based on focal delivery of a therapeutic agent. Second, as mentioned above, abnormal gene expression at local vascular sites possibly plays a major role in the development of atherosclerotic coronary artery disease. Given that abnormalities in gene expression may foster local vascular disease, it is logical to attempt both to prevent and to treat vascular disease through the modification of gene expression at the site of vessel-wall pathology.

The local approach to vascular therapy provided by gene transfer may be contrasted to currently employed vascular therapeutic approaches using vasoactive, antithrombotic or interventional strategies. Vasoactive drug treatment regimens consist mainly in oral delivery of agents such as receptor antagonists (e.g. *β*-blockers), vasodilators (e.g. nitrates) and enzyme inhibitors (e.g. angiotensin converting-enzyme inhibitors). These agents are delivered systemically, with accompanying potential for systemic toxicity. In addition, they are not principally targeted at preventing the development of local vascular pathology. As with vasoactive agents, antithrombotic drugs such as heparin and tissue plasminogen activator are also delivered systemically; they are not targeted at specific sites of the vasculature. The systemic toxicities of these two agents, principally increased bleeding, are well known. Finally, mechanical interventional revascularization procedures, while performed locally, are in general palliative in nature and do not attempt to alter basic underlying disease processes.

In contrast to these currently employed therapeutic approaches, vascular gene transfer permits local delivery of therapeutic agents and is theoretically capable of modulating and reversing disease processes at a basic biologic level. With this promise in view, we will discuss present approaches to the delivery of genetic material into the vessel wall.

Methods of vascular gene transfer

Cell-based gene transfer

There are two methods by which new genetic material may be transferred into the vessel wall: (1) indirect, cell-based, *ex vivo* gene transfer and (2) direct, vector-based, *in vivo* gene transfer. Cell-based gene transfer involves transfer of recombinant genes into the vessel wall by implanting cells that have been genetically modified *ex vivo* to express new genetic material. With this approach, cells are harvested from the wall of an explanted peripheral vessel such as a saphenous or jugular vein, modified by insertion of new genetic material *ex vivo*, then reintroduced into the vasculature, either along a denuded vessel or on a prosthetic vascular device.[15–18] The vector-based approach involves the transfer of genetic material directly into the vasculature, obviating the need for cell harvesting and reimplantation.[19–21]

The cell-based approach was common in initial attempts at vascular gene transfer, as it is a direct extension of initial *in vitro* gene-transfer experiments with cultured cells. This approach has certain theoretical advantages over the direct *in vivo* gene-transfer approach:

1. Transfer and expression of the inserted gene can be easily confirmed and can be optimized *in vitro*.
2. The identity of the target cells is more certain since harvested cells can be characterized extensively and purified prior to reimplantation.
3. The potential effect of gene transfer on the target-cell phenotype can be monitored *in vitro* prior to reimplantation.
4. The possibility of ectopic gene transfer into nontarget organs is drastically decreased, and most likely is eliminated entirely.

A cell-based vascular gene-transfer approach, in which the genetically modified cells are implanted onto the surface of denuded vessels, was first described by Nabel *et al.*[19] Endothelial cells were harvested from the jugular vein of a pig, established in culture, and genetically engineered with a retroviral vector to express a β-galactosidase marker gene (expression of this marker gene is easily detected with a specific histochemical stain in which cells expressing the gene turn blue[22]). These genetically marked cells were reimplanted on the surface of balloon-denuded porcine iliofemoral arteries. Initially, a significant percentage of introduced cells (2–11%) successfully attached to the denuded vessel. Appreciable numbers of these initially attached cells (20–100%) remained attached 2–4 weeks following re-establishment of flow, as judged by histochemical staining. In a more recent study, Conte *et al.* reported high-efficiency initial seeding of transduced endothelial cells on denuded rabbit carotids (approximately 90% coverage) but only variable persistence of the transduced cells at 14 days (from zero to over 85% coverage with transduced cells).

A cell-based gene-transfer approach has also been used to introduce genetically modified smooth-muscle cells into the vasculature. Smooth-muscle cells marked with a reporter gene have been introduced into porcine iliofemoral arteries[23] and rat carotid arteries.[24] In the latter experiments, long-term expression of the inserted gene was demonstrated for over one year (Figure 8.1).[25]

A second approach to the transfer of genetically modified vascular cells *in vivo* is to attach the cells to a prosthetic device rather than to the surface of a denuded vessel. This strategy is aimed at improving the performance of the device either by decreasing thrombogenicity or preventing neointimal hyperplasia through the introduction of therapeutic genes. Either endothelial or smooth-muscle cells are

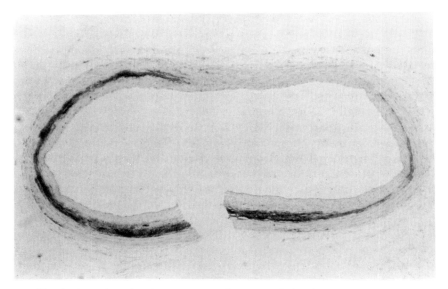

Figure 8.1 Histologic section taken from a rat carotid artery seeded with smooth-muscle cells transduced *ex vivo* with a retroviral vector. This section was taken 12 months after implantation of the cells, which are detected with a histochemical stain for recombinant alkaline phosphatase. The dark band of stained cells within the artery wall confirms persistent recombinant gene expression. (From Clowes, M. M., Lynch, C. M., Miller, A. D. *et al.* (1994) Long-term biological response of injured rat carotid artery seeded with smooth muscle cells expressing retrovirally introduced human genes. *J. Clin. Invest.*, **93**, 649, with permission.)

harvested from explanted vessels, genetically modified *in vitro*, then seeded onto a device which is implanted either within a vessel (in the case of seeded intravascular stents) or between two vessels (in the case of seeded vascular grafts). This approach could eventually be applicable to the placement of stents within the coronary vasculature or the construction of genetically engineered aortocoronary bypass grafts.

Coating of prosthetic devices with genetically modified endothelial cells was first proposed by Wilson *et al.*[15] and Dichek *et al.*[26] In the first of these studies, genetically modified autologous canine endothelial cells were seeded onto Dacron grafts and implanted as carotid interposition grafts. Cell retention was documented by staining for recombinant β-galactosidase expression and confirmed to persist for at least five weeks.[15] In the second study, sheep endothelial cells were modified to express either *Escherichia coli* β-galactosidase (as a marker gene) or human tissue plasminogen activator (as a potential therapeutic agent) and were seeded onto balloon expandable stents *in vitro*. Complete coverage of stent surfaces could be achieved after several days in culture. A subsequent study on seeded stents[27] described the development of a clinically applicable protocol to deliver genetic materials into the vessel using a stent seeded with autologous, genetically modified endothelial cells. In this protocol, endothelial cells were harvested from saphenous veins with survival of donor sheep. Harvested cells were transduced with a retroviral vector containing a marker gene (β-galactosidase) and seeded onto catheter-mounted stents. Examination of the

stents revealed complete coverage of the visible stent surfaces with seeded endothelial cells (Figure 8.2). The stents were deployed in a pulsatile flow system and
exposed to flow at 150 ml min^{-1} for 2 hours. Significant numbers of viable seeded
cells remained on the stent surface as demonstrated by histochemical staining as
well as by recovery of the cells from the stent followed by counting and propagation
in vitro. This study demonstrated that autologous endothelial cells can be harvested,
transduced and seeded onto stents, and that these seeded stents can then be
deployed with significant retention and survival of the seeded cells.

These initial experiments showed that transfer of genetic material into the vessel
wall using a cell-mediated gene-transfer technique is feasible. However, several
factors limit the potential utility of these techniques for the treatment of ischemic
heart disease. First, there is an obligatory time delay from autologous cell harvesting
to the implantation of cells. In the seeded stent studies,[27] the time from cell harvest to
stent deployment was 2–3 months. This time delay was improved upon by Conte
et al. in experiments involving seeding of denuded rabbit vessels;[18] however, the
mean 17-day lag period between cell harvest and implantation reported by these
authors continues to mandate a two-step procedure for local gene transfer: cell
harvest with *in vitro* culture then cell reimplantation.

A major factor necessitating a delay in transduced-cell reimplantation is the
relatively low transduction efficiency of retroviral vectors. Zwiebel *et al.*[28] reported
transduction efficiencies of 0.5–1% in rabbit endothelial cells, as determined by a
neomycin resistance assay. Wilson *et al.*[15] reported a somewhat higher transduction
efficiency of 5–60% as determined by histochemical staining for β-galactosidase. In
our laboratory, the transduction efficiency into a variety of endothelial cells has been
shown initially to be 1–15%; however, improvements in *in vitro* gene transfer
protocols have increased this percentage to 50–90%.[29] Still, in order to obtain
routinely a purified population of 100% retrovirally-transduced endothelial cells,
the use of vectors containing a selectable marker gene (such as the neomycin
phosphotransferase (*neo*) gene) may be required.

While prolonged *in vitro* culture and selection may allow production of a purified
population of transduced cells, this procedure also creates potential hazards. The *in*

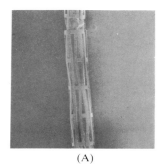
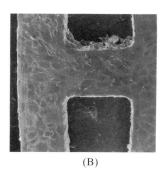
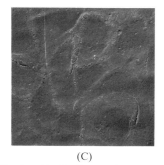

(A)   (B)   (C)

Figure 8.2 Scanning electron micrographs taken at increasing magnification (A–C) of a stainless-steel
intravascular stent seeded with genetically engineered endothelial cells. A confluent layer of endothelial
cells covers the stent surface. (From Flugelman, M. Y., Virmani, R., Leon, M. B. *et al.* (1992) Genetically
engineered endothelial cells remain adherent and viable after stent deployment and exposure to flow *in
vitro*. *Circ. Res.*, **70**, 348, with permission.)

vitro selection period lasts at least 10 days, which places the cells at continued risk of microbial contamination. In addition, both endothelial cells and smooth-muscle cells may develop an altered phenotype during *in vitro* culture,[30–33] which may affect their ability to perform normal cellular functions on return *in vitro*. Reimplantation of dysfunctional cells, expressing genes that might initiate or propagate thrombosis or intimal proliferation, would not be desirable.

Another technical difficulty that potentially limits the success of the reimplantation of genetically modified cells *in vivo* is the achievement of complete coverage of denuded vascular surfaces. This issue is particularly important since the current protocols of cell-based gene transfer onto native vessels require injury to the vessel wall. This vascular injury might result in local thrombosis or hyperplasia as a result of the cell implantation protocol. Relevant to this concern, Conte *et al.* reported the presence of intimal thickening following implantation of endothelial cells along balloon-denuded rabbit arteries.[18] Future studies are needed to address this potential hazard of cell-based arterial gene transfer.

A third potentially problematic aspect of cell-based gene transfer is the loss of either recombinant gene expression or of the transduced cells themselves following cell reimplantation. As mentioned above, the latest time point at which recombinant gene expression from implanted transduced vascular cells has been documented is five weeks. The recent report of Conte *et al.* wherein coverage of seeded vessels decreased from a mean of over 90% at days 4–7 to well below 50% at day 14 suggests that either loss of expression or cell death may be a significant problem. This result contrasts with the 12-month expression data of Clowes *et al.*, mentioned above.[25] Future studies may define the mechanisms by which long-term expression of recombinant genes from transduced, implanted cells may be routinely achieved.

In summary, for the cell-based gene-transfer technique to be useful in the treatment of ischemic heart disease, each of the steps of cell harvest, *in vitro* gene transfer and cell implantation must be optimized and the questions of vessel injury and long-term expression must be addressed. When these technical issues have been satisfactorily resolved, the real challenge – choice of an appropriate therapeutic gene to intervene in the complex biologic processes of atherosclerosis and thrombosis – will begin.

Vector-based gene transfer

Because of the difficulties associated with *ex vivo* gene transfer, many groups have developed direct *in vivo* vascular gene-transfer protocols. The principal clinical advantage of *in vivo* gene transfer is that the same gene-transfer reagent can be prepared in bulk and aliquotted for individual use. This is in contrast to *ex vivo*, cell-based gene transfer in which, because of the potential for rejection, each individual recipient must have cells removed, transduced, then reimplanted. An *in vivo* gene-transfer reagent can potentially be stored like any other drug, then used as needed with no advance cell harvesting, growth and *in vitro* gene transfer. The practical advantages of *in vivo* gene transfer are therefore substantial.

Both viral and nonviral vectors have been used to perform *in vivo* arterial gene transfer. Nonviral methods include naked DNA,[34] liposome–DNA complexes (lipofection)[20,35-37] and liposome–virus–DNA complexes.[38,39] Viral methods include retroviral and adenoviral vectors. Prior to discussing the results of *in vivo* gene-transfer experiments, certain terms need to be standardized. We will use 'efficiency' to denote the number of cells or percentage of target cells into which successful gene transfer has occurred. 'Level of expression' refers to the amount of transgene protein product found following successful gene transfer.

Successful direct *in vivo* gene transfer into the vessel wall was first reported in 1990.[37] Retroviral vectors and lipofection were used to transfer a β-galactosidase reporter gene into pig iliofemoral arteries via a double-balloon catheter (Figure 8.3B). Using this reporter gene, Nabel *et al.*[37] reported evidence of successful *in vivo* gene transfer at time points ranging from 10 days to 21 weeks after introduction of genetic material. Photographs of blue vessels suggested that both high efficiency of gene transfer and high levels of transgene expression were attained in all layers of the vessel wall. The efficiency and level of transgene expression were not specifically measured and quantitated. Subsequent reports of false positivity consequent to use of a cytoplasmic β-galactosidase reporter gene in vascular tissue[20,21,24] as well as the failure of several groups to achieve appreciable levels of gene expression following either retroviral or plasmid-mediated gene transfer[20,36,40] have cast doubt on the efficiency of these vectors.

More quantitative assessments of the efficiency of gene transfer following retro-viral vector-mediated gene transfer and lipofection have been performed by at least two groups. Flugelman *et al.*[21] used a perforated balloon catheter to deliver genetic material into the vessel wall (Figure 8.3A). The authors estimated transduction efficiency using a semiquantitative polymerase chain reaction method following injection of retroviral vectors into the rabbit aorta (Figure 8.4). The number of transduced cells was typically <100 cells in a 2-cm length of a rabbit aorta (approxi-mately 1 in 100 000 cells in the full-thickness rabbit aortic specimens). Leclerc *et al.*[36] used *in situ* hybridization to assess the efficiency of gene transfer following lipofec-tion of atherosclerotic rabbit vessels and estimated the efficiency of gene transfer at fewer than 1 in 1000 cells of the neointima. The overall percentage of transduced cells in the entire vessel wall was certainly lower, given the relatively small percentage of arterial cells in the intima.

These initial studies suggested that retroviral vector-mediated gene transfer and lipofection into the vessel wall are extremely inefficient and the level of transgene expression consequent to these procedures is low. Several factors might explain both the low efficiency of *in vivo* arterial gene transfer by retroviral vectors and the low likelihood that this can easily be improved upon. Retrovirus-mediated gene transfer requires actively dividing cells for integration and expression of the viral genome.[41] Estimates of the percentage of proliferating cells in the normal vessel wall are in the range 0.01–0.1%.[42,43] In addition, retroviral virions can be propagated only to moderately high titers (10^5–10^7 infectious virions ml^{-1}, compared to 10^{11} to 10^{12} for adenovirus vectors; see below). Finally, retrovirus is rapidly inactivated by complement-mediated processes in primates *in vivo*,[44,45] a phenomenon that may limit the extension of any successful animal protocols to the level of human studies. Reasons for the inefficiency of *in vivo* liposome-mediated gene transfer are less clear.

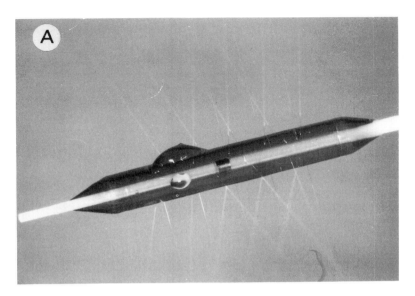

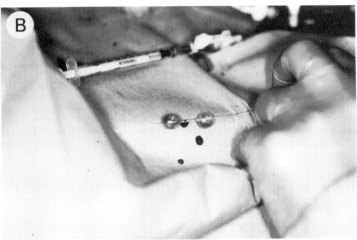

Figure 8.3 (A) Tip of a porous balloon catheter, with dye injected through the balloon. The two oval masses on the catheter surface are drops of liquid. The catheter surface is uniformly smooth. (B) A double-balloon infusion catheter. The balloons are inflated and dye is injected out the port between the balloons. When deployed *in vivo* the balloons occlude the arterial lumen and isolate a segment of artery into which a gene-transfer solution can be infused. (From Dichek, D. A. (1994) Interventional approaches to the introduction of genetic material into the vasculature. In: Topol, E. J. (ed.) *Textbook of Interventional Cardiology*, vol. 2, pp. 991, 998. Philadelphia: Saunders, with permission.)

Concerted efforts of several groups to obtain high-level, reproducible, liposome-mediated arterial gene transfer have not yet been successful.[20,34,36,40]

The deficiencies of retroviral vector- and liposome-mediated gene transfer have led to new approaches to optimize both transduction efficiency and the level of

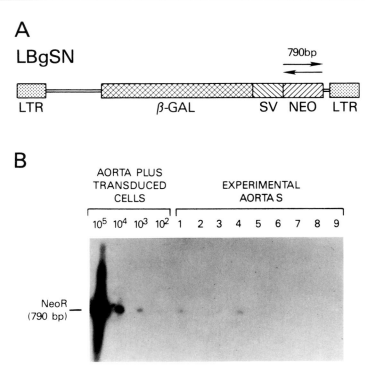

Figure 8.4 Detection of direct *in vivo* retroviral vector-mediated gene transfer by the polymerase chain reaction. A 790 basepair sequence contained in the neomycin phosphotransferase gene was amplified from DNA extracted from arteries subjected to gene transfer with the LBgSN vector.[29] Southern blotting and detection with a cDNA probe, and comparison with a standard curve constructed with known numbers of transduced cells permits a semiquantitative assessment of the efficiency of *in vivo* gene transfer. Approximately 100–1000 transduced cells are present in experimental aortas 1, 3 and 4. This experiment was repeated several times, with positive amplifications typically giving bands indicative of the presence of fewer than 100 cells per vessel. (From Dichek, D. A. (1994) Interventional approaches to the introduction of genetic material into the vasculature. In: Topol, E. J. (ed.) *Textbook of Interventional Cardiology*, vol. 2, p. 2000. Philadelphia: Saunders, with permission.)

recombinant gene expression. The use of two new vector systems, 'HVJ–liposome' complexes and adenoviral vectors, has generated much exciting *in vivo* vascular gene-transfer data.

HVJ–liposome-mediated gene transfer

HVJ–liposome-mediated gene transfer (named after the hemagglutinating virus of Japan, HVJ) was first described by Kaneda *et al.*[46] for *in vitro* and *in vivo* transfection of hepatocytes. This technique takes advantages of properties of HVJ viral envelope proteins that permit associated DNA to escape endosomal degradation. Additional incorporation of high mobility group-1 nuclear protein into the HVJ–liposome complex facilitates targeting of the DNA to the nucleus, once the DNA has escaped from the endosome. Morishita *et al.* first described use of this method in vascular cells both *in vitro*[47] and *in vivo*.[38] The efficiency of HVJ–liposome-mediated gene transfer was reported to be 10-fold greater than that attained with cationic liposomes alone. In injured and noninjured rat carotid arteries, a plasmid expressing the SV40 large T antigen was introduced into the vessel wall using the HVJ–liposome system. Successful gene transfer was documented by immunohistochemical staining. At one week after transduction, 9 of 11 injured and 7 of 11 noninjured experimental arteries still showed evidence of transgene expression. The efficiency and level of transgene expression were not, however, reported.

While these initial studies suggest that HVJ–liposome-mediated gene transfer may be a very useful technique for direct arterial *in vivo* transfer, it will be important to obtain more extensive quantitative assessments of recombinant gene expression following HVJ–liposome-mediated gene transfer. In addition, the duration of expression following *in vivo* gene transfer requires further definition. Finally, it will be important to address the possibility of a host immune response to the viral proteins.

Recombinant adenoviral vectors

Recombinant adenoviral vectors are a second vector system capable of highly efficient *in vivo* arterial gene transfer. Adenoviral vectors have a wide range of target-cell tropism and have been shown to be efficient at transferring genetic material into many target organs *in vivo* including lungs,[48] liver[49,50] and brain.[51–53] Unlike retroviruses, adenoviral vectors do not require active replication of target cells for infection, and can be propagated and concentrated to very high titers. Since the vessel wall is composed largely of quiescent cells[42,43] and only small volumes of vector-containing solutions can be placed in proximity to the vessel wall, adenoviral vectors are well suited for direct *in vivo* arterial gene transfer.

Adenoviral vector-mediated gene transfer into vascular cells was first reported by Lemarchand *et al.*[54] Human umbilical veins were exposed to adenoviral vectors containing either a β-galactosidase reporter gene, a human α_1-antitrypsin gene or a human cystic fibrosis transmembrane conductance regulator gene. More recently, this same group extended their *in vitro* findings by performing adenoviral vector-mediated gene transfer *in vivo*.[55] Normal sheep jugular veins and carotid arteries were surgically exposed and infused with adenoviral vectors. Highly efficient gene transfer to the luminal endothelium was demonstrated by histochemical staining and recombinant gene expression was further documented by Northern analysis and by immunoprecipitation of secreted α_1-antitrypsin.

These initial findings of high-efficiency adenovirus-mediated arterial gene transfer were extended to injured arteries by our group.[56] In the first of these studies, balloon-injured rat carotid arteries were infused with an adenoviral vector expressing a nuclear targeted β-galactosidase marker gene (Figure 8.5). The efficiency of gene transfer into medial smooth-muscle cells was approximately 30%, as determined by histochemical staining. The level of transgene expression was quantitated by measuring the amount of β-galactosidase antigen and activity in tissue extracts (Figure 8.6). Recombinant β-galactosidase was present in tissue extracts at approximately 100 ng mg^{-1} of protein or 25 ng per 10 mm segment of rat carotid artery. This level of expression was at least two-to-three orders of magnitude higher than that previously reported for liposome-mediated gene transfer, and resulted in recombinant protein levels that were similar to those of certain endogenous arterial proteins,

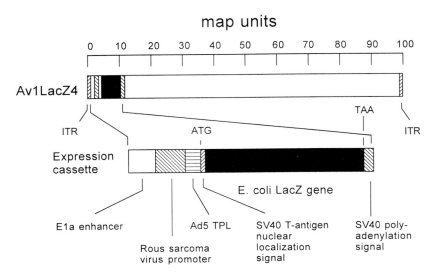

Figure 8.5   The Av1LacZ4 adenoviral vector, used in arterial gene transfer studies. The vector (provided by Genetic Therapy Incorporated, Gaithersburg, MD, USA) was generated by homologous recombination between a plasmid containing the expression cassette (lower part of figure) and an adenovirus 5 deletion mutant, Ad d1327. Important structural features of the vector are labeled: ITR, inverted terminal repeats; E1a enhancer, enhancer sequences preceding the viral *E1a* gene; Ad5 TPL, adenovirus 5 tripartite leader; SV40, simian virus-40. The start (ATG) and stop codons (TAA) of the *Escherichia coli β*-galactosidase gene '*E. coli lacZ* gene' are indicated. The *lacZ* gene has been modified by addition of sequences from the SV40 T-antigen nuclear localization signal so that expression of the protein is directed to the target-cell nucleus. (From Lee, S. W., Trapnell, B. C., Rade, J. J. *et al*. (1993) *In vivo* adenoviral vector-mediated gene transfer into balloon-injured rat carotid arteries. *Circ. Res.*, **73**, 802, with permission.)

including tissue plasminogen activator and basic fibroblast growth factor.[56] In a subsequent study, Guzman *et al.*[57] reported *in vivo* adenovirus-mediated gene transfer of apparently similar efficiency into the neointima of previously injured rat carotid arteries. Taken together, these experiments demonstrated that high levels of both transgene expression and transduction efficiency can be achieved using adenoviral vector-mediated gene transfer. For the first time *in vivo* gene transfer appeared to be sufficiently efficient that one might reasonably contemplate the introduction of therapeutic genes into the vessel wall.

Critical issues in vascular gene transfer: target cells, duration of expression, safety

Three issues have emerged in the development of *in vivo* vascular gene-transfer approaches, each of which is critical to consider in the design of gene-therapy strategies for the treatment of ischemic heart disease: (1) identification of the location and identity of the cellular targets of gene transfer, (2) duration of expression and (3) safety concerns.

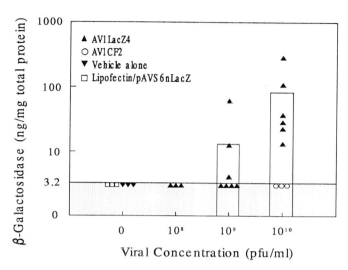

Figure 8.6 β-galactosidase antigen expression following *in vivo* gene transfer. Injured rat carotid arteries were exposed to either increasing concentrations of a β-galactosidase-containing adenoviral vector (Av1LacZ4), vehicle alone, Lipofectin®–plasmid DNA complex or an adenoviral vector (Av1Cf2) expressing the human cystic fibrosis transmembrane conductance regulator (at a concentration of 10^{10} pfu ml^{-1}). At 3 days after transduction, β-galactosidase expression was measured from tissue lysate using an ELISA. Each data point represents a single animal. Bars indicate the mean β-galactosidase antigen in each group. (From Lee, S. W., Trapnell, B. C., Rade, J. J. *et al.* (1993) *In vivo* adenoviral vector-mediated gene transfer into balloon-injured rat carotid arteries. *Circ. Res.*, **73**, 802, with permission.)

Gene-transfer cellular targets

Potential target cells in the normal vessel wall include endothelial cells in the intima, smooth-muscle cells in the media and several cell types in the adventitia including endothelial cells and fibroblasts. Initial studies using a cytoplasmic β-galactosidase reporter gene identified gene transfer into all layers of the vessel wall.[37] This report could not be independently confirmed due to widespread problems with false positivity using the cytoplasmic β-galactosidase reporter gene. These problems forced many groups to use a luciferase reporter gene; however, since expression of luciferase is not detectable histochemically, the location of the transduced cells remained unclear.[20,34,36,40]

The advent of more reliable histochemical markers of recombinant gene expression such as nuclear-targeted β-galactosidase[58] and alkaline phosphatase[25] has permitted confident identification of transduced cells while eliminating concerns of false positivity. Use of these reporter genes has yielded the following general conclusions regarding the location of gene transfer:

1. Gene transfer into normal arteries results predominantly in expression in luminal endothelial cells.[58,59] If branch vessels and vasa vasorum are present, gene transfer and expression can be found in the adventitia as well.[58]
2. In balloon-injured normal vessels, gene transfer occurs in smooth-muscle cells in the superficial layers of the media, which are exposed secondary to denudation of the endothelium.[59,60] If the media of a denuded artery is very thin (for

example in the rat carotid there are only three or four layers of medial smooth-muscle cells), or alternatively if a high-pressure porous balloon catheter is used to infuse vectors into a thicker artery, then gene transfer and expression can occur throughout the full thickness of the media.[56,58]
3. In vessels in which a neointima is present, gene transfer and expression occurs primarily in the neointima.[36,57]

These findings suggest that arterial anatomy may impose important constraints on the delivery of genetic material to vascular cells. Vectors do not appear to penetrate the arterial wall indiscriminately; they follow the path of least resistance and do not routinely accumulate and transduce cells in all three layers of the vessel wall. The distribution of gene transfer in severely diseased arteries (with calcified plaques, cholesterol deposits and neovascularization) is likely to be even more complex. Factors that may influence the distribution of gene transfer into diseased arteries will likely include the presence of branch vessels, the thickness of the neointima, the presence or absence of denuding injury and the type of catheter used to infuse the gene-transfer reagent, particularly the amount of pressure used to drive the infusion. It is not likely that any presently described technique will achieve evenly distributed gene transfer into all layers of the vessel wall. Data generated by attempts at gene transfer in animal models of severe coronary pathology will be extremely valuable in the design of future gene-therapy protocols involving atherosclerotic human coronary arteries.

Duration of expression

Duration of expression following *in vivo* gene transfer is another critical issue to be considered in the design of vascular gene-transfer approaches. While it may be argued that short-term recombinant gene expression is sufficient for the prevention of restenosis after angioplasty (which occurs over a defined time period of weeks to months), it would seem that a therapy aimed at prevention or correction of ischemic heart disease would be required to persist for decades. It is in this context that duration of expression data should be critically evaluated. Theoretically, vectors that result in chromosomal integration into target-cell genome, such as retroviral vectors, should offer the most persistent gene expression, while vectors that do not integrate, such as plasmids and adenoviral vectors, should result in a shorter duration of expression, particularly in dividing cells in which nonchromosomal DNA is diluted with each cell division.

Initial data on duration of expression following *in vivo* gene transfer is found in the work of Nabel *et al.*[37] These authors reported *in vivo* expression of retrovirally encoded β-galactosidase for up to 21 weeks following infection. Other studies using retroviral vectors either did not address the issue of duration of expression[21] or even failed completely to show evidence of gene transfer.[24] Virtually no groups are currently reporting data using retroviral vectors for vascular gene transfer, most likely because the efficiency of *in vivo* retrovirus-mediated gene transfer is so low. Therefore, the issue of duration of expression of retroviral vectors is somewhat moot in the arterial gene-transfer field.

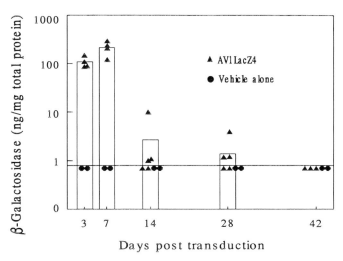

Figure 8.7 Duration of β-galactosidase expression following *in vivo* gene transfer. Injured rat carotid arteries were exposed to either a β-galactosidase-containing adenoviral vector (Av1LacZ4 at a concentration of 10^{10} pfu ml^{-1}) or to vehicle alone. At the indicated number of days following transduction, levels of β-galactosidase antigen were measured in carotid artery lysates. Antigen levels are expressed as ng mg total protein^{-1} in the tissue extracts. Each data point represents a single animal. Bars indicate the mean β-galactosidase expression in each group. The lower limit of detection of the β-galactosidase antigen in the experiments illustrated in this figure was 0.7 ng mg^{-1}. (From Lee, S. W., Trapnell, B. C., Rade, J. J. *et al.* (1993) *In vivo* adenoviral vector-mediated gene transfer into balloon-injured rat carotid arteries. *Circ. Res.*, **73**, 802, with permission.)

Several groups have reported data on the duration of expression following liposome-mediated gene transfer. Nabel *et al.* reported *in vivo* expression of β-galactosidase for up to six weeks following lipofection of plasmids.[37] Subsequent studies, using the more reliable luciferase reporter gene, have reported shorter-term expression, limited to a few days to 2–3 weeks.[36,40] It is likely that *in vivo* expression following plasmid-mediated gene transfer into blood vessels is transient.

In vivo expression following adenovirus-mediated vascular gene transfer also appears to be transient. Lemarchand *et al.*[55] reported expression of α_1-antitrypsin at 1–14 days, but not at 28 days following gene transfer. Our studies of duration of expression following adenoviral vector-mediated gene transfer[56,61] produced similar data. Expression of β-galactosidase in either injured rat carotids or noninjured sheep carotids peaked at 3–7 days and declined rapidly to background levels by 42 days following gene transfer (Figure 8.7). In summary no vector system is yet capable of achieving measurable levels of long-term expression following *in vivo* gene transfer into the adult vasculature.

Safety

A final issue that must be considered in the design of vascular gene therapy protocols is safety. Potential complications and toxic effects can occur locally at the site of gene transfer as well as systemically. Local toxicity due to gene transfer into the vessel wall might include direct vascular injury leading to focal vascular proliferation, stenosis, thrombosis – and in extreme cases – vascular perforation as well as unexpected pathogenic effects of expression of the transferred gene.

Direct vascular injury could potentially occur from the vector/vehicle preparation itself or from the catheter used to deliver the vector. For example, liposomes are quite toxic to vascular cells when delivered *in vitro* and might also be toxic *in vivo*. Adenoviral vector-mediated gene transfer at high multiplicity of infection *in vitro* also causes significant acute cell death. Preliminary observations in our laboratory indicate this may also be true *in vivo*.[56] Catheter-induced injury during gene delivery was documented by Flugelman *et al.*,[21] who reported focal excavations of the vessel wall following *in vivo* gene transfer using the porous balloon catheter. In addition to these potentially deleterious effects of gene-delivery systems, vascular injury might be caused by the expression of specific transgenes that are intended to be therapeutic. For example, antiproliferative molecules could possibly interfere with normal growth and repair processes, as was found by Casscells *et al.* following the infusion of an antiproliferative toxin into injured rat arterial walls.[62] Overall, the issue of potential local toxicity should not be ignored in the development of arterial gene-therapy protocols.

Few data are available regarding potential systemic toxicities and side effects of arterial gene transfer. Barr *et al.* reported evidence of systemic gene transfer following intracoronary infusion of adenoviral vectors. Vector DNA was found in the brain, testes and several other organs.[63] Data from *in vivo* gene transfer performed in other organ systems is also informative. Roessler *et al.* reported a systemic immune response both to adenoviral antigens and to an inserted β-galactosidase transgene following synovial gene transfer in rabbits.[64] Yang *et al.* reported hepatitis, hepatic necrosis and a systemic cellular immune response to adenoviral antigens following intrabiliary infusion of adenoviral vectors.[65] Injection of replication-competent retrovirus into immune-compromised monkeys resulted in T-cell lymphoma, due most likely to activation of oncogenes following integration of the retrovirus into chromosomal DNA.[66] While this scenario is far less likely with adenovirus-based vectors, which integrate only at a very low frequency, it is not impossible. As the therapeutic potential of direct *in vivo* gene transfer becomes more apparent and specific therapeutic genes are identified and introduced, a more extensive assessment of local and systemic toxicity of gene transfer will be appropriate.

Thrombosis: a specific target for vascular gene transfer

Thrombus formation plays an important role in the generation and progression of atherosclerotic plaques and acute coronary syndromes. Recurrent plaque rupture and thrombus formation is thought to lead to rapid progression of plaques.[67] Acute coronary syndromes such as unstable angina or acute myocardial infarction are thought to be primarily due to formation of thrombus on a ruptured plaque. In accordance with the pivotal role of thrombosis in the pathogenesis of myocardial ischemia and infarction, current pharmacologic strategies for both the prevention and treatment of myocardial infarction rely heavily on the systemic administration of antithrombotic and fibrinolytic drugs such as aspirin, heparin and tissue plasminogen activator (t-PA).

The systemic administration of antithrombotic and fibrinolytic drugs is associated with systemic side effects, most notably bleeding. Gene transfer provides a unique means to deliver antithrombotic or fibrinolytic agents to a site that is prone to thrombosis without creating systemic complications. If an antithrombotic or fibrinolytic agent could be delivered to a segment of the vasculature by means of gene transfer either proximal to, or within, that segment, then this agent would be in highest concentration at the point at which it is most required. Distal to this site, the agent would be diluted in the total blood volume, most likely to a point below which any side effects would be found. It should be emphasized that this local gene-transfer approach is not intended as a therapy for acute myocardial infarction, in which an occluding thrombus is most appropriately treated with an immediate systemic dose of a thrombolytic agent. Rather, the gene-transfer approach proposes that continuous local delivery might shift the balance between coagulation and fibrinolysis sufficiently that progression of plaques is retarded and occlusive thrombi never form.

Efforts to develop a focal gene-transfer approach to the prevention of intravascular thrombosis have focused on the development of vectors expressing recombinant plasminogen activators. A retroviral vector expressing human t-PA was used to transduce sheep,[68] bovine[69] and human[70] endothelial cells *in vitro*. In all cases, increased t-PA production was measured, demonstrating the feasibility of a strategy that increases plasminogen activator production by gene transfer.

These initial studies on overexpression of t-PA from endothelial cells revealed substantial binding and inactivation of the recombinant t-PA by endothelial-derived plasminogen activator inhibitor type 1 (PAI-1). Because of a concern that PAI-1 might limit the effectiveness of recombinant plasminogen activators *in vivo*, vectors were designed that expressed single-chain urokinase, a plasminogen activator that is resistant to PAI-1. Retroviral vectors were constructed that expressed both wild-type single-chain urokinase and a novel form of urokinase that was anchored to the apical endothelial cell surface so as to achieve particularly high concentrations of plasminogen activator activity at the cell surface.[71] Localization of plasminogen activators to the cell surface has certain theoretical advantages over secreted plasminogen activators:

1. Plasminogen activators that are attached to the cell surface would not be cleared from the site of production by blood flow.
2. Cell-surface localization would potentially permit optimal interactions with other components of the cell-surface fibrinolytic system, particularly bound plasminogen.[72–74]
3. Cell-surface localization could confine particularly high concentrations of plasminogen activators to a specific site and thereby might limit systemic fibrinolysis.

To achieve cell-surface localization of a plasminogen activator, we constructed a single-chain urokinase molecule fused to a carboxyl terminal glycolipid anchoring signal (Figure 8.8).[71] When this recombinant urokinase molecule was expressed in endothelial cells, it was targeted to the apical cell surface. *In vitro* testing of this recombinant anchored urokinase revealed enhancement of cell-associated fibrino-lytic activity not only due to the high concentration of cell-surface urokinase (1×10^6 molecules cell^{-1}) but also due to favorable interactions of the anchored urokinase molecule with cell-surface plasminogen.[75] This anchored single-chain urokinase molecule might be expressed by a gene-transfer strategy on the surface of endo-thelial cells near an area prone to thrombosis. When plasmin is generated in the setting of early thrombus formation, the accumulated single-chain urokinase would be activated to the enzymatically active two chain urokinase and might significantly enhance local fibrinolysis. While *in vivo* studies will be required to demonstrate that this salutary chain of events will indeed occur, the possibility that a fibrinolytic proenzyme could be stored on the luminal endothelial surface of a blood vessel to be activated following the initiation of thrombus formation is theoretically attractive.

Other groups have also reported results of attempts to prevent thrombosis by gene-transfer strategies. Podrazik *et al.*[76] demonstrated high-level t-PA secretion following retroviral vector-mediated transfer of a human t-PA cDNA into canine endothelial cells. Eskin *et al.* found antithrombotic effects following implantation of canine endothelial cells expressing a mutant form of t-PA.[77] An antithrombotic gene-transfer strategy involving overproduction of prostacyclin was reported by Xu *et al.*,[78] showing a significant increase in prostacyclin secretion by endothelial cells consequent to retroviral vector-mediated expression of prostaglandin H synthase. A preliminary report[79] extends these findings *in vivo*, also reporting an antithrombotic effect. Rade *et al.*[80] expressed hirudin, a potent inhibitor of thrombin, in endothelial cells by both retroviral and adenoviral vector-mediated gene transfer. These data are particularly noteworthy as thrombin may play a role in the progression of vascular lesion formation[81] in addition to its well-known role in thrombus formation.

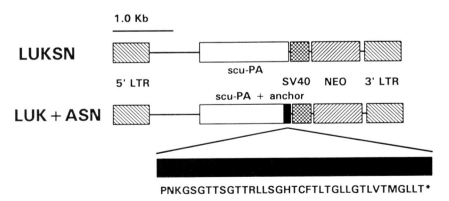

Figure 8.8 Retroviral vectors LUKSN, containing a wild-type scu-PA cDNA and LUK + ASN, containing a scu-PA cDNA fused to a membrane anchoring signal at the carboxyl terminus. The amino acid sequence of this anchoring signal is given, using single-letter symbols; ∗ = Stop. The early promoter of simian virus-40 (SV40), the neomycin phosphotransferase gene (NEO), and the 5′ and 3′ viral long terminal repeats (LTR) are shown. Approximate size is shown in kilobases (kb). (From Lee, S. W., Kahn, M. L. and Dichek, D. A. (1992) Expression of an anchored urokinase in the apical endothelial cell membrane. *J. Biol. Chem.*, **267**, 13020–7, with permission.)

In summary, thrombosis is an attractive target for vascular gene-transfer strategies designed to combat ischemic heart disease. Several groups have proposed the transfer of candidate molecules into the vessel wall for the purpose of preventing thrombus formation or enhancing fibrinolysis. Initial *in vitro* studies have documented the feasibility of increasing both fibrinolytic and antithrombotic activity, and preliminary *in vivo* data are promising. The challenge for the future, in applying this approach to the prevention of ischemic and thrombotic heart disease, will be the efficient introduction of therapeutic genes into the coronary vasculature and the careful testing of the ability of these genes to prevent plaque progression and coronary thrombosis.

Hepatic gene transfer for manipulation of plasma lipids and lipoproteins

Hypercholesterolemia plays a role both in the initiation and progression of atherosclerosis. The importance of hypercholesterolemia in the pathogenesis of coronary artery disease and the massive amount of data supporting efforts to reduce cholesterol as a means of preventing or reversing coronary artery disease are summarized elsewhere.[82]

As the genetic basis of hypercholesterolemia becomes more clearly defined, gene transfer is becoming recognized as an extremely powerful tool for reprogramming the genes that control cholesterol metabolism, thereby treating hypercholesterolemia at its source. The liver is the principal organ involved in lipid, lipoprotein, and cholesterol metabolism; therefore gene-therapy strategies for the treatment of hypercholesterolemia make use of liver-directed gene-transfer approaches. To date, these approaches have involved attempts both to decrease low-density lipoprotein (LDL) cholesterol and increase high-density lipoprotein (HDL) cholesterol.

Initial gene-therapy efforts to lower plasma LDL have focused on extreme cases of LDL elevation, specifically in the case of homozygous LDL-receptor deficiency. When present in humans, homozygous LDL-receptor deficiency is known as familial hypercholesterolemia and is associated with severe coronary artery disease before the age of 10 years.[83,84] There is no adequate medical or surgical therapy for this condition, therefore raising the exciting possibility that gene-transfer techniques might provide a uniquely successful therapeutic approach.

Initial gene-therapy studies for the treatment of homozygous LDL-receptor deficiency have been performed in authentic animal models of the disease (rabbits[85] and mice[86]). Wilson *et al.* first reported successful correction of LDL-receptor deficiency in rabbit hepatocytes *in vitro* by retroviral vector-mediated gene transfer.[85] A subsequent study by Chowdhury *et al.* extended these findings *in vivo*.[87] In these *in vivo* studies, autologous rabbit hepatocytes were harvested, transduced *in vitro* with a retroviral vector expressing the rabbit LDL receptor and infused into the spleens of the donor rabbits. Migration of the infused hepatocytes into the liver via the portal circulation was documented, and successful implantation of viable genetically modified hepatocytes was demonstrated by ribonuclease protection assay. Transplantation of hepatocytes expressing LDL receptors resulted in a

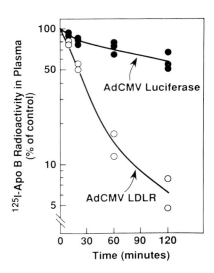

Figure 8.9   Disappearance of labeled very low-density lipoprotein (VLDL) cholesterol from the circulation of LDL-receptor-deficient mice after treatment with an adenoviral vector expressing a human LDL-receptor cDNA (AdCMV LDLR) or a luciferase cDNA, as a control (AdCMV luciferase). There is rapid clearance of VLDL in mice treated with the adenoviral vector expressing a human LDL-receptor cDNA. (From Ishibashi, S., Brown, M. S., Goldstein, J. L. *et al*. (1993) Hypercholesterolemia in low density lipoprotein receptor knockout mice and its reversal by adenovirus-mediated gene delivery. *J. Clin. Invest.*, **92**, 883, with permission.)

lowering of total serum cholesterol to approximately 30–50% of pretreatment values for up to 120 days after infusion.

More recently, Ishibashi *et al.* described the use of a 'knockout' mouse model of homozygous LDL-receptor deficiency to demonstrate the capacity of *in vivo* adenoviral-mediated gene transfer to reverse this genetically based form of hypercholesterolemia. The rate of clearance of VLDL from the circulation, which is severely impaired consequent to the absence of LDL receptors, was returned essentially to normal four days after injection of an adenoviral vector expressing a mouse LDL-receptor cDNA (Figure 8.9). In addition, the lipoprotein cholesterol profiles of the mice receiving this gene therapy demonstrated a dramatic shift towards normal, with a large predominance of HDL over LDL cholesterol.

Perhaps of greater relevance to the potential for human gene therapy for hypercholesterolemia, Herz and Gerard used a similar technique of adenovirus-mediated gene transfer to demonstrate an increase in LDL clearance and a decrease in plasma cholesterol in normal mice.[50] The possibility that gene transfer might be capable of altering cholesterol levels in humans without a known genetic defect widens the therapeutic potential of this tool immensely.

The feasibility of LDL-receptor gene transfer for the treatment of human familial hypercholesterolemia was demonstrated by Grossman *et al.*, who used an *ex vivo* retrovirus-mediated gene-therapy strategy, with subsequent reinfusion of transduced hepatocytes, to express functional LDL receptors in a patient with the condition.[88] Four months after gene therapy, percutaneous liver biopsy and *in situ* hybridization confirmed the presence of the normal LDL-receptor transgene. LDL

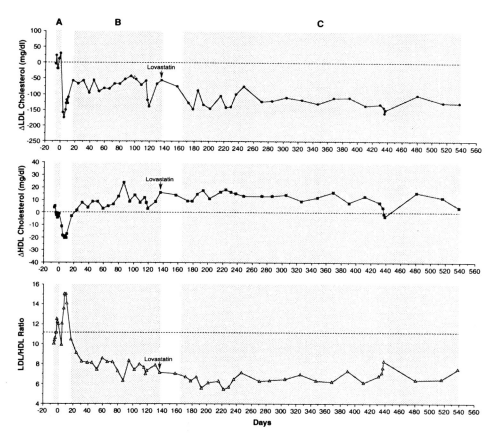

Figure 8.10 Lipid profiles of a patient with familial hypercholesterolemia following *ex vivo* gene therapy. Period A represents a period prior to gene therapy. Period B represents a 131-day interval after gene therapy, prior to institution of lovastatin therapy. Period C represents a 15-month interval following period B during which the patient was treated with lovastatin. The top panel illustrates change in the level of LDL from the baseline level, the middle panel the level of HDL and the bottom panel the ratio of LDL to HDL cholesterol. (From Grossman M., Raper, S. E., Kozarsky, K. *et al.* (1994) Successful *ex vivo* gene therapy directed to liver in a patient with familial hypercholesterolaemia. *Nature-Genetics*, **6**, 335, with permission.)

cholesterol dropped by approximately $100\,\mathrm{mg\,dl^{-1}}$ and HDL increased by 10–$20\,\mathrm{mg\,dl^{-1}}$ (Figure 8.10). The LDL:HDL ratio dropped from 10:13 to 5:8, which would predict a significant decrease in cardiovascular risk. In accordance with this, the authors reported that the patient's coronary artery disease did not progress during the 18-month study period, as evaluated by serial angiography. This pioneering study, the first to demonstrate long-term phenotypic amelioration of a genetic defect in a human following gene transfer, reveals the tremendous potential of gene therapy to alter the incidence and the course of coronary artery disease.

While most groups interested in gene therapy for hyperlipidemia have focused on LDL-receptor gene transfer, others have proposed a second, potentially complementary approach: overexpression of apolipoprotein AI (ApoAI). ApoAI is the major lipoprotein component of plasma HDL, and epidemiologic studies have revealed an inverse correlation between HDL levels and risk for coronary artery disease.[89,90] The protective action of HDL may be mediated through enhanced reverse cholesterol transport. While the potential protective effect of high levels of HDL is evident, potential means for reliably modifying this level in humans have been difficult to identify. Again, as with the LDL receptor for decreasing LDL cholesterol, gene transfer may provide the key technology to increase levels of HDL.

An experimental approach to genetic manipulation of ApoAI levels was first reported by Rubin et al.[91] A strain of mice with a hereditary susceptibility to diet-induced atherosclerosis was used to generate lines of mice that were transgenic with a human ApoAI allele. These transgenic mice had elevations of plasma HDL, and were significantly protected from diet-induced fatty streak formation. Aortic fatty-streak lesions were completely absent in transgenic mice fed a moderately atherogenic diet, and were reduced by seven-fold in mice placed on a more atherogenic diet. While it is important to note that this study addresses only the formation of early fatty-streak lesions, it is intriguing to speculate that manipulation of ApoAI levels in adults might retard, or even reverse, the progression of more advanced atherosclerotic lesions. Further data that address this possibility will be of great interest.

Human ApoAI and HDL levels are clearly not amenable to manipulation by germline transgenic technology, for both ethical and practical reasons. However, *somatic* transgenic manipulations are already being applied to the treatment of human disease. The work on LDL-receptor gene transfer in familial hypercholesterolemia discussed above provides the most relevant example of human somatic-cell gene therapy. A recent report by Kopfler et al.[92] suggests that somatic gene transfer may eventually be an effective way to increase HDL levels in humans. These workers used a recombinant adenovirus to transfer a human ApoAI cDNA into the livers of mice. Plasma ApoAI and HDL levels were significantly elevated (35% increase for HDL) to levels adequate to be associated with a decreased cardiovascular risk. As with other *in vivo* studies using first-generation adenoviral vectors, however, expression was transient with a loss of both RNA and protein expression by 2–3 weeks. Longer-term expression will be required to assess the potential of ApoAI gene transfer to affect the development or progression of atherosclerosis.

In summary, somatic-cell gene transfer of genes that control lipid metabolism is already being used as a therapeutic tool in humans, at least partially with the goal of retarding the progression of the severe ischemic heart disease associated with familial hypercholesterolemia. The technical aspects of this particular therapeutic protocol are daunting, however, involving partial hepatectomy, massive *in vitro* manipulation of harvested hepatocytes and a prolonged hospital stay. If gene therapy for lipid abnormalities is to become a widespread clinical tool, then more simple gene-transfer protocols will be required. Injectable vectors such as the adenovirus are promising agents for *in vivo* gene transfer, but are currently not appropriate for human use for two principal reasons:

1. Both humoral and cellular immune responses to the vector and inserted transgenes, with associated hepatitis, have been reported following adenoviral vector injection.[64,65]

2. Expression is transient, so that it is has not yet been possible either to examine long-term vector safety profiles or to demonstrate long-term effects of vector-encoded transgenes on atherosclerosis progression.

Given that atherosclerosis has a time course of decades, the development and testing of vector systems that can convincingly modify atherosclerotic risk in the general population represents a significant and exciting challenge.

Gene transfer into the myocardium for the enhancement of collateral formation

A third potential target of gene-transfer strategies for the treatment of ischemic heart disease is the myocardium itself. The viability and function of the myocardium in the setting of severe coronary stenoses and occlusions is highly dependent on the presence of collateral vessels. The importance of the coronary collateral circulation is highlighted by studies demonstrating that the presence of collateral circulation at the time of myocardial infarction is associated with improved patient survival[93] as well as preservation of left-ventricular function and viability.[94-97]

Extreme examples of the value of coronary collateral vessels are provided by patients who are found at catheterization to have complete coronary occlusions but who have no evidence of myocardial infarction or left-ventricular dysfunction. In many of these cases, myocardial ischemia can be identified with provocative techniques, demonstrating that the collateral circulation is not able to compensate completely for the occluded arteries. In both these patients and in those with subtotal occlusions, aortocoronary artery bypass surgery is often performed to create new collaterals to the ischemic areas. The molecular approach to myocardial ischemia proposes to create these collaterals with a biochemical or genetic rather than a surgical approach.

Yanagisawa-Miwa *et al.* were the first to demonstrate beneficial effects consequent to the injection of an angiogenic growth factor into the coronary circulation.[98] Recombinant human basic fibroblast growth factor (bFGF) was infused into the left circumflex coronary artery of dogs following experimental occlusion of the left anterior descending artery. One week later, dogs that had received the growth factor had relatively preserved left-ventricular function, decreased infarct size and an increased density of capillaries and arterioles in the peri-infarct area. These findings were extended by Unger and colleagues, who demonstrated that intracoronary infusion of either bFGF or the related angiogenic peptide vascular endothelial cell growth factor (VEGF) in a canine model of ischemia (rather than infarction) also increased both collateral flow and density of distribution vessels in the ischemic zone.[99,100] While promising, these protocols have a practical limitation of requiring continuous physical access to the coronary circulation for several weeks. For this reason, delivery of genes to the myocardium with consequent synthesis and release of angiogenic factors *in situ* offers an attractive alternative approach. This approach may indeed be simply an application of a lesson of nature. The successful extraction of an angiogenic factor from infarcted human myocardial tissue[101] suggests that

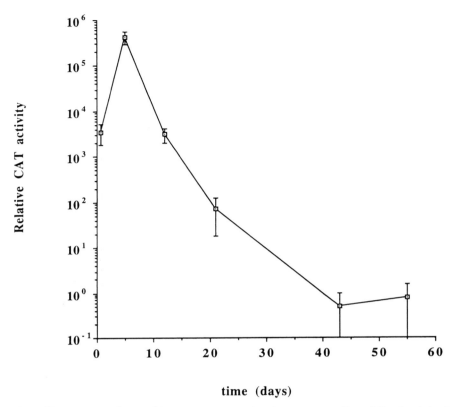

Figure 8.11 Time course of recombinant gene expression in rat myocardium following injection of 6×10^7 pfu of adenovirus expressing chloramphenicol acetyltransferase (CAT). Between two and four animals were sacrificed at each of the indicated time points, and CAT activity measured in extracts of left ventricles. (From Kass-Eisler, A., Falck-Pedersen, E., Alvira, M. *et al.* (1993) Quantitative determination of adenovirus-mediated gene delivery to rat cardiac myocytes *in vitro* and *in vivo*. *Proc. Natl Acad. Sci. USA*, **90**, 11500, with permission.)

local growth-factor expression production is nature's own means of engendering the growth of coronary collaterals. The delivery and expression of growth-factor genes would merely replicate and enhance this natural process.

The feasibility of *in vivo* gene transfer into the myocardium was first demonstrated by Lin *et al.*[102] and Acsadi *et al.*[103] These workers injected plasmid DNA directly into rat myocardium and demonstrated expression of a β-galactosidase marker gene in small numbers of myocardial cells for 2–4 weeks. More recently, the use of adenoviral vectors[104,105] has resulted in dramatic increases in efficiency of gene transfer and levels of recombinant gene expression. Kass-Eisler *et al.*[105] injected adenoviral vectors directly into the myocardium of rats. Recombinant gene expression was again transient, peaking within one week (Figure 8.11); however, these levels of gene expression were one-to-two orders of magnitude above those reported by the same group following injection of plasmid DNA. Using both injected plasmid DNA and injected virus, recombinant gene expression was primarily localized to the

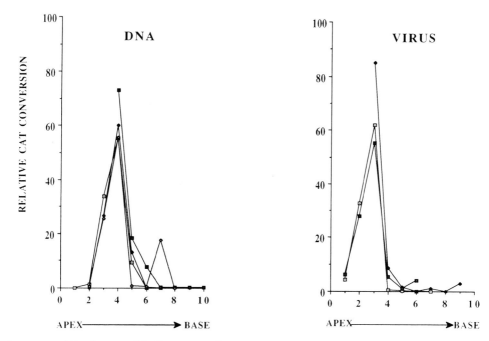

Figure 8.12 Distribution of CAT activity in hearts injected with plasmid DNA or adenovirus vectors. Hearts were harvested 5 days following injection, and sliced into seven 1.5-mm transverse sections. Each section appears as a data point; sections from the same animal are connected by lines. Total CAT activity from hearts injected with DNA (10 μg) or adenovirus vectors (6 × 10^7 pfu) in relative units were 2799 ± 1353 and 117 501 ± 15 944, respectively. Based on 75 ng of CAT DNA present in 6 × 10^7 pfu of virus, the adenovirus is approximately 5000-fold more efficient than plasmid DNA, yet the distribution of activity is nearly identical for the two techniques. (From Kass-Eisler, A., Falck-Pedersen, E., Alvira, M. _et al._ (1993) Quantitative determination of adenovirus-mediated gene delivery to rat cardiac myocytes _in vitro_ and _in vivo. Proc. Natl Acad. Sci. USA,_ **90**, 11500, with permission.)

site of injection (Figure 8.12), demonstrating the potential to target gene delivery to specific areas of myocardium that might benefit from increases in local growth-factor production.

The means are now at hand for testing the hypothesis that overexpression of growth factor genes in ischemic myocardium will increase collateral formation. If this hypothesis is borne out, as was suggested in a preliminary report by Barr _et al._,[106] it will be important to demonstrate relief of ischemia and protection from myocardial damage at the time of subsequent coronary occlusions, as these are the putative salutary effects of increasing the coronary collateral circulation. Simultaneous with these efficacy studies, the issue of whether growth-factor expression causes either progression of proliferative cardiac and extracardiac vascular lesions or proliferative disease in other organs such as the kidney[107] will need to be addressed. A preliminary study suggests that intracardiac growth-factor infusion may indeed increase vascular proliferation at distant sites.[108]

Future directions

Progress in somatic-cell gene transfer and gene-therapy approaches for the treatment of ischemic heart disease has been extremely rapid. The first abstract presentations in this area were presented at the American Heart Association Scientific Sessions in 1989. This year an entire abstract submission category is devoted to *in vivo* gene transfer/gene therapy. The initial studies of gene transfer were focused on demonstrations of feasibility as well as optimization of gene-transfer efficiency and level of recombinant gene expression. Current studies are aimed at the achievement of well-defined therapeutic endpoints: retardation of plaque progression, decrease in vessel thrombogenicity, lowering of lipid levels, enhancement of coronary collaterals and protection against the consequences of myocardial ischemia.

Progress in gene therapy for ischemic heart disease has reached the stage of human trials, in the case of LDL-receptor gene replacement for familial hypercholesterolemia.[88] Our eagerness to extend the application of this new and exciting therapeutic modality to other settings should be tempered by the realization that virtually all cases of ischemic heart disease have a more complex etiology and a more prolonged and varied natural history than does this condition. Proposed gene therapies for these types of ischemic heart disease will require comparison with other treatments as to therapeutic efficacy, safety and cost effectiveness. Nevertheless, the molecular genetic approach to ischemic heart disease may well eventually hold the day, for it is uniquely capable of manipulating vascular, hepatic and cardiac gene expression so as to correct and reprogram cardiovascular disease at its biologic source.

References

1. *Gene Transfer and Expression Protocols* (1991), pp. 16–17. Clifton, NJ: Humana Press.
2. Miller, A. D. (1992) Human gene therapy comes of age. *Nature*, **357**, 455–60.
3. Hoogerbrugge, P. M., Vossen, J. M., Beusechem, V. W. and Valerio, D. (1992) Treatment of patients with severe combined immunodeficiency due to adenosine deaminase (ADA) deficiency by autologous transplantation of genetically modified bone marrow cells. *Human Gene Ther.*, **3**, 553–8.
4. Blaese, R. M., Culver, K. W., Chang, L. *et al.* (1992) Treatment of severe combined immunodeficiency disease (SCID) due to adenosine deaminase deficiency with CD34+ selected autologous peripheral blood cells transduced with a human ADA gene. Amendment to clinical research project, Project 90-C-195, January 10, 1992. *Human Gene Ther.*, **4**, 521–7.
5. Wilson, J. M., Grossman, M., Raper, S. E. *et al.* (1992) *Ex vivo* gene therapy of familial hypercholesterolemia. *Human Gene Ther.*, **3**, 179–222.
6. Welsh, M. J., Smith, A. E., Zabner, J. *et al.* (1994) Cystic fibrosis gene therapy using an adenovirus vector: *in vivo* safety and efficacy in nasal epithelium. *Human Gene Ther.*, **5**, 209–19.
7. Ross, R. (1993) The pathogenesis of atherosclerosis: a perspective for the 1990s. *Nature*, **362**, 801–9.
8. Fuster, V., Badimon, L., Badimon, J. J. and Chesebro, J. H. (1992) The pathophysiology of coronary artery disease and the acute coronary syndromes. *N. Engl. J. Med.*, **326**, 310–18.
9. Levin, E. G. (1983) Latent tissue plasminogen activator produced by human endothelial cells in culture. *Proc. Natl Acad. Sci. USA*, **80**, 6804–8.

10. Cooke, J. P., Singer, A. H., Tsao, P. *et al.* (1992) Antiatherogenic effects of L-arginine in the hypercholesterolemic rabbit. *J. Clin. Ivest.*, **90**, 1168–72.
11. Radomski, M. W., Palmer, R. M. and Moncada, S. (1987) Endogenous nitric oxide inhibits human platelet adhesion to vascular endothelium. *Lancet*, **ii**, 1057–8.
12. Quax, P. H. A., van den Hoogen, M., Verheijen, J. H. *et al.* (1990) Endotoxin induction of plasminogen activator and plasminogen activator inhibitor type 1 mRNA in rat tissues *in vivo*. *J. Biol. Chem.*, **265**, 15560–3.
13. Sawdey, M. S. and Loskutoff, D. J. (1991) Regulation of murine type 1 plasminogen activator inhibitor gene expression *in vivo*: tissue specificity and induction by lipopolysaccharide, tumor necrosis factor-alpha, and transforming growth factor-beta. *J. Clin. Invest.*, **88**, 1346–53.
14. Moore, K. L., Andreoli, S. P., Esmon, N. L. *et al.* (1987) Endotoxin enhances tissue factor and suppresses thrombomodulin expression *in vitro*. *J. Clin. Invest.*, **79**, 124–30.
15. Wilson, J. M., Birinyi, L. K., Salomon, R. N. *et al.* (1989) Implantation of vascular grafts lined with genetically modified endothelial cells. *Science*, **244**, 1344–6.
16. Dichek, D. A., Neville, R. F., Zwiebel, J. A. *et al.* (1989) Seeding of intravascular stents with genetically engineered endothelial cells. *Circulation*, **80**, 1347–53.
17. Geary, R. L., Clowes, A. W., Lau, S. *et al.* (1994) Gene transfer in baboons using prosthetic vascular grafts seeded with retrovirally transduced smooth muscle cells: a model for local and systemic gene therapy. *Human Gene Ther.*, **5**, 1211–16.
18. Conte, M. S., Birinyi, L. K., Miyata, T. *et al.* (1994) Efficient repopulation of denuded rabbit arteries with autologous genetically modified endothelial cells. *Circulation*, **89**, 2161–9.
19. Nabel, E. G., Plautz, G., Boyce, F. M. *et al.* (1989) Recombinant gene expression *in vivo* within endothelial cells of the arterial wall. *Science*, **244**, 1342–4.
20. Lim, C. S., Chapman, G. D., Gammon, R. S. *et al.* (1991) *In vivo* gene transfer into canine coronary and peripheral arteries. *Circulation*, **83**, 2007–11.
21. Flugelman, M. Y., Jaklitsch, M. T., Newman, K. D. *et al.* (1992) Low level *in vivo* gene transfer into the arterial wall through a perforated balloon catheter. *Circulation*, **85**, 1110–17.
22. Sanes, J. R., Rubenstein, J. L. R. and Nicolas, J. F. (1986) Use of a recombinant retrovirus to study post-implantation cell lineage in mouse embryos. *EMBO J.*, **5**, 3133–42.
23. Plautz, G., Nabel, E. G. and Nabel, G. J. (1991) Introduction of vascular smooth muscle cells expressing recombinant genes *in vivo*. *Circulation*, **83**, 578–83.
24. Lynch, C. M., Clowes, M. M., Osborne, W. R. *et al.* (1992) Long-term expression of human adenosine deaminase in vascular smooth muscle cells of rats: a model for gene therapy. *Proc. Natl Acad. Sci. USA*, **89**, 1138–42.
25. Clowes, M. M., Lynch, C. M., Miller, A. D. *et al.* (1994) Long-term biological response of injured rat carotid artery seeded with smooth muscle cells expressing retrovirally introduced human genes. *J. Clin. Invest.*, **93**, 644–51.
26. Dichek, D. A., Neville, R. F., Zwiebel, J. A. *et al.* (1989) Seeding of intravascular stents with genetically engineered endothelial cells. *Circulation*, **80**, 1347–53.
27. Flugelman, M. Y., Virmani, R., Leon, M. B. *et al.* (1992) Genetically engineered endothelial cells remain adherent and viable after stent deployment and exposure to flow *in vitro*. *Circ. Res.*, **70**, 348–54.
28. Zwiebel, J. A., Freeman, S. M., Kantoff, P. W. *et al.* (1989) High-level recombinant gene expression in rabbit endothelial cells transduced by retroviral vectors. *Science*, **243**, 220–2.
29. Kahn, M. L., Lee, S. W. and Dichek, D. A. (1992) Optimization of retroviral vector-mediated gene transfer into endothelial cells *in vitro*. *Circ. Res.*, **71**, 1508–17.
30. Dichek, D. A. and Quertermous, T. (1989) Variability in messenger RNA levels in human umbilical vein endothelial cells of different lineage and time in culture. *In Vitro Cell. Dev. Biol.*, **25**, 289–92.
31. Chamley-Campbell, J. H. and Campbell, G. R. (1981) What controls smooth muscle phenotype? *Atherosclerosis*, **40**, 347–57.

32. Kocher, O., Skalli, O., Bloom, W. S. and Gabbiani, G. (1984) Cytoskeleton of rat aortic smooth muscle cells. *Lab. Invest.*, **50**, 645–52.
33. Rovner, A. S., Murphy, R. A. and Owens, G. K. (1986) Expression of smooth muscle and nonmuscle myosin heavy chains in cultured vascular smooth muscle cells. *J. Biol. Chem.*, **261**, 14740–5.
34. Chapman, G. D., Lim, C. S., Gammon, R. S. *et al.* (1992) Gene transfer into coronary arteries of intact animals with a percutaneous balloon catheter. *Circ. Res.*, **71**, 27–33.
35. Leclerc, G., Gal, D., Nikol, S. *et al.* (1991) *In vivo* arterial gene transfer in the normal rabbit: characterization of long-term expression following liposome-mediated transfection. *Circulation*, **84**, II-295 (Abstract).
36. Leclerc, G., Gal, D., Takeshita, S. *et al.* (1992) Percutaneous arterial gene transfer in a rabbit model. *J. Clin. Invest.*, **90**, 936–44.
37. Nabel, E. G., Plautz, G. and Nabel, G. J. (1990) Site-specific gene expression *in vivo* by direct gene transfer into the arterial wall. *Science*, **249**, 1285–8.
38. Morishita, R., Gibbons, G. H., Kaneda, Y., Ogihara, T. and Dzau, V. J. (1993) Novel and effective gene transfer technique for study of vascular renin angiotensin system. *J. Clin. Invest.*, **91**, 2580–5.
39. Kupfer, J. M., Ruan, X. M., Liu, G. *et al.* (1994) High-efficiency gene transfer to autologous rabbit jugular vein grafts using adenovirus-transferrin/polylysine-DNA complexes. *Human Gene Ther.*, **5**, 1437–44.
40. Barbee, R. W., Stapleton, D. D., Perry, B. D. *et al.* (1993) Prior arterial injury enhances luciferase expression following *in vivo* gene transfer. *Biochem. Biophys. Res. Commun.*, **190**, 70–8.
41. Miller, D. G., Adam, M. A. and Miller, A. D. (1990) Gene transfer by retrovirus vectors occurs only in cells that are actively replicating at the time of infection. *Mol. Cell. Biol.*, **10**, 4239–42.
42. Clowes, A. W., Reidy, M. A. and Clowes, M. M. (1983) Kinetics of cellular proliferation after arterial injury I. Smooth muscle cell growth in the absence of endothelium. *Lab. Invest.*, **49**, 327–33.
43. Gordon, D., Reidy, M. A., Benditt, E. P. and Schwartz, S. M. (1990) Cell proliferation in human coronary arteries. *Proc. Natl Acad. Sci. USA*, **87**, 4600–4.
44. Cornetta, K., Moen, R. C., Culver, K. *et al.* (1990) Amphotropic murine leukemia retrovirus is not an acute pathogen for primates, *Human Gene Ther.*, **1**, 15–30.
45. Cooper, N. R., Jensen, F. C., Welsh, R. M. and Oldstone, M. B. A. (1976) Lysis of RNA tumor viruses by human serum: direct antibody-independent triggering of the classical complement pathway. *J. Exp. Med.*, **144**, 970–84.
46. Kaneda, Y., Iwai, K. and Uchida, T. (1989) Increased expression of DNA cointroduced with nuclear protein in adult rat liver. *Science*, **243**, 375–8.
47. Morishita, R., Gibbons, G. H., Kaneda, Y. *et al.* (1993) Novel and effective gene transfer technique for study of vascular reinin–angiotensin system. *J. Clin. Invest.*, **91**, 2580–5.
48. Rosenfeld, M. A., Yoshimura, K., Trapnell, B. C. *et al.* (1992) *In vivo* transfer of the human cystic fibrosis transmembrane conductance regulator gene to the airway epithelium. *Cell*, **68**, 143–55.
49. Jaffe, H. A., Danel, C., Longenecker, M. *et al.* (1992) Adenovirus-mediated *in vivo* gene transfer and expression in normal rat liver. *Nature-Genetics*, **1**, 372–8.
50. Herz, J. and Gerard, R. D. (1993) Adenovirus-mediated transfer of low density lipoprotein receptor gene acutely accelerates cholesterol clearance in normal mice. *Proc. Natl Acad. Sci. USA*, **90**, 2812–16.
51. Breakefield, X. O. (1993) Gene delivery into the brain using virus vectors. *Nature-Genetics*, **3**, 187–9.
52. Akli, S., Caillaud, C., Vigne, E. *et al.* (1993) Transfer of a foreign gene into the brain using adenovirus vectors. *Nature-Genetics*, **3**, 224–8.
53. Bajocchi, G., Feldman, S. H., Crystal, R. G. and Mastrangeli, A. (1993) Direct *in vivo* gene transfer to ependymal cells in the central nervous system using recombinant adenovirus vectors. *Nature-Genetics*, **3**, 229–34.

54. Lemarchand, P., Jaffe, H. A., Danel, C. *et al.* (1992) Adenovirus-mediated transfer of a recombinant human alpha-1 antitrypsin cDNA to human endothelial cells. *Proc. Natl Acad. Sci. USA*, **89**, 6482–6.
55. Lemarchand, P., Jones, M., Yamada, I. and Crystal, R. G. (1993) *In vivo* gene transfer and expression in normal, uninjured blood vessels using replication deficient recombinant adenovirus vectors. *Circ. Res.*, **72**, 1132–8.
56. Lee, S. W., Trapnell, B. C., Rade, J. J. *et al.* (1993) *In vivo* adenoviral vector-mediated gene transfer into balloon-injured rat carotid arteries. *Circ. Res.*, **73**, 797–807.
57. Guzman, R. J., Lemarchand, P., Crystal, R. G. *et al.* (1993) Efficient and selective adenovirus-mediated gene transfer into vascular neointima. *Circulation*, **88**, 2838–48.
58. Rome, J. J., Shayani, V., Flugelman, M. Y. *et al.* (1994) Anatomic barriers influence the distribution of *in vivo* gene transfer into the arterial wall: modeling with microscopic tracer particles and verification with a recombinant adenoviral vector. *Arterioscler. Thromb.*, **14**, 148–61.
59. Willard, J. E., Landau, C., Glamann, D. B. *et al.* (1994) Genetic modification of the vessel wall. Comparison of surgical and catheter-basd techniques for delivery of recombinant adenovirus. *Circulation*, **89**, 2190–7.
60. Riessen, R., Rahimizadeh, H., Blessing, E. *et al.* (1993) Arterial gene transfer using pure DNA applied directly to a hydrogel-coated angioplasty balloon. *Human Gene Ther.*, **4**, 749–58.
61. Rome, J. J., Shayani, V., Farrell, K. D. *et al.* (1994) Adenoviral vector-mediated gene transfer into sheep arteries using a double balloon catheter. *Human Gene Ther.*, 1249–58.
62. Casscells, W., Lappi, D. A., Olwin, B. B. *et al.* (1992) Elimination of smooth muscle cells in experimental restenosis: targeting of fibroblast growth factor receptors. *Proc. Natl Acad. Sci. USA*, **89**, 7159–63.
63. Barr, E., Carroll, J., Kalynych, A. M. *et al.* (1994) Efficient catheter-mediated gene transfer into the heart using replication-defective adenovirus. *Gene Ther.*, **1**, 51–8.
64. Roessler, B. J., Allen, E. D., Wilson, J, M. *et al.* (1993) Adenoviral-mediated gene transfer to rabbit synovium *in vivo*. *J. Clin. Invest.*, **92**, 1085–92.
65. Yang, Y., Nunes, F. A., Berencsi, K. *et al.* (1994) Cellular immunity to viral antigens limits E1-deleted adenoviruses for gene therapy. *Proc. Natl Acad. Sci. USA*, **91**, 4407–11.
66. Donahue, R. E., Kessler, S. W., Bodine, D. M. *et al.* (1992) Helper virus induced T cell lymphoma in nonhuman primates after retroviral mediated gene transfer. *J. Exp. Med.*, **176**, 1125–35.
67. Fuster, V., Badimon, L., Badimon, J. J. and Chesebro, J. H. (1992) The pathophysiology of coronary artery disease and the acute coronary syndromes. *N. Engl. J. Med.*, **326**, 242–50.
68. Dichek, D. A., Nussbaum, O., Degen, S. J. F. and Anderson, W. F. (1991) Enhancement of the fibrinolytic activity of sheep endothelial cells by retroviral vector-mediated gene transfer. *Blood*, **77**, 533–41.
69. Jaklitsch, M. T., Biro, S., Casscells, W. and Dichek, D. A. (1993) Transduced endothelial cells expressing high levels of tissue plasminogen activator have an unaltered phenotype *in vitro*. *J. Cell. Physiol.*, **154**, 207–16.
70. Dichek, D. A. (1991) Retroviral vector-mediated gene transfer into endothelial cells. *Mol. Biol. Med.*, **8**, 257–66.
71. Lee, S. W., Kahn, M. L. and Dichek, D. A. (1992) Expression of anchored urokinase in the apical endothelial cell membrane. *J. Biol. Chem.*, **267**, 13020–7.
72. Nachman, R. L. and Hajjar, K. A. (1991) Endothelial cell fibrinolytic assembly. *Ann. NY Acad. Sci.*, **614**, 240–9.
73. Plow, E. F., Felez, J. and Miles, L. A. (1991) Cellular regulation of fibrinolysis. *Thromb. Haemost.*, **66**, 32–6.
74. Ellis, V., Behrendt, N. and Dano, K. (1991) Plasminogen activation by receptor-bound urokinase; a kinetic study with both cell-associated and isolated receptor. *J. Biol. Chem.*, **266**, 12752–8.
75. Lee, S. W., Ellis, V. and Dichek, D. A. (1994) Characterization of plasminogen activation by glycosylphosphatidylinositol-anchored urokinase. *J. Biol. Chem.*, **269**, 2411–18.

76. Podrazik, R., Whitehill, T. A., Ekhterae, D. *et al*. (1992) High-level expression of recombinant human t-PA in cultivated canine endothelial cells under varying conditions of retroviral gene transfer. *Ann. Surg.*, **216**, 446–53.

77. Eskin, S. G., Meidell, R. S., McNatt, J. *et al*. (1991) Protective effect of mutant tissue plasminogen activator expressed from endothelial cells seeded on implanted stents. *Circulation*, **84**, II-399 (Abstract).

78. Xu, X-M., Ohashi, K., Sanduja, S. K. *et al*. (1993) Enhanced prostacyclin synthesis in endothelial cells by retrovirus-mediated transfer of prostaglandin H. synthase cDNA. *J. Clin. Invest.*, **91**, 1843–9.

79. Zoldhelyi, P., Xu, X-M., Meidell, R. *et al*. (1993) Enhancement of prostacyclin synthesis *in vitro* and *in vivo* by adenovirus-mediated transfer of prostaglandin-H synthase cDNA. *Circulation*, **88**, 476 (Abstract).

80. Rade, J. J., Lee, S. W. and Dichek, D. A. (1994) Viral vector-mediated expression of biologically active hirudin in cultured endothelial cells. *Circulation*, **88**, I-418 (Abstract).

81. Schwartz, S. M. (1993) Serum-derived growth factor is thrombin? *J. Clin. Invest.*, **91**, 4.

82. Schwartz, C. J., Valente, A. J., Sprague, E. A. *et al*. (1992) Atherosclerosis. Potential targets for stabilization and regression. *Circulation*, **86**, III-117–III-23.

83. Bilheimer, D. W., Goldstein, J. L., Grundy, S. M. *et al*. (1984) Liver transplantation to provide low density lipoprotein receptors and lower plasma cholesterol in a child with homozygous familial hypercholesterolemia. *N. Engl. J. Med.*, **311**, 1658–64.

84. Goldstein, J. L. and Brown, M. S. (1983) Familial hypercholesterolemia. In: Stanbury, J. B., Wyngaarden, J. B., Fredrickson, D. S., Goldstein, J. L. and Brown, M. S. (eds) *The Metabolic Basis of Inherited Disease*, 5th edn, pp. 672–712. New York: McGraw-Hill.

85. Wilson, J. M., Chowdhury, N. R., Grossman, M. *et al*. (1990) Temporary amelioration of hyperlipidemia in low density lipoprotein receptor-deficient rabbits transplanted with genetically modified hepatocytes. *Proc. Natl Acad. Sci. USA*, **87**, 8437–41.

86. Ishibashi, S., Brown, M. S., Goldstein, J. L. *et al*. (1993) Hypercholesterolemia in low density lipoprotein receptor knockout mice and its reversal by adenovirus-mediated gene delivery. *J. Clin. Invest.*, **92**, 883–93.

87. Chowdhury, J. R., Grossman, M., Gupta, S. *et al*. (1991) Long term improvement of hypercholesterolemia after *ex vivo* gene therapy in LDLR-deficient rabbits. *Science*, **254**, 1802–4.

88. Grossman, M., Raper, S. E., Kozarsky, K. *et al*. (1994) Successful *ex vivo* gene therapy directed to liver in a patient with familial hypercholesterolaemia. *Nature-Genetics*, **6**, 335–41.

89. Castelli, W. P., Doyle, J. T., Gordon, T. *et al*. (1977) HDL cholesterol and other lipids in coronary artery disease: the Cooperative Lipoprotein Phenotyping study. *Circulation*, **55**, 767–72.

90. Gordon, T., Castelli, W. P., Hjortland, M. C. *et al*. (1977) High density lipoprotein as a protective factor against coronary heart disease: the Framingham Study. *Am. J. Med.*, **62**, 707–14.

91. Rubin, E. M., Krauss, R. M., Spangler, E. A. *et al*. (1991) Inhibition of early atherogenesis in transgenic mice by human apolipoprotein A1. *Nature*, **353**, 265–7.

92. Kopfler, W. P., Willard, M., Betz, T. *et al*. (1994) Adenovirus-mediated transfer of a gene encoding human apolipoprotein A-I into normal mice increases circulating high-density lipoprotein cholesterol. *Circulation*, **90**, 1319–27.

93. Webster, J. S., Moberg, C. and Rincon, G. (1974) Natural history of severe proximal coronary artery disease as documented by coronary cineangiography. *Am. J. Cardiol.*, **33**, 195–200.

94. Rentrop, K. P., Feit, F., Sherman, W. *et al*. (1989) Late thrombolytic therapy preserves left ventricular function in patients with collateralized total coronary occlusion: primary end point findings of the Second Mount Sinai–New York University Reperfusion Trial. *J. Am. Coll. Cardiol.*, **14**, 58–64.

95. Rogers, W. J., Hood, W. P., Jr, Mantle, J. A. *et al.* (1984) Return of left ventricular function after reperfusion in patients with myocardial infarction: importance of subtotal stenoses or intact collaterals. *Circulation*, **69**, 338–49.
96. Saito, Y., Yasuno, M., Ishida, M. *et al.* (1985) Importance of coronary collaterals for restoration of left ventricular function after intracoronary thrombolysis. *Am. J. Cardiol.*, **55**, 1259–63.
97. Schuler, G., Schwarz, F., Hofmann, M. *et al.* (1982) Thrombolysis in acute myocardial infarction using intracoronary streptokinase: assessment by thallium-201 scintigraphy. *Circulation*, **66**, 658–64.
98. Yanagisawa-Miwa, A., Uchida, Y., Nakamura, F. *et al.* (1992) Salvage of infarcted myocardium by angiogenic action of basic fibroblast growth factor. *Science*, **257**, 1401–3.
99. Unger, E. F., Banai, S., Shou, M. *et al.* (1994) Basic fibroblast growth factor enhances myocardial collateral flow in a canine model. *Am. J. Physiol.*, **266**, H1588–H1595.
100. Banai, S., Jaklitsch, M. T., Shou, M. *et al.* (1994) Angiogenic-induced enhancement of collateral blood flow to ischemic myocardium by vascular endothelial growth factor in dogs. *Circulation*, **89**, 2183–9.
101. Kumar, S., West, D., Shahabuddin, S. *et al.* (1983) Angiogenesis factor from human myocardial infarcts. *Lancet*, **ii**, 364–8.
102. Lin, H., Parmacek, M. S., Morle, G. *et al.* (1990) Expression of recombinant genes in myocardium *in vivo* after direct injection of DNA. *Circulation*, **82**, 2217–21.
103. Acsadi, G., Jiao, S., Jani, A., *et al.* (1991) Direct gene transfer and expression into rat heart *in vivo*. *New Biologist*, **3**, 71–81.
104. Guzman, R. J., Lemarchand, P., Crystal, R. G. *et al.* (1993) Efficient gene-transfer into myocardium by direct injection of adenovirus vectors. *Circ. Res.*, **73**, 1202–7.
105. Kass-Eisler, A., Falck-Pedersen, E., Alvira, M. *et al.* (1993) Quantitative determination of adenovirus-mediated gene delivery to rat cardiac myocytes *in vitro* and *in vivo*. *Proc. Natl Acad. Sci. USA*, **90**, 11498–502.
106. Barr, E., Lin, H., Bolling, S. *et al.* (1991) Induction of angiogenesis following *in vivo* gene transfer into myocardium. *Circulation*, **84**, II-420 (Abstract).
107. Isaka, Y., Fujiwara, Y., Ueda, N. *et al.* (1993) Glomerulosclerosis induced by *in vivo* transfection of transforming growth factor-beta or platelet-derived growth factor gene into the rat kidney. *J. Clin. Invest.*, **92**, 2597–601.
108. Lazarous, D. F., Scheinowitz, M., Shou, M. *et al.* (1995) Effects of chronic systemic administration of basic fibroblast growth factor on collateral development in the canine heart. *Circulation*, **91**, 145–53.

9

Endothelium and Vasoreactive Diseases

Andrew P. Selwyn
Peter Ganz

Introduction

The vasomotor control of the coronary circulation has been investigated by physiologists and clinicians with special regard to autoregulation, metabolic regulation and the balance between sympathetic and parasympathetic control of vascular smooth-muscle tone. For example, this classic physiology has described the role of the coronary resistance vessels in maintaining perfusion during changes in blood pressure (autoregulation), heart rate and cardiac output, and the regulation of regional myocardial perfusion to meet the needs of the myocardium for oxygen and substrate (metabolic regulation).[1] Since 1977 we must add to this body of knowledge evidence that the vasomotor control of epicardial and resistance coronary vessels is also regulated locally by physical, neural and humoral influences,[2,3] on the interaction of vascular endothelium and the subjacent smooth-muscle cells.

The function of the endothelium as it pertains to the interactions with smooth-muscle cells during constriction or dilation appears to be greatly influenced by risk factors for atherosclerosis and the growth of this pathology. There are several severe consequences of endothelial cell dysfunction in this setting that appear to contribute to abnormal coronary constriction and myocardial ischemia.[4] Therefore, this introduction will focus on the interactions between the endothelium and smooth-muscle cells, characteristic disturbances that occur in coronary atherosclerosis and the clinical consequences in patients. New therapies aimed at these cell dysfunctions and coronary events in patients will be discussed.

Physiology of the healthy endothelium and vascular smooth-muscle cells

The healthy vascular endothelium has many functions including the maintenance of a permeability barrier, control of appropriate growth of smooth-muscle cells and matrix, preservation of an anticoagulant surface and regulation of local coronary vasomotion.[3,5] The healthy endothelial cell surface also controls and severely limits platelet adhesion and the adhesion of inflammatory cells through expression of adhesion molecules.[6–10] There are endothelial cell-surface receptors and ion channels that can respond to circulating hormones or local neurotransmitters (acetylcholine, norepinephrine, histamine, substance P, bradykinin), the products of thrombosis (thrombin), platelet aggregation (serotonin, ADP) and changes in shear stress, pulse pressure and blood pressure. This response is transduced through intracellular second-messenger pathways which lead to endothelial cell production of vasoconstrictor and vasodilator compounds that exert profound local effects.[4]

In this regard, the endothelium produces short-lived and locally acting vasodilators (nitric oxide or its derivatives such as nitrosothiol, and also prostacyclin and hyperpolarizing factor) and vasoconstrictor substances such as endothelin and free radicals of oxygen. Acetylcholine can stimulate endothelial cell-surface muscarinic receptors that interact with a second-messenger system involving G proteins that stimulate nitric oxide synthase to catalyze the cleavage of nitric oxide from L-arginine. The local diffusion of nitric oxide increases the activity of cyclic GMP in smooth-muscle cells that is followed by vasodilation. Interestingly, in the absence of a functioning endothelium, many of the compounds that induce endothelium-dependent dilation in health will act directly on smooth-muscle cells, leading to an opposite or vasoconstrictor response.[11–14]

The control of coronary endothelium-dependent vasodilation in humans can be examined using local infusions of agonists such as acetylcholine, serotonin, substance P or by inducing local increases in coronary blood flow (i.e. flow-mediated dilation).[15–17]

Infusion in the left anterior descending coronary artery of acetylcholine at 10^{-8} to 10^{-6} M produces dose-dependent dilation that is blocked by a specific inhibitor of nitric oxide synthase (L-monomethylarginine) or by free hemoglobin (that inactivates nitric oxide).[18,19] The endothelium can mediate constriction by the local production of endothelin, again in response to a wide range of stimuli. Oxygen free radicals and thromboxane A_2 can produce the same effect.[4] The physiologic control systems that involve these various constrictor mechanisms in the human coronary arteries are not well understood. Nevertheless, there is ample evidence in patients that the healthy endothelium and smooth-muscle cells together control a local homeostatic system of vasodilation and vasoconstriction. This control system is responsive to influences that change shear stress outside of a particular physiologic range and to signals that promote thrombosis. Therefore, this local system appears to preserve vessel patency and control physical forces acting on the endothelium. It is interesting to note that one of the most important local mediators of vasodilation (nitric oxide) also diminishes atherogenesis by inhibiting platelet adhesion, smooth-muscle cell proliferation, adhesion of inflammatory cells and accumulation of oxygen free radicals.[4]

Dysfunction of the endothelium and smooth-muscle cell

Endothelial damage

Early experiments which employed isolated rings of rabbit aorta showed that removal of the endothelium abolishes endothelium-dependent dilation in response to acetylcholine.[3,20] More elaborate models in rabbits, pigs, monkeys and dogs (with or without hypercholesterolemia) have shown that angioplasty of an epicardial coronary artery results in loss of endothelium-dependent dilation and development of constriction in response to acetylcholine, serotonin and aggregating platelets.[10,13,21–23] In the monkey, chronic stress caused by repeated social disruption leads to worsening or failure to recover endothelial function in models of atherosclerosis.[24] Interestingly, most of the above models have demonstrated profound and early loss of endothelium-dependent vasodilator function, preservation of smooth-muscle cell constrictor responses, and finally prolonged impairment of the function of the endothelium that regenerates after arterial injury.[23] This evidence will be relevant when considering the response of atherosclerotic arterial segments to different interventions and the implantation of foreign materials.

Risk factors and arterial dysfunction

Early experimental models have demonstrated that hypercholesterolemia increases constriction of arterial strips in response to ergonovine.[25] Shortly thereafter, similar models in dogs, cats, monkeys, rabbits and pigs have all demonstrated that induction of hypercholesterolemia, an increase in the plasma low-density lipoprotein (LDL), transient or established hypertension and hyperglycemia can all induce loss of endothelium-dependent dilation which is replaced by paradoxical constriction before the development of intimal atherosclerosis.[25–30]

In experiments using arterial strips, oxidized LDL was the most potent agent causing early loss of endothelial function. This probably occurs because of the toxic effects of lysophosphatidylcholine that is released during the metabolism of oxidized LDL, dysfunction of a G protein involved in signal transduction, toxic effects of oxygen free radicals and finally inactivation of nitric oxide.[4] Clinical studies in patients have examined the vasomotor response of angiographically smooth coronary arteries following the local infusion of acetylcholine. The loss of endothelium-dependent vasomotor function in these studies is related to the presence of well-known risk factors for coronary atherosclerosis and ischemic heart disease.[31,32] For example, the loss of endothelium-dependent dilation and development of constriction in patients has been found in association with a raised plasma cholesterol, raised plasma LDL, increased plasma levels of small dense LDL particles, systemic hypertension, increasing age and diabetes.[4,33] Preservation or loss of endothelium-dependent vasomotor function can also be examined in the forearm resistance vessels and the brachial artery using noninvasive techniques. In younger subjects, these studies have also shown early loss of endothelium-dependent vasomotor function in patients with hypercholesterolemia, smokers, hypertension and diabetes.[34] Although coronary angiography cannot rule out the presence of some subintimal atherosclerosis without vessel narrowing, these observations in patients extend and validate the notion from experimental studies that the presence and severity of the well-known risk factors for atherosclerosis will, in themselves, lead to dysfunction of the vascular endothelium before or very early in the development of atherosclerosis. Further studies in patients have revealed important functional consequences. Seiler *et al.* have shown in patients that the vasomotor response of epicardial coronary arteries to physical exercise is related to the level of plasma cholesterol and patients with raised cholesterol show failure of coronary dilation and development of abnormal constriction.[35]

Vascular dysfunction in atherosclerosis: experimental studies

The characteristic pathology of atherosclerosis includes intimal growth, thrombosis and vasoconstriction.[4,36] The early loss of endothelial function(s) is an important pathogenic feature of this disease. Experimental models of atherosclerosis in rabbits, pigs and monkeys have all shown that endothelium-dependent dilation in response to a wide range of stimuli is lost in all stages of atherosclerosis.[4,23,25,26] This loss of function occurs in response to stimuli such as acetylcholine, serotonin, substance P and aggregating platelets. There is conflicting evidence regarding the cellular and molecular mechanisms that cause this loss of function. Different animal models have demonstrated decreased formation of nitric oxide, in part related to defective coupling of endothelial receptors to G protein, while others have emphasized enhanced degradation of the available nitric oxide by a reaction with excess oxygen free radicals, forming vasoinactive peroxynitrite.[36,37] The experimental models have also shown that the dysfunctional endothelium in atherosclerosis develops an abnormal procoagulant surface, exhibits increased adhesion of inflammatory cells to specific cell-membrane receptor sites and finally, becomes growth promoting instead of growth inhibiting.[8,9,36,38]

Vascular dysfunction in patients with atherosclerosis

The relationship between risk factors, atherosclerosis and the presence of endothelial dysfunction with a loss of endothelium-dependent vasodilation and development of constriction has been thoroughly investigated in patients. The loss of endothelium-dependent dilation occurs very early and before the appearance of atherosclerotic vessel narrowing in the epicardial arteries of patients studied in the cardiac catheterization laboratory. The loss of this function is patchy, and appears to be more severe at arterial branchpoints.[39] Studies that have examined the loss of endothelial function during the development of atherosclerosis have shown that the receptor-mediated endothelium-dependent dilation in response to acetylcholine is lost first followed by flow-mediated responses and finally dilator responses to sympathetic arousal caused by exposure to cold.[32] Vasodilator responses are lost and replaced by abnormal constriction. Interestingly, endothelial function is lost in relation to different systemic risk factors and yet the development of atherosclerosis is patchy. As a result, the abnormal constriction of arterial segments to acetylcholine is only partially related to the severity of atherosclerotic stenoses.

Patients with entirely smooth coronary arteries and no risk factors will frequently demonstrate dilation of epicardial arteries in response to sympathetic arousal that occurs during exposure to cold, mental stimulation or physical exercise.[4,40–43] These studies in patients in the catheterization laboratory have demonstrated that any early or late evidence of atherosclerosis in these large epicardial vessels is associated with the loss of this normal dilator function and replacement by abnormal constriction.[17] The normal response to stress and abnormal constriction in atherosclerotic arteries is mirrored by the response of the same arterial segments to tests of endothelial function using acetylcholine. Therefore, the functional state of the coronary endothelium appears to govern the net vasomotor response of epicardial arteries to stress. When superimposed on important atherosclerotic stenoses, this paradoxical and abnormal constriction with stress interferes with coronary blood supply and plays an important role in causing episodes of transient myocardial ischemia.[40–44] In this regard, Vita and colleagues have demonstrated that epicardial arteries in patients with endothelial dysfunction in response to acetylcholine are abnormally sensitive to the constrictor effect of a catecholamine (phenylephrine).[44]

In patients with unstable angina and myocardial infarction, frequently one atherosclerotic stenosis in an epicardial artery is complicated by varying degrees of plaque disruption and thrombosis. Both platelet aggregation and thrombosis can trigger segmental constriction when the endothelium is dysfunctional and cannot mediate appropriate dilator responses. Products of platelet aggregation (serotonin) and thrombosis (thrombin) lead to dilation of normal but constriction of atherosclerotic arteries. In these circumstances, the plaque is lipid-rich, infiltrated by macrophages and inflammatory cells at their boundaries and each plaque is subject to fracture at sites of rapidly changing strain and distortion in response to the stress of arterial blood pressure, shear forces or vasomotion.[7,23,26,45–47]

Treatment of arterial dysfunction

While all therapies in patients with coronary artery disease aim to relieve symptoms, prevention of coronary events is equally important. There is little evidence at present that therapeutic manipulation of coronary blood supply and myocardial demand by β-adrenoreceptor blocking drugs, calcium blockers and nitrates for the treatment of angina and ischemia will necessarily improve patient outcomes. At the same time, controlled clinical trials have not yet clearly shown that coronary angioplasty or other new interventions can reduce coronary event rates and prolong life. Interestingly, many of the causes and consequences of endothelial dysfunction in coronary atherosclerosis under investigation are also risk factors well known to be associated with coronary atherosclerosis, myocardial infarction and sudden coronary death.[4] What is the relationship between the treatment of coronary risk factors and the cell dysfunctions in atherosclerotic coronary arteries? A few aspects of this relationship are discussed below.

Cholesterol

Plasma cholesterol and LDL clearly play important roles in causing endothelial dysfunction and in the development of atherosclerosis. In the monkey with dietary atherosclerosis, therapeutic lowering of cholesterol results in improvements in vasodilator function, disappearance of inflammatory cells in the intimal space and eventually physical regression of atheroma.[48] In patients undergoing cardiac catheterization, loss of endothelium-dependent dilation in atherosclerotic coronary arteries has been measured using intracoronary acetylcholine. Plasma cholesterol and LDL were then treated for a year and evidence found on retesting of improvement in endothelial vasomotor function.[49] Interestingly, trials of cholesterol lowering show very little physical regression of atheroma but a gratifying reduction in adverse coronary event rates.[50]

Oxidation of lipids

Experimental studies have confirmed that in the development of atherosclerosis, the inflammatory cells, smooth-muscle cells and endothelial cells all produce an excess of oxygen free radicals that appear to be damaging and partly responsible for the loss of endothelium-dependent dilation by inactivating the available nitric oxide.[51] In the rabbit with atherosclerosis inhibition of oxygen free radicals using superoxide dismutase partially restores endothelium-derived nitric oxide and vasodilation. At the same time, inhibition of LDL oxidation using probucol also improves endothelium-dependent vasodilation and diminishes the growth of atherosclerosis in cholesterol-fed animals.[52–54] In patients with atherosclerosis, the intracoronary infusion of superoxide dismutase results in improvement in the endothelium-dependent vasomotor responses in atherosclerotic coronary arteries tested in the cardiac catheterization laboratory.[55] Treatment in these patients for one year by lowering LDL with lovastatin and inhibition of LDL oxidation with probucol results in significant improvements in endothelium-dependent vasomotor function.[49] The studies in patients indicate that preventing the oxidation of LDL seems to be a promising therapeutic option that needs further examination.

Hormones and arterial function

Administration of hormone-replacement therapy to postmenopausal women results in a gratifying 50% reduction in adverse coronary outcomes.[55] This is only partly due to favorable changes in plasma lipids. Administration of estrogens to surgically ovariectomized female monkeys with diet-induced hypercholesterolemia and atherosclerosis improves endothelium-dependent vasomotor function in affected arteries.[56] The estrogen appears to restore endothelium-dependent dilation but only in the estrogen-deficient state. In postmenopausal women with coronary atherosclerosis and endothelial dysfunction, the constrictor response to intracoronary acetylcholine is improved by the administration of 17β-estradiol or premarin.[57] The basic mechanisms of action of estrogen, the time course of the effects and the minimum effective dose need to be much better understood in order to maximize the well-known beneficial effects of hormone-replacement therapy in postmenopausal women.

Substrate supply and endothelial function

There is encouraging evidence that an excess supply of substrate (L-arginine) for nitric oxide production can improve endothelial function in cholesterol-fed rabbits and possibly inhibit smooth-muscle cell proliferation and the growth of athero-sclerosis. Although L-arginine can improve the endothelium-dependent vasomotor responses of coronary resistance vessels in patients, there is no evidence yet for a role in the treatment of coronary atherosclerosis and prevention of adverse clinical events.[58–59]

Summary and conclusions

Experimental and clinical studies have better defined certain characteristic cell dysfunctions in coronary atherosclerosis. As a result, important questions have arisen:

1. Is there a systematic and useful relationship between the various dysfunctions affecting the endothelium such as control of dilation, anticoagulant function, the control of inflammatory cells and the growth of atherosclerosis?
2. What are the underlying molecular mechanisms that control the loss of these normal endothelial functions very early in the native disease or following coronary interventions in the cardiac catheterization laboratory?
3. How can new therapies be developed that exploit these new mechanistic insights and that would be aimed at reversal of these cell dysfunctions?

It is encouraging that the risk factors involved in the growth of atherosclerosis and coronary events in patients also appear to directly cause the cell dysfunctions in atherosclerotic coronary arteries. Treatment by reversal of risk factors appears to partially correct these dysfunctions in experimental studies and in patients while they also appear to cut coronary event rates in large-scale clinical trials. The treatment of risk factors used to be applied as a long-term measure in order to cause regression of atheroma and reduce adverse coronary outcomes. In the future, targeted and aggressive treatment of risk factors will likely be used in the short and intermediate term as well in an attempt to improve endothelial function (less constriction and more dilation), preserve an anticoagulant surface, inhibit inflamma-tory cell adhesion and infiltration and finally inhibit inappropriate growth of atheroma and development of unstable plaque. Simple manipulation of risk factors has not solved the problems of restenosis following coronary interventions. These procedures and particularly implantation of devices into the coronary arteries will also have to consider additional molecular mechanisms that translate arterial injury into restenosis.

References

1. Braunwald, E. and Sobel B. E. (1980) Coronary blood flow and myocardial ischemia. In: *Heart Disease: A Textbook of Cardiovascular Medicine*, 4th edn, pp. 1191–221. New York: W. B. Saunders.
2. Vane, J. R., Anggard, E. E. and Botting, R. M. (1990) Regulatory functions of the vascular endothelium. *N. Engl. J. Med.*, **323**, 27–36.

3. Furchgott, R. F. (1990) The 1989 Ulf von Euler Lecture: studies on endothelium-derived relaxing factor. *Acta Physiol. Scand.*, **19**, 3–16.
4. Meredith, I. T., Yeung, A. C., Weidinger, F. R. *et al.* (1993) Role of impaired endothelium-dependent vasodilation in ischemic manifestations of coronary artery disease. *Circulation*, **87**, 56–66.
5. Furchgott, R. F. and Zawadzki, J. V. (1980) The obligatory role of endothelial cells in the relaxation of arterial smooth muscle by acetylcholine. *Nature*, **288**, 373–6.
6. Gerlach, H., Esposito, C. and Stern, D. M. (1990) Modulation of endothelial hemostatic properties: an active role in the host response. *Annu. Rev. Med.*, **41**, 15–24.
7. Gertler, J. P. and Abbott, W. M. (1992) Prothrombotic and fibrinolytic function of normal and perturbed endothelium. *J. Surg. Res.*, **52**, 89–95.
8. Becker, R. C. (1991) Seminars in thrombosis, thrombolysis and vascular biology: 1. The vascular endothelium. *Cardiology*, **78**, 13–22.
9. Cybulski, M. I. and Gimbrone, M. A. Jr. (1991) Endothelial expression of a mononuclear leukocyte adhesion molecule during atherogenesis. *Science*, **251**, 788–91.
10. Harlan, J. M., Vedder, N. B., Winn, R. K. *et al.* (1991) Mechanisms and consequences of leukocyte–endothelial interaction. *West. J. Med.*, **155**, 365–9.
11. Ingarro, L. J. (1990) Biosynthesis and metabolism of endothelium-derived nitric oxide. *Annu. Rev. Pharmacol. Toxicol.* **30**, 535–60.
12. Moncada, S., Radomski, M. W. and Palmer, R. M. (1988) Endothelium-derived relaxing factor: identification as nitric oxide and role in the control of vascular tone and platelet function. *Biochem. Pharmacol.*, **37**, 2495–501.
13. Vanhoutte, P. M. (1990) Endothelium-derived relaxing and contracting factors. *Adv. Nephrol. Necker Hosp.*, **139**, 257–70.
14. Gryglewski, R., Bunting, S. and Vane, J. R. (1976) An enzyme isolated from arteries transforms prostaglandin endoperoxidase to an unstable substance that inhibits platelet aggregation. *Nature*, **263**, 663–5.
15. Cox, D. A., Vita, J. A., Treasure, C. B. *et al.* (1989) Atherosclerosis impairs flow-mediated dilation of coronary arteries in humans. *Circulation*, **80**, 458–65.
16. Nabel, E. G., Selwyn, A. P. and Ganz, P. (1990) Large coronary arteries in humans are responsive to changing blood flow: an endothelium dependent mechanism that fails in patients with atherosclerosis. *J. Am. Coll. Cardiol.*, **16**, 349–56.
17. Ludmer, P. L., Selwyn, A. P., Shook, T. L. *et al.* (1986) Paradoxical vasoconstriction induced by acetylcholine in atherosclerotic coronary arteries. *N. Engl. J. Med.*, **315**, 1046–51.
18. Lefroy, D. C., Crane, T., Uren, N. G. *et al.* (1992) Effect of nitric oxide in the human coronary circulation (Abstract). *Circulation*, **86**(Supp. 1), I-118.
19. Collins, P. and Fox, K. (1991) Haemoglobin inhibits endothelium-dependent relaxation *in vivo* (Abstract). *Eur. J. Cardiol.*, **12**(Supp.), 203.
20. Harrison, D. G. (1991) Endothelial modulation of vascular tone: relevance to coronary angioplasty and restenosis. *J. Am. Coll. Cardiol.*, **17**, 71B–76B.
21. Luscher, T. F. (1991) Endothelium-derived nitric oxide: the endogenous nitrovasodilator in the human cardiovascular system. *Eur. Heart J.*, **12,** (Supp. E), 2–11.
22. Vanhoutte, P. M. and Shimokawa, H. (1989) Endothelium-derived relaxing factor and coronary vasospasm. *Circulation*, **80**, 1–9.
23. Shimokawa, H., Aarhis, L. L. and Vanhoutte, P. M. (1987) Porcine coronary arteries with regenerated endothelium have reduced endothelium-dependent responsiveness to aggregating platelets and serotonin. *Circ. Res.*, **61**, 256–70.
24. Kaplan, J. R., Manuck, S. B., Clarkson, T. B. *et al.* (1983) Social stress and atherosclerosis in normocholesterolemic monkeys. *Science*, **220**, 733–5.
25. Heistad, D. D., Armstrong, M. L., Marcus, M. L. *et al.* (1984) Augmented responses to vasoconstrictor stimuli in hypercholesterolemic and atherosclerotic monkeys. *Circ. Res.*, **54**, 711–18.

26. Freiman, P. C., Mitchell, G. C., Heistad, D. D. *et al.* (1986) Atherosclerosis impairs endothelium-dependent vascular relaxation to acetylcholine and thrombin in primates. *Circ. Res.*, **58**, 783–9.
27. Brush, J. E. Jr, Faoxon, D. P., Salmon, S. *et al.* (1992) Abnormal endothelium-dependent vasomotion in hypertensive patients. *J. Am. Coll. Cardiol.*, **19**, 809–15.
28. Treasure, C. B., Manoukian, S. V., Klein, J. L. *et al.* (1992) Epicardial coronary artery responses to acetylcholine are impaired in hypertensive patients. *Circ. Res.*, **71**, 776–81.
29. Hodgson, J. McB., Ravi, N., Sheehan, H. M. *et al.* (1992) Endothelial dysfunction in coronary arteries precedes ultrasonic or angiographic evidence of atherosclerosis in patients with risk factors. *J. Am. Coll. Cardiol.*, **19**(Supp. A), 323A.
30. Panza, J. A., Quyumi, A. A., Brush, J. E. *et al.* (1990) Abnormal endothelium-dependent vascular relaxation in patients with essential hypertension. *N. Engl. J. Med.*, **323**, 22–7.
31. Zeiher, A. M., Drexler, H., Wollschlager, H. *et al.* (1991) Modulation of coronary vasomotor tone in humans: progressive endothelial dysfunction with different early stages of coronary atherosclerosis. *Circulation*, **83**, 391–401.
32. Vita, J. A., Vekshtein, V. I., Selwyn, A. P. *et al.* (1990) The coronary vasomotor response to acetylcholine relates to risk factors for coronary artery disease. *Circulation*, **81**, 491–7.
33. Dyce, M. C., Anderson, T. J., Yeung, A. C. *et al.* (1993) Indices of LDL particle size closely relate to endothelial dysfunction. *Circulation*, **88**, I-466.
34. Celermajer, D. S., Sorensen, K. E., Bull, C. *et al.* (1994) Endothelium-dependent dilation in the systemic arteries of asymptomatic subjects relates to coronary risk factors and their interaction. *J. Am. Coll. Cardiol.*, **24**, 1468–74.
35. Seiler, C., Hess, O. M., Beuchi, M. *et al.* (1993) Influence of serum cholesterol and other coronary risk factors on vasomotion of angiographically normal coronary arteries. *Circulation*, **88**, 2139–48.
36. Mitchinson, M. J. and Ball, R. Y. (1987) Macrophages and atherogenesis. *Lancet*, **ii**, 146–8.
37. Henning, B. and Chow, C. K. (1988) Lipid peroxidation and endothelial cell injury: implication in atherosclerosis. *Free Radical Biol. Med.*, **4**, 99–106.
38. Flavahan, N. A. (1992) Atherosclerosis or lipoprotein-induced endothelial dysfunction: Potential mechanisms underlying reduction in EDRF/nitric oxide activity. *Circulation*, **85**, 1927–38.
39. McLenachan, J. M., Vita, J. A., Fish, R. D. *et al.* (1990) Early evidence of endothelial vasodilator dysfunction at coronary branchpoints. *Circulation*, **82**, 1169–73.
40. Gage, J. E., Hess, O. M., Murakami, T. *et al.* (1986) Vasoconstriction of stenotic coronary arteries during dynamic exercise in patients with classic angina pectoris: reversibility by nitroglycerin. *Circulation*, **73**, 865–76.
41. Gordon, J. B., Ganz, P., Nabel, E. G. *et al.* (1989) Atherosclerosis and endothelial function influence the coronary vasomotor response to exercise. *J. Clin. Invest.*, **83**, 1046–52.
42. Zeiher, A. M., Drexler, H., Wollschlager, H. *et al.* (1989) Coronary vasomotion in response to sympathetic stimulation in humans: importance of the functional integrity of the endothelium. *J. Am. Coll. Cardiol.*, **14**, 1181–90.
43. Yeung, A. C., Vekshtein, V. I., Krantz, D. S. *et al.* (1991) The effect of atherosclerosis on the vasomotor response of coronary arteries to mental stress. *N. Engl. J. Med.*, **325**, 1551–6.
44. Vita, J. A., Treasure, C. B., Yeung, A. C. *et al.* (1992) Patients with evidence of coronary endothelial dysfunction as assessed by acetylcholine infusion demonstrate marked increase in sensitivity to constrictor effects of catecholamines. *Circulation*, **85**, 1390–7.
45. Fuster, V., Stein, B., Ambrose, J. A. *et al.* (1990) Atherosclerotic plaque rupture and thrombosis: evolving concepts. *Circulation*, **82** (Supp. 2), II-47–II-59.
46. Golino, P., Piscion, F., Willerson, J. T. *et al.* (1991) Divergent effects of serotonin on coronary artery dimensions and blood flow in patients with coronary atherosclerosis and control patients. *N. Engl. J. Med.*, **324**, 641–8.
47. McFadden, E. P., Clarke, J. G., Davis, G. J. *et al.* (1991) Effect of intracoronary serotonin on coronary vessels in patients with stable angina and patients with variant angina. *N. Engl. J. Med.*, **324**, 648–54.

48. Harrison, D. G., Armstrong, M. L., Freiman, P. C. and Heistad, D. D. (1987) Restoration of endothelium-dependent relaxation by dietary treatment of atherosclerosis. *J. Clin. Invest.*, **80**, 1808–11.

49. Anderson, T. J., Meredith, I. T., Yeung, A. C. *et al.* (1995) The effect of cholesterol lowering and antioxidant therapy on endothelium-dependent coronary vasomotion. *N. Engl. J. Med.*, **332**(8), 488–93.

50. Brown, B. G., Albers, J. J., Fisher, L. D. *et al.* (1990) Regression of coronary artery disease as a result of intensive lipid-lowering therapy in men with high levels of apolipoprotein B. *N. Engl. J. Med.*, **323**, 1289–98.

51. Steinberg, D., Parthasarathy, S., Carew, T. E. *et al.* (1989) Beyond cholesterol: modification of low-density lipoproteins that increase atherogenicity. *N. Engl. J. Med.*, **320**, 915–24.

52. Keaney, J. R. Jr, Shwaery, G. T., Xu, A. *et al.* (1994) 17β-Estradiol preserves endothelial vasodilator function and limits low-density lipoprotein oxidation in hypercholesterolemic swine. *Circulation*, **89**, 2251–9.

53. Omar, H. A., Cheryy, R. D., Mortelliti, M. P. *et al.* (1991) Inhibition of coronary artery superoxide dismutase attenuates endothelium-dependent and -independent nitrovasodilator relaxation. *Circ. Res.*, **69**, 601–8.

54. Schneider, J. E., Berk, B. C., Gravanis, M. B. *et al.* (1993) Probucol decreases neointimal formation in a swine model of coronary artery balloon injury. A possible role for antioxidants in restenosis. *Circulation*, **88**, 628–37.

55. Barrett-Connor, E. and Bush, T. L. (1991) Estrogen and coronary heart disease in women. *JAMA*, **265**, 1861–7.

56. Williams, J. K., Adams, M. R., Herrington, D. M. *et al.* (1992) Short-term administration of estrogen and vascular responses of atherosclerotic coronary arteries. *J. Am. Coll. Cardiol.*, **20**, 452–7.

57. Bing, R. J. and Conforto, A. (1992) Reversal of acetylcholine effect on atherosclerotic coronary arteries by estrogen: pharmacologic phenomenon of clinical importance? *J. Am. Coll. Cardiol.*, **20**, 458–9.

58. Drexler, H., Zeiher, A. M., Meinzer, K. *et al.* (1991) Correction of endothelial dysfunction in coronary microcirculation of hypercholesterolaemic patients by L-arginine. *Lancet*, **338**, 1546–50.

59. Cooke, J. P., Andon, N. A., Girerd, X. J. *et al.* (1991) Arginine restores cholinergic relaxation of hypercholesterolemic rabbit thoracic aorta. *Circulation*, **83**, 1057–62.

10

Vasoreactive Diseases: Molecular Approach

David Marks
Joseph Loscalzo

Introduction

Over the past fifteen years, an understanding of the physiologic and pathophysiologic determinants of vasomotion has increased dramatically. Under normal circumstances, endothelial products, including notably endothelium-derived relaxing factor (EDRF) maintain resting vascular tone in the basal state. Disturbances in vasomotion, by contrast, accompany many vascular diseases and are themselves early markers of vascular pathology, contributing directly to evolution of these common disorders. In this chapter, we will discuss the pathophysiology of disturbances of vasomotion and review current attempts to intervene in the local manifestations of these abnormalities.

Many common diseases affect vasomotor function. Prior to the development of frank atherosclerosis, risk factors, including hypertension, diabetes and hypercholesterolemia, profoundly affect the normal responses of blood vessels to various vasodilator stimuli. A common, early manifestation of these diseases is local vasomotor perturbation leading either to attenuated endothelium-dependent vasodilator responses or frank, 'paradoxical' vasoconstriction. These changes in vasomotor function often precede overt structural manifestations of vascular diseases and escape diagnostic testing, including angiography.[1]

Atherosclerotic plaques are subject to local mechanical and paracrine perturbations that contribute to plaque rupture. Rupture exposes the richly thrombogenic subendothelium, which promotes deposition of platelets and activation of the hemostatic system.[2] The acute thrombus that forms abruptly narrows the artery lumen, both by its mass and by elaborating substances that directly constrict the vessel. This constriction of the blood vessel by thrombus-derived factors, such as thrombin, further reduces blood flow and exacerbates the clinical sequelae of acute vascular syndromes.

Given their central pathophysiologic role, local atherothrombotic lesions are, therefore, important targets for intervention. In this chapter, we will review the vascular factors that are likely candidates for molecular intervention at the local level, and describe the progress to date on efforts to use this logical therapeutic approach to improve vascular function.

The molecular control of vasomotion

A variety of local and systemic forces interact to modulate vasomotor tone.[3] Given the complex interplay among these determinants and the observation that responses mediated by the normal endothelium may in its absence be attenuated or reversed through direct responses of the smooth-muscle cell, categorization is somewhat artificial. A list of the most commonly recognized endogenous vasoactive substances is presented in Table 10.1.

Vasomotor tone is important in the routine homeostatic responses of the vasculature. Tone influences local blood flow to specific tissue beds. Vascular tone also accounts, in part, for the maintenance of blood pressure. The principal organ responsible for the control of vasomotion is the endothelium. Endothelial cells manifest a number of important effects that control local vasomotion. The primary endothelial mediator of vasoregulation is endothelium-derived relaxation factor (EDRF).[4] This substance is either nitric oxide (NO) or a closely related NO-containing molecule.[5]

Under normal circumstances, blood vessels are maintained in a constant tone of relative relaxation mediated by EDRF, an effect that occurs as a consequence of NO-mediated activation of guanylyl cyclase in the vascular smooth-muscle cell.[6,7] When blood vessels dilate in response to a number of physiologic stimuli, they do so through EDRF-mediated mechanisms. These biologic vasodilator agonists are clinically relevant biochemical[7] and mechanical[8] stimuli that promote vessel patency under normal conditions through stimulating synthesis of EDRF in the endothelial cell. Commonly recognized agonists in this category include serotonin, thrombin, adenosine-3'5'-diphosphate, acetylcholine, bradykinin, substance P and shear stress.[9]

Table 10.1 Endogenous vasoactive mediators*

Vasoconstriction	Vasodilation
Acetylcholine†	Acetylcholine†
Adenosine diphosphate†	Adenosine diphosphate†
Angiotensin II	Atrial natriuretic peptide
Arginine vasopressin	EDHF
Endothelin	EDRF
Epinephrine†	Epinephrine†
Hemoglobin	Glucagon
Histamine	Insulin
Norepinephrine†	Prostacyclin
Serotonin†	Norepinephrine†
Superoxide anion	Serotonin†
Thromboxane A_2	Substance P

*That certain agonists are capable of evincing both vasoconstricting and vasodilatory effects is a consequence of their contrasting direct effects on (normal) endothelium and vascular smooth muscle, respectively. These are indicated †.

In addition to its vasodilatory role, EDRF possesses other functions relevant to vascular homeostasis. EDRF inhibits platelet activation and aggregation, binding to the heme moiety of guanylyl cyclase and increasing the concentration of cyclic guanosine 5'-monophosphate in the platelet.[10] EDRF inhibits the *in vitro* proliferation of vascular smooth-muscle cells,[11] and modulates leukocyte adhesion to the subendothelium by downregulating expression of adhesion molecules.[12] Evidence has also been recently presented that EDRF modulates vascular permeability.[13] Given the free-radical nature of NO, this simple diatomic molecule has the capacity to quench pathogenic free-radical oxidants, such as superoxide anion.[14,15] Thus, EDRF functions to maintain blood flow through a variety of closely related mechanisms in addition to its vasodilator action.

Mechanical removal of the endothelium abolishes the vasodilator responses to endothelium-dependent vasoactive stimuli while leaving the direct smooth-muscle vasoconstrictor effects of these agonists unopposed.[16] This observation is relevant to several clinical scenarios, including the mechanical denudation of the endothelial surface that occurs with balloon angioplasty and the direct exposure of subendothelial structures that occurs with atheromatous plaque rupture. In addition to these straightforward effects of structural alterations in the vasculature, regenerated endothelium is often functionally abnormal,[17] and changes in proximal vessel function may affect the more distal microvasculature resulting in inappropriate constriction.[18]

Endothelium-dependent vasodilation is abnormal in many disease states, and 'paradoxical' vasoconstriction in response to agonists with vasodilator actions under normal conditions has been clearly documented in a variety of ischemic syndromes.[19–21] Prior to the development of overt ischemic syndromes, this endothelial dysfunction has been demonstrated in hypercholesterolemia,[22] atherosclerosis,[23] hypertension[24] and diabetes mellitus.[25] Moreover, the number of risk factors for atherosclerosis in a given individual correlates with the quantitative extent of endothelial dysfunction.[26] In that the risk of clinical vascular events in individuals with atherosclerosis does not correlate with the physical severity of the lesions[27] dynamic vasomotor responses likely play an important role in the pathophysiology of these acute vascular syndromes. Furthermore, impairment of EDRF action may also play a direct role in preclinical atherogenesis.[28] These observations underscore the importance of vasomotion and the factors which control it in many pathologic vascular syndromes.

Molecular approaches for restoration of vascular function

As with the other systems of local delivery discussed in this book the selection of the agent to deliver and the mode of delivery are of paramount importance. The principal promise of the current molecular 'revolution' is that any gene product can potentially be transferred to a local volume of tissue and be expressed at that site exclusively, thereby mitigating unwanted systemic side effects. Similarly, it is possible to populate a local area of vessel with genetically altered cells that contain molecular 'vectors' which express a desired gene product. It is also possible to interrupt the production of an unwanted gene through the delivery of antisense oligonucleotides or specific antibodies to a protein. Hence, the molecular approach to delivery allows for the expression, enhancement, or inhibition of conceivably any endogenous vasoactive molecule or the enzymatic machinery required for its synthesis.

Exogenous vasoactive agents may also be delivered locally using both mechanical and molecularly targeted delivery approaches. Examples of mechanical delivery include molecule-eluting stents or drug-delivery catheters (see Chapter 2). Larger molecules can also be fashioned to deliver drugs to 'vasoactive sites' locally. Examples of these carrier molecules include antibodies directed against basement-membrane components,[29] proliferating smooth-muscle cells,[30] platelets,[31] unique epitopes in atheromatous plaques or a combination of these elements.[32] While this diversity of carrier molecules provides many opportunities for tailored therapeutic approaches, defining the optimal carrier and the ideal delivery regimen remain elusive problems.

EDRF/NO

The endothelium plays a key role in the maintenance of vascular homeostasis, and this function is mediated by several molecules elaborated directly by the endothelial cell, principal among which is EDRF. EDRF is not only a potent vasodilator, but also inhibits local platelet deposition, leukocyte adherence, smooth-muscle cell proliferation and endothelial permeability.

Nitric oxide, the principal determinant of EDRF action, has been used systemically for many years in the form of pharmacologic nitrovasodilators. Brunton first described the clinical use of amyl nitrite for angina pectoris in 1867 and since that time, organic nitrovasodilators have been used extensively in patients with coronary disease. Systemic nitroglycerin, in particular, has enjoyed widespread application owing to its principal venodilating effects,[33] lowering myocardial-wall tension and reducing myocardial oxygen consumption. Nitroglycerin also inhibits platelet aggregation, and this effect is potentiated by thiol groups.[34] Early work suggested the systemic delivery of NO donors in acute myocardial infarction may be beneficial; however, recently published studies have failed to support this view. The ESPRIM group found that lisidomine followed by molsidomine did not change the short-term clinical endpoints of patients with myocardial infarction,[35] and the recently published results of the ISIS-4 Trial confirm the lack of direct benefit of nitrates on survival following acute myocardial infarction.[36]

Despite this lack of benefit with systemic delivery of nitrovasodilators in acute myocardial infarction, more encouraging results have been reported with the use of NO donors in angioplasty. Groves and colleagues[37] have demonstrated reduced local platelet adhesion and thrombus formation after systemic administration of SIN-1, an NO donor and metabolite of molsidomine. In humans, a preliminary report from the ACCORD trial suggests that NO donors might be an effective adjunctive therapy in angioplasty.[38] This group randomized patients to receive lisidomine and molsidomine for a total of six months and compared outcomes to those treated with diltiazem. They found no acute difference between groups, but at six months a reduction in restenosis rates was achieved.

Attempts to normalize endothelial function by providing excess substrate for nitric oxide synthase (L-arginine) have also been published by several groups. Indeed, investigators have shown improvement in endothelium-dependent vasodilation in hypercholesterolemic pigs[39] and rabbits with infusion of L-arginine,[40] and recent evidence suggests that L-arginine may improve vasomotion in hyperlipidemic patients, as well.[41] L-Arginine supplementation has also been shown to reduce lesion surface area and intimal thickness in aortae from cholesterol-fed rabbits.[42] Preliminary evidence suggests that dietary supplementation of L-arginine may be useful in reducing intimal hyperplasia independent of smooth-muscle cell proliferation,[43] an effect that is also mediated by nitric oxide.[44] In contrast to these beneficial effects among hypercholesterolemic and atherosclerotic individuals, L-arginine supplementation is not effective in essential hypertensive patients,[45] suggesting that the mechanisms of endothelial dysfunction may differ in different vascular disease states.[46]

NO adducts/S-nitrosothiols

Nitric oxide is a reactive free radical that can readily form adducts with biologic nucleophiles, principal among which are thiols. Thiols potentiate the action of nitric oxide and EDRF, and likely do so by forming thionitrites or S-nitrosothiols. Mellion and colleagues first demonstrated the effects of synthetic S-nitroso-compounds as platelet inhibitors.[47,48] Loscalzo demonstrated that the thiol, *N*-acetylcysteine, potentiates the inhibitory effect of nitroglycerin on platelets by forming an S-nitrosothiol, *S*-nitroso-*N*-acetylcysteine. We subsequently demonstrated the importance and efficacy of synthetically nitrosating thiols for pharmacologic effect.[49] The observations of the importance of thiols in EDRF metabolism were further extended by Cooke and colleagues[50] who demonstrated that shear stress, a known stimulus for EDRF release, is potentiated by thiols.

Building on these previous observations, Stamler *et al.*[51] investigated the reactions of various sulfhydryl-containing proteins with NO and EDRF. We demonstrated that S-nitrosoproteins are readily formed under physiologic conditions and that these molecules, acting through a cyclic GMP-dependent mechanism, possess significant vasodilatory and platelet inhibitory properties. Subsequently, we described the presence and reservoir function of endogenous S-nitrosoproteins in plasma, primarily an S-nitroso adduct of serum albumin (S-NO-BSA (Bovine Serum Albumin)).[52] Moreover, nitrosation was found to modulate the activity of enzymes with thiol groups suggesting a possible novel mechanism of posttranslational modification of proteins and, thus, of biologic signaling.[53]

EDRF has a short half-life in biologic buffers (0.1–1 s).[54] The discovery of biologic adducts of EDRF, S-nitrosothiols, revealed a class of molecules with EDRF-like properties of vasorelaxation and platelet inhibition having a substantially longer half-life.[57] The half-life of S-NO-BSA is 12 h at 37°C, pH 7.4.[57] S-NO-BSA has a prolonged duration of action as compared to lower-molecular-weight

S-nitrosothiols, e.g. S-nitrosocysteine, but is less potent as a vasodilator.[55] S-nitrosothiols can be viewed as nitrosonium (NO^+) carriers under physiologic conditions,[58] and low-molecular-weight thiols likely undergo transnitrosation reactions with NO complexed to protein thiols, especially S-NO-BSA.

Keaney et al.[55] subsequently investigated the in vivo properties of S-NO-BSA and found dose-dependent changes in coronary blood flow, coronary artery diameter and mean arterial pressure in response to S-NO-BSA infusion in dogs.[54] In addition, S-NO-BSA produced significant dose-dependent inhibition of bleeding time and ex vivo platelet aggregation in these animals. Given these observations on the vasodilator and antiplatelet properties of S-NO-BSA, we chose to extend our studies to an investigation of the possible role that S-nitrosothiols play as modulators of the response to vascular injury.

We recently investigated the role of S-NO-BSA as an adduct for delivery of NO to injured rabbit femoral arteries. Owing to the observation that serum albumin binds avidly to subendothelium following acute denuding injury and, thereby, 'passivates' the surface, we hypothesized that S-NO-BSA would target NO delivery to the site of injury. Using a model of vascular injury modified after Rogers and co-workers,[57] we first used New Zealand white rabbits to assess the avidity of the injured subendothelium for albumin and the efficacy of nitrosated albumin (S-NO-BSA) to inhibit intimal proliferation. We occluded a 1.5–2.0-cm segment of a femoral artery with stainless-steel clips, ligated all side branches, and denuded the vessel with a 2F Fogarty catheter (Baxter Healthcare Corp., Edwards Division, Santa Ana, CA, USA) inflated and withdrawn three times from the vessel. S-NO-BSA (115 nmol)[58] was then instilled in the vessel for 15 minutes, after which flow was re-established by removal of the vascular clips and ligation of the superficial femoral artery. Blood was allowed to recirculate for 15 minutes and the vessels were harvested. The contralateral femoral artery served as a matched control to examine the effects of vehicle.

The binding of S-NO-BSA to the injured vessel was first assayed using ^{125}I-labeled S-NO-BSA. Albumin was shown to bind to de-endothelialized arterial segments 30-fold more efficiently with local delivery compared to systemic delivery. Virtually no albumin was deposited on intact arterial segments harvested as controls (Figure 10.1). Approximately 0.15% of the total S-NO-BSA mass administered bound to the injured vessel segment. This study confirmed that S-NO-BSA is adequate for the local vascular delivery of NO. Systemically administered S-NO-BSA, by contrast, would likely have a low rate of deposition at the site of injury given the sizable dilution effects that accompany systemic administration.

We next investigated the effects of local delivery of S-NO-BSA on intimal proliferation in this rabbit model. We used the same experimental protocol of balloon injury and local instillation of either S-NO-BSA or bovine serum albumin (BSA), with the latter control administered to the contralateral artery. After two weeks, arterial segments were pressure-fixed for pathologic analysis. Calculations of intimal:medial ratio were performed using computer-assisted planimetry on segments stained for elastin, and these results are shown in Figure 10.2. The local delivery of S-NO-BSA failed to achieve a statistically significant reduction in the intimal:medial

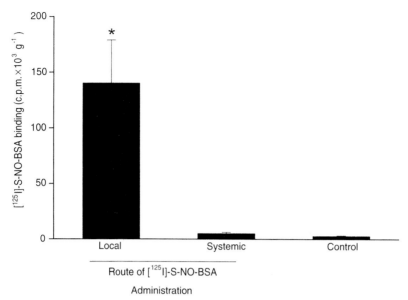

Figure 10.1 Local delivery of ^{125}I-labeled S-NO-BSA to balloon-injured New Zealand white rabbit femoral arteries. *$P < 0.05$ vs systemic and control.

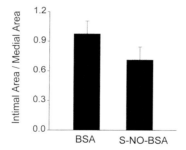

Figure 10.2 Local delivery of S-NO-BSA to balloon-injured New Zealand white rabbit femoral arteries and effects on neointimal proliferation.

ratio compared with control, although intimal proliferation was reduced by 27% (intima:media = 0.715 ± 0.12 vs 0.975 ± 0.16).

Given the possibility that insufficient NO was delivered by this S-NO-BSA adduct, we modified the albumin by thiolation using N-acetyl-D,L-homocysteine thiolactone,[59] which yielded 3.2 ± 1.3 thiol groups per albumin molecule. These groups were then S-nitrosated, leading to the synthesis of a polythiolated, poly-S-nitrosated albumin (pS-NO-BSA).

Repeating the balloon-injury protocol with local delivery, we next compared the effect of local administration of pS-NO-BSA with that of control, polythiolated BSA

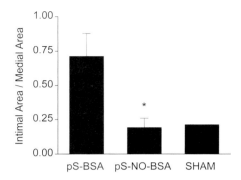

Figure 10.3 Local delivery of pS-NO-BSA to balloon-injured New Zealand white rabbit femoral arteries and effects on neointimal proliferation. *$P < 0.05$ vs pS-NO-BSA.

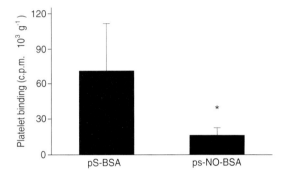

Figure 10.4 Local delivery of pS-NO-BSA to balloon-injured New Zealand white rabbit femoral arteries inhibits [111] In-labeled platelet binding. *$P < 0.05$.

(pBSA). The results of these studies are shown in Figure 10.3. pS-NO-BSA significantly inhibited intimal proliferation (intima:media = 0.192 ± 0.07 vs 0.714 ± 0.16, $P = 0.025$), and did so essentially completely; the intima:media ratio for pS-NO-BSA was essentially identical to that of sham controls. Importantly, a single administration of this molecule at the time of injury was effective, suggesting that the effect was long-lived, perhaps as a consequence of the affinity of albumin for subendothelial protein(s).

To investigate inhibition of platelet binding as a potential effect of local delivery of pS-NO-BSA, we conducted the following experiments. Using the rabbit model of balloon injury and local delivery, pS-NO-BSA was infused into the femoral arteries of normal New Zealand white rabbits; pBSA was infused into paired contralateral controls. Immediately after delivery, ^{111}In-labeled platelets were systemically administered and blood allowed to recirculate within the segments for 15 minutes. Arterial segments were harvested after an additional 15 minutes for analysis. The results of these studies are shown in Figure 10.4. The local delivery of pS-NO-BSA inhibited platelet binding nearly fourfold compared to the contralateral control: $1.8 \pm 0.6 \times 10^4$ c.p.m. mg tissue^{-1} vs $8.6 \pm 3.8 \times 10^4$ c.p.m. mg tissue^{-1}; $P = 0.02$. This finding is intriguing since deposited platelets contribute to the proliferative and cell-migratory response following injury through release of growth factors. Thus, pS-NO-BSA may have biologic effects in disease states characterized by platelet deposition. Unstable angina, myocardial infarction and transluminal angioplasty are, therefore, possible targets for intervention using this approach.

Exogenous replacement

The use of S-nitrosated thiols as local, vasoactive pharmaceuticals offers many unique possibilities as delivery vehicles. While albumin forms an active adduct with NO, we have shown that it binds to damaged arterial vessels with limited efficacy. Covalent modification of the molecule with multiple thiol functionalities available for S-nitrosation yields a product with much higher specific NO activity than the native protein. In addition to increasing NO:albumin stoichiometry, it is possible that NO delivery could also be enhanced by using site-specific target molecules as carriers, such as antibodies against cellular elements of the atherosclerotic plaque, platelets, thrombin or other locally expressed antigens. Molecules of this general type may increase the local concentration and half-life of NO leading to more profound biologic effects, and may also alleviate the need for local mechanical delivery.

Endogenous replacement

Arterial injury is a complex process involving numerous interactive elements in the vascular wall. While the deposition of platelets on the injured wall may lead to increased NO liberated from the platelets themselves following calcium-dependent activation of their constitutive (i.e., endothelial or isoform III) nitric oxide synthase (cNOS), arterial injury is also accompanied by increased transcription of another isoform of NOS with further increases in NO formation.[60] This increase in NO production involves the enhanced transcription of inducible nitric oxide synthase (iNOS) by inflammatory cytokines, such as interleukin-1, and by endotoxin.[61] While this process may be adaptive, induction of transcription takes several hours and is synergistic with cyclic AMP-elevating agents, most notably forskolin.[62] This latter observation is particularly important given the preliminary work using forskolin-eluting stents in vascular intervention.

Nitric oxide synthase, the enzyme responsible for the elaboration of NO from L-arginine, exists in several isoforms. The constitutive forms of the enzyme are found in brain, endothelium and platelets, and are the products of a distinct gene family.[63] cNOS is tightly regulated by the calcium–calmodulin complex.[64] Inducible NOS is not calcium-regulated because calmodulin[65] remains essentially irreversibly bound to it; this enzyme has also been purified and cloned from macrophages and hepatocytes.[66] The transfer or delivery of this enzyme, which remains active for hours, in vascular smooth-muscle cells also represents a possible mechanism for local delivery of an endogenous vasoactive molecule. Since regenerating endothelial cells are phenotypically abnormal,[67] genetically altered endothelial cells, which actively produce NO from L-arginine, could be mechanically delivered to a site of arterial injury to repopulate or 'seed' the site of injury with 'normal' endothelial cells.

Not only could cNOS be overexpressed using this approach, but other beneficial gene products could also potentially be expressed in the seeded cells. Dzau's group has recently demonstrated in a rat model of arterial injury that cNOS can be transfected and expressed in vascular smooth-muscle cells following vascular injury.[68] A significant biologic effect was demonstrated with reduced neointima formation in the transfected vessels. While he examined intimal proliferation as an endpoint, he did not examine the effects of this intervention on vasomotion. Thus, this preliminary report demonstrates that endogenous vasoactive molecules can be delivered either directly or indirectly as gene products and can have important biologic effects.

Prostacyclin

Prostacyclin (PGI_2) is an active metabolite of arachidonic acid produced by the cyclooxygenase pathway. Prostacyclin is thought to oppose the prothrombotic effects of thromboxane A_2, which is also a metabolite of arachidonic acid synthesized in platelets. PGI_2 is a product of endothelial cells; it is a potent vasodilator and platelet inhibitor,[69] an effect exerted through elevations in intracellular cAMP.

Similar to EDRF, cell-culture studies have demonstrated increased production of prostacyclin in response to a variety of physiologic endothelial stimuli including fibrin,[70] shear stress,[71] and HDL;[72] conversely, elaboration of prostacyclin is inhibited by cigarette smoke.[73]

The systemic use of prostacyclin has been associated with intolerable systemic side effects. Flushing, headache and hypotension are seen with the use of this agent and its synthetic analogs, thus arguing for local-delivery approaches. In five patients with advanced vascular disease, intra-arterial administration of prostacyclin was associated with clinical improvement.[74,75] In addition, prostacyclin produced by blood vessels and cardiac tissue tends to be increased in patients receiving fish oil rich in omega-3 fatty acids,[76] as a result of which *ex vivo* aggregation studies demonstrated inhibition of platelet function without systemic side effects reported.

Recently, Banning and colleagues reported preliminary work on the local delivery of iloprost, a stable prostacyclin derivative, to sites of angioplasty using electroporation of platelets and a double-balloon catheter.[77] This study showed a significant reduction in neointima formation in vessels that were superficially injured by balloon angioplasty. It is interesting to note that the effect was not observed in vessels in which the internal elastic membrane was ruptured, suggesting a true limitation to this approach.

Forskolin

Forskolin is a lipophilic adenylyl cyclase activator that acts by a mechanism similar to PGI_2. By increasing intracellular cAMP, cAMP-dependent protein kinases are activated leading to phosphorylation of specific intracellular proteins. This cascade eventually leads to the sequestering of cytosolic calcium and the relaxation of vascular smooth muscle. Forskolin has also been shown to inhibit platelet activation by interfering with the calcium-dependent binding of fibrinogen and von Wille-brand factor to ADP- or thrombin-activated platelets.[78] Given its long-term stability and hydrophobic nature, it is a suitable candidate for local drug delivery, particularly as part of an eluting stent. A forskolin-eluting, polymer-coated, metallic stent has been shown to increase the time to *in situ* thrombosis,[79] improve flow and increase the time to cyclic flow variations compared with a control stent, suggesting a powerful local antiplatelet effect.[80]

Angiopeptin

Angiopeptin is a synthetic cyclic octapeptide and an analog of somatostatin. This peptide has multiple biologic effects including the inhibition of growth hormone release[81] and of vascular smooth-muscle proliferation.[82] Intrinsic vasomotor proper-ties have not been observed with this molecule. Normal and atherosclerotic animal models of vascular injury have shown a significant reduction in intimal thickness after therapy with angiopeptin.[83,84] The mechanism by which angiopeptin inhibits intimal growth is unknown; evidence does not suggest that this effect occurs by inhibition of growth factor release or action.[85] In an important study, Light and colleagues[86] investigated the effects of angiopeptin on the vasoactive properties of New Zealand white rabbit aortae. They found no difference in the amount of prostacyclin elaborated after arachidonic acid stimulation. In contrast, relaxation to acetylcholine was markedly improved, although significantly different from normal controls. These data suggest that while not a vasodilator itself, angiopeptin can improve endothelial function.

Two recent clinical trials have been preliminarily reported in which angiopeptin was used to limit restenosis following angioplasty. Eriksen and coworkers[87] reported in a randomized, placebo-controlled trial of 112 patients that angiopeptin (750 mg day^{-1}, s.c.) reduced the binary restenosis rate from 37.8% in the control group to 7.5% in the treatment group. Conversely, Kent and colleagues[88] reported no difference in restenosis rate after angiopeptin administration (190, 750, 3000 mg day^{-1}). Neither abstract nor presentation reported vasomotor effects in these trials. These conflicting results will need to be reconciled in further studies. In addition, possible effects on vasomotion need to be addressed.

Endothelin

In addition to its important role in vasodilation, the endothelium also synthesizes and releases a potent vasoconstrictor, endothelin (ET). ET is a potent mitogen for smooth-muscle cells.[89] First described in 1985,[90] endothelin is a 21-amino acid peptide[91] subsequently shown to be a member of a family of peptides[92] connected by two disulfide bridges that have significant vasoconstrictive properties.[93] Three isoforms of ET are known,[94] with ET-1 produced by endothelial cells.

The vascular effects of ET-1 are mediated by two receptors, ETA and ETB, which have been characterized and cloned.[95,96] ET-1 is translated as a 203-amino acid prepropeptide that is cleaved to proendothelin. Proendothelin is converted by endothelin converting enzyme (ECE)[97] to the final mature 21-amino acid product. After binding to the ET receptor, phospholipase C is activated initiating a cascade that promotes the intracellular release and extracellular influx of Ca^{2+} leading to contraction of smooth muscle.[98] Given that the release of ET is polarized to the basolateral side of the endothelial cell, it is suspected that endothelin functions as a paracrine signal molecule.[99] This observation is exceedingly important in considering the potential for local delivery of ET antagonists. Since the systemic concentrations of ET do not reflect the local concentrations of the substance, antagonists are needed, first to study the effects of inhibition of this agent and, second, to attempt to mitigate the associated pathologic actions of the molecule.

Elevation of endothelin in the systemic circulation accompany many disease states, including hypertension,[100] atherosclerosis,[101] coronary artery spasm,[102] myocardial infarction,[103] congestive heart failure[104] and renal failure.[105] Elevated plasma endothelin levels at the time of myocardial infarction are associated with a poor one-year survival.[106] Local endothelin release within the coronary artery bed after angioplasty has also been documented.[107]

Many inhibitors of endothelin binding to ETA are known, including an orally active ETA receptor antagonist.[108] This molecule (Ro 46-2005) has been shown to bind ETA avidly and to compete well with ET for its receptor. While these molecules are useful tools, the recent observations of Seo and colleagues[109] may hinder clinical trials of this molecule. This group found that, unlike various reported animal models, antagonism of both the ETA and ETB receptors is required for inhibition of ET-1-mediated vasoconstriction in humans. While a combined ETA/ETB receptor antagonist has been described,[110] it is possible that this inhibitor will antagonize ET-1 effects on nitric oxide and prostacyclin release from endothelial cells, potentially limiting its clinical applicability.[111] Further studies are needed to dissect the efficacy of manipulation of this complex pathway. There are, as yet, no reports of the effect of local delivery of any ET antagonist. Given that the molecule likely acts as a local agent, it may be well suited to local interventional approaches.

Other therapies that block the biologic effects of ET-1 will soon be available. As ET must be converted by ECE to the active molecule, ECE inhibitors are being synthesized that will circumvent the problems highlighted by Seo and coworkers. Similarly, as an endogenous vasoconstrictor, ET is a target for local delivery of antisense oligonucleotides that inhibit the translation of the molecule. In addition to these direct methods of decreasing the local concentration of ET, an indirect method has also been described. Endothelin receptors have been shown to be downregulated by steroids.[112] Local delivery of dexamethasone by an eluting stent has preliminarily been shown not to affect intima hyperplasia significantly in a porcine model,[113] but has been shown to inhibit neointimal proliferation significantly in an injured rat carotid artery model.[114]

Hemostatic elements

Platelets, while important in the early hemostatic response, are likely important mediators of inappropriate vasomotion, as well. Thromboxane A_2 and serotonin are two important mediators of vasoconstriction derived from platelets, serving important homeostatic mechanisms against hemorrhage. Yet, the interaction of platelets with the atherosclerotic plaque and the damaged vessel wall can lead to significant vascular pathology.[115] Platelet aggregation is increased cyclically and in a coordinated pattern following acute vascular injury;[116] similarly, spontaneous platelet aggregation is associated with an increased risk of further vascular events in a cohort of survivors of acute myocardial infarction.[117] Platelet-derived growth factor (PDGF), is a potent determinant for vascular cell migration following injury.[118] Investigation into the manipulation of the vasoactive properties of platelet products is proceeding, although an exploration of local modulation has not yet been conducted. One can theoretically exploit the propensity of platelets to localize at a site of vascular injury by using these anuclear cells to deliver a drug of interest directly. Rybak's use of 'plateletsomes' represents one example of this approach.[119]

Thromboxane A_2 is formed from arachidonic acid in platelets. The half-life of this eicosanoid is approximately 30 s, and its principal effects are to cause vasoconstriction[120] and to activate other platelets.[121] Vasospasm induced by this molecule is augmented in animal models of atherosclerosis.[122] Metabolites of thromboxane A_2 are elevated in acute vascular syndromes, such as unstable angina,[123] reinforcing the concept of platelet activation in these disorders. Aspirin irreversibly inhibits platelets by acetylating cyclooxygenase/Prostaglandin G/H synthase. The inhibition of platelets by aspirin has been shown not to be effective in limiting restenosis[124] despite its efficacy as a platelet inhibitor and usefulness in acute vascular syndromes.

Prostacyclin synthesis in endothelial cells is also inhibited by the administration of aspirin. Attempts at modulating the delivery of aspirin, either by the development of a continuous release preparation[125] or by use of a lower dose,[126] have met with some success. The systemic delivery of a specific thromboxane A_2 synthase inhibitor has been shown to be effective in animal models of unstable vascular syndromes.[127] Similarly, specific systemic administration of a thromboxane A_2 receptor antagonist has been shown to be efficacious in comparison to either diltiazem or nitroglycerin as a platelet inhibitor at sites of injury.[128] In combination, synthase inhibition and receptor antagonism synergistically abolish platelet-dependent effects on the vessel wall following vascular injury; in an animal model, combined synthase inhibition and receptor blockade are more potent than the systemic administration of aspirin.[129] Local delivery of either receptor antagonist or thromboxane synthase inhibitor has not been reported.

Serotonin is another platelet product that is reasonably vasoactive. Similar to thromboxane A_2, this molecule not only has vascular effects, but also activates other platelets. Serotonin may also directly affect smooth-muscle growth.[130] In normal arteries, serotonin is a stimulus for the endothelial release of EDRF and, thus, vasorelaxation.[131] When isolated vascular smooth-muscle cells are exposed to serotonin, constriction generally occurs[132] and this effect can be antagonized by blockade of 5-HT$_2$ serotonergic receptors. After vascular injury, the regenerated endothelial cells lose their capacity to respond appropriately to serotonergic stimulation.[133,134] Recently, preliminary evidence in a canine model suggests that the addition of an inhibitor of ADP-mediated platelet inhibition to a regimen of inhibition of thromboxane A_2 synthesis and serotonin prevents neointimal proliferation after endothelial injury.[135]

Summary

Vasomotion and vasoactive molecules play a pivotal role in both vascular biology and in many vascular disease states. The categorization of molecules as purely 'vasoactive' is likely an artificial denotation owing to the myriad of biologic processes in which traditionally 'vasoactive' molecules participate. The plasticity of the local molecular approaches described here cannot be overemphasized. Targeted delivery of genes or of carrier molecules that facilitate the local expression of a desired bioactivity will doubtless continue to develop and will clearly represent a viable therapeutic strategy in the near future in a wide range of vascular disorders.

References

1. Roberts, W. C., Curry, R. C., Isner, J. M. *et al.* (1982) Sudden death in Prinzmetal's angina with coronary spasm documented by angiography: analysis of three necropsy patients. *Am. J. Cardiol.*, **50**, 203–10.
2. Collins, P. and Fox, K. M. (1990) Pathophysiology of angina. *Lancet*, **i**, 94–6.
3. O'Rourke, S. and Vanhoutte, P. M. (1992) Vascular pharmacology. In: Loscalzo, J., Creager, M. and Dzau, V. (eds) *Vascular Medicine*, 1st edn, pp. 133–56. Boston: Little, Brown.
4. Furchgott, R. F. and Zawadzki, J. F. (1980) The obligatory role of endothelial cells in the relaxation of arterial smooth muscle by acetylcholine. *Nature*, **288**, 373–6.
5. Moncada, S., Palmer, R. M. and Higgs, E. A. (1991) Nitric oxide: physiology, pathophysiology and pharmacology. *Pharmacol. Rev.*, **43**, 109–42.
6. Rees, D. D., Palmer, R. M. and Moncada, S. (1989) Role of endothelium-derived nitric oxide in the regulation of blood pressure. *Proc. Natl Acad. Sci. USA*, **86**, 3375–8.
7. Vallance, P., Collier, J. and Moncada, S. (1989) Effects of endothelium-derived nitric oxide on peripheral arteriolar tone in man [see comments]. *Lancet*, **ii**, 997–1000.
8. Furchgott, R. (1983) Role of endothelium in responses of vascular smooth muscle. *Circ. Res.*, **35**, 557–73.
9. Rubanyi, G. M., Romero, J. C. and Vanhoutte, P. M. (1986) Flow-induced release of endothelium-derived relaxation factor. *Am. J. Physiol.*, **250**, H1145–H1149.
10. Radomski, R. A., Palmer, R. M. J. and Moncada, S. (1987) Comparative physiology of endothelium-derived relaxing factor, nitric oxide, and prostacyclin in platelets. *Br. J. Pharmacol.*, **92**, 181–7.
11. Garg, U. C. and Hassid, A. (1986) Nitric oxide-generating vasodilators and 8-bromo-cyclic guanosine monophosphate inhibit mitogenesis and proliferation of cultured rat vascular smooth muscle cells. *J. Clin. Invest.*, **83**, 1774–7.
12. Kubes, P., Suzuki, M. and Granger, D. N. (1991) Nitric oxide: an endogenous modulator of leukocyte adhesion. *Proc. Natl. Acad. Sci. USA*, **88**, 4651–5.
13. Kubes, P. and Granger, D. N. (1993) Nitric oxide modulates microvascular permeability. *Am. J. Physiol.*, **262**, H611–H615.
14. Feigl, O. E. (1988) EDRF – a protective factor. *Nature*, **331**, 490–1.
15. Saran, M., Michael, C. and Bars, W. (1990) Reaction of NO with O_2. Implications for the reaction of endothelium-derived relaxing factor (EDRF). *Free Radical Res. Commun.*, **10**, 221–6.

16. Furchgott, R. F. and Zawadzki, J. F. (1980) The obligatory role of endothelial cells in the relaxation of arterial smooth muscle by acetylcholine. *Nature*, **288**, 373–6.

17. Weidinger, F. F., McLenachan, J. M., Cybulsky, M. I. *et al.* (1990) Persistent dysfunction of regenerated endothelium after balloon angioplasty of rabbit iliac artery. *Circulation*, **81**, 1667–79.

18. Harrison, D. G. (1991) Endothelial modulation of vascular tone: relevance to coronary angioplasty and restenosis. *J. Am. Coll. Cardiol.*, **17**, 71B–76B.

19. Brown, G. B., Bolson, E. L. and Dodge, H. T. (1984) Dynamic mechanism in human coronary stenosis. *Circulation*, **70**, 917–22.

20. Fuster, V. (1988) Insights into the pathogenesis of acute ischemic syndromes. *Circulation*, **77**, 1213–20.

21. Ganz, P., Abben, R. P. and Barry, W. H. (1987) Dynamic variations in resistance of coronary arterial narrowings in angina pectoris at rest. *Am. J. Cardiol.*, **59**, 66–70.

22. Vita, J. A., Treasure, C. B., Nabel, E. G. *et al.* (1990) Coronary vasomotor response to acetylcholine relates to risk factors for coronary artery disease. *Circulation*, **81**, 491–7.

23. Ludmer, P. L., Selwyn, A. P., Shook, T. L. *et al.* (1986) Paradoxical vasoconstriction induced by acetylcholine in atherosclerotic coronary arteries. *N. Engl. J. Med.*, **315**, 1046–51.

24. Treasure, C. B., Manoukian, S. V., Klein, J. L. *et al.* (1992) Epicardial coronary artery responses to acetylcholine are impaired in hypertensive patients. *Circ. Res.*, **71**, 776–81.

25. Nitenberg, A., Valersi, P., Sachs, R., Dali, M., Aptecar, E. and Attali, J. R. (1993) Impairment of coronary vascular reserve in an ACH-induced coronary vasodilation in diabetic patients with angiographically normal coronary arteries and normal left ventricular systolic function. *Diabetes*, **42**, 1017–25.

26. Vita, J. A., Treasure, C. B., Nabel, E. G. *et al.* (1990) Coronary vasomotor response to acetylcholine relates to risk factors for coronary artery disease. *Circulation*, **81**, 491–7.

27. Ambrose, J. A., Winters, S. L., Stern, A. *et al.* (1985) Angiographic morphology and the pathogenesis of unstable angina pectoris. *J. Am. Coll. Cardiol.*, **5**, 609–16.

28. Cooke, J. P., Songer, A. H., Tsao, P. *et al.* (1992) Antiatherogenic effects of L-arginine in hypercholesterolemic rabbits. *J. Clin. Invest.*, **90**, 1168–72.

29. Ragni, M., Cirillo, P., Ezekowitz, M. D. *et al.* (1993) Anti-tissue factor antibody shortens lysis time by t-PA and prevents reocclusion in a rabbit model of carotid artery thrombosis. *Circulation*, **88**, I-615.

30. Narula, J., Petrov, A., Ditlow, C. *et al.* (1993) Localization of experimental atherosclerotic lesions with negatively-charged polymer-modified chimeric antibody specific for proliferating neointimal smooth muscle cells. *Circulation*, **88**, I-250.

31. Bode, C., Freitag, M., Mewald, P. *et al.* (1993) Fibrin-targeted or platelet-targeted recombinant hirudin inhibits fibrin deposition on experimental clots more efficiently than untargeted hirudin. *Circulation*, **88**, I-417.

32. More, R. S., Underwood, M., Brack, M. *et al.* (1993) Inhibition of *in vivo* thrombus formation by locally delivered antibody targeted antiplatelet–fibrinolytic conjugate. *Circulation*, **88**, I-265.

33. Brown, B. G., Bolson, E., Petersen, R. B. *et al.* (1981) The mechanisms of nitroglycerin action: stenosis vasodilation as a major component of the drug response. *Circulation*, **64**, 1089–97.

34. Loscalzo, J. (1985) N-Acetylcysteine potentiates inhibition of platelet aggregation by nitroglycerin. *J. Clin. Invest.*, **76**, 703–8.

35. Leizorovicz, A. (1993) Can NO donors improve the prognosis of acute MI patients? Results from a large scale placebo controlled study. *Circulation*, **88**, I-394.

36. ISIS 4 (1994) Randomized study of oral isosorbide mononitrate in over 50 000 patients with suspected acute myocardial infarction. *Circulation*, **88**, I-394.

37. Groves, P. H., Lewis, M. J., Cheadle, H. A. and Penny, W. J. (1993) SIN-1 reduces platelet adhesion and platelet thrombus formation in a porcine model of balloon angioplasty. *Circulation*, **87**, 590–7.

38. The ACCORD Study Investigators (1994) Nitric oxide donors reduce restenosis after coronary angioplasty: the ACCORD study. *J. Am. Coll. Cardiol.*, **23** (Supp. 1), 59A.
39. Tanner, F. C., Noli, G., Boulanger, C. M. and Luscher, T. F. (1991) Oxidized low-density lipoproteins inhibit relaxations of porcine coronary arteries: role of scavenger receptor and endothelium-derived nitric oxide. *Circulation*, **83**, 2012–20.
40. Girerd, X. J., Hirsch, A. T., Cooke, J. P. *et al.* (1990) L-Arginine augments endothelium-dependent vasodilation in cholesterol fed rabbits. *Circ. Res.*, **67**, 1301–8.
41. Creager, M. A., Gallagher, S. H., Gierd, X. J. *et al.* (1992) L-Arginine improves endothelium-dependent vasodilation in hypercholesterolemic patients. *J. Clin. Invest.*, **90**, 1248–53.
42. Cooke, J. P., Singer, A. H., Tsao, P. *et al.* (1992) Antiatherogenic effects of L-arginine in the hypercholesterolemic rabbit. *J. Clin. Invest.*, **90**, 1168–72.
43. Tarry, W. C., Bettinger, D. A. and Makhoul, R. G. (1993) L-Arginine, the nitric oxide precursor, reduces intimal hyperplasia following endothelial injury independent of early smooth muscle proliferation. *Circulation*, **88**, I-367.
44. McNamara, N. B., Ignarro, L. J. and Akers, D. L. (1993) L-Arginine inhibits balloon catheter-induced intimal hyperplasia without improving neoendothelial-dependent acetylcholine-induced relaxation. *Circulation*, **88**, I-371.
45. Panza, J. A., Casino, P. R., Badar, D. M. and Quyyumi, A. A. (1993) Effect of increased availability of endothelium-derived nitric oxide precursor on endothelium-dependent vascular relaxation in normal subjects and in patients with essential hypertension. *Circulation*, **87**, 1475–81.
46. Luscher, T. F. and Haefeli, W. E. (1993) L-Arginine in the clinical arena: tool or remedy? *Circulation*, **87**, 1746–8.
47. Mellion, B. T., Ignarro, L. J., Ohlstein, E. H. *et al.* (1981) Evidence for the inhibitory role of guanosine 3',5'-monophosphate in ADP-induced human platelet aggregation in the presence of nitric oxide and related vasodilators. *Blood*, **57**, 946–55.
48. Mellion, B. T., Ignarro, J. L., Myers, C. B. *et al.* (1983) Inhibition of platelet aggregation of S-nitrosothiols: heme-dependent activation of soluble guanylate cyclase and stimulation of cyclic GMP accumulation. *Mol. Pharmacol.*, **23**, 653–64.
49. Loscalzo, J., Smick, D., Andon, N. and Cooke, J. (1989) S-Nitrosocaptopril. I. Molecular characterization and effects on the vasculature and on platelets. *J. Pharmacol. Expl Ther.*, **249**, 726–9.
50. Cooke, J. P., Stamler, J., Andon, N. *et al.* (1990) Flow stimulates endothelial cells to release a nitrovasodilator that is potentiated by reduced thiol. *Am. J. Physiol.*, **259**, H804–H812.
51. Stamler, J. S., Simon, D. I., Osborne, J. A. *et al.* (1992) S-nitrosylation of proteins with nitric oxide: synthesis and characterization of biologically active compounds. *Proc. Natl Acad. Sci. USA*, **89**, 444–8.
52. Stamler, J. S., Jaraki, O., Osborne, J. *et al.* (1992) Nitric oxide circulates in mammalian plasma primarily as an S-nitroso adduct of serum albumin. *Proc. Natl Acad. Sci. USA*, **89**, 7674–7.
53. Stamler, J. S., Simon, D. I., Jaraki, O. *et al.* (1992) S-nitrosylation of tissue-type plasminogen activator confers vasodilatory and antiplatelet properties on the enzyme. *Proc. Natl Acad. Sci. USA*, **89**, 8087–91.
54. Kelm, M. and Schrader, J. (1990) Control of coronary vascular tone by nitric oxide. *Circ. Res.*, **66**, 1561–75.
55. Keaney, J. F. Jr, Simon, D. I., Stamler, J. S. *et al.* (1993) NO forms an adduct with serum albumin that has endothelium-derived relaxing factor-like properties. *J. Clin. Invest.*, **91**, 1582–9.
56. Stamler, J. S., Singel, D. J. and Loscalzo, J. (1992) Biochemistry of nitric oxide and its redox-activated forms. *Science*, **258**, 1898–902.
57. Rogers, S., Karnovsky, M. J. and Edelman, E. R. (1993) Inhibition of experimental neointimal hyperplasia and thrombosis depends on the type of vascular injury and the site of drug administration. *Circulation*, **88**, 1215–21.

58. Saville, B. (1958) A scheme for the colorimetric determination of microgram amounts of thiols. *Analyst*, **83**, 670–2.
59. Benesch, R. and Benesch, R. E. (1958) Thiolation of proteins. *Proc. Natl Acad. Sci. USA*, **44**, 848–53.
60. Hansson, G. K., Holm, J., Geng, Y. *et al.* (1993) Vascular expression of inducible nitric oxide synthase *in vivo* in response to endothelial injury in rats. *Circulation*, **88**, I-383.
61. Joly, G. A., Schini, V. B. and Vanhoutte, P. M. (1992) Balloon injury and interleukin-1 beta induce nitric oxide synthase activity in rat carotid arteries. *Circ. Res.*, **71**, 331–8.
62. Koide, M., Kawahara, Y., Nakayama, I. *et al.* (1993) Cyclic AMP-elevating agents induce an inducible type of nitric oxide synthase in cultured vascular smooth muscle cells. *J. Biol. Chem.*, **33**, 24949.
63. Lamas, S., Marsden, P. A., Li, G. K. *et al.* (1992) Endothelial nitric oxide synthase: molecular cloning and characterization of a distinct constitutive isoform. *Proc. Natl Acad. Sci. USA*, **89**, 6384–52.
64. Abu-Soud, H. M. and Stuehr, D. J. (1993) Nitric oxide synthases reveal a role for calmodulin in controlling electron transfer. *Proc. Natl Acad. Sci. USA*, **90**, 10769–72.
65. Cho, H. J., Xie, Q-W., Calaycay J. *et al.* (1992) Calmodulin is a subunit of nitric oxide synthase from macrophages. *J. Exptl Med.*, **176**, 599–604.
66. Gellers, D. A., Lowenstein, C. J., Shapiro, R. A. *et al.* (1993) Molecular cloning and expression of inducible nitric oxide synthetase from human hepatocytes. *Proc. Natl Acad. Sci. USA*, **90**, 3491–5.
67. Weidinger, F. F., McLenachan, J. M., Cybulsky, M. I. *et al.* (1990) Persistent dysfunction of regenerated endothelium after balloon angioplasty of rabbit iliac artery. *Circulation*, **81**, 1667–79.
68. von der Leyen, H., Gibbons, G. H., Morishita, R. *et al.* (1994) Overexpression of constitutive endothelial-type nitric oxide synthase to an in vivo gene transfer approach to prevent neointima formation after vascular injury. *Clin. Res.*, **42**, 180a.
69. Dzau at AFCR 71. Bunting, S., Gryglewski, R., Moncada, A. S. and Vane, J. R. (1976) Arterial walls generate from prostaglandin endoperoxides a substance (prostaglandin X) which relaxes strips of mesenteric and coeliac arteries and inhibits platelet aggregation. *Prostaglandins*, **12**, 8967–73.
70. Kaplan, K. L., Mather, T., DeMarcol, L. and Soloma, S. (1989) Effect of fibrin on endothelial cell production of prostacyclin and tissue plasminogen activator. *Atherosclerosis*, **9**, 43–9.
71. Grabowski, E. F., Jaffe, E. A. and Weksler, B. B. (1985) Prostacyclin production by cultured endothelial cell monolayers exposed to step increases in sheer stress. *J. Lab. Clin. Med.*, **105**, 36–43.
72. Fleisher, L. N., Tall, A. R., Witte, L. D. *et al.* (1982) Stimulation of arterial endothelial cell prostacyclin synthesis by high density of lipoproteins. *J. Biol. Chem.*, **257**, 6653–5.
73. Reinders, J. H., Brinkman, H. M., van Mourik, J. A. and DeGroot, P. G. (1986) Cigarette smoke impairs endothelial cell prostacyclin production. *Arteriosclerosis*, **6**, 15–23.
74. Szczeklik, A., Skawinski, S., Gluszko, P. *et al.* (1979) Successful therapy of advanced arteriosclerosis obliterans with prostacyclin. *Lancet*, **i**, 1111–14.
75. Belch, J. J. F., McArdle, B., Pollock, J. G. *et al.* (1983) Epoprostenol (prostacyclin) and severe arterial disease: a double blind trial. *Lancet*, **i**, 315–19.
76. DeCanterina, R., Giannessi, D., Mazzone, A. *et al.* (1990) Vascular prostacyclin is increased in patients ingesting omega-3 polyunsaturated fatty acids before coronary artery bypass graft surgery. *Circulation*, **82**, 428–38.
77. Banning, A. P., Groves, P. H., Brewer, L. *et al.* (1994) Locally delivered platelet encapsulated iloprost inhibits carotid neo-intimal hyperplasia following balloon angioplasty in pigs. *J. Am. Coll. Cardiol.*, **23** (Supp. 1), 19A.
78. Hawiger, J. (1993) The interaction of platelets and other cellular elements with the vessel wall. In: Loscalzo, J., Creager, M. and Dzau, V. (eds) *Vascular Medicine: A Textbook of Vascular Biology and Diseases*, pp. 205–31. Boston: Little, Brown.

79. Lambert, T., Dev, V., Litvack, F. *et al.* (1993) Localized arterial drug delivery from a polymer coated removable metallic stent: kinetics and bioactivity of forskolin. *Circulation*, **88**, I-310.
80. Eigler, N. L., Lambert, T. L., Dev, V. *et al.* (1994) Local arterial wall drug delivery from a polymer coated removable metallic stent: kinetics, distribution, and bioactivity of forskolin. *J. Am. Coll. Cardiol.*, **23** (Supp. 1), 4A.
81. Pan, M. G., Florio, T. and Stork, P. J. S. (1992) G protein activation of a hormone-stimulated phosphatase in human tumor cells. *Science*, **256**, 1215–17.
82. Dicorleto, P. E., Bowen, F. and Poke, D. F. (1983) Cultured endothelial cells produces a platelet derived growth factor-like protein. *Proc. Natl Acad. Sci. USA*, **80**, 1919–23.
83. Lundergan, C. F., Foegh, M. L. and Ramwell, P. W. (1991) Peptide inhibition of myointima proliferation by angiopeptin, a somatostatin analogue. *J. Am. Coll. Cardiol.*, **17**(6B), 132B–136B.
84. Santoian, E. C., Schneider, J. E., Gravanis, M. B. *et al.* (1993) Angiopeptin inhibits intimal hyperplasia in porcine coronary arteries. *Circulation*, **88**, 11–14.
85. Lundergan, C., Loegh, M. L., Vargas, R. *et al.* (1989) Inhibition of myointimal proliferation of the rat carotid artery by the peptides angiopeptin and BIM23034. *Atherosclerosis*, **80**, 49–55.
86. Light, J. T., Bellan, J. A., Chen, I. L. *et al.* (1993) Angiopeptin enhances acetylcholine-induced relaxation and inhibits intimal hyperplasia after vascular injury. *Am. J. Physiol.*, **265**, H1265.
87. Eriksen, U. H., Amtorp, O., Bagger, J. P. *et al.* (1993) Continuous angiopeptin infusion reduces coronary restenosis following balloon angioplasty. *Circulation*, **88**, I-594.
88. Kent, K. M., Williams, D. O., Cassagneau, B. *et al.* (1993) Double blind, controlled trial of the effect of angiopeptin on coronary restenosis following balloon angioplasty. *Circulation*, **88**, I-506.
89. Komuro, I., Kurihara, H., Sugiyama, T. *et al.* (1988) Endothelin stimulates c-*fos* and c-*myc* expression and proliferation of vascular smooth muscle cells. *FEBS Lett.*, **238**, 249–52.
90. Rubanyi, G. M. and Vanhoutte, P. M. (1985) Hypoxia releases a vasoconstrictor substance from the canine vascular endothelium. *J. Physiol.*, **364**, 45–56.
91. Yanagisawa, M., Kurihara, H., Kimura, S. *et al.* (1988) A novel potent vasoconstrictor peptide produced by vascular endothelial cells. *Nature*, **322**, 411–15.
92. Inoue, A., Yanagisawa, M., Kimura, S. *et al.* (1989) The human endothelin family: three structurally and pharmacologically distinct isopeptides predicted by three separate genes. *Proc. Natl Acad. Sci. USA*, **86**, 2863–7.
93. Miller, W. L., Redfield, M. M. and Burnett, J. C. (1989) Integrated cardiac, renal, and endocrine actions of endothelin. *J. Clin. Invest.*, **83**, 317–20.
94. Masaki, T. (1994) Endothelin in vascular biology. *Ann. NY Acad. Sci.*, **714**, 101–108.
95. Arai, H., Hori, S., Aramori, I. *et al.* (1990) Cloning and expression of a cDNA encoding an endothelin receptor. *Nature*, **348**, 730–2.
96. Sakurai, T., Yanagisawa, M., Takuwa, Y. *et al.* (1990) Cloning of a cDNA encoding a non-isopeptide selective subtype of the endothelin receptor. *Nature*, **348**, 732–5.
97. Opgenorth, T. J., Wu-Wong, J. R. and Shiosaki, K. (1992) Endothelin-converting enzymes. *FASEB J.*, **6**, 2653–9.
98. Marsden, P. A., Danthuluri, N. R., Brenner, B. M. *et al.* (1989) Endothelin action on vascular smooth muscle cells involves inositol triphosphate and calcium mobilization. *Biochem. Biophys. Res. Commun.*, **158**, 86–93.
99. Yoshimoto, J., Ishizaki, Y., Mori, A. *et al.* (1991) The role of cerebral microvessel endothelium in regulation of cerebral blood flow through production of endothelin-1. *J. Cardiovasc. Pharmacol.*, **17** (Supp. 7), S260–S263.
100. Saito, Y., Nakao, K., Mukoyama, M. and Imura, H. (1990) Increased plasma endothelin level in patients with essential hypertension. *N. Engl. J. Med.*, **322**, 205.
101. Luscher, T. F., Yang, Z., Diederich, D. and Buhler, F. R. (1989) Endothelium-derived vasoactive substances: potential role in hypertension, atherosclerosis, and vascular occlusion. *J. Cardiovasc. Pharmacol.*, **14** (Supp. 6), S63–S69.

102. Toyo-oka, T., Aizawa, T., Suzuki, N. *et al.* (1991) Increased plasma level of endothelin-1 and coronary spasm induction in patients with vasospastic angina pectoris. *Circulation*, **83**, 476–83.
103. Stewart, D. J., Kubag, G., Costello, K. B. and Cernacek, P. (1991) Increased plasma endothelin-1 in early hours of acute myocardial infarction. *J. Am. Coll. Cardiol.*, **18**, 38–43.
104. Cernacek, P. and Stewart, D. J. (1989) Immunoreactive endothelin in human plasma: marked elevations in patients in cardiogenic shock. *Biochem. Biophys. Res. Commun.*, **161**, 562–7.
105. Koyama, H., Tabata, T., Nishzawa, Y. *et al.* (1989) Plasma endothelin level in patients with uraemia. *Lancet*, **i**, 991–2.
106. Omland, T., Lie, R. T., Aakvaag, A. *et al.* (1993) Prognostic value of plasma endothelin determination in acute myocardial infarction. *Circulation*, **88**, I-153.
107. Lerman, A., Holmes, D. R. Jr., Garratt, K. N. *et al.* (1994) Local release of endothelin in human coronary arteries in response to balloon angioplasty. *J. Am. Coll. Cardiol.*, **23** (Supp. 1), 124A.
108. Clozel, M., Breu, V., Burri, K. *et al.* (1993) Pathophysiological role of endothelin revealed by the first orally active endothelin receptor antagonist. *Nature*, **365**, 759–61.
109. Seo, B., Oemar, B. S., Siebenmann, R. *et al.* (1994) Both ETA and ETB receptors mediate contraction to endothelin-1 in human blood vessels. *Circulation*, **89**, 1203–8.
110. Clozel, M., Clozel, J. P. and Hess, P. (1993) Endothelin receptor antagonism, a new therapeutic approach in experimental hypertension. *Circulation*, **88**, I-316.
111. Koiwski, W., Luscher, T. F., Linder, L. and Buhler, F. R. (1991) Endothelin-1-induced vasoconstriction in humans: reversal by calcium channel blockade but not by nitrovaso-dilators or endothelium-derived relaxing factor. *Circulation*, **83**, 469–75.
112. Nambi, P., Pullen, M., Wu, H. *et al.* (1992) Dexamethasone down-regulates the expression of endothelin receptors in vascular smooth muscle cells. *J. Biol. Chem.*, **267**, 19555–9.
113. Linncoff, M. A., Furst, J. G. and Lee, P. (1993) Local delivery of dexamethasone by an eluting stent attenuates the adverse response to biodegradable polymer in the porcine coronary artery. *Circulation*, **88**, I-655.
114. Villa, A. E., Guzman, L. A., Chen, W. *et al.* (1994) Local delivery of dexamethasone for prevention of neointimal proliferation in a rat model of balloon angioplasty. *J. Clin. Invest.*, **93**, 1243–9.
115. Hawiger, J. (1992) The interaction of platelets and other cellular elements with the vessel wall. In: Loscalzo, J., Creager, M. A. and Dzau, V. (eds) *Vascular Medicine: A Textbook of Vascular Biology and Diseases*, pp. 205–31. Boston: Little, Brown.
116. Tofler, G. H., Brezinski, D., Schafer, A. I. *et al.* (1987) Concurrent morning increase in platelet aggregability and the risk of myocardial infarction and sudden cardiac death. *N. Engl. J. Med.*, **316**, 1514–18.
117. Trip, M. K., Cats, V. M., van Capelle, F. J. L. and Vreeken, J. (1990) Platelet hyperreactivity and prognosis in survivors of myocardial infarction. *N. Engl. J. Med.*, **322**, 1549–54.
118. Ross, R., Glomset, J., Kariya, B. and Harker, L. (1974) A platelet-dependent serum factor that stimulates the proliferation of arterial smooth muscle cells *in vitro*. *Proc. Natl Acad. Sci. USA*, **71**, 1207–10.
119. Rybak, M. E. and Renzulli, L. A. (1993) A liposome based platelet substrate, the plateletsome, with hemostatic efficiency. *Biomat. Arter. Cell. Immobil. Biotechnol.*, **21**, 101–18.
120. Smith, W. L. (1989) The eicosanoids and their biochemical mechanisms of action. *Biochem. J.*, **259**, 315–24.
121. FitzGerald, G. A. (1991) Mechanisms of platelet activation: thromboxane A_2 as an amplifying signal for other agonists. *Am. J. Cardiol.*, **68**, 11B–15B.
122. Lopez, J. A. G., Armstrong, M. L., Piegors, D. J. and Heistad, D. D. (1989) Effects of early and advanced atherosclerosis on vascular responses to serotonin, thromboxane A_2 and ADP. *Circulation*, **79**, 698–705.

123. Vejar, M., Fragasso, G., Hackett, D. *et al.* (1990) Dissociation of platelet activation and spontaneous myocardial ischemia in unstable angina. *Thromb. Haemost.*, **63**, 163–8.
124. Schwartz, L., Bourassa, M. G., Lesperance, J. *et al.* (1988) Aspirin and dipyridamole in the prevention of restenosis after percutaneous transluminal coronary angioplasty. *N. Engl. J. Med.*, **318**, 1714–19.
125. Clarke, R. J., Mayo, G., Price, P. and Fitzgerald, G. A. (1991) Suppression of thromboxane A$_2$ but not of systemic prostacyclin by controlled-release aspirin. *N. Engl. J. Med.*, **325**, 1137–41.
126. Fitzgerald, G. A., Lupinetti, M. D., Charman, S. and Charman, W. (1991) Presystemic acetylation of platelets by aspirin: reduction in dose and rate of drug delivery to improve biochemical selectivity for thromboxane A$_2$. *J. Pharmacol. Exptl Ther.*, **259**, 1043–9.
127. Bush, L. R., Campbell, W. B., Buja, L. M. *et al.* (1984) Effects of the selective thromboxane synthetase inhibitor dazoxiben on variations in cyclic blood flow in stenosed canine coronary arteries. *Circulation*, **69**, 1161–70.
128. Golino, P., Buja, L. M., Yao, S. *et al.* (1990) Failure of nitroglycerine and diltiazem to reduce platelet-mediated vasoconstriction in dogs with coronary artery stenosis and endothelial injury: further evidence for thromboxane A$_2$ and serotonin as mediators of coronary artery vasoconstriction *in vivo*. *J. Am. Coll. Cardiol.*, **15**, 718–26.
129. Yao, S., Rosolowsky, M., Anderson, H. V. *et al.* (1990) Combined thromboxane A$_2$ synthetase inhibition and receptor blockade are more effective in preventing spontaneous and epinephrine-induced canine coronary cyclic flow variations. *J. Am. Coll. Cardiol.*, **16**, 705–13.
130. Zander, J. F., Aarhus, L. L., Katuskic, Z. S. *et al.* (1986) Effects of naftidrofuryl on adrenergic nerves, endothelium and smooth muscle in isolated canine blood vessels. *J. Pharmacol. Exp. Ther.*, **239**, 760–7.
131. Vanhoutte, P. M., Cohen, R. A. and VanNueter, J. M. (1984) Serotonin and arterial vessels. *J. Cardiovasc. Pharmacol.*, **6** (Supp. 2), S421–S421–S428.
132. Vanhoutte, P. M. (1991) Platelet-derived serotonin, the endothelium, and cardiovascular disease. *J. Cardiovasc. Pharmacol.*, **17** (Supp. 5), S6–S12.
133. Shimokawa, H., Aarhus, A. A. and Vanhoutte, P. M. (1987) Porcine coronary arteries with regenerated endothelium have a reduced endothelium-dependent responsiveness to aggregating platelets and serotonin. *Circ. Res.*, **61**, 256–70.
134. Heistad, D. D., Armstrong, M. L., Marcus, M. L. *et al.* (1984) Augmented responses to vasoconstrictor stimuli in hypercholesterolemic and atherosclerotic monkeys. *Circ. Res.*, **54**, 711–18.
135. Willerson, J. J., McNatt, J., Yao, S. *et al.* (1994) Pretreatment with antagonists to thromboxane A$_2$, serotonin, and ADP reduces neointimal proliferation in canine coronary arteries after endothelial injury. *J. Am. Coll. Cardiol.*, **23** (Supp. 1), 234A.

11

Molecular Basis of Vasoreactive Diseases: Angiotensin II as a Paradigm

Gary H. Gibbons

Introduction

It has become increasingly clear that the vasculature is a complex, integrated organ capable of regulating the delicate homeostatic balance that governs vessel function and structure. In general, the maintenance of homeostasis appears to involve a dynamic balance of countervailing forces. The vasculature produces a wide spectrum of biologic mediators including vasodilators and vasoconstrictors, procoagulants and anticoagulants, leukocyte adhesion molecules that promote inflammation and endogenous inhibitors of inflammation, as well as growth stimulatory factors and growth inhibitors. The complex interplay between this 'yin–yang' balance of mediators is a critical determinant of the clinical manifestations of vascular disease such as vasospasm, thrombosis, atherogenesis, plaque rupture and hypertension. It is intriguing that many of the vasoreactive mediators generated by the vasculature are pleiotropic in their capacity to regulate both vessel tone and vessel structure. For example, vasodilators generated by the vasculature such as nitric oxide, prostaglandins and natriuretic peptides tend to be inhibitors of vascular cell growth whereas vasoconstrictors such as angiotensin II and endothelin are growth promoters.[1,2] Similarly, vasoactive substances modulate platelet aggregation, the thrombolytic capacity of the vasculature, leukocyte adhesion to the endothelium, and govern vascular-cell migration, matrix production and growth.[3–6] These observations indicate that the yin–yang balance of vasoreactive factors may determine the pathogenesis of vascular disease by influencing thrombogenicity and vessel structure in addition to regulating vessel tone. Furthermore, it is postulated that therapies directed at modifying the local expression of vasoreactive substances may have particular efficacy in altering the natural history of human vascular disease. This chapter will focus on angiotensin II as a paradigmatic vasoreactive factor produced within the vasculature that appears to play an important role in the pathogenesis of vascular disease.

Circulating and tissue angiotensin systems

One hundred years have now passed since the discovery of renin by Tigerstedt and Bergman. This seminal observation was followed by the discoveries of angiotensinogen, the liver-derived substrate for renin, as well as angiotensin converting enzyme (ACE), the proteinase that converts angiotensin I to angiotensin II. Eventually, the important linkage between this enzymatic cascade and the induction of aldosterone production also became established. It is now recognized that the renin–angiotensin–aldosterone system is an endocrine system that is a major determinant of blood-pressure regulation and sodium balance.[7]

More recently, it has also become clear that there are local tissue angiotensin systems within various organs that appear to complement the role of the circulating endocrine renin–angiotensin system.[8,9] In addition, there are other enzymes such as the cathepsins that have renin-like activity as well as enzymes such as chymase[10] that also have the capacity to generate angiotensin II from angiotensin I and thereby bypass the role of ACE. Although some controversy persists,[11,12] a growing body of evidence indicates that increased levels of angiotensin II can be generated locally within tissues independent of the circulating level of renin.[8,9,12] The generation of angiotensin II independent of the circulation has been documented in isolated blood vessels as well as in isolated heart preparations.[13–15] Moreover, molecular analysis with polymerase chain reaction, *in situ* hybridization as well as immunohistochemical and biochemical analyses have defined the expression of various components of the angiotensin system within the heart and vasculature as well as other organs.[9,12,16] Furthermore, several studies in both animal models and in humans have documented tissue-specific activation of these local paracrine angiotensin systems in response to pathologic stimuli such as myocardial infarction, heart failure, hypertension and vascular injury.[9,15,17–21]

The evolution of both the circulating and tissue angiotensin systems in parallel provides a mechanism for tissue-specific changes in angiotensin II expression within the organism without perturbing systemic homeostasis. It is intriguing that in pathobiologic circumstances such as myocardial infarction and hypertension, the activation of the tissue angiotensin system within the heart and vasculature appears to be associated with long-term structural changes within the myocardium or blood vessel. Indeed, there appears to be a judicious division of labor between the circulating and tissue angiotensin systems insofar as the classical endocrine system is well suited to short-term regulation of vascular tone and sodium balance whereas the tissue systems appear to be more adapted to long-term changes in organ function as well as ventricular and vascular remodeling.

The precise role of the tissue angiotensin system versus the circulating angiotensin system in the pathogenesis of human vascular disease remains to be further elucidated. In retrospect, one of the early clues of the potential clinical importance of the tissue angiotensin system was suggested by the observation that ACE inhibitors have broad efficacy as antihypertensive agents despite the fact that most patients have normal or low circulating renin levels. This clinical observation was recapitulated in studies of rats with genetic hypertension in which the activity of the circulating angiotensin system is suppressed. Despite the low activity of the circulating system, ACE inhibitors proved to be effective in lowering blood pressure to normotensive levels. Unger *et al.*[22] extended this observation by assessing the effect of discontinuing the ACE inhibitor treatment after two weeks of therapy. As expected, shortly after discontinuing the administration of the ACE inhibitor, plasma ACE activity was restored to baseline levels. However, despite the fact that the activity of the circulating angiotensin system was no longer inhibited, the blood pressure remained significantly reduced compared to placebo controls. Indeed, these investigators observed that the persistence of the antihypertensive response after discontinuation of drug administration correlated with a persistent inhibition of the tissue ACE activity within the vasculature. Thus the efficacy of ACE inhibitors as antihypertensive agents in this model correlated best with inhibition of tissue angiotensin generation rather than the activity of the circulating system. If the tissue angiotensin systems play an important role in tissue remodeling and the pathogenesis of cardiovascular disease, it is conceivable that the natural history of cardiovascular disease can be modified by developing more effective pharmacotherapeutic and drug-delivery strategies for modulating the activity of these paracrine angiotensin systems.

Pathogenic role of angiotensin II

Insights from molecular genetics

The traditional approach to defining the pathogenesis of vascular diseases has depended on epidemiologic studies that have characterized risk factors such as hyperlipidemia, obesity or diet. However, recent advances in molecular genetics have begun to transform our capacity to define the genetic basis of disease and establish causal links between biologic mediators and human disease. A rapidly emerging body of evidence suggests that the renin–angiotensin system may be an important determinant of the natural history of human vascular disease.

In addition to conventional risk factors for cardiovascular disease, epidemiologic studies indicate that the level of activation of the renin–angiotensin system may be an independent risk factor for the complications of vascular disease such as myocardial infarction in hypertensive patients[23] but not in normotensive subjects.[24] Similarly, patients with elevated plasma ACE levels appear to be at increased risk of developing significant carotid artery vascular pathology as detected by ultrasound.[25] Recently, Cambien and colleagues[26] have reported that increased plasma ACE levels are associated with a deletion polymorphism of the angiotensin converting-enzyme gene (*ACE*) and an increased risk of myocardial infarction in patients with hypertension. Furthermore, diabetic patients with this *ACE* genotype are at significantly increased risk of cardiovascular complications compared to those with a normal *ACE* genotype.[27] The mechanistic basis of this correlative observation remains to be clarified. However, as discussed below, there is increasing evidence that angiotensin II may be involved in the pathogenesis of atherosclerosis. In this regard, it is noteworthy that the *ACE* gene deletion polymorphism is associated with increased ACE expression within T-lymphocytes and monocyte/macrophages, two cell types that are major constituents of atherosclerotic plaques.[28] Taken together, these observations provide a suggestive potential link between the *ACE* genotype, vascular ACE expression and the natural history of atherosclerotic vascular disease. Although these observations do not establish causality, the growing weight of evidence is consistent with the postulate that genetic factors that modulate angiotensin II generation may influence the pathogenesis of human vascular disease.

Epidemiologic studies have clearly established a genetic basis for hypertension as well as atherosclerotic vascular disease. A critical element in the pursuit of characterizing the genetic basis of hypertension has involved selective breeding techniques to develop appropriate animal models. It is interesting that genetic loci associated with the hypertensive phenotype in several different animal strains appear to be in proximity to components of the renin–angiotensin system as evidenced in the Dahl salt-sensitive hypertensive model,[29] the Lyon hypertensive rat,[30] as well as the stroke-prone spontaneously hypertensive rat.[31] Moreover, transgenic animals that overexpress components of the renin–angiotensin system either in the systemic circulation[32] or limited to a tissue angiotensin system[33] also exhibit a hypertensive phenotype. Utilizing transgenic technology in rats, Mullins and coworkers[33] have developed a novel model that demonstrates that selective upregulation of the tissue angiotensin system while maintaining normal activity of the endocrine renin–angiotensin system is associated with fulminant hypertension. These studies are consistent with the postulate that activation of local-tissue angiotensin systems present within the vasculature, adrenal gland, heart or brain may play important roles in cardiovascular physiology. Moreover, these findings in animal models suggest that genetic abnormalities that influence the regulation of either the circulating or tissue angiotensin systems may play an important mediating role in genetic hypertension.

In parallel with the analysis of genetic loci that determine the hypertensive phenotype in animal models, molecular genetic studies have also attempted to further characterize the genetic basis of human essential hypertension. Recently, studies of human hypertensives have established a genetic linkage between the angiotensinogen gene and essential hypertension in ethnic groups derived from Europe[34,35] as well as Asian populations.[36] In addition, this same genetic locus is associated with a predisposition to develop pregnancy-induced hypertension.[37] Overall, these studies provide additional supportive evidence that angiotensin II may play an important pathogenic role in human vascular disease. It is speculated that there may be a subset of patients that are genetically predisposed to vascular disease and its complications based upon abnormalities in the regulation of angiotensin activity. Future studies are necessary to further define the causal relationships between the factors that determine angiotensin II expression and the natural history of human vascular disease.

Vascular remodeling

The pathogenesis of vascular disease involves a process of vascular remodeling in which changes in vascular cell growth, programmed cell death, cell migration as well as matrix production and degradation induce dramatic alterations in vessel architecture. This process of vascular remodeling occurs in a variety of clinical contexts including: hypertension, atherosclerosis, vein bypass grafts as well as restenosis after angioplasty. Vascular remodeling is governed by the interplay between the expression of autocrine–paracrine mediators produced within the blood vessel itself as well as systemic hemodynamic and neurohumoral stimuli.[38] It is postulated that angiotensin II generated within the heart and vasculature is an important determinant of both ventricular and vascular remodeling. In this brief discussion, focus will be on the potential role of angiotensin II in the vascular remodeling of hypertension and atherosclerosis.

Studies of vascular structure in animal models as well as human hypertensives have documented that vascular remodeling is a common pathogenic process regardless of the inciting mechanism of the hypertension. The nature of the remodeling process often involves an increase in the wall:lumen ratio that potentiates vascular reactivity and promotes an increase in vascular resistance and tissue ischemia. This process of vascular remodeling in hypertension appears to involve changes in vascular cell growth, migration, matrix production as well as matrix degradation. The changes in vessel architecture that ensue appear to perpetuate the state of hypertension despite normal levels of vasoconstrictor factors. Studies in animal models and in humans have documented that hypertensive vascular remodeling can be reversed by treatment with antihypertensive agents and that blockade of angiotensin II generation has particular efficacy in reversing these structural changes.[38–40] Furthermore, treatment with ACE inhibitors for a limited time period during the incipient stages of remodeling aborts the process and results in a long-term effect of lowering the blood pressure and altering the natural history of the disease in animal models.[41] These data suggest that angiotensin II generation may play a critical role in the vascular remodeling process of hypertension and that blockade of angiotensin generation may alter the natural history of hypertensive vascular disease. It remains to be demonstrated whether long-term ACE inhibition initiated in the early phases of the disease will have similar effects on the natural history of human essential hypertensive vascular disease.

However, the mechanisms by which angiotensin II influences vessel structure as well as vessel tone remain to be further elucidated. Conventional pharmacologic studies in animal models and in patients with hypertension involve a multiplicity of variables that may also influence vascular structure including effects on systemic hemodynamics, the activity of the sympathetic nervous system and nitric oxide generation induced by ACE inhibition. To further elucidate the potential role of angiotensin II as a determinant of vascular remodeling, our laboratory has employed two alternative experimental strategies: (1) the characterization of molecular mechanisms in *in vitro* model systems of vascular cell-growth regulation and (2) the use of *in vivo* genetic engineering to test postulates characterized in the *in vitro* models.

Characterization of the molecular mechanisms by which angiotensin II modulates vessel structure has been advanced by elucidating the cellular events triggered by ligand–receptor interactions. The coupling between angiotensin II and vascular cell behavior is mediated by at least three receptor subtypes – AT-1A, AT-1B and the AT-2 receptor. The biologic role of the recently cloned AT-2 receptor remains somewhat mysterious because it appears to be upregulated during development and perhaps during vascular remodeling, yet is quite distinct from the AT-1 receptors based on the lack of coupling to well-described signal-transduction mechanisms such as the phosphoinositol pathway or adenylate cyclase.[42] Recent studies indicate that it may be involved in angiogenesis[43] or the regulation of vascular cell growth (Nakajima *et al.*, pers. commun.). Further characterization of the biologic role of the AT-2 receptor will be advanced with the advent of more effective and specific receptor antagonists.

A large body of evidence has documented a wide spectrum of effects of angiotensin II on vascular cell behavior. Its pleiotropic properties relate in part to its capacity to activate several cellular signaling mechanisms via the AT-1 receptor including activation of phosphoinositol hydrolysis, protein kinase C, the Na^+–H^+ exchanger, a protein-tyrosine phosphatase, tyrosine phosphorylation of raf-1 and phospholipase C-γl, as well as the regulation of intracellular calcium and adenylate cyclase activity. In addition, angiotensin II activates immediate early genes and transcription factors such as c-*fos*, c-*jun* and c-*myc*.[44–48] The activation of these various cellular signaling molecules results in a cascade of events that modify cell behavior.

Studies of angiotensin II infusion in animals have documented that this factor induces vascular cell growth.[49] However, these studies are limited by confounding changes in blood pressure and the expression of other neurohumoral factors that accompany systemic angiotensin II infusion. To further characterize the growth-regulatory properties of angiotensin II, several groups have documented in *in vitro* models that angiotensin II induces vascular smooth muscle cell hypertrophy.[47,48,50] Our laboratory has further demonstrated that the growth response to angiotensin II involves an interplay between growth stimulatory versus growth inhibitory autocrine factors produced by the vascular smooth muscle cells in response to angiotensin II. We have demonstrated that angiotensin II induces increased mRNA expression of platelet-derived growth factor (PDGF)-A, basic fibroblast growth factor (bFGF) and transforming growth factor-β_1 (TGF-β_1). Utilizing neutralizing antibodies and antisense oligonucleotides, we have selectively inhibited the biologic activity of each factor and documented that the net growth response to angiotensin II involves a balance between growth stimulatory effects predominantly mediated by bFGF versus an antiproliferative effect mediated by TGF-β_1. Under most conditions, both proliferative (bFGF) and antiproliferative (TGF-β_1) pathways are activated and the net growth response is cellular hypertrophy without hyperplasia. However, under conditions in which the antiproliferative pathway is inactivated, angiotensin II is capable of inducing mitogenesis.[48,51,52] Moreover, we have observed that under certain *in vitro* conditions in which plasmin generation is inhibited, TGF-β_1 expression is induced but remains in a latent biologically inactive form and therefore angiotensin II is mitogenic.[53] Alternatively, in certain vascular smooth-muscle cell phenotypes such as those derived from the spontaneously hypertensive rat in which TGF-β_1 is a mitogen, angiotensin II is also mitogenic.[54] Therefore, the growth response to angiotensin II may be either cellular hypertrophy or hyperplasia depending on the cell phenotype and the balance of proliferative versus antiproliferative autocrine factors.

In addition, it has recently been observed that angiotensin induces the expression of other growth modulatory molecules such as insulin-like growth factor-I,[55] heparin-binding epidermal growth factor[56] and another vasoreactive factor endothelin-1.[57] It appears likely that the proliferative growth response to angiotensin II involves a synergistic interaction between these various growth stimulatory molecules. Thus, autocrine–paracrine growth factors appear to play a critical mediator role in regulating the vascular smooth muscle cell growth response to angiotensin II stimulation.

The process of vascular remodeling not only involves changes in vascular cell growth, but also changes in cell migration and invasion as well as dynamic changes in matrix composition and structure. In addition to its effects on vascular growth, angiotensin II stimulates vascular smooth muscle cell migration,[58] matrix production (e.g. fibronectin and tenascin),[59] and modulates the balance of proteinases and endogenous proteinase inhibitors that regulate the degradation of extracellular matrix.[60] Furthermore, these effects of angiotensin II on vascular cell growth and matrix composition appear to be potentiated by the direct effects of hemodynamic stimuli on these same cellular parameters. Indeed, *in vitro* models have documented that exposure of vascular smooth-muscle cells to increased mechanical strain markedly enhances the growth stimulatory effects of angiotensin II on cell growth.[61] It is postulated that the integrative interplay between hemodynamic stimuli and locally generated vasoreactive factors induce changes in cell growth, migration and matrix composition that promote the process of vascular remodeling in hypertension.

In addition to hypertensive vascular disease, the process of vascular remodeling is also observed in other forms of vascular disease such as atherosclerosis.[38] As described above, clinical studies have provided suggestive evidence that the expression of angiotensin II is associated with the progression of human vascular disease and its complications. It is interesting that atherogenesis involves the accumulation of intimal smooth muscle cells and that the phenotypic modulation that occurs during the formation of a neointimal lesion is associated with a marked upregulation of ACE activity.[20] In addition to the accumulation of intimal smooth-muscle cells that express ACE, inflammatory T-cells and monocyte/macrophages that invade the vessel intima also have the capacity to express ACE and generate angiotensin II.[28,62] The potential atherogenic role of angiotensin II can be inferred by the fact that angiotensin II increases the avidity of these leukocytes for adhesion to the endothelium, modulates the migratory behavior of T cells and monocyte/macrophages[63] and induces the autocrine expression of cytokines such as tumor necrosis factor-α by leukocytes.[5] Indeed, in recent preliminary studies we have observed that monocyte/macrophages within human atherosclerotic plaques express high levels of ACE (Diet *et al.*, pers. commun.). Thus, the atherosclerotic lesion appears to have increased capacity for local generation of angiotensin II and this activated vascular angiotensin system may potentiate atherosclerotic lesion formation via its effects on monocyte/macrophage activation and vascular cell growth and matrix production.

This vascular angiotensin system may also modulate the biologic activity of the plaque as well as promote its formation. It is now recognized that an atherosclerotic plaque is more than an ossified fibrotic scar, it is a dynamic lesion capable of dramatic changes such as plaque rupture that precipitate acute ischemic syndromes. There is increasing evidence that the dynamic character of plaques relate to changes in oxidative stress and the balance of forces regulating hemostasis. In this regard it is noteworthy that recent studies indicate that angiotensin II may modify the redox state within the vessel wall by inducing the generation of superoxide anion in vascular smooth-muscle cells.[64] Increased generation of superoxide anion is associated with a dysfunctional endothelium[65] and increased capacity to generate the atherogenic particle – oxidized low-density lipoprotein cholesterol. Given these findings, it is not surprising that pharmacologic studies with ACE inhibitors in rabbit, pig and primate models of atherogenesis have documented that blockade of angiotensin II generation is associated with the inhibition of atherosclerosis independent of the potential hemodynamic effects of these agents.[66–68]

In addition to the foam-cell accumulation and lipid oxidation, the progression of atherosclerotic plaque formation is potentiated by recurrent thrombosis. Moreover, the process of recurrent thrombosis also plays a critical role in the acute ischemic syndromes of vascular disease. In accordance with this postulate, it is of interest that angiotensin II appears to promote thrombosis by increasing the expression of plasminogen activator inhibitor.[4] It is speculated that this angiotensin-mediated effect on inhibiting endogenous thrombolytic capacity may also play a role in inciting acuted ischemic syndromes such as myocardial infarction. Indeed, this postulate is consistent with the recent finding of the SAVE trial that the administration of ACE inhibitors postmyocardial infarction prevents a subsequent reinfarction.[69] One may speculate that the efficacy of ACE inhibition in preventing myocardial infarction is related to its potential effect on the progression of human coronary vascular disease and acute thrombosis rather than an effect on afterload reduction or ventricular remodeling. Given the effects of angiotensin II on growth factor expression, vascular cell migration, growth and matrix production, as well as its effect on monocyte/macrophage adhesion and activation, and vessel thrombolytic capacity, it appears likely that the activity of the vascular angiotensin system may influence the natural history of atherosclerotic vascular disease. Future studies are needed to further test this hypothesis in animal models and in patients with atherosclerotic vascular disease.

In vivo genetic engineering by local delivery systems

It has become increasingly clear that the characterization of the biologic role of autocrine–paracrine systems in the pathogenesis of vascular disease is an important research problem with profound clinical implications. However, the current experimental paradigm of utilizing systemic administration of pharmacologic inhibitors has significant limitations in addressing this question. As an alternative approach we have utilized a novel molecular delivery system composed of an inactivated Sendai virus (Hemagglutinating Virus of Japan, HVJ) coupled to a liposome complex to deploy DNA molecules within the vessel wall that are capable of modulating gene expression within vascular cells. This is a high-efficiency transfection system based upon the intrinsic fusogenic properties of the viral protein coat that promotes the cellular uptake of DNA and targets the DNA to the cell nucleus thereby bypassing the degradative lysosomal pathways for DNA that limit the efficacy of conventional DNA delivery systems. The transfection of DNA into the vessel wall via the HVJ–liposome delivery system is capable of inducing marked changes in gene expression within the vasculature. The HVJ–liposome delivery system is at least as efficient as current adenoviral vectors yet retains the simplicity of standard plasmid expression vectors and oligonucleotides and avoids the cytotoxicity associated with the immune response induced by adenoviral infection.[70-72]

We have utilized two antigene approaches to inhibit the expression of a target protein: (1) transfection of antisense oligonucleotides that selectively bind to the targeted mRNA, block translation and promote the degradation of the targeted mRNA; and (2) transfection of *cis* element decoy oligonucleotides into vascular cells to selectively inhibit gene transcription by competitive antagonism with the endogenous gene promoter elements for binding of the targeted transcription factor. To test the feasibility of utilizing this *in vivo* genetic engineering experimental approach, we initially employed the HVJ–liposome delivery system to inhibit the expression of cell-cycle regulatory genes and thereby inhibit cell proliferation in response to balloon injury in the rat carotid model. We observed that the HVJ–liposome molecular delivery system was highly efficient in delivering oligonucleotides throughout the vessel wall and markedly enhanced the kinetics of intracellular oligonucleotide stability by targeting the DNA to the nucleus and avoiding lysosomal degradation *in vivo*. This resulted in more effective and sustained inhibition of the expression of the targeted genes in the intact animal. We have documented that a single intraluminal delivery of antisense oligonucleotides directed against the cell-cycle genes cdc2 kinase, proliferating cell nuclear antigen and/or cdk2 kinase inhibits DNA synthesis and neointima formation for up to eight weeks after local delivery.[70,71]

Recent studies of cell growth control have shown that cell-cycle progression is a highly regulated genetic program involving sequential activation of the gene transcription of cell-cycle regulatory molecules. Based on these observations, we postulated that blockade of the transcription factor that coordinates this programmed activation of each of these genes would be a more effective strategy of inhibiting cell proliferation. We therefore targeted the transcription factor E2F which plays a critical role in transactivating a series of cell-cycle regulatory genes essential for cell-cycle progression and mitogenesis. Recently, we have observed that HVJ-mediated transfection of E2F-binding *cis* element decoys into the balloon-injured rat carotid artery inhibits the capacity of E2F to transactivate endogenous cell-cycle regulatory genes and thereby inhibits DNA synthesis and neointima formation.[73] Taken together, these studies establish the feasibility of using the HVJ–liposome molecular delivery system for *in vivo* genetic engineering within the vasculature.

Based on these studies, it is clear that the HVJ–liposome method is an effective molecular delivery system capable of modulating gene expression within a discrete segment of the vessel wall. This experimental approach has many advantages: (1) it facilitates defining the role of a gene product within the vessel by selectively inactivating it without influencing the expression of that gene in other tissues,(2) it allows the assessment of the biologic function of an autocrine–paracrine factor by augmenting its expression locally while utilizing another vessel as an internal control, and (3) all of the effects of the *in vivo* genetic engineering are within the context of normal adult physiology and therefore a paracrine system can be manipulated locally without confounding systemic effects or the interfering influence of developmental factors frequently encountered in transgenic animal engineering.

Based upon these feasibility studies, we have recently utilized this approach to further define the role of the vascular angiotensin system in vascular remodeling in the intact animal. As described above, in response to balloon injury in the rat carotid artery model, there is an upregulation of ACE activity and angiotensinogen expression within the vessel wall in association with neointima formation.[20,21] Moreover, several groups of investigators have shown that the administration of either ACE inhibitors or AT-1 receptor antagonists inhibits neointima formation in this model system.[74] However, based on this conventional pharmacologic approach, it remained unclear whether the upregulation of the local vascular angiotensin system was essential for neointima formation or whether the efficacy of systemically administered angiotensin inhibitors was due to blockade of the endocrine renin–angiotensin system. To directly address this question, we used the HVJ–liposome molecular delivery system to selectively and locally modulate the activity of the vascular angiotensin system. In recent studies, we have observed that local delivery of antisense oligonucleotides directed against ACE expression within the balloon-injured vessel wall inhibits the upregulation of ACE activity after vascular injury and also inhibits neointima formation after vascular injury in the rat carotid model.[75] These studies support the postulate that local ACE expression is a rate-limiting step in local angiotensin generation and that locally generated angiotensin plays an important role in promoting neointima formation in the rat carotid model.

Although these results support the importance of the tissue angiotensin system in the rat model, it is important to point out that clinical trials of ACE-inhibition therapy for restenosis after angioplasty have failed to document any therapeutic efficacy in human restenosis.[76] There are a multiplicity of potential reasons for these negative results including the limitations of animal models in simulating human restenosis, species differences and pathobiologic differences (e.g. the relative role of thrombosis versus cell migration versus proliferation). However, it is also conceivable that the design of the clinical trials failed to adequately block the tissue angiotensin system within the vasculature. Our studies of local molecular delivery indicate that a more effective therapeutic strategy may involve sustained local delivery of inhibitors of the vascular angiotensin system. Future studies are needed to further test this postulate.

As discussed above, the vascular angiotensin system is also activated in association with the vascular remodeling of hypertension, and systemic blockade of angiotensin II generation reverses this remodeling process.[6,40,41] These animal model studies provide indirect evidence that angiotensin II is an important mediator of vascular remodeling in hypertension, but fail to define the relative role of the vascular angiotensin system in this process. Studies from our laboratory and others have documented that angiotensin can induce vascular cell growth in *in vitro* systems, but it has become increasingly clear that the growth response to angiotensin II is dependent on the cellular context – the cell phenotype and the milieu of autocrine–paracrine growth factors. It is therefore impossible to extrapolate from the observations derived from *in vitro* models to various *in vivo* contexts. To address this issue, we utilized the *in vivo* genetic engineering approach of local molecular delivery to increase ACE expression within a segment of the uninjured rat carotid artery. We postulated that this *in vivo* genetic engineering experiment would simulate the increased ACE expression observed in hypertensive vessels undergoing vascular remodeling and determine whether the upregulation of vascular ACE is sufficient to induce the characteristic changes in vessel architecture.

Indeed, we have recently shown that transfection of the *ACE* gene into the carotid artery results in a twofold increase in ACE activity above control arteries and was associated with growth stimulation *in vivo* as reflected in a two- to threefold increase in DNA synthesis. Furthermore, when we assessed the effect of selectively upregulating the expression of vascular ACE on vessel structure two weeks after transfection, we observed an increase in vessel-wall protein content, medial thickness and an increased wall:lumen ratio without neointima formation. Moreover, these effects on vascular cell growth and vessel hypertrophy were abolished by the administration of an AT-1 receptor antagonist. Furthermore, *ACE* gene transfection into the vessel wall had no influence on the activity of the circulating renin–angiotensin system or systemic hemodynamics and the changes in vessel architecture were limited to the transfected region of the vessel.[77] Thus, these studies provide the first evidence that increased activity of the vascular angiotensin system is sufficient to induce changes in vessel architecture characteristic of the vascular remodeling of hypertension. We speculate that the presence of an intact endothelium may be an important determinant of whether the activation of the vascular angiotensin system induces vessel hypertrophy versus neointima formation.

The use of local molecular delivery systems such as HVJ–liposomes for *in vivo* genetic engineering has great potential for defining the role of autocrine–paracrine systems and cellular processes in the pathogenesis of vascular disease. Indeed, recent studies in our laboratory have documented that transfection of the endothelial cell-type nitric oxide synthase gene into the balloon injured vessel wall restores nitric oxide generation and vessel vasorelaxation in addition to inhibiting neointima formation.[78] These data are consistent with the postulate that the regulation of both vessel tone and structure involves the interplay of countervailing vasoreactive molecules such as nitric oxide and angiotensin II.[38,79]

In addition to providing new biologic insights such as the role of paracrine vasoreactive systems, the *in vivo* genetic engineering experimental approach is useful for defining the feasibility of using local delivery strategies as therapeutic approaches to treat vascular conditions. We anticipate that further development of these technologies will foster novel clinical strategies to more effectively prevent and treat human vascular disease.

Conclusions and future directions

Although this review has focused on angiotensin II as a paradigm for the role of vasoreactive factors in the pathogenesis of vascular disease, it should be clear that vascular remodeling involves a complex interaction of many mediators as well as an interaction with hemodynamic stimuli. As detailed elsewhere in this book, other vasoreactive factors such as nitric oxide, endothelin and natriuretic peptides undoubtedly play significant contributory roles to vascular remodeling. It is postulated that a complex interplay between countervailing influences such as nitric oxide and angiotensin II are part of a delicate homeostatic balance that regulates vessel tone and structure. We are just beginning to understand the mechanisms by which these paracrine systems regulate the vasculature and participate in the pathogenesis of vascular disease.

The ongoing challenge is to link advances in our understanding of physiology, pathobiology, pharmacology and molecular genetics with the treatment of human disease. The fruitfulness of this task is evidenced by two recent clinical trials which have documented that blockade of angiotension II generation favorably alters the natural history of human cardiovascular disease. The SAVE trial has established that blockade of this system prevents deleterious ventricular remodeling postmyocardial infarction and thereby reduces morbidity and mortality.[69] Furthermore, ACE inhibitors appear to prevent the vascular remodeling that results in diabetic nephropathy and thereby changes the natural history of this devastating disease.[80] It is noteworthy that both of these seminal clinical studies were based on many years of research using animal models that simulate human disease in which local tissue angiotensin systems appear to play an important pathogenic role in tissue remodeling and the progression to end-organ failure.[17,81] It is anticipated that future studies will continue to extend our understanding of the role of these local vasoreactive systems in atherogenesis, angiogenesis, pulmonary hypertension and other vascular diseases. We are in an era in which an exciting confluence of insights are merging between studies of the genetic basis of disease and the technology of *in vivo* genetic engineering and transgenic animal models. We anticipate that future studies will continue to characterize the genetic basis of vascular diseases such as hypertension and atherosclerosis and further define the role of vasoreactive molecules as determinants of the natural history of vascular disease. The combination of advances in molecular genetics combined with new technologies in molecular delivery hold great promise for the development of novel approaches to human vascular disease.

Acknowledgments

The author is indebted to Richard Pratt and Victor Dzau for many useful discussions. This work is supported by funding from the Pew Scholar Program in Biomedical Sciences, the Baxter Foundation and the California Tobacco-related Research Surtax Fund.

References

1. Dzau, V. J. and Gibbons, G. H. (1991) Endothelium and growth factors in vascular remodeling of hypertension. *Hypertension*, **18**(Supp. 3), III-115–21.
2. Jackson, C. L. and Schwartz, S. M. (1992) Pharmacology of smooth muscle cell replication. *Hypertension*, **20**, 713–36.

3. Touyz, R. M. and Schiffrin, E. L. (1993) Effects of angiotensin II and endothelin-1 on platelet aggregation and cytosolic pH and free Ca^{2+} concentrations in essential hypertension. *Hypertension*, **22**, 853–62.
4. Ridker, P. M., Gaboury, C. L., Conlin, P. R. *et al.* (1993) Stimulation of plasminogen activator inhibitor *in vivo* by infusion of angiotensin II. Evidence of a potential interaction between the renin–angiotensin system and fibrinolytic function. *Circulation*, **87**, 1969–73.
5. Hahn, A. W. A., Jonas, U., Buhler, F. R. and Resink, T. J. (1994) Activation of human peripheral monocytes by angiotensin II. *FEBS Lett.*, **347**, 178–80.
6. Gibbons, G. H. (1993) Autocrine–paracrine factors and vascular remodeling in hypertension. *Curr. Opin. Nephrol. Hyperten.*, **2**, 291–8.
7. Gibbons, G. H., Dzau, V. J., Farhi, E. and Barger, A. C. (1984) Interaction of signals influencing renin release. *Annu. Rev. Physiol.*, **46**, 291–308.
8. Dzau, V. J. (1988) Circulating versus local renin–angiotensin system in cardiovascular homeostasis. *Circulation*, **77**(Supp. 1), I-4–I-13.
9. Lee, M. A., Bohm, M., Paul, M. and Ganten, D. (1993) Tissue renin–angiotensin systems. Their role in cardiovascular disease. *Circulation*, **87**(Supp. 5), IV-7–13.
10. Urata, H., Boehm, K. D., Philip, A. *et al.* (1993) Cellular localization and regional distribution of an angiotensin II-forming chymase in the heart. *J. Clin. Invest.*, **91**, 1269–81.
11. von Lutterotti, N., Catanzaro, D. F., Sealey, J. E. Z. and Laragh, J. H. (1994) Renin is not synthesized by cardiac and extrarenal vascular tissues. A review of experimental evidence. *Circulation*, **89**, 458–70.
12. Dzau, V. J. and Re, R. (1994) Tissue angiotensin system in cardiovascular medicine: a paradigm shift? *Circulation*, **89**, 493–8.
13. Oliver, J. A. and Sciacca, R. R. (1984) Local generation of angiotensin II as a mechanism of regulation of peripheral vascular tone in the rat. *J. Clin. Invest.*, **74**, 1247–51.
14. Hilgers, K. F., Peters, J., Veelken, R. *et al.* (1992) Increased vascular angiotensin formation in female rats harboring the mouse *Ren-2* gene. *Hypertension*, **19**, 687–91.
15. Schunkert, H., Jackson, B., Tang, S. S. *et al.* (1993) Distribution and functional significance of cardiac angiotensin converting enzyme in hypertrophied rat hearts. *Circulation*, **87**, 1328–39.
16. Paul, M., Wagner, J. and Dzau, V. J. (1993) Gene expression of the renin–angiotensin system in human tissues: quantitative analysis by the polymerase chain reaction. *J. Clin. Invest.*, **1**, 2058–64.
17. Hirsch, A. T., Talsness, C. E., Schunkert, H. *et al.* (1991) Tissue-specific activation of cardiac angiotensin converting enzyme in experimental heart failure. *Circ. Res.*, **69**, 475–82.
18. Studer, R., Reinecke, H., Muller, B. *et al.* (1994) Increased angiotensin-I converting enzyme gene expression in the failing human heart: quantitation by competitive RNA polymerase chain reaction. *J. Clin. Invest.*, **94**, 301–10.
19. Shiota, N., Miyazaki, M. and Okunishi, H. (1992) Increase of angiotensin converting enzyme gene expression in the hypertensive aorta. *Hypertension*, **20**, 168–74.
20. Rakugi, H., Kim, D. K., Krieger, J. E. *et al.* (1994) Induction of angiotensin converting enzyme in the neointima after vascular injury. Possible role in restenosis. *J. Clin. Invest.*, **93**, 339–46.
21. Rakugi, H., Jacob, H. J., Krieger, J. E. *et al.* (1993) Vascular injury induces angiotensinogen gene expression in the media and neointima. *Circulation*, **87**, 283–90.
22. Unger, T., Ganten, D., Lang, R. E. and Scholkens, B. A. (1985) Persistent tissue converting enzyme inhibition following chronic treatment with Hoe498 and MK421 in spontaneously hypertensive rats. *J. Cardiovasc. Pharmacol.*, **7**, 36–41.
23. Alderman, M. H., Madhavan, S., Ooi, W. L. *et al.* (1991) Association of the renin–sodium profile with the risk of myocardial infarction in patients with hypertension. *N. Engl. J. Med.*, **324**, 1098–104.
24. Meade, T. W., Cooper, J. A. and Peart, W. S. (1993) Plasma renin activity and ischemic heart disease. *N. Engl. J. Med.*, **329**, 616–19.

25. Bonithon-Kopp, C., Ducimetiere, P., Touboul, P. J. *et al.* (1994) Plasma angiotensin-converting enzyme activity and carotid wall thickening. *Circulation*, **89**, 952–4.
26. Cambien, F., Poirier, O., Lecerf, L. *et al.* (1992) Deletion polymorphism in the gene for angiotensin converting enzyme is a potent risk factor for myocardial infarction. *Nature*, **359**, 641–4.
27. Ruiz, J., Blanche, H., Cohen, N. *et al.* (1994) Insertion/deletion polymorphism of the angiotensin-converting enzyme gene is strongly associated with coronary heart disease in non-insulin-dependent diabetes mellitus. *Proc. Natl Acad. Sci. USA*, **91**, 3662–5.
28. Cousterousse, C., Allegrini, J., Lopez, M. and Alhenc-Gelas, F. (1991) Angiotensin I-converting enzyme in human circulating mononuclear cells: genetic polymorphism of expression in T-lymphocytes. *Biochem. J.*, **56**, 689.
29. Rapp, J. P., Wang, S. and Dene, H. (1989) A genetic polymorphism in the renin gene of Dahl rats cosegregates with blood pressure. *Science*, **243**, 542–3.
30. Dubay, C., Vincent, M., Samani, N. J. *et al.* (1993) Genetic determinants of diastolic and pulse pressure man to different loci in Lyon hypertensive rats. *Nature-Genetics*, **3**, 354–7.
31. Jacob, H. J., Lindpainter, K., Lincoln, S. E. *et al.* (1991) Genetic mapping of a gene causing hypertension in the stroke-prone spontaneously hypertensive rat. *Cell*, **67**, 213–24.
32. Ohkubo, H., Kawakami, H., Kekehi, Y. *et al.* (1990) Generation of transgenic mice with elevated blood pressure by introduction of the rat renin and angiotensinogen genes. *Proc. Natl Acad. Sci. USA*, **87**, 5153–7.
33. Mullins, J. J., Peters, J. and Ganten, D. (1990) Fulminant hypertension in transgenic rats harbouring the mouse *Ren-2* gene. *Nature*, **344**, 541–4.
34. Jeunemaitre, X., Soubrier, F., Kotelevtsev, Y. V. *et al.* (1992) Molecular basis of human hypertension: role of angiotensinogen. *Cell*, **71**, 169–80.
35. Caulfield, M., Lavender, P., Farrall, M. *et al.* (1994) Linkage of the angiotensinogen gene to essential hypertension. *N. Engl. J. Med.*, **330**, 1629–33.
36. Hata, A., Namikawa, C., Sasaki, M. *et al.* (1994) Angiotensinogen as a risk factor for essential hypertension in Japan. *J. Clin. Invest.*, **93**, 1285–7.
37. Ward, K., Hata, A., Jeunemaitre, X. *et al.* (1993) A molecular variant of angiotensinogen associated with preeclampsia. *Nature Genetics*, **4**, 59–61.
38. Gibbons, G. H. and Dzau, V. J. (1994) The emerging concept of vascular remodeling. *N. Engl. J. Med.*, **330**, 1431–8.
39. Heagerty, A. M., Aalkjaer, C., Bund, S. J. *et al.* (1993) Small artery structure in hypertension: dual processes of remodeling and growth. *Hypertension*, **21**, 391–7.
40. Limas, C., Westrum, B. and Limas, C. J. (1984) Comparative effects of hydralazine and captopril on the cardiovascular changes in spontaneously hypertensive rats. *Am. J. Pathol.*, **117**, 360–71.
41. Harrap, S. B., van der Merwe, W. M., Griffin, S. A. *et al.* (1990) Brief angiotensin converting enzyme inhibitor treatment in young spontaneously hypertensive rats reduces blood pressure long-term. *Hypertension*, **16**, 603–14.
42. Mukoyama, M., Nakajima, M., Horiuchi, M. *et al.* (1993) Expression cloning of type 2 angiotensin II receptor reveals a unique class of seven-transmembrane receptors. *J. Biol. Chem.*, **268**, 24539–42.
43. Le Noble, F. A., Schreurs, N. H., van Straaten, H. W. *et al.* (1993) Evidence for a novel angiotensin II receptor involved in angiogenesis in chick embryo chorioallantoic membrane. *Am. J. Physiol.*, **264**, R460–5.
44. Griendling, K. K. and Alexander, R. W. (1993) The angiotensin (AT1) receptor. *Semin. Nephrol.*, **13**, 558–66.
45. Marrero, M. B., Paxton, W. G., Duff, J. L. *et al.* (1994) Angiotensin II stimulates tyrosine phosphorylation of phospholipase C-γ1 in vascular smooth muscle cells. *J. Biol. Chem.*, **269**, 10935–9.
46. Butcher, R. D., Schollmann, C. and Marne, D. (1993) Angiotensin II mediates intracellular signalling in vascular smooth muscle cells by activation of tyrosine-specific protein kinases and c-*raf*-1. *Biochem. Biophys. Res. Commun.*, **196**, 1280–7.

47. Taubman, M. B., Berk, B. C., Izumo, S. *et al.* (1989) Angiotensin II induces c-*fos* mRNA in aortic smooth muscle: role of Ca^{2+} mobilization and protein kinase C activation. *J. Biol. Chem.*, **264**, 526–30.
48. Naftilan, A. J., Pratt, R. E. and Dzau, V. J. (1989) Induction of platelet-derived growth factor A-chain and c-*myc* gene expressions by angiotensin II in cultured rat vascular smooth muscle cells. *J. Clin. Invest.*, **83**, 1419–24.
49. van Kleef, E. M., Smits, J. F. M., De Mey, J. G. R., *et al.* (1992) α_1-Adrenergic blockade reduces the angiotensin II-induced vascular smooth muscle cell DNA synthesis in the rat thoracic aorta and carotid artery. *Circ. Res.*, **70**, 1122–7.
50. Geisterfer, A. A. T., Peach, M. J. and Owens, G. K. (1988) Angiotensin II induces hypertrophy, not hyperplasia, of cultured rat aortic smooth muscle cells. *Circ. Res.*, **62**, 749–56.
51. Gibbons, G. H., Pratt, R. E. and Dzau, V. J. (1992) Vascular smooth muscle cell hypertrophy vs hyperplasia: Autocrine transforming growth factor-beta expression determines growth response to angiotensin II. *J. Clin. Invest.*, **90**, 456–61.
52. Itoh, H., Mukoyama, M., Pratt, R. E. *et al.* (1993) Multiple autocrine growth factors modulate vascular smooth muscle cell growth response to angiotensin II. *J. Clin. Invest.*, **91**, 2268–74.
53. Koibuchi, Y., Lee, W. S., Gibbons, G. H. and Pratt, R. E. (1993) Role of TGFb1 in the cellular growth response to angiotensin II. *Hypertension*, **21**, 1046–50.
54. Stouffer, G. A. and Owens, G. K. (1992) Angiotensin II-induced mitogenesis of spontaneously hypertensive rat-derived cultured smooth muscle cells is dependent on autocrine production of transforming growth factor-β. *Circ. Res.*, **170**, 820–8.
55. Delafontaine, P. and Lou, H. (1993) Angiotensin II regulates insulin-like growth factor I gene expression in vascular smooth muscle cells. *J. Biol. Chem.*, **268**, 16866–70.
56. Temizer, D. H., Yoshizumi, M., Perrella, M. A. *et al.* (1992) Induction of heparin-binding epidermal growth factor-like growth factor mRNA by phorbol ester and angiotensin II in rat aortic smooth muscle cells. *J. Biol. Chem.*, **267**, 24892–6.
57. Scott-Burden, T., Resink, T. J., Hahn, A. W. and Vanhoutte, P. M. (1991) Induction of endothelin secretion by angiotensin II: effects on growth and synthetic activity of vascular smooth muscle cells. *J. Cardiovasc. Pharmacol.*, **17**(Supp. 7), S96–S100.
58. Bell, L. and Madri, J. A. (1990) Influence of the angiotensin system on endothelial and smooth muscle cell migration. *Am. J. Pathol.*, **137**, 7–12.
59. Sharifi, B. G., Lafleur, D. W., Pirola, C. J. *et al.* (1992) Angiotensin II regulates tenascin gene expression in vascular smooth muscle cells. *J. Biol. Chem.*, **267**, 23910–15.
60. van Leeuwen, R. T. J., Kol, A., Andreotti, F. *et al.* (1994) Angiotensin II increases plasminogen activator inhibitor type 1 and tissue-type plasminogen activator messenger RNA in cultured rat aortic smooth muscle cells. *Circulation*, **90**, 362–8.
61. Sudhir, K., Wilson, E., Chatterjee, K. and Ives, H. E. (1993) Mechanical strain and collagen potentiate mitogenic activity of angiotensin II in rat vascular smooth muscle cells. *J. Clin. Invest.*, **92**, 3003–7.
62. Weinstock, J. V. and Blum, A. M. (1987) Synthesis of angiotensins by cultured granuloma macrophages in murine Schistosomiasis mansoni. *Cell. Immunol.*, **107**, 273–80.
63. Weinstock, J. V., Blum, A. M. and Kassab, J. T. (1987) Angiotensin II is chemotactic for a T-cell subset which can express migration inhibition factor activity in murine Schistosomiasis mansoni. *Cell. Immunol.*, **107**, 180–7.
64. Griendling, K. K., Minieri, C. A. Ollerenshaw, J. D. and Alexander, R. W. (1994) Angiotensin II stimulates NADH and NADPH oxidase activity in cultured vascular smooth muscle cells. *Circ. Res.*, **74**, 1141–48.
65. Ohara, Y., Peterson, T. E. and Harrison, D. G. (1993) Hypercholesterolemia increases endothelial superoxide anion production. *J. Clin. Invest.*, **91**, 2546–51.
66. Chobanian, A. V., Haudenschild, C. C., Nickerson, C. and Hope, S. (1992) Trandolapril inhibits atherosclerosis in the Watanabe heritable hyperlipidemic rabbit. *Hypertension*, **20**, 473–7.

67. Schuh, J. R., Blehm, D. J., Frierdich, G. E. *et al.* (1993) Differential effects of renin–angiotensin system blockade on atherogenesis in cholesterol-fed rabbits. *J. Clin. Invest.*, **91**, 1453–8.

68. Sharpe, N. (1993) The effects of ACE inhibition on progression of atherosclerosis. *J. Cardiovasc. Pharmacol.*, **22**(Supp. 9), S9–S12.

69. Pfeffer, M. A., Braunwald, E., Moye, L. A. *et al.* (1992) Effect of captopril on mortality and morbidity in patients with left ventricular dysfunction after myocardial infarction: results of the survival and ventricular enlargement trial. *N. Engl. J. Med.*, **327**, 669–677.

70. Morishita, R., Gibbons, G. H., Ellison, K. E. *et al.* (1993) Single intraluminal delivery of antisense cdc2 kinase and PCNA oligonucleotides results in chronic inhibition of neointimal hyperplasia. *Proc. Natl Acad. Sci. USA*, **90**, 8474–8.

71. Morishita, R., Gibbons, G. H., Ellison, K. E. *et al.* (1994) Intimal hyperplasia after vascular injury is inhibited by antisense cdk2 kinase oligonucleotides. *J. Clin. Invest.*, **93**, 1458–64.

72. Engelhardt, J. F., Ye, X., Doranz, B. and Wilson, J. M. (1994) Ablation of E2A in recombinant adenoviruses improves transgene persistence and decreases inflammatory response in mouse liver. *Proc. Natl Acad. Sci. USA*, **91**, 6196–200.

73. Morishita, R., Gibbons, G. H., Ellison, K. E. *et al.* (1995) A molecular strategy using cis element 'decoy' of E2F binding site inhibits smooth muscle proliferation *in vivo*. *Proc. Natl Acad. Sci. USA*, in press.

74. Powell, J. S., Clozel, J. P., Müller, R. K. M. *et al.* (1989) Inhibitors of angiotensin-converting enzyme prevent myointimal proliferation after vascular injury. *Science*, **245**, 186–8.

75. Morishita, R., Kaneda, Y., Tomita, N. *et al.* (1994) Antisense oligonucleotide inhibition of local angiotensin converting enzyme resulted in the inhibition of neointima formation after vascular injury. *Circulation*, **90**, I–142.

76. The MERCATOR Study Group (1992) Does the new angiotensin converting enzyme inhibitor cilazapril prevent restenosis after percutaneous transluminal coronary angioplasty? Results of the MERCATOR study: a multicenter, randomized, double-blind placebo-controlled trial. *Circulation*, **86**, 100–10.

77. Morishita, R., Gibbons, G. H., Nakajima, M. *et al.* (1994) Evidence for direct local effect of angiotensin in vascular hypertrophy: *in vivo* gene transfer of angiotensin converting enzyme. *J. Clin. Invest.*, **94**, 978–984.

78. von der Leyen, H., Gibbons, G. H., Morishita, R. *et al.* (1995) Gene therapy inhibiting neointimal vascular lesion: *in vivo* transfer of endothelial cell nitric oxide synthase gene. *Proc. Natl Acad. Sci. USA*, **92**, 1137–41.

79. Cooke, J. P. and Tsao, P. S. (1994) Is NO an endogenous antiatherogenic molecule? *Arterioscler. Thromb.*, **14**, 653–5.

80. Lewis, E. J., Hunsicker, L. G., Bain, R. P. and Roihde, R. D., and the Collaborative Study Group (1993) The effect of angiotensin converting enzyme inhibition on diabetic nephropathy. *N. Engl. J. Med.*, **329**, 1456–62.

81. Zatz, R., Dunn, B. R., Meyer, T. W. *et al.* (1986) Prevention of diabetic glomerulopathy by pharmacological amelioration of glomerular capillary hypertension. *J. Clin. Invest.*, **77**, 1925–30.

12

Pulmonary Vasoreactive Diseases: Inhaled Nitric Oxide

William E. Hurford
Warren M. Zapol

The treatment of pulmonary hypertension has been limited severely by the unavailability of selective pulmonary vasodilators. Nonselective pulmonary vasodilation may produce severe systemic hypotension and worsen arterial hypoxemia by altering the matching of ventilation to pulmonary perfusion. This effect may be particularly pronounced in patients with acute lung injury.[1–3] In 1991, however, nitric oxide (NO) was reported to selectively vasodilate the pulmonary circulation when the gas was administered by inhalation.[4–6] Significant systemic hypotension did not occur because NO is inactivated by rapid binding to hemoglobin in the blood. In an injured lung with pulmonary hypertension, inhaled NO was found to produce local vasodilation of well-ventilated lung regions.[7,8] This reduced intrapulmonary shunting of venous blood and improved systemic arterial oxygenation. The possible use of NO and related compounds for treating pulmonary hypertensive states is therefore receiving intense examination.

Nitric oxide

Nitric oxide is a gaseous endogenous vasodilator and has been identified as an endothelium-derived relaxing factor (EDRF).[9–12] It is an ideal local transcellular messenger because of its small size, lipophilic nature and short duration of action.[13] Nitric oxide is synthesized from the terminal guanidino nitrogen of L-arginine and diffuses rapidly into subjacent cells.[14,15] In vascular smooth muscle, NO binds to the heme iron complex of soluble guanylate cyclase. The resulting nitrosyl-heme activates guanylate cyclase, stimulating the production of cyclic guanosine 3',5'-monophosphate (cGMP) and subsequent relaxation of vascular smooth muscle.[14,16,17] When NO diffuses into the intravascular space, its biologic activity is limited by avid binding to hemoglobin.[18] Commonly used chemical nitrosovasodilators, such as nitroglycerin and nitroprusside, appear to act by releasing NO.[19]

Nitric oxide has diverse physiologic functions besides smooth-muscle relaxation, including neurotransmission, immunoregulation and inhibition of platelet aggregation. These functions have been reviewed extensively.[17,20,21] Distinct NO synthases regulate these functions. Multiple isozymes of NO synthase, homologous to cytochrome P450 reductase, have been isolated and/or cloned from various tissues.[22-25] These NO synthase enzymes have been grouped into two types on the basis of cofactor requirements and structure. A Ca^{2+}-dependent enzyme is constitutively expressed in vascular endothelium, cerebellum, adrenal tissue, and platelets. An inducible Ca^{2+}-independent form is present in lung, hepatic Kupffer cells, and macrophages.[23] Endotoxin stimulates and glucocorticoids inhibit the inducible form of this enzyme.[26] Inhibitors of NO synthesis, such as N^G-monomethyl-L-arginine, decrease the production of endogenous nitric oxide by the intact lung and enhance hypoxic pulmonary vasoconstriction of isolated pulmonary artery rings.[27] Similarly, chemical inhibitors of guanylate cyclase activation such as methylene blue inhibit the action of NO, whereas specific cGMP phosphodiesterase inhibitors such as Zaprinast can enhance or potentiate some of the biologic actions of NO.[13,17,28,29]

Endothelium-dependent relaxation of pulmonary arteries occurs in response to a variety of physical and pharmacologic stimuli.[30,31] Endogenous NO has been measured in the exhaled air of rabbits, guinea pigs, and humans.[32,33] In patients and volunteers, relatively high levels of nitric oxide (0.07–0.13 ppm) appear to be produced in the nasopharynx, possibly by colonizing bacteria.[33] The NO produced in the nasopharynx subsequently is inhaled and approximately 50–70% of the inhaled gas is absorbed. When the tracheas of patients were intubated, bypassing the nasopharynx, NO levels were greatly reduced in inhaled and exhaled gas. It is possible that the inhaled endogenous NO might have a role in the regulation of ventilation/perfusion matching. In normal lungs, however, baseline pulmonary vascular tone is very low and the administration of acetylcholine or the addition of exogenous NO has little effect on pulmonary vascular resistance.[4,34-36] In patients with pulmonary hypertension, on the other hand, acetylcholine infusion or NO inhalation can reduce pulmonary vascular resistance.[4,34,35] It is possible that in some pulmonary hypertensive states, such as adult respiratory distress syndrome (ARDS), the production of endogenous NO is impaired.[37,38] This might produce further vasoconstriction and foster platelet aggregation. Evidence supporting this hypothesis is indirect at this time. Dinh Xuan and coworkers reported that patients with cor pulmonale secondary to congenital heart disease had an impaired pulmonary vasodilatory response to acetylcholine.[39] The same group also studied 18 patients with chronic obstructive pulmonary disease and reported that impairment of acetylcholine-induced relaxation was correlated with lower arterial oxygen tensions and greater intimal thickening of pulmonary blood vessels.[37] Such patients may have an intact response to exogenously administered NO even though their response to intravenous acetylcholine is impaired.[40]

Zapol and coworkers hypothesized that inhaled NO should diffuse into the pulmonary vasculature of ventilated lung regions and cause relaxation of pulmonary vascular smooth muscle, thereby decreasing pulmonary hypertension.[5,6] Since the NO is inhaled, the gas should be distributed predominantly to well-ventilated alveoli and not to collapsed or fluid-filled areas of the lung. In the presence of increased vasomotor tone, local vasodilation of well-ventilated lung regions should cause a 'steal' or diversion of pulmonary artery blood flow towards well-ventilated alveoli, improving the matching of ventilation to perfusion and improving arterial oxygenation during ARDS. Such an effect would be in marked contrast to the effects of intravenously administered conventional vasodilators (such as nitroprusside, nitroglycerin or prostacyclin). These intravenous agents also decrease pulmonary artery pressure, but by nonselectively dilating the pulmonary vasculature, they augment blood flow to nonventilated areas, thereby increasing right-to-left shunting and reducing the PaO_2. Also unlike available intravenous vasodilators, inhaled NO, because it is avidly bound to hemoglobin and rapidly inactivated, should not produce systemic vasodilation.

Acute pulmonary vasoreactive diseases

Two diseases, the adult respiratory distress syndrome (ARDS) and persistent pulmonary hypertension of the newborn (PPHN), are notable for the presence of severe acute pulmonary hypertension. These two disease states are both important clinical problems and excellent models for the study of pulmonary vascular regulation.

Adult respiratory distress syndrome

Acute pulmonary hypertension consistently occurs in severe ARDS. In survivors, pulmonary vascular resistance progressively decreases over time. Nonsurvivors tend to have a persistently increased pulmonary vascular resistance. The increased pulmonary artery pressure is independent of changes of cardiac output and persists after the correction of systemic hypoxemia.[41]

The pulmonary vascular changes in ARDS are produced by a complex combination of primary lung injury (i.e. aspiration, trauma, infection), the consequences of the pulmonary inflammatory response to injury (hypoxia, acidosis, release of cytokines and components of the complement system and the arachidonic acid pathway, as well as inhibitors of fibrinolysis), and the iatrogenic complications of intensive care therapy (oxygen toxicity and barotrauma). In severe ARDS, thromboembolic occlusion of the pulmonary vasculature is also common.[42]

Various vasodilator therapies aimed at reducing pulmonary hypertension have been tested in patients with ARDS. Systemic vasodilation and hypotension occur with the use of all currently available intravenous vasodilators tested in dosages sufficient to reduce the pulmonary artery pressure. Intravenous infusion of systemic vasodilators such as nitroprusside or prostacyclin (PGl_2) also markedly increases the venous admixture and may decrease oxygen delivery to peripheral tissues.[1–3,43]

Persistent pulmonary hypertension of the newborn

At birth, there is a sustained decrease of pulmonary vascular resistance and an increase of pulmonary blood flow, in part due to increasing oxygen tensions. If this does not occur, PPHN may result. This syndrome is characterized by an increased pulmonary vascular resistance, increased right-to-left shunting across the ductus arteriosus and foramen ovale, and severe hypoxemia. Extracorporeal membrane oxygenation (ECMO) is often used to support these infants, because conventional vasodilator therapy is limited by severe hypotension. Hypotension may reduce PaO_2 further by increasing right-to-left shunting. It has been hypothesized that endogenous production of NO by the pulmonary vasculature might be decreased in PPHN. If so, then inhaled NO might provide an effective therapy for these severely ill infants.[44–48]

Laboratory and clinical studies of inhaled nitric oxide

Acute pulmonary hypertension

Inhaled NO decreases pulmonary hypertension without altering the systemic vascular resistance.[5,6] In studies of normal awake lambs without pulmonary hypertension, inhaling 80 ppm NO had no hemodynamic effect. The pulmonary artery pressure, cardiac output, systemic arterial pressure and systemic vascular resistance were unchanged. When the pulmonary artery pressure was acutely increased, either by hypoxia, infusing the thromboxane endoperoxide analog U46619, or producing the heparin–protamine reaction, the pulmonary hypertension was reversed by inhalation of 40–80 ppm NO.[5,6] Pulmonary vasodilation occurred within three minutes, lasted throughout the duration of the inhalation, and disappeared within three minutes after the discontinuation of NO (Figure 12.1). Importantly, the systemic vascular resistance was unchanged. The pulmonary vasodilator effect occurred at low levels of inhaled NO (i.e. 5 ppm). Potent vasodilation (65% of the maximal effect) occurred at 20 ppm inhaled NO. This concentration is less than the NIOSH standard for eight-hour working exposures (25 ppm). During continuous inhalation of 80 ppm NO for one hour, no tolerance was observed. That inhaled NO reverses hypoxic pulmonary vasoconstriction has been confirmed by others.[7,49,50] Pison and coworkers studied the matching of ventilation to perfusion using the multiple inert gas technique in mechanically-ventilated normal sheep.[7] They reported that inhaling 20 ppm NO redistributed blood flow to better ventilated alveoli and reversed the pulmonary hypertension caused by breathing a hypoxic gas mixture.

Frostell *et al.* subsequently studied the effects of breathing 40 ppm NO for 10 minutes in nine awake, healthy human volunteers exposed to hypoxic conditions.[35] During air breathing, 40 ppm NO had no pulmonary or systemic vasodilatory effect. When the subjects breathed 12% oxygen, causing mild pulmonary hypertension, 40 ppm NO completely reversed the hypoxia-induced increase of pulmonary artery pressure and vascular resistance. Systemic blood pressure and vascular resistance were unchanged and methemoglobin levels remained below 1%.

The effects of inhaled NO on endotoxin-induced pulmonary hypertension are more complex. Inhaled NO at a concentration of 10 ppm selectively decreased the acute pulmonary hypertension occurring at least 30 min after the intravenous

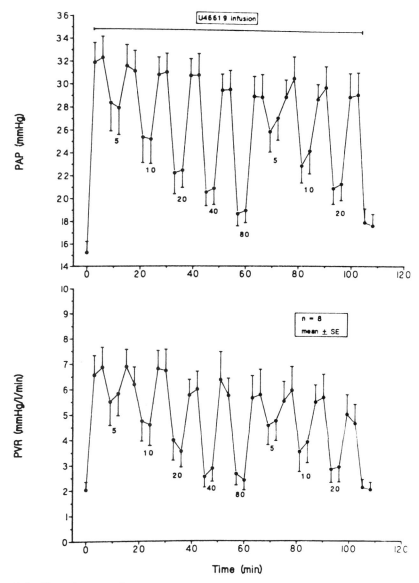

Figure 12.1 Plots of mean pulmonary artery pressure (PAP) and pulmonary vascular resistance (PVR) during a continuous infusion of U46619. Lambs breathed various levels of NO (5–80 ppm) at FiO_2 0.6 for 6 min, then breathed a gas mixture at FiO_2 0.6 for 6 min without NO ($n = 8$, mean ± SEM). (After Frostell et al., 1991.[5])

administration of *Escherichia coli* endotoxin in anesthetized pigs.[51] Arterial oxygenation and pH were also improved during NO inhalation. The early increase in pulmonary artery pressure (within 30 min after endotoxin administration), however, was unaffected by this low NO dose. Thromboxane A_2 is believed to cause the early increase of pulmonary artery pressure observed following endotoxin infusion. In models of acute pulmonary hypertension characterized by an increased plasma thromboxane A_2 level, high doses of inhaled NO effectively block the vasoconstriction. In a study by Fratacci and coworkers, for example, the acute and transient pulmonary hypertension caused by the heparin–protamine reaction in the awake sheep was blocked by inhaling 180 ppm NO.[6] The reasons for differing dose–response relationships in different species and in different models of acute pulmonary hypertension are not yet understood.

Inhaled NO probably mediates pulmonary vasodilation during lung injury by increasing cGMP levels within smooth muscle. This increase may be reflected by increased plasma cGMP concentrations. Rovira and coworkers studied a model of acute lung injury induced by bilateral lung lavage in anesthetized lambs.[52] When endogenous NO production was inhibited by infusing N^G-nitro-L-arginine methyl ester (L-NAME), a consistent increase of aortic, as compared with pulmonary arterial, plasma cGMP concentration could be measured within 5 min of breathing 60 ppm NO. Increased aortic plasma cGMP levels were associated with selective pulmonary vasodilation, reduced venous admixture, and increased PaO_2. Levels of plasma cGMP returned to baseline within 10 min of discontinuing NO breathing.

Nitric oxide inhalation in ARDS

Rossaint and coworkers compared the effects of NO inhalation (18 and 36 ppm) to intravenously infused prostacyclin in nine patients with ARDS.[8] Nitric oxide selectively reduced mean pulmonary artery pressure from 37 ± 3 to 30 ± 2 mmHg (mean $\pm$ SE). Oxygenation improved due to decreased venous admixture ($\dot{Q}_{VA}/\dot{Q}_t$). During NO breathing, the PaO_2/FiO_2 ratio increased from 152 ± 15 mmHg to 199 ± 23 mmHg (Figure 12.2). While the intravenous infusion of prostacyclin also reduced pulmonary artery pressure, mean arterial pressure and PaO_2 decreased as $\dot{Q}_{VA}/\dot{Q}_t$ increased. Subsequent reports documented that inhalation of lower concentrations of NO (<20 ppm) effectively reduced pulmonary artery pressure and improved PaO_2.[53–56] Even very small inhaled concentrations (as low as 250 ppb NO) may be effective in some patients.[57] Right ventricular ejection fraction may increase in some patients responding to inhaled NO, suggesting that the observed decreases of pulmonary artery pressure may be hemodynamically important.[55,56] Interestingly, improvement of oxygenation may occur at inhaled NO levels (as low as 60 ppb) which do not cause significant changes of pulmonary vascular resistance.[58]

A marked variation has been reported for the hemodynamic and respiratory effects of NO inhalation, both among patients and within the same patient at different times in their illness.[53,59,60] It is possible that pre-existing pulmonary disease as well as the concomitant administration of other vasoactive drugs may contribute the observed variability. In general, the baseline level of pulmonary vascular resistance appears to predict the degree of pulmonary vasoconstriction reversible by NO inhalation. Those with the greatest degree of pulmonary hypertension appear to respond best to NO inhalation.[53,60] In addition, the concomitant

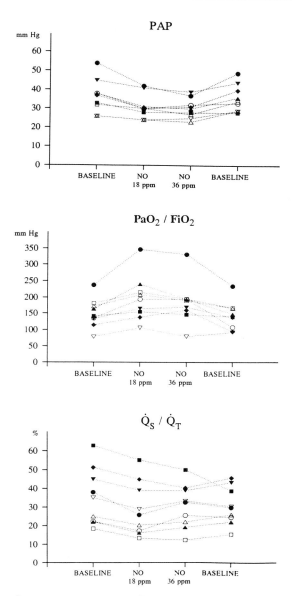

Figure 12.2 Mean pulmonary artery pressure (PAP), arterial oxygenation efficiency (PaO_2/FiO_2), and intrapulmonary shunting $\dot{Q}_S/\dot{Q}_T$ in nine patients with ARDS during inhalation of NO. (After Rossaint *et al.*, 1993.[8])

intravenous infusion of a novel vasoconstricting drug, almitrine, which increases the degree of hypoxic vasoconstriction in the lung, has been reported to enhance the beneficial effect of inhaled NO on PaO_2.[61] Almitrine, however, also increased mean pulmonary artery pressure and cardiac output.

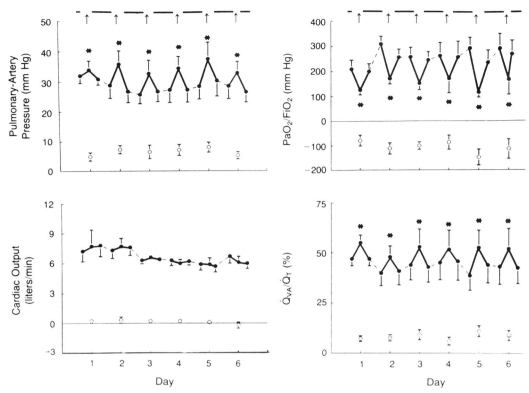

Figure 12.3 Hemodynamic function and gas exchange before, during and after brief interruptions (arrows) of NO inhalation (bars) during the first six days of treatment in seven patients with ARDS. Values are means ± SE (solid symbols); also shown (open symbols) are the means ± SE of the individual differences between the values for the effect of treatment and the means of the values determined before and after interrupting NO therapy. The standard errors for the treatment effects were small, indicating that the effects of withdrawal of NO were clear and precisely estimated. Each asterisk denotes a significant difference from the mean of the values determined before and after interrupting NO therapy (After Rossaint *et al.*, 1993.[8])

Tachyphylaxis has not been observed even when NO inhalation was continued for up to 53 days.[8] Pulmonary artery pressure and PaO_2 quickly return to baseline values, however, after discontinuation of the gas (Figure 12.3). Occasionally, sudden discontinuation of inhaled NO can produce problematic transient pulmonary vasoconstriction and possibly bronchoconstriction.[53,62,63] The reason for this is unclear. Possibly, the addition of exogenous NO may decrease NO synthase activity[64] or increase tissue cGMP phosphodiesterase activity.

Inhaled NO in persistent pulmonary hypertension of the newborn

Several investigators have studied the effects of inhaled NO on the neonatal pulmonary circulation. In hypoxic newborn lambs studied by Roberts and co-workers, NO inhalation decreased pulmonary artery pressure and increased pulmonary blood flow without reducing systemic vascular resistance.[65] Ventilation with 80 ppm NO at an FiO_2 of 0.21 caused a threefold increase of both lung and preductal plasma cGMP concentrations. Severe respiratory acidosis did not attenuate the pulmonary vasodilation caused by inhaled NO. Zayek and coworkers studied the effects of inhaled NO (6–100 ppm) in a model of PPHN created by prenatal ligation of the ductus arteriosus in lambs.[48] They reported that inhaled NO caused dose-dependent decreases of pulmonary artery pressure and pulmonary vascular resistance. Decreased right-to-left shunting of blood flow through the foramen ovale during NO inhalation resulted in an increased PaO_2 (from 43 ± 16 mmHg to 185 ± 72 mmHg, mean ± SEM, while breathing 100 ppm NO) and arterial oxygen saturation (from 74 ± 8 to 96 ± 2%) and a decreased PaO_2. Systemic blood pressure was unaffected by breathing NO.[48] Using this model, Zayek and coworkers subsequently documented an increased survival rate with NO therapy.[66] After prenatal ligation of the ductus arteriosus and delivery 13 days later, newborn lambs were ventilated at FiO_2 of 0.92 and randomly allocated to breathe 80 ppm NO for 23 hours or receive no additional treatment. All seven control lambs died before the end of the study, whereas five of six lambs treated with NO survived. Arterial oxygenation was increased in the NO-breathing lambs, compared with controls. Interestingly, blood methemoglobin concentration increased to 3% after four hours of NO breathing, but did not increase further over the 23 hours of the study. DeMarco and coworkers also reported that inhaled NO reversed acute pulmonary artery hypertension induced by hypoxia or U46619 in the newborn lamb. This group also reported slightly increased methemoglobin levels after 80 ppm NO breathing for three hours.[67] In a piglet model of Group B *Streptococcus* sepsis, a common cause of neonatal respiratory failure that was studied by Berger and coworkers, inhalation of 150 ppm NO for 30 minutes reversed the pulmonary hypertension caused by the infusion of Group B *Streptococcus*.[50] The inhalation of NO did not alter ventilation/perfusion abnormalities caused by Group B *Streptococcus* sepsis or affect systemic hemodynamics in this study.

In clinical studies by Roberts and coworkers, critically ill infants with PPHN rapidly increased preductal oxygen saturation in response to NO inhalation at concentrations up to 80 ppm. In five of six infants studied, postductal oxygen saturation also increased. In one newborn, the resulting improvement in PaO_2 persisted after the discontinuation of NO, eliminating the need for ECMO.[46]

Kinsella and coworkers reported the effects of inhaling 10–20 ppm NO in nine infants with severe PPHN. All nine showed a rapid improvement in oxygenation without systemic hypotension. Clinical improvement continued during treatment with 6 ppm NO for 24 hours in six of the infants.[44] Subsequently, this group has reported that 13 of 15 patients with PPHN who were candidates for support with ECMO were successfully treated with inhaled NO. ECMO therapy was avoided in these patients.[47,68] Successful treatment of a 1180-g premature newborn with pulmonary hypertension caused by Group B *Streptococcus* sepsis has also been reported by this group.[69] Nitric oxide inhalation in babies with PPHN currently is being studied in several blinded randomized multicenter trials.

Inhaled NO in other pulmonary hypertensive states

Chronic pulmonary hypertension

Clinical studies of brief periods of NO inhalation have been performed in patients with chronic pulmonary hypertension. In 18 patients with either chronic pulmonary hypertension or cardiac disease, Pepke-Zaba and coworkers reported that inhalation of 40 ppm NO in air decreased pulmonary vascular resistance by 5–68% without affecting systemic vascular resistance.[4] Similar hemodynamic effects have been reported in response to inhaled NO in six patients with pulmonary hypertension following mitral-valve replacement for mitral stenosis,[70] in patients with chronic obstructive lung disease complicated by pulmonary hypertension,[40,71] and in a 5-month-old child with idiopathic pulmonary hypertension which was unresponsive to intravenous vasodilators.[72]

Congenital and acquired heart disease

Inhaled NO has been evaluated as potential therapy for patients with pulmonary hypertension due to cardiac disease. Roberts and coworkers studied 10 children from 3 months to 6.5 years of age with chronic pulmonary hypertension due to congenital heart defects. Inhaling 20–80 ppm NO at FiO_2 0.9 for 10 min promptly decreased pulmonary artery pressure and pulmonary vascular resistance.[73] Compared to breathing 0 ppm NO at FiO_2 0.9, NO decreased the mean pulmonary artery pressure from 48 ± 19 mmHg to 37 ± 11 mmHg (mean ± SD). Under the same conditions, NO decreased the pulmonary vascular resistance from 536 ± 376 to 308 ± 260 dyne s cm^{-5} m^{-2}, while systemic arterial pressure and resistance remained unchanged. Inhaling 80 ppm NO at FiO_2 0.9 increased pulmonary blood flow in all of the six patients with intracardiac shunts. Similar results have been reported when inhaled NO was used to decrease acute pulmonary hypertension in the perioperative period.[74–77]

In adult patients, Rich and coworkers have studied the effects of inhaling 20 ppm NO in 20 patients undergoing various types of cardiac surgery requiring cardiopulmonary bypass and five patients requiring ventricular assist devices.[60] Nitric oxide inhalation decreased the pulmonary artery pressure from 36 ± 3 (mean ± SEM) to 29 ± 2 mmHg and 32 ± 2 to 27 ± 1 mmHg, before and after cardiopulmonary bypass, respectively, and from 68 ± 12 to 55 ± 9 mmHg in patients requiring ventricular assist devices. The decrease of pulmonary vascular resistance during NO breathing was proportional to patients' baseline pulmonary vascular resistance. Once again, systemic hemodynamics were unaffected.

Toxicity of nitric oxide

The interest generated by reports of the successful therapeutic use of inhaled NO is tempered by concerns over its toxicity. Nitric oxide is a common pollutant. It is produced in nature by lightning and the burning of fossil fuels and exists in the

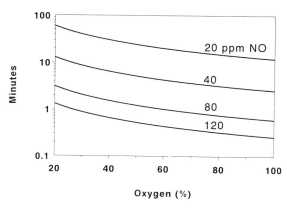

Figure 12.4 Time in minutes to yield 5 ppm NO with differing mixtures of NO and oxygen. (Adapted from Petros *et al.*, 1992.[104])

atmosphere at levels near 10 ppb. Its major atmospheric breakdown pathway at these low levels is via combination with ozone.[78] Nitric oxide is present in cigarette smoke and is routinely inhaled for short periods in concentrations of 400–1000 ppm by millions of people.[79] Although the US Occupational Safety and Health Administration has set an NO exposure limit of 25 ppm when breathed for 8 hours per day in the workplace, long-term studies of NO toxicology have not been conducted.[80]

Nitric oxide may form several toxic products. In oxygen mixtures, NO is oxidized to nitrogen dioxide (NO_2). The rate of oxidation is dependent upon the oxygen concentration and the square of the NO concentration (Figure 12.4).[81] Nitrogen dioxide is clearly cytotoxic[82] and is converted in aqueous solutions to nitric and nitrous acids. Occupational safety and health standards limit the exposure of workers to NO_2 to 5 ppm.[80] In aqueous solutions, NO reacts rapidly with O_2^- to form peroxynitrite $OONO^-$.[83] This species is also highly cytotoxic. In addition, NO forms complexes with transition-metal complexes, including those in metalloproteins such as hemoglobin. In tissues, nitrosation of iron-containing enzymes and iron-sulfur proteins of target cells may be responsible for the cytotoxic action of NO generated by activated macrophages.[84,85] In the circulation, NO combines extremely rapidly with hemoglobin to form nitrosyl Fe(II)-hemoglobin and then methemoglobin.[18] Endogenous NO production probably accounts for the methemoglobin levels found in the blood of nonsmokers.[86] S-nitrosothiols, mostly S-nitrosoproteins, are also formed in plasma. S-nitrosothiols have been identified in human airway lining fluid and in the plasma of normal subjects[87] and patients inhaling NO mixtures.[88] The formation of relatively stable iron–nitrosyl complexes and S-nitrosothiols may provide ways of tailoring the duration of action and transport properties of NO and a means of detoxifying NO in tissues.[87,89] High levels of intracellular NO have been reported to cause DNA damage and mutations in human cell preparations.[90]

High inhaled concentrations of NO have been reported to cause acute pulmonary injury, methemoglobinemia, decreased platelet adhesion, asphyxia and death.[82,91,92] Greenbaum *et al.* exposed anesthetized dogs to 5000–20 000 ppm NO. Death ensued secondary to methemoglobinemia, acidemia and alveolar edema.[93]

Subsequent controlled studies demonstrated that much of the direct pulmonary toxicity in inhaled NO is due to the NO_2 contained in the gas mixtures. In studies which meticulously controlled for the presence of NO_2 during NO exposure, rats breathing 1000 ppm NO for 30 min or 1500 ppm for 15 min showed no changes of lung wet weight or histologic structure.[82] Histologic evidence of lung injury, however, was found when the animals were exposed to 25 ppm NO_2 for 30 min and lung wet weight was increased after 30 min exposures to 50 ppm NO_2 as well as after 5–15-min exposures to 100 ppm NO_2.[82] In studies of low-level NO exposure, rabbits breathing 43 ppm NO and 3.6 ppm NO_2 for six days showed no pulmonary pathologic changes by light or electron microscopy or gravimetric techniques.[94]

Methemoglobinemia may occur if its production is increased or its reduction via the NADH-diaphorase (methemogloblin reductase) system is diminished.[95] Clinically significant methemoglobinemia has not been reported following low-level NO exposure. For example, mice exposed to 10 ppm NO for six months had a methemoglobin concentration up to 0.3%, identical to unexposed animals.[96] Also, von Nieding and coworkers found that methemoglobin levels did not rise above 0.7% in 48 normal volunteers breathing 40 ppm NO for up to 15 min.[97] Furthermore, Frostell and coworkers recently reported that breathing 80 ppm NO for three hours did not increase blood methemoglobin levels in awake spontaneously ventilating lambs.[5] It is possible, however, that certain patients with decreased NADH-diaphorase activity may develop methemoglobinemia in the face of an increased rate of hemoglobin oxidation. The activity of NADH-diaphorase may be decreased as a result of a hereditary deficiency and is normally low in newborn infants.[95]

Damage to erythrocyte membranes may occur following long-term low-level exposure to NO. Oda and coworkers reported enlarged spleens and increased bilirubin levels, suggestive of increased erythrocyte turnover, in mice following six months of exposure to 10 ppm NO.[96] Nitric oxide also inhibits platelet adhesion to endothelial cells and reverses platelet aggregation *in vitro*.[98] Prolongation of the bleeding time during experimental NO inhalation has been reported[99] but the clinical significance of this effect is uncertain.

Technical considerations for NO inhalation

Inhalation circuits designed to deliver NO must ensure the accurate continuous delivery of NO while minimizing levels of NO_2. Sudden discontinuation of inhaled NO may produce severe arterial desaturation and pulmonary hypertension in some patients.[53,63] Breathing circuits capable of delivering inhaled NO should therefore be available to allow manual ventilation of the patient during tracheal suctioning, transport, etc. Concentrations within a breathing circuit will vary with the NO and oxygen concentrations used and the residence time of NO within the lungs and breathing circuit.[100] Because conversion of NO to NO_2 is offset by minimizing the residence time of NO in the inhaled gas mixture, mixing of a stock gas of NO in nitrogen with the carrier gases (usually oxygen and air) should take place immediately before inhalation. Several studies have used large gas collection bags to store and deliver NO mixed with oxygen-containing gases. Such $NO–O_2$ mixtures produce steadily increasing levels of NO_2 with concomitantly decreasing levels of NO.[101] This method of administration is unsuitable for clinical application because it does not allow prolonged breathing of constant levels of NO with minimal levels of NO_2. Soda lime may be useful in removing NO_2 from the breathing circuit.[102] but will not eliminate the production of higher oxides of nitrogens within the lung. Continuous or intermittent monitoring of NO and NO_2 gas concentrations can be performed with commercially available chemiluminescence[103] or electrochemical analyzers.[104]

At present, NO inhalation therapy remains experimental. Several important areas remain to be studied: for how long and at what levels is it safe for the normal or acutely injured lung to breathe NO? What is the effect of inhaled NO on pulmonary structure and function? What are the best methods to deliver NO to the critically ill patient? Will NO inhalation therapy measurably change outcome in patients with pulmonary hypertension? The study of NO biology has already provided us with many new insights into pulmonary vascular function and control. Potentially, the use of inhaled NO is just one of several therapies based upon these studies which may benefit patients with lung disease.

References

1. Radermacher, P., Santak, B. and Falke, K. J. (1989) Comparison of prostaglandin E_1 and nitroglycerin in patients with ARDS. *Prog. Clin. Biol. Res.*, **301**, 267–70.
2. Radermacher, P., Santak, B., Wust, H. J. *et al.* (1990) Prostacyclin for the treatment of pulmonary hypertension in the adult respiratory distress syndrome: effects on pulmonary capillary pressure and ventilation–perfusion distributions. *Anesthesiology*, **72**, 238–44.
3. Radermacher, P., Santak, B., Wust, H. J. *et al.* (1990) Prostacyclin and right ventricular function in patients with pulmonary hypertension associated with ARDS. *Intensive Care Med.*, **16**, 227–32.
4. Pepke-Zaba, J., Higenbottam, T. W., Dinh-Xuan, A. T. *et al.* (1991) Inhaled nitric oxide as a cause of selective pulmonary vasodilation in pulmonary hypertension. *Lancet*, **338**, 1173–4.
5. Frostell, C., Fratacci, M-D., Wain, J. C. *et al.* (1991) Inhaled nitric oxide: a selective pulmonary vasodilator reversing hypoxic pulmonary vasoconstriction. *Circulation*, **83**, 2038–47.
6. Fratacci, M. D., Frostell, C., Chen, T-Y. *et al.* (1991) Inhaled nitric oxide: a selective pulmonary vasodilator of heparin–protamine vasoconstriction in sheep. *Anesthesiology*, **75**, 990–9.
7. Pison, U., Lopez, F. A., Heidelmeyer, C. F. *et al.* (1993) Inhaled nitric oxide reverses hypoxic pulmonary vasoconstriction without impairing gas exchange. *J. Appl. Physiol.*, **74**, 1287–92.
8. Rossaint, R., Falke, K. F., Lopez, F. *et al.* (1993) Inhaled nitric oxide for the adult respiratory distress syndrome. *N. Engl. J. Med.*, **328**, 399–405.
9. Ignarro, L. J., Buga, G. M., Wood, K. S. *et al.* (1987) Endothelium-derived relaxing factor produced and released from artery and vein is nitric oxide. *Proc. Natl Acad. Sci. USA*, **84**, 9265–9.
10. Palmer, R. M. J., Ferrige, A. G. and Moncada, S. (1987) Nitric oxide release accounts for the biological activity of endothelium-derived relaxation factor. *Nature*, **327**, 524–6.
11. Ignarro, L. J., Buga, G. M., Byrns, R. E. *et al.* (1988) Endothelium-derived relaxing factor and nitric oxide possess identical pharmacologic properties as relaxants of bovine arterial and venous smooth muscle. *J. Pharmacol. Exptl Ther.*, **246**, 218–26.

12. Archer, S. L., Rist, K., Nelson, D. P. *et al.* (1990) Comparison of the hemodynamic effects of nitric oxide and endothelium-dependent vasodilators in intact lungs. *J. Appl. Physiol,* **68**, 735–47.

13. Ignarro, L. J. (1991) Signal transduction mechanisms involving nitric oxide. *Biochem. Pharmacol.,* **41**, 485–90.

14. Palmer, R. M. J., Ashton, D. S. and Moncada, S. (1988) Vascular endothelial cells synthesize nitric oxide from L-arginine. *Nature,* **333**, 664–6.

15. Moncada, S., Palmer, R. M. J. and Higgs, E. A. (1989) Biosynthesis of nitric oxide for L-arginine. A pathway for the regulation of cell function and communication. *Biochem. Pharmacol.,* **38**, 1709–15.

16. Furchgott, R. F. and Vanhoutte, P. M. (1989) Endothelium-derived relaxing and contracting factors. *FASEB J.,* **3**, 2007–18.

17. Ignarro, L. J. (1989) Biological actions and properties of endothelium-derived nitric oxide formed and released from artery and vein. *Circ. Res.,* **65**, 1–21.

18. Doyle, M. L. and Hoekstra, J. W. (1981) Oxidation of nitrogen oxides by bound dyoxygen in hemoproteins. *J. Inorg. Biochem.,* **14**, 351–8.

19. Gruetter, C. A., Gruetter, D. Y., Lyon, J. E. *et al.*, (1981) Relationship between cyclic guanosine 3':5'-monophosphate formation and relaxation of coronary artery arterial smooth muscle by glyceryl trinitrate, nitroprusside, nitrite and nitric oxide. *J. Pharmacol. Exptl Ther.,* **219**, 181–6.

20. Ignarro, L. J. (1989) Endothelium-derived nitric oxide: actions and properties. *FASEB J.,* **3**, 31–6.

21. Snyder, S. H. and Bredt, D. S. (1992) Biologic roles of nitric oxide. *Sci. Am.,* **266**, 68–77.

22. Pollock, J. S., Forstermann, U., Mitchell, J. A. *et al.* (1991) Purification and characterization of particulate endothelium-derived relaxing factor synthase from cultured and native bovine aortic endothelial cells. *Proc. Natl Acad. Sci. USA,* **88**, 10480–4.

23. Janssens, S. P., Shimouchi, A., Quertermous, T. *et al.* (1992) Cloning and expression of a cDNA encoding human endothelium-derived relaxing factor/nitric oxide synthase. *J. Biol. Chem.,* **267**, 14519–22.

24. Bredt, D. S., Hwang, P. M., Glatt, C. E. *et al.* (1991) Cloned and expressed nitric oxide synthase structurally resembles cytochrome P-450 reductase. *Nature,* **351**, 714–18.

25. Xie, Q-W., Cho, H. J., Calaycay, J. *et al.* (1992) Cloning and characterization of inducible nitric oxide synthase from mouse macrophages. *Science,* **256**, 225–8.

26. Knowles, R. G., Salter, M., Brooks, S. L. *et al.* (1990) Anti-inflammatory glucocorticoids inhibit the induction by endotoxin of nitric oxide synthase in the lung, liver and aorta of the rat. *Biochem. Biophys. Res. Commun.,* **172**, 1042–8.

27. Rees, D. D., Palmer, R. M. J., Schulz, R. *et al.* (1990) Characterization of three inhibitors of endothelium nitric oxide synthase *in vitro* and *in vivo*. *Br. J. Pharmacol.,* **101**, 746–52.

28. Ignarro, L. J. and Kadowitz, P. J. (1985) The pharmacological and physiological role of cyclic GMP in vascular smooth muscle relaxation. *Annu. Rev. Pharmacol. Toxicol.,* **25**, 171–91.

29. Martin, W., Furchgott, R. F., Villani, G. M. *et al.* (1986) Phosphodiesterase inhibitors induce endothelium-dependent relaxation of rat and rabbit aorta by potentiating the effects of spontaneously released endothelium-derived relaxing factor. *J. Pharmacol. Exptl Ther.,* **237**, 539–47.

30. Chand, N. and Altura, B. M. (1981) Acetylcholine and bradykinin relax intrapulmonary arteries by acting on endothelial cells: role in lung vascular disease. *Science,* **213**, 1376–9.

31. Dinh Xuan, A. T., Higenbottam, T. W., Clelland, C. *et al.* (1990) Acetylcholine and adenosine disphosphate cause endothelium-dependent relaxation of isolated human pulmonary arteries. *Eur. Resp. J.,* **3**, 633–8.

32. Gustafsson, L. E., Leone, A. M., Persson, M. G. *et al.* (1991) Endogenous nitric oxide is present in the exhaled air of rabbits, guinea pigs and humans. *Biochem. Biophys. Res. Commun.,* **181**, 852–7.

33. Gerlach, H., Rossaint, R. and Pappert, D. (1994) Autoinhalation of nitric oxide after endogenous synthesis in nasopharynx. *Lancet*, **343**, 518–19.
34. Fritts, A. W., Harris, P., Clauss, H. *et al.* (1958) The effect of acetylcholine on the human pulmonary circulation under normal and hypoxic conditions. *J. Clin. Invest.*, **37**, 99–108.
35. Frostell, C. G., Blomqvist, H., Hedenstierna, G. *et al.* (1993) Inhaled nitric oxide selectively reverses human hypoxic pulmonary vasoconstriction without causing systemic vasodilation. *Anesthesiology*, **78**, 427–35.
36. Högman, M., Frostell, C., Amberg, H. *et al.* (1993) Inhalation of nitric oxide modulates methacholine-induced bronchoconstriction in the rabbit. *Eur. Resp. J.*, **6**, 177–80.
37. Cremona, G., Dinh Xuan, A. T. and Higenbottam, T. W. (1991) Endothelium-derived relaxing factor and the pulmonary circulation. *Lung*, **169**, 185–202.
38. Dinh Xuan, A. T., Higenbottam, T. W., Clelland, C. *et al.* (1991) Impairment of endothelium-dependent pulmonary artery relaxation in chronic obstructive lung disease. *N. Engl. J. Med.*, **324**, 1539–47.
39. Dinh Xuan, A. T., Higenbottam, T. W., Clelland, C. *et al.* (1990) Impairment of pulmonary endothelium-dependent relaxation in patients with Eisenmenger's syndrome. *Br. J. Pharmacol.*, **99**, 9–10.
40. Adatia, I., Thompson, J., Landzberg, M. and Wessel, D. L. (1993) Inhaled nitric oxide in chronic obstructive lung disease. *Lancet*, **341**, 307–8.
41. Zapol, W. M. and Snider, M. T. (1977) Pulmonary hypertension in severe acute respiratory failure. *N. Engl. J. Med.*, **296**, 476–80.
42. Zapol, W. M. and Jones, R. (1987) Vascular components of ARDS: clinical pulmonary hemodynamics and morphology. *Am. Rev. Respir. Dis.*, **136**, 471–4.
43. Zapol, W. M. (1985) Pulmonary circulation during adult respiratory distress syndrome. In: Zapol, W. M. and Falke, K. J. (eds) *Acute Respiratory Failure*, pp. 241–70. New York: Marcel Dekker.
44. Kinsella, J. P., Neish, S. R., Shaffer, E. *et al.* (1992) Low-dose inhalational nitric oxide in persistent pulmonary hypertension of the newborn. *Lancet*, **340**, 819–20.
45. Kinsella, J. P., McQueston, J. A., Rosenberg, A. A. and Abman, S. H. (1992) Hemodynamic effects of exogenous nitric oxide in ovine transitional pulmonary circulation. *Am. J. Physiol.*, **263**, H875–H880.
46. Roberts, J. D., Jr., Polaner, D. M., Lang, P. *et al.* (1992) Inhaled nitric oxide in persistent pulmonary hypertension of the newborn. *Lancet*, **340**, 818–19.
47. Kinsella, J. P. and Abman, S. H. (1993) Inhalational nitric oxide therapy for persistent pulmonary hypertension of the newborn. *Pediatrics*, **91**, 997–8.
48. Zayek, M., Cleveland, D., Morin, F. C. III *et al.* (1993) Treatment of persistent pulmonary hypertension in the newborn lamb by inhaled nitric oxide. *J. Pediatr.*, **122**, 743–50.
49. Tönz, M., von-Segesser, L. K. and Turina, M. (1993) Selective pulmonary vasodilation with inhaled nitric oxide. *J. Thorac. Cardiovasc. Surg.*, **105**, 760–2.
50. Berger, J. I., Gibson, R. L., Redding, G. J. *et al.* (1993) Effect of inhaled nitric oxide during Group B Streptococcal sepsis in piglets. *Am. Rev. Respir. Dis.*, **147**, 1080–6.
51. Weitzberg, E., Rudehill, A. and Lundberg, J. M. (1993) Nitric oxide inhalation attenuates pulmonary hypertension and improves gas exchange in endotoxin shock. *Eur. J. Pharmacol.*, **233**, 85–94.
52. Rovira, I., Chen, T-Y., Winkler, M. *et al.* (1994) Effects of inhaled nitric oxide on pulmonary hemodynamics and gas exchange in an ovine model of ARDS. *J. Appl. Physiol.*, **76**, 345–55.
53. Bigatello, L. M., Hurford, W. E., Kacmarek, R. M. *et al.* (1994) Prolonged inhalation of low concentrations of nitric oxide in patients with severe adult respiratory distress syndrome. *Anesthesiology*, **80**, 761–70.
54. Payen, D., Gatecel, C. and Guinard, N. (1993) Inhalation of low dose of nitric oxide (NO) and i.v. L-arg in ARDS: effect on pulmonary hemodynamic, gas exchange and NO metabolites. *Am. Rev. Respir. Dis.*, **147**, A720.

55. Grover, R., Smithies, M. and Bihari, D. (1993) A dose profile of the physiological effects of inhaled nitric oxide in acute lung injury. *Am. Rev. Respir. Dis.*, **147**, A350.
56. Wysocki, M., Vignon, P., Roupie, E. *et al.* (1993) Improvement in right ventricular function with inhaled nitric oxide in patients with the adult respiratory distress syndrome (ARDS) and permissive hypercapnia. *Am. Rev. Respir. Dis.*, **147**, A350.
57. Zapol, W. M., Falke, K. J. and Rossaint, R. (1993) Inhaled nitric oxide for the adult respiratory distress syndrome. *N. Engl. J. Med.*, **329**, 207.
58. Gerlach, H., Pappert, D., Lewandowski, K. *et al.* (1993) Long-term inhalation with evaluated low doses of nitric oxide for selective improvement of oxygenation in patients with adult respiratory distress syndrome. *Intensive Care Med.*, **19**, 443–9.
59. Ricou, B. and Suter, P. M. (1993) Variable effects of nitric oxide (NO) in ARDS patients. *Am. Rev. Respir. Dis.*, **147**, A350.
60. Rich, G. F., Murphy, G. D., Roos, C. M. and Johns, R. A. (1993) Inhaled nitric oxide: selective pulmonary vasodilation in cardiac surgical patients. *Anesthesiology*, **78**, 1028–35.
61. Payen, D. M., Gatecel, C. and Plaisance, P. (1993) Almitrine effect on nitric oxide inhalation in adult respiratory distress syndrome. *Lancet*, **341**, 1664.
62. Dupuy, P. M., Shore, S. A., Drazen, J. M. *et al.* (1992) Bronchodilator action of inhaled nitric oxide in guinea pigs. *J. Clin. Invest.*, **90**, 421–8.
63. Grover, R., Murdoch, I., Smithies, M. *et al.* (1992) Nitric oxide during hand ventilation in patient with acute respiratory failure. *Lancet*, **340**, 1038–9.
64. Rengasamy, A. and Johns, R. A. (1993) Regulation of nitric oxide synthase by nitric oxide. *Mol. Pharmacol.*, **44**, 124–8.
65. Roberts, J. D., Jr., Chen, T. Y. and Kawai, N. (1993) Inhaled nitric oxide reverses pulmonary vasoconstriction in the hypoxic and acidotic newborn lamb. *Circ. Res.*, **72**, 246–54.
66. Zayek, M., Wild, L., Roberts, J. D. and Morin, F. C. III (1993) Effect of nitric oxide on the survival rate and incidence of lung injury in newborn lambs with persistent pulmonary hypertension. *J. Pediatr.*, **123**, 947–52.
67. DeMarco, V., Skimming, J., Ellis, T. M. and Cassin, S. (1994) Nitric oxide inhalation: effects on the ovine neonatal pulmonary and systemic circulations. *Chest*, **105**, 91S–92S.
68. Kinsella, J. P. and Abman, S. H. (1994) Efficacy of inhalational nitric oxide therapy in the clinical management of persistent pulmonary hypertension of the newborn. *Chest*, **105**, 92S–94S.
69. Abman, S. H., Kinsella, J. P., Schaffer, M. S. and Wilkening, R. B. (1993) Inhaled nitric oxide in the management of a premature newborn with severe respiratory distress and pulmonary hypertension. *Pediatrics*, **92**, 606–9.
70. Girard, C., Lehot, J. J., Pannetier, J. C. *et al.* (1992) Inhaled nitric oxide after mitral valve replacement in patients with chronic pulmonary artery hypertension. *Anesthesiology*, **77**, 880–3.
71. Adnot, S., Kouyoumdjian, C., Defouilloy, C. *et al.* (1993) Hemodynamic and gas exchange responses to infusion of acetylcholine and inhalation of nitric oxide in patients with chronic obstructive lung disease and pulmonary hypertension. *Am. Rev. Respir. Dis.*, **148**, 310–16.
72. Kinsella, J. P., Toews, W. H., Henry, D. *et al.* (1993) Selective and sustained pulmonary vasodilation with inhalational nitric oxide therapy in a child with idiopathic pulmonary hypertension. *J. Pediatr.*, **122**, 803–6.
73. Roberts, J. D., Jr., Lang, P., Bigatello, L. M. *et al.* (1993) Inhaled nitric oxide in congenital heart disease. *Circulation*, **87**, 447–53.
74. Haydar, A., Malhere, T., Mauriat, P. *et al.* (1992) Inhaled nitric oxide for postoperative pulmonary hypertension in patients with congenital heart defects. *Lancet*, **340**, 1545.
75. Sellden, H., Winberg, P., Gustafsson, L. E. *et al.* (1993) Inhalation of nitric oxide reduced pulmonary hypertension after cardiac surgery in a 3.2-kg infant. *Anesthesiology*, **78**, 577–80.
76. Miller, O. I., James, J. and Elliott, M. J. (1993) Intraoperative use of inhaled low-dose nitric oxide. *J. Thorac. Cardiovasc. Surg.*, **105**, 550–1.

77. Berner, M., Beghetti, M., Ricou, B. *et al.* (1993) Relief of severe pulmonary hypertension after closure of a large ventricular septal defect using low dose inhaled nitric oxide. *Intensive Care Med.*, **19**, 75–7.
78. Levine, J. S. (1989) Photochemistry of biogenic gases. In: Rambler, M. B., Margulis, L. and Fester, R. (eds) *Global Ecology*, pp. 51–74. New York: Academic Press.
79. Norman, V. and Keith, C. (1965) Nitrogen oxides in tobacco smoke. *Nature*, **205**, 915–16.
80. NIOSH Recommendations for Occupational Safety and Health Standards (1988) *MMWR Morb. Mortal. Wkly Rep.*, **37**(Supp. S–7), 21.
81. Glasson, W. A. and Tuesday, C. S. (1963) The atmospheric thermal oxidation of nitric oxide. *J. Am. Chem. Soc.*, **85**, 2901–4.
82. Stavert, D. M. and Lehnert, B. E. (1990) Nitric oxide and nitrogen dioxide as inducers of acute pulmonary injury when inhaled at relatively high concentrations for brief periods. *Inhal. Toxicol.*, **2**, 53–67.
83. Beckman, J. S., Beckman, T. W., Chen, J. *et al.* (1990) Apparent hydroxyl radical production by peroxynitrite: implications for endothelial injury from nitric oxide and superoxide. *Proc. Natl Acad. Sci. USA*, **87**, 1620–4.
84. Hibbs, J. B., Taintor, R. R., Vavrin, Z. and Rachlin, E. M. (1988) Nitric oxide: a cytotoxic activated macrophage effector molecule. *Biochem. Biophys. Res. Commun.*, **157**, 87–94.
85. Stuehr, D. J. and Nathan, C. F. (1989) Nitric oxide: a macrophage product responsible for cytostasis and respiratory inhibition in tumor target cells. *J. Exptl Med.*, **169**, 1543–55.
86. Borland, C. D. R., Harmes, K., Cracknell, N. *et al.* (1985) Methaemoglobin levels in smokers and non-smokers. *Arch. Environ. Health*, **40**, 330–3.
87. Stamler, J. S., Jaraki, O., Osborne, J. *et al.* (1992) Nitric oxide circulates in mammalian plasma primarily as an S-nitroso adduct of serum albumin. *Proc. Natl Acad. Sci. USA*, **89**, 7674–7.
88. Payen, D. (1993) Inhaled NO in severe ARDS. In: *International Conference on Recent Advances in the Treatment of the Adult Respiratory Distress Syndrome*. Tutzing, Germany, July 5–8.
89. Stamler, J. S., Singel, D. J. and Loscalzo, J. (1993) Biochemistry of nitric oxide and its redox-activated forms. *Science*, **258**, 1898–1902.
90. Nguyen, T., Brunson, D., Crespi, C. L. *et al.* (1992) DNA damage and mutation in human cells exposed to nitric oxide *in vitro*. *Proc. Natl Acad. Sci. USA*, **89**, 3030–4.
91. Clutton-Brock, J. (1967) Two cases of poisoning by contamination of nitrous oxide with higher oxides of nitrogen during anaesthesia. *Br. J. Anaesth.*, **39**, 388–92.
92. Austin, A. T. (1967) The chemistry of higher oxides of nitrogen as related to the manufacture, storage and administration of nitrous oxide. *Br. J. Anaesth.*, **39**, 345–50.
93. Greenbaum, R., Bay, J., Hargreaves, M. D. *et al.* (1967) Effects of higher oxides of nitrogen on the anesthestized dog. *Br. J. Anaesth.*, **39**, 393–404.
94. Hugod, C. (1979) Effect of exposure to 43 ppm nitric oxide and 3.6 ppm nitrogen dioxide on rabbit lung. *Int. Arch. Occup. Environ. Health*, **42**, 159–67.
95. Beutler, E. (1977) Methemoglobinemia and sulfhemoglobinemia. In: Williams, W. J., Beutler, E., Erslev, A. J. and Rundles, R. W. (eds) *Hematology*, 2nd edn, pp. 491–4. New York: McGraw-Hill.
96. Oda, H., Nogami, H., Kusumoto, S. *et al.* (1976) Long-term exposure to nitric oxide in mice. *J. Jpn. Soc. Air Pollut.*, **11**, 150–60.
97. von Nieding, G., Wagner, H., and Kockeler, H. (1975) Investigation of the acute effects of nitrogen monoxide on lung function in man. *Staub-Reinhalt Luft*, **35**, 175–8.
98. Radomski, M. W., Palmer, R. M. J. and Moncada, S. (1987) Endogenous nitric oxide inhibits human platelet adhesion to vascular endothelium. *Lancet*, **ii**, 1057–8.
99. Högman, M., Frostell, C., Amberg, H. and Hedenstierna, G. (1993) Bleeding time prolongation and NO inhalation. *Lancet*, **341**, 1664–5.
100. Foubert, L., Fleming, B., Latimer, R. *et al.* (1992) Safety guidelines for use of nitric oxide. *Lancet*, **339**, 1615–16.
101. Bouchet, M., Renaudin, M. H., Raveau, C. *et al.* (1993) Safety requirement for use of inhaled nitric oxide in neonates. *Lancet*, **341** 968–9.

102. Oda, H., Kusumoto, S. and Nakajima, T. (1975) Nitrosyl-hemoglobin formation in the blood of animals exposed to nitric oxide. *Arch. Environ. Health*, **30**, 453–6.
103. Fontijin, A., Sabadell, A. J. and Ronco, R. J. (1970) Homogeneous chemiluminescent measurement of nitric oxide and ozone. *Anal. Chem.*, **42**, 575–9.
104. Petros, A. J., Cox, P. B. and Bohn, D. (1992) Simple method for monitoring concentration of inhaled nitric oxide. *Lancet*, **340**, 1167.

13

Secondary Molecular Alterations in Failing Human Myocardium

Wilson S. Colucci

Cardiac failure occurs when global myocardial function is not sufficient to meet the metabolic needs of the body. There are numerous causes of myocardial dysfunction, but in the United States the large majority of cases are the result of coronary artery disease, and to a lesser extent, so-called 'idiopathic' dilated cardiomyopathy. A growing body of data, based on observations in failing human myocardium obtained at the time of cardiac transplantation, indicates that myocardial failure is associated with numerous molecular and cellular alterations (Table 13.1). In contrast to genetic forms of myocardial disease (e.g. familial hypertrophic cardiomyopathy) in which a genetic abnormality is the primary cause of myocardial dysfunction, in most patients myocardial failure occurs because normal myocardium is subjected to abnormal environmental stresses. These stresses result in secondary molecular and cellular alterations which can have deleterious effects on the structure and function of the previously normal myocardium.

Myocardial failure may develop in the hours and days immediately following a large myocardial infarction. However, in the majority of cases, myocardial failure develops over a period of months or years. Although the patient is often asymptomatic during this interval, the noninfarcted myocardium is undergoing major

Table 13.1 Molecular alterations observed in failing human myocardium

β_1-Adrenergic receptors (number/mRNA)	↓/↓
β_2-Adrenergic receptors (number/mRNA)	↔/↔
β-Adrenergic receptor kinase (activity/mRNA)	↑/↑
G_i (activity/mRNA)	↑/↔
G_s (activity/mRNA)	↔/↔
Sarcoplasmic reticulum Ca^{2+}-ATPase (activity/mRNA)	↓/↓
Phospholamban (mRNA)	↓
Voltage-dependent calcium channel (number/mRNA)	↓/↓
Calcium release channel (mRNA, idiopathic/ischemic)	↔/↓
Calsequestrin (mRNA)	↔
Atrial natriuretic peptide (mRNA)	↑
Brain natriuretic peptide (mRNA)	↑
β-Myosin heavy chain (mRNA)	↔
Troponin-T_2 (protein)	↑

structural and functional changes, which collectively are referred to as 'remodeling'. Remodeling also occurs in myocardium that is chronically exposed to abnormal hemodynamic stresses as may result from regurgitant valvular lesions, hypertension, or any process that impairs myocyte function (e.g. myocarditis or idiopathic cardiomyopathy) and thereby increases the work of unaffected myocytes. Thus, remodeling is a generalized secondary response of the myocardium to a variety of environmental stresses and stimuli. Morphologically, remodeling involves changes in chamber size, wall thickness, the ratio of wall thickness to chamber size, myocyte size and shape, and both the quantity and quality of the extracellular matrix. At the molecular level, these morphologic changes are associated with alterations in excitation–contraction coupling, contractile and regulatory proteins, growth factors and signaling pathways. Collectively, these secondary molecular alterations can lead to progressive abnormalities of systolic and diastolic function.

Ventricular remodeling

Ventricular remodeling refers to the changes in cardiac structure that occur in response to any of a number of extrinsic stimuli. Although remodeling of the heart can be a useful adaptation, in many cases, the form and/or extent of remodeling are either maladaptive or insufficient. The most common stimulus for myocardial hypertrophy and remodeling is hemodynamic overload.

Based on Laplace's law myocardial wall stress can be approximated by the relationship, $Pr/2h$, where P is left ventricular intra-cavitary pressure, h is left ventricular wall thickness, and r is the chamber radius. An increase in systolic wall stress is most often the result of an increase in left-ventricular systolic pressure, as may occur in patients with hypertension or aortic stenosis, but may also occur with a normal or reduced systolic pressure if systolic chamber volume is increased. Diastolic wall stress is generally increased as the result of chamber dilation and/or an increase in diastolic filling pressure.

An important cause of ventricular remodeling is myocardial infarction.[1] Diastolic wall stress can be markedly increased after an infarction as a result of increases in ventricular volume (due to expansion of the infarcted tissue) and filling pressures (due to reduced global contractile function). If sufficient compensatory hypertrophy occurs, the increase in ventricular wall thickness may normalize systolic and diastolic wall stresses. However, if additional chamber dilation occurs and/or the increase in wall thickness is insufficient, systolic and/or diastolic wall stresses remain abnormally elevated, and there may be further chamber dilation, eventually leading to hemodynamic failure.

At the gross morphologic level, the characteristics of the response to hemodynamic overload depend on the nature of the stimulus.[2] With pure systolic pressure overload, the increase in systolic wall stress results in the parallel addition of sarcomeres and widening of cardiac myocytes. At the gross morphologic level, there is concentric hypertrophy. Alternatively, if the hemodynamic stimulus consists primarily of an increase in ventricular diastolic volume (e.g. with mitral regurgitation prior to an increase in end-systolic volume), there is series addition of

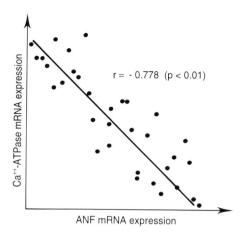

Figure 13.1 Relationship between the levels of mRNA for Ca^{2+}-ATPase and atrial natriuretic factor (ANF) in myocardium from right and left ventricles obtained from 17 patients with various forms of cardiomyopathy. There is a striking inverse relationship between the expression of mRNAs for Ca^{2+}-ATPase, an adult muscle-specific gene, and ANF, a fetal gene. These reciprocal changes in the expression of adult and fetal genes are typical of hypertrophied and failing myocardium. (Adapted from Arai *et al.*, 1993.[5])

sarcomeres and a lengthening of cardiac myocytes. At the gross morphologic level there is eccentric hypertrophy. Clinically, both systolic and diastolic wall stresses are commonly elevated in the same ventricle, and at the microscopic level there is generally both series and parallel addition of sarcomeres, which are otherwise organized in a normal pattern.

Although the sarcomeres in remodeled myocardium retain a normal gross morphologic appearance, the expression of several functionally important proteins is altered. A hallmark of the ventricular remodeling response to hemodynamic overload is the reinduction of fetal genes that are normally not expressed in adult myocardium, and a reciprocal decrease in the expression of several adult, muscle-specific genes.[3,4] For example, mRNA levels for atrial natriuretic peptide (ANP) and brain natriuretic peptide (BNP), which are normally expressed in fetal cardiac tissue but not normal adult ventricular tissue, are re-expressed in left-ventricular myocardium from patients with heart failure. Conversely, the amount of mRNA for cardiac sarcoplasmic reticulum Ca^{2+}-ATPase (SERCA2), a protein which is important for excitation–contraction coupling and normally expressed in abundance in normal adult myocardium, is reduced in ventricular myocardium from patients with heart failure. The reciprocal nature of these changes in adult and fetal gene expression is illustrated by the observation that in severely failing myocardium obtained at the time of cardiac transplantation, the decrease in SERCA2 mRNA level bears a striking inverse relationship to the increase in ANP mRNA level[5] (Figure 13.1).

In addition to myocytes, ventricular myocardium consists of several other cell types including fibroblasts, endothelial cells and vascular smooth-muscle cells. Not surprisingly, remodeling of the ventricle in response to hypertrophic stimuli involves adaptations in both the myocyte and nonmyocyte compartments of the heart.

Cardiac myocytes, which are terminally differentiated and therefore unable to divide, respond to hypertrophic stimuli by increasing in size (hypertrophy). In contrast, nonmyocytes in the myocardium, primarily fibroblasts, respond to hypertrophic stimuli by proliferating (hyperplasia) and elaborating increased amounts of interstitial matrix, an important consequence of which may be the development of interstitial fibrosis which contributes to abnormal myocardial function by decreasing diastolic compliance and impairing the supply of nutrients to myocytes.

Calcium regulation

The regulation of the intracellular concentration of calcium involves several sarcolemmal and sarcoplasmic reticulum proteins.[6] Membrane depolarization stimulates the influx of calcium by way of voltage-dependent calcium channels. The resulting influx of Ca^{2+} causes the sarcoplasmic reticulum to release of a large pool of Ca^{2+} which transiently increases the intracellular free Ca^{2+} concentration. Calcium ions bind to troponin-C, a component of a complex of regulatory proteins consisting of troponin-I, troponin-T and tropomyosin, and thereby promote the development of contractile force by favoring the interaction of actin and myosin filaments. Stimulation of β-adrenergic receptors coupled to adenylate cyclase increases the availability of cAMP, which increases influx of calcium via voltage-dependent calcium channels.

Calcium handling is deranged in the myocardium of patients with end-stage heart failure.[6,7] In single ventricular myocardial cells obtained from patients with dilated cardiomyopathy, the action potential is substantially prolonged (Figure 13.2A). Likewise, intracellular calcium transients, as assessed by the fura-2 technique in myocytes prepared in a similar manner from patients with dilated cardiomyopathy, fail to rise normally after stimulation and remain elevated for a prolonged time (Figure 13.2B). Such abnormalities in calcium transients probably contribute to both systolic and diastolic ventricular dysfunction.

Abnormal calcium handling in failing myocardium is associated with altered expression of several important calcium-handling proteins. The mRNA levels for voltage-dependent Ca^{2+} channels (VDCC), SERCA2 and phospholamban are depressed in myocardium obtained from patients with both idiopathic dilated and ischemic cardiomyopathy,[5,8,9] whereas the mRNA level for calsequestrin, a protein which binds calcium within the sarcoplasmic reticulum is normal. Another potential site for altered calcium handling is the calcium release channel (CRC), which mediates the release of calcium by the sarcoplasmic reticulum. Interestingly, in contrast to SERCA2 and VDCC mRNA expression, which appears to be depressed in both ischemic and primary cardiomyopathies, mRNA levels for the CRC are reduced in myocardium obtained from patients with ischemic, but not idiopathic cardiomyopathy.[10]

Although these observations are noteworthy, it should be appreciated that the relationship between the observed decreases in mRNA levels for various calcium-handling proteins and abnormal myocyte function has not been clearly demonstrated. Nevertheless, given the central role of SERCA2, VDCC and CRC in the

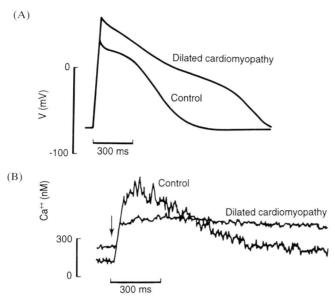

Figure 13.2 **A**. Action potential recorded in a single cardiac myocyte isolated from the ventricular myocardium of a patient with end-stage dilated cardiomyopathy. Compared to the action potential in a cell from a normal ventricle (control), the action potential in the myopathic cell is markedly prolonged. **B**. The intracellular calcium transient, as demonstrated using the fluorescent indicator fura 2, in a ventricular myocyte obtained as in (**A**) from a patient with dilated cardiomyopathy. Compared to a normal control cell, the signal in the myopathic cell is reduced in amplitude and markedly prolonged. These observations are consistent with reduced expression and/or abnormal function of one or more calcium-handling proteins including sarcoplasmic reticulum Ca^{2+}-ATPase, phospholamban, voltage-dependent calcium channels and the calcium-release channel. (Adapted from Beuckelmann *et al.*, 1992.[7])

regulation of excitation–contraction coupling, it seems likely that one or more of these molecular alterations contributes to the pathophysiology of myocardial failure.

Contractile apparatus

The contractile apparatus consists of the force generating proteins actin and myosin, and a complex of regulatory proteins consisting of tropomyosin, and troponin C, troponin I and troponin T.[11] The maximal ATPase activity that can be stimulated by calcium is significantly reduced in myofibrils obtained from hearts of patients with idiopathic cardiomyopathy, as compared to control subjects with normal ventricular function, suggesting that in addition to deranged calcium handling, there may be abnormalities in the function of the contractile apparatus in cardiomyopathy.

Myosin consists of three isoenzymes designated V_1, V_2 and V_3. The V_2 and V_3 isoforms are associated with reduced myofibrillar ATPase activity and a slower velocity of shortening, and in the rat it can be shown that in pressure overload hypertrophy the quantity of the V_2 and V_3 isoenzymes is increased. Conversely, in rats chronically trained by swimming, the V_2 and V_3 isoforms are decreased, and ATPase activity and the velocity of shortening are increased. Although observations such as these in rats have suggested that a shift in myosin isoforms may contribute to myocardial dysfunction in man, myosin in human myocardium consists predominantly of the slow V_3 isoform, and studies to date suggest that in humans the myosin isoform distribution is not affected by the development of hypertrophy or cardiomyopathy.[9]

Alterations in contractile apparatus regulatory proteins are another potential locus for abnormal contractile function. Troponin T is one such protein that regulates the interaction of actin and myosin. In myocardium from patients with normal ventricular function, there is a single predominant isoform, referred to as troponin T_1. A second isoform referred to as troponin T_2 (TnT_2) normally accounts for only about 2% of the total troponin T. In contrast, in myocardium obtained from patients with heart failure, there is increased expression of the TnT_2 isoform.[12] Although the functional significance of the shift in TnT isoforms is not known, this observation is important because it implicates changes in regulatory elements of the contractile apparatus as a potential site of functional abnormalities in the failing myocardium.

Autonomic effector pathways

A characteristic physiologic abnormality in patients with heart failure is a reduction in the inotropic and chronotropic responses to exercise and other types of sympathetic stimulation. The responsiveness of trabeculae from normal hearts and hearts with end-stage failure has been examined by determining the development of contractile tension in response to several agonists. Using this approach, it was shown that although the contractile response to calcium is preserved in failing myocardium, the contractile responses to the β-adrenergic agonists isoproterenol and dobutamine are significantly reduced, as is the response to enoximone, a phosphodiesterase inhibitor which is dependent on the availability of cAMP.[13] In contrast, forskolin, a substance which directly activates adenylate cyclase, thereby bypassing the β-adrenergic receptor, elicited a normal response in failing myocardium. These observations suggest that reduced adrenergic responsiveness of the myocardium in heart failure is relatively specific for the β-adrenergic receptor pathway.[13]

The expression of various autonomic receptors has been measured in tissue samples by the binding of isotopically-labeled ligands specific for each receptor.[13] In normal human myocardium, β_1- and β_2-adrenergic receptors are present in a ratio of approximately 4:1 (Figure 13.3). In myocardium obtained from patients with end-stage heart failure, there is a marked reduction in the number of β_1-adrenergic receptors (on the order of 50–70%), but not β_2-adrenergic receptors (Figure 13.3). In contrast, the numbers of muscarinic and α_1-adrenergic receptors are unchanged in failing human myocardium.

Regulation of β-adrenergic responsiveness involves molecular events at multiple loci.[14] Phosphorylation of the β-adrenergic receptor by protein kinase-A, β-adrenergic receptor kinase (βARK) or tyrosine kinase (TK) may result in rapid desensitization due to uncoupling of the receptor from G_s. Uncoupled receptors may be internalized in vesicles from which they may be degraded or recycled to the cell

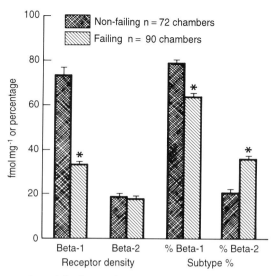

Figure 13.3 The expression of β-adrenergic receptors in normal and failing human ventricular myocardium. In normal myocardium (black bars), the β_1-adrenergic receptors outnumber the β_2-subtype by about 4:1. In failing hearts (hatched bars), there is an approximately 50% decrease in the density of β_1-receptors, but no change in the density of β_2-receptors, with an increase in the proportion of total receptors that are β_2. Muscarinic cholinergic and α_1-adrenergic receptor densities are not altered in failing myocardium. * = $P < 0.05$ vs. nonfailing (Adapted from Bristow, 1993.[13])

surface. The rate of receptor synthesis may also be regulated at the level of mRNA transcription and degradation. The functional responsiveness to β-adrenergic receptor stimulation thus depends on several regulatable factors including the level of receptor phosphorylation, the partitioning of receptors between surface and sequestered sites, and the balance between the rates of receptor synthesis and degradation.

In myocardium obtained from patients with end-stage heart failure, as compared to control tissue from patients without failure, the level of β-adrenergic kinase (βARK) mRNA is increased (Figure 13.4A) and the level of β_1-adrenergic receptor mRNA is reduced (Figure 13.4B), whereas the level of mRNA for β_2-adrenergic receptors is unchanged (Figure 13.4C).[15] These observations provide the molecular basis for the observation that the number of β_1-adrenergic receptors, but not β_2-adrenergic receptors, is reduced in failing myocardium. The increased expression of βARK may also explain the observation that the responsiveness to both β_1- and β_2-adrenergic agonists can be depressed out of proportion to the decrease in receptor number.

Growth signaling signals

Several signaling pathways have the potential to regulate the growth and phenotype of cardiac cells. *In vitro*, it can be shown that several hormones and/or neurotransmitters, including the α-adrenergic agonist norepinephrine, angiotensin and endothelin, can induce hypertrophy and fetal gene expression in cardiac myocytes. The receptors for these substances couple to phospholipase-C (PL-C) and calcium influx

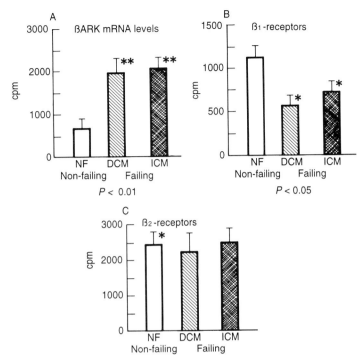

Figure 13.4 Levels of mRNA for β-adrenergic receptor kinase or βARK (A), β_1-adrenergic receptors (B) and β_2-adrenergic receptors (C) in ventricular myocardium from nonfailing control hearts (NF, open bars), and hearts of patients with end-stage dilated cardiomyopathy (DCM, hatched bars) and ischemic cardiomyopathy (ICM, solid bar). (Adapted from Ungerer et al., 1993.[15])

channels by way of G proteins. Activation of PL-C results in the generation of two second messengers, inositol trisphosphate (IP$_3$) and diacylglycerol (DAG). IP$_3$ causes the release of calcium from intracellular stores, and DAG activates protein kinase-C (PK-C). Both calcium and PK-C have important effects on the regulation of gene expression. Peptide growth factors (e.g. transforming growth factor-β, fibroblast growth factor, etc.) can be elaborated by various cells within the heart and may act in an autocrine or paracrine manner.[16] These growth factors activate cellular receptors which generally possess tyrosine kinase activity and are coupled to a cascade of protein kinases leading to the activation of mitogen-activated protein kinase (MAPK), an important convergence point for several growth-related signaling pathways. Mechanical deformation of cardiac myocytes (and other cell types) can activate and/or modulate several cellular signaling pathways involving the regulation of ion channels (e.g. calcium, sodium), cell volume, pH, adenylate cyclase and PL-C, PK-C and MAPK.[17,18] Although the relative roles of mechanical forces, hormones and various other growth factors in causing myocardial remodeling remains to be learned, it is likely that multiple factors are involved and vary in importance depending on the nature of the pathologic stimulus (e.g. aortic stenosis vs myocardial infarction).

Mechanical stresses

Abnormal mechanical stresses on cardiac myocytes appear to be a fundamental stimulus for myocardial remodeling. Relatively little is known about how mechanical stresses are coupled to signaling pathways. In cardiac myocytes cultured from neonatal rat hearts and grown on a deformable silastic membrane it is possible to study the effect of a linear stretch on secondary events. Cells that are stretched to increase their length by 20% for 48 hours show an approximately 30% increase in cellular protein content indicative of hypertrophy.[18] Under these conditions, there is activation of a large number of second-messenger pathways including calcium influx, inositol phosphate generation and activation of PK-C and MAPK, and the induction of a variety of early response genes (e.g. c-*fos*) and fetal genes (e.g. prepro-ANF). Since no other cell types or extrinsic growth factors are present in these *in vitro* experiments, these findings suggest that mechanical deformation of the myocyte, *per se*, can be an important determinant of myocyte growth and phenotype.

Catecholamines

Innervation is another extrinsic factor that has been implicated in the regulation of cell growth and differentiation. For example, norepinephrine, the primary sympathetic neurotransmitter, can be shown to stimulate the growth of cardiac myocytes.[19,20] Exposure of neonatal rat cardiac myocytes in culture dishes to norepinephrine (NE) for 24 hours causes cellular hypertrophy, as indicated by an increase in cell size and protein content, associated with the induction of several early response and fetal genes. These effects are inhibited by an α_1-selective antagonist, but not a β-adrenergic antagonist, indicating that the hypertrophic effect of norepinephrine is mediated by an α_1-adrenergic receptor located on the cardiac myocyte.

Neonatal cardiac myocytes express at least three subtypes of α_1-adrenergic receptors. Interestingly, the growth effect of NE is mediated predominantly by one subtype which can be selectively inhibited by a variety of pharmacologic agents including niguldipine and 5-methylurapidil.[21] This observation suggests that the coupling of α_1-adrenergic receptor subtypes is heterogeneous with regard to growth signaling pathways, and thus may offer a potential site for pharmacologic and/or molecular intervention.

An increase in the activity of the sympathetic nervous system is a common secondary response to cardiac failure.[22] Under normal conditions, inhibitory afferent input from arterial and cardiopulmonary baroreceptors reduces sympathetic tone so that the predominant autonomic activity is parasympathetic. Inhibitory afferent activity from arterial and cardiopulmonary baroreceptors is reduced and excitatory input increased in patients with heart failure, resulting in a net withdrawal of parasympathetic activity and an increase in sympathetic outflow. Although sympathetic activity is most elevated in severe decompensated heart failure, there is also evidence that sympathetic tone is increased even in patients with asymptomatic left-ventricular dysfunction, at a time prior to activation of the circulating renin–angiotensin system. Increased sympathetic activity may thus be an early stimulus for remodeling of the myocardium in response to hemodynamic stresses. In addition, increased agonist levels appear to play a primary role in the downregulation of adrenergic receptor effector pathways (e.g. β-adrenergic receptors, G proteins, etc.), thereby causing myocardial hyporesponsiveness to adrenergic stimulation.

Renin–angiotensin system

The circulating renin–angiotensin system (RAS) is frequently activated in patients with heart failure, particularly in more advanced disease. In addition, both myocardial and vascular tissues contain all of the requisite components for an active RAS, and there is evidence for activation of the tissue RAS in heart failure.[23] The relative contributions of the circulating and tissue renin–angiotensin systems vary during the acute, compensated and decompensated phases of myocardial failure. Although serum RAS activity often returns to relatively normal levels in well-compensated heart failure, it has been suggested that tissue RAS activity may remain elevated in the myocardium, vasculature and elsewhere, and could thereby contribute importantly to the progression of cardiac and vascular remodeling.[23]

Several components of the tissue RAS, including angiotensin-converting enzyme activity, the level of angiotensinogen mRNA and the density of angiotensin-II receptors, are upregulated in the noninfarcted myocardium of rats following myocardial infarction.[24–26] Taken together, these observations suggest that there may be both increased activity of the tissue RAS, resulting in more available angiotensin, and increased responsiveness of the tissue to angiotensin.

Angiotensin has been implicated as a causative factor in myocardial hypertrophy, independent of its effect on vascular tone and cardiac loading conditions.[27] Angiotensin has been shown to increase [^{3}H]-phenylalanine incorporation in both cardiac myocytes and nonmyocytes, but to increase [^{3}H]-thymidine incorporation only in the nonmyocytes. These effects on nonmyocytes suggest that, in addition to causing myocyte hypertrophy, angiotensin could play a role in causing proliferation of fibroblasts and the development of interstitial fibrosis, an important component of cardiac remodeling.

There is also evidence that in addition to being a target, cardiac myocytes may be a source of tissue angiotensin II. Fluorescence staining of rat ventricular myocytes with an antibody directed against angiotensin II reveals focal areas of staining within the cell indicative of intracellular angiotensin II.[28] It was observed that stretching of cultured neonatal rat cardiac myocytes on a silicone membrane induced the expression of fetal genes and increased protein synthesis, and that these effects were blocked by the angiotensin-receptor antagonist losartan.[28] These observations led to the suggestion that angiotensin II is released from cardiac myocytes by mechanical stress and plays an autocrine role in the cardiac myocyte growth response to hemodynamic overload.

Endothelin

Endothelin-1 can have important effects on cardiac myocyte growth and phenotype.[29] In neonatal rat cardiac myocytes in culture, exposure to endothelin for $\geqslant 24$

hours causes an increase in size, and increased expression of myosin light chain-2 which is organized into contractile units. Recent observations have suggested that endothelin-1, which can be produced by a variety of cells in the myocardium, may serve as an autocrine/paracrine regulator of the molecular and cellular effects of angiotensin II (and potentially, other hypertrophic stimuli) on cardiac myocytes.[30] In cultured neonatal rat cardiac myocytes, angiotensin II (Ang II) induces the expression of ET-1. By using an antisense oligonucleotide directed against preproendothelin-1 mRNA (ppET-1, the precursor of ET-1), it was shown that cells treated with antisense to ppET-1 have a significantly reduced growth response to Ang II, as reflected by leucine incorporation into protein. In other experiments, an antagonist for ET-1 receptors was similarly shown to inhibit the growth effects of angiotensin II. These observations raise the intriguing possibility that in cardiac myocytes ET-1 plays a critical autocrine role in the cellular response to Ang II.

Peptide growth factors

There is increasing evidence that peptide growth factors are expressed in the heart and play an important role in myocardial development and/or remodeling.[16,31,32] Peptide growth factors can have potent effects on the growth and phenotype of several cell types in the myocardium and have a major influence on the composition of the extracellular matrix.

Several peptide growth factors can stimulate the growth and phenotype of cardiac myocytes. In cultured neonatal rat ventricular myocytes, acidic fibroblast growth factor (aFGF), basic fibroblast growth factor (bFGF), tumor necrosis factor (TNFα), transforming growth factor-β_1 (TGFβ_1) and platelet-derived growth factor (PDGF) each increase myocyte protein synthesis.[33] In addition, several peptide growth factors can regulate the expression of mRNA for adult and fetal cardiac contractile proteins[34] (Figure 13.5). In general, peptide growth factors have been shown to decrease the expression of adult contractile protein isoforms (e.g. α-myosin heavy chain and α-cardiac actin) and to increase the expression of fetal isoforms (e.g. α-skeletal actin, α-smooth muscle actin and β-myosin heavy chain). This re-expression of a fetal gene pattern is characteristic of hypertrophied and failing myocardium.

TGF-β plays a central role in the regulation of extracellular matrix formation and cellular differentiation in a variety of tissues, and can be demonstrated in the myocardium.[32] Following myocardial infarction there is an increase in the expression of TGF-β_1 mRNA in both the area of the infarct and the noninfarcted myocardium.[35] It can also be shown that TGF-β_1 mRNA is induced in rat cardiac myocytes *in vitro* or by exposing the animal to an infusion of norepinephrine or aortic banding[36] (Figure 13.6). Taken together, these observations suggest that TGF-β may play a role in remodeling of the myocardium in response to a variety of hypertrophic stimuli.

Extracellular matrix

Although myocytes are the major component of the heart on the basis of mass, they represent only a minority of the cells on the basis of number. Nonmyocyte cellular

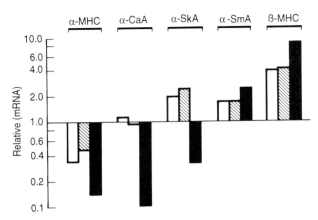

Figure 13.5 Effects of three peptide growth factors, transforming growth factor-β_1 (TGF-β_1, open bars), basic fibroblast growth factor (bFGF, hatched bars) and acidic fibroblast growth factor (aFGF, solid bars) on the expression of mRNAs for several adult and fetal isoforms of contractile proteins in cultured cardiac myocytes from neonatal rats. In general, these growth factors induced the expression of the fetal isoforms, β-myosin heavy chain (β-MHC), α-smooth muscle actin (α-SmA) and α-skeletal actin (α-SkA), and reduced the expression of the adult isoforms, α-myosin heavy chain (α-MHC) and α-cardiac actin (α-CaA). (Adapted from Parker *et al.*, 1990.[34])

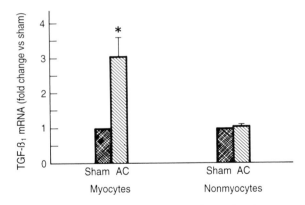

Figure 13.6 Effect of pressure overload on the expression of transforming growth factor-β_1 (TGF-β_1) mRNA in the rat heart. Rats were subjected to aortic constriction for three days and the left ventricles were dissociated into myocyte-rich and nonmyocyte-rich fractions, the latter consisting primarily of fibroblasts. Pressure overload caused a threefold induction of TGF-β_1 mRNA in the myocyte-rich fraction, but had no effect on the nonmyocytes. These data suggest that the cardiac myocyte may play a central role, via the elaboration of peptide growth factors, in orchestrating the remodeling of the ventricle in response to hemodynamic stimuli. (Adapted from Takahashi *et al.*, 1994.[36])

constituents of the myocardium include fibroblasts, arterioles containing smooth-muscle cells and capillaries containing endothelial cells. Myocytes and nonmyocytes are interconnected by a complex of connective tissue and extracellular matrix. Components of the extracellular matrix include collagens, proteoglycans, glyco-proteins such as fibronectin, several peptide growth factors and proteases such as plasminogen activators. There is increasing appreciation that by regulating the nature and quantity of the extracellular matrix, nonmyocytes in the heart play an important role in determining the response of the myocardium to pathologic stimuli.[37] A characteristic feature of pathologic myocardial hypertrophy is an abnormal accumulation of interstitial connective tissue resulting in interstitial fibrosis which may affect the mechanical properties of the myocardium (e.g. impairing relaxation) and restrict the delivery of nutrients to myocytes.

Implications for therapy

Secondary molecular alterations in remodeled and failing myocardium may have an important impact on the clinical course of the patient. As our understanding of the basic biology of these events advances, it is likely that additional new diagnostic and therapeutic approaches will emerge. For instance, the ability to assess the 'molecular status' of the myocardium may allow for a better tracking of the disease progression, earlier detection of asymptomatic patients, improved prognostication, and the design of therapeutic regimens that are tailored at the molecular level. New classes of therapeutic agents will emerge. Drugs which block cytokine or growth factor receptors already exist and offer prospects. It is now reasonable to consider the development of molecular strategies (e.g. utilizing the transfer of genes or antisense oligonucleotides) aimed at reversing molecular abnormalities in the failing myocardium and/or preventing their occurrence in myocardium exposed to pathologic stresses. Finally, new approaches for the local delivery of drugs, peptides and nucleotides may provide mechanisms for the specific targeting of pharmacologic and molecular agents.

References

1. Pfeffer, J. M. (1991) Progressive ventricular dilation in experimental myocardial infarction and its attenuation by angiotensin-converting enzyme inhibition. *Am. J. Cardiol.*, **68**, 17D–25D.
2. Anversa, P., Ricci, R. and Olivetti, G. (1986) Quantitative structural analysis of the myocardium during growth and induced cardiac hypertrophy: a review. *J. Am. Coll. Cardiol.*, **7**, 1140–9.
3. van Bilsen, M. and Chien, K. R. (1993) Growth and hypertrophy of the heart: towards an understanding of the cardiac specific and inducible gene expression. *Cardiovas. Res.*, **27**, 1140–9.
4. Takahashi, T., Allen, P. D. and Izumo, S. (1992) Expression of A-, B-, and C-type natriuretic peptide genes in failing and developing human ventricles. *Circ. Res.*, **71**, 9–17.
5. Arai, M., Alpert, N. R., MacLennan, D. H. *et al.* (1993) Alterations in sarcoplasmic reticulum gene expression in human heart failure. *Circ. Res.*, **72**, 463–9.
6. Morgan, J. P. (1991) Abnormal intracellular modulation of calcium as a major cause of cardiac contractile dysfunction. *N. Engl. J. Med.*, **325**, 625–32.
7. Beuckelmann, D. J., Nabauer, M. and Erdmann, E. (1992) Intracellular calcium handling in isolated ventricular myocytes from patients with terminal heart failure. *Circulation*, **85**, 1046–55.
8. Takahashi, T., Allen, P. D., Lacro, R. V. *et al*, (1992) Expression of dihydropyridine receptor (Ca^{2+} channel) and calsequestrin genes in the myocardium of patients with end-stage heart failure. *J. Clin. Invest.*, **90**, 927–35.

9. Feldman, A. M., Ray, P. E., Silan, C. M. *et al.* (1991) Selective gene expression in failing human heart. Quantification of steady-state levels of messenger RNA in endomyocardial biopsies using the polymerase chain reaction. *Circulation,* **83**, 1866–72.
10. Brillantes, A.-M., Allen, P., Takahashi, T. *et al.* (1992) Differences in cardiac calcium release channel (ryanodine receptor) expression in myocardium from patients with end-stage heart failure caused by ischemic versus dilated cardiomyopathy. *Circ. Res.,* **71**, 18–26.
11. Solaro, R. J., Powers, F. M., Gao, L and Gwathmey, J. K. (1993) Control of myofilament activation in heart failure. *Circulation,* **87**, VII-38–VII-43.
12. Anderson, P. A. W., Malouf, N. N., Oakeley, A. E. *et al.* (1992) Troponin T isoform expression in the normal and failing human left ventricle: a correlation with myofibrillar ATPase activity. *Basic Res. Cardiol.,* **87**, 117–27.
13. Bristow, M. R. (1993) Changes in myocardial and vascular receptors in heart failure. *J. Am. Coll. Cardiol.,* **22**, 61A–71A.
14. Hausdorff, W. P., Caron, M. G. and Lefkowitz, R. J. (1990) Turning off the signal: desensitization of β-adrenergic receptor function. *FASEB J.,* **4**, 2881–89.
15. Ungerer, M., Bohm, M., Elce, J. S. *et al.* (1993) Altered expression of β-adrenergic receptor kinase and β-adrenergic receptors in the failing heart. *Circulation,* **87**, 454–63.
16. Schneider, M. D. and Parker, T. G. (1990) Cardiac myocytes as targets for the action of peptide growth factors. *Circulation,* **81**, 1443–56.
17. Watson, P. A. (1991) Function follows form: generation of intracellular signals by cell deformation. *FASEB J.,* **5**, 2013–19.
18. Sadoshima, J.-I., Jahn, L., Takahashi, T. *et al.* (1992) Molecular characterizations of the stretch-induced adaptation of cultured cardiac cells. An *in vitro* model of load-induced cardiac hypertrophy. *J. Biol. Chem.* **267**, 10551–60.
19. Simpson, P. and McGrath, A. (1983) Norepinephrine-stimulated hypertrophy of cultured rat myocardial cells is an alpha$_1$ adrenergic response. *J. Clin. Invest.,* **72**, 732–8.
20. Iwaki, K., Sukhatme, V. P., Shubeita, H. E. and Chien, K. R. (1990) α- and β-adrenergic stimulation induces distinct patterns of immediate early gene expression in neonatal rat myocardial cells. *fos/jun* Expression is associated with sarcomere assembly; *Egr-1* induction is primarily an α$_1$-mediated response. *J. Biol. Chem.,* **265**, 13809–17.
21. Knowlton, K. U., Michel, M. C., Itani, M. *et al.* (1993) The α$_{1A}$ adrenergic receptor subtype mediates biochemical, molecular, and morphologic features of cultured myocardial cell hypertrophy. *J. Biol. Chem.,* **268**, 15374–80.
22. Floras, J. S. (1993) Clinical aspects of sympathetic activation and parasympathetic withdrawal in heart failure. *J. Am. Coll. Cardiol.,* **22**, 72A–84A.
23. Dzau, V. J. (1993) Tissue renin–angiotensin system in myocardial hypertrophy and failure. *Arch. Intern. Med.,* **153**, 937–42.
24. Hirsch, A. T., Talsness, C. E., Schunkert, H. *et al.* (1991) Tissue-specific activation of cardiac angiotensin converting enzyme in experimental heart failure. *Circ. Res.,* **69**, 475–82.
25. Lindpaintner, K., Lu, W., Niedermajer, N. *et al.* (1993) Selective activation of cardiac angiotensinogen gene expression in post-infarction ventricular remodeling in the rat. *J. Mol. Cell. Cardiol.,* **25**, 133–43.
26. Meggs, L. G., Coupet, J., Huang, H. *et al.* (1993) Regulation of angiotensin II receptors on ventricular myocytes after myocardial infarction in rats. *Circ. Res.,* **72**, 1149–62.
27. Sadoshima, J.-I. and Izumo, S. (1993) Molecular characterization of angiotensin II-induced hypertrophy of cardiac myocytes and hyperplasia of cardiac fibroblasts. Critical role of the AT$_1$ receptor subtype. *Circ. Res.,* **73**, 413–23.
28. Sadoshima, J.-I., Xu, Y., Slayter, H. S. and Izumo, S. (1993) Autocrine release of angiotensin II mediates stretch-induced hypertrophy of cardiac myocytes *in vitro. Cell,* **75**, 977–84.
29. Shubeita, H. E., McDonough, P. M., Harris, A. N. *et al.* (1990) Endothelin induction of inositol phospholipid hydrolysis, sarcomere assembly, and cardiac gene expression in ventricular myocytes. A paracrine mechanism for myocardial cell hypertrophy. *J. Biol. Chem.,* **265**, 20555–62.

30. Ito, H., Hirata, Y., Adachi, S. *et al.* (1993) Endothelin-1 is an autocrine/paracrine factor in the mechanism of angiotensin II-induced hypertrophy in cultured rat cardiomyocytes. *J. Clin. Invest.*, **92**, 398–403.
31. Engelmann, G. L., Dionne, C. A. and Jaye, M. C. (1993) Acidic fibroblast growth factor and heart development. Role in myocyte proliferation and capillary angiogenesis. *Circ. Res.*, **72**, 7–19.
32. Thompson, N. L., Flanders, K. C., Smith, J. M. *et al.* (1989) Expression of transforming growth factor-β_1 in specific cells and tissues of adult and neonatal mice. *J. Cell Biol.*, **108**, 661–9.
33. Long, C. S., Henrich, C. J. and Simpson, P. C. (1991) A growth factor for cardiac myocytes is produced by cardiac nonmyocytes. *Cell Regul.*, **2** 1081–95.
34. Parker, T. G., Packer, S. E. and Schneider, M. D. (1990) Peptide growth factors can provide 'fetal' contractile protein gene expression in rat cardiac myocytes. *J. Clin. Invest.*, **85**, 507–14.
35. Casscells, W., Bazoberry, F., Speir, E. *et al.* (1990) Transforming growth factor-β_1 in normal heart and in myocardial infarction. *Ann. NY Acad. Sci.*, **593**, 148–60.
36. Takahashi, N., Calderone, A., Izzo, N. J., Jr. *et al.* (1994) Hypertrophic stimuli-induced transforming growth factor-β_1 expression in rat ventricular myocytes. *J. Clin. Invest.*, **94**, 1470–6.
37. Weber, K. T. and Brilla, C. G. (1991) Pathological hypertrophy and cardiac interstitium. Fibrosis and renin–angiotensin–aldosterone system. *Circulation*, **83**, 1849–65.

14

Congestive Heart Failure: Molecular Approach and Transplantation

John A. Jarcho

Introduction

Cardiac transplantation is the treatment of last resort for end-stage congestive heart failure. Since the first successful human heart transplant was performed in 1967, use of this procedure has grown nationwide and worldwide; in the United States approximately 2000 heart transplants are performed annually at more than 150 centers.[1,2] The clinical outcome for carefully managed patients has improved dramatically since the first operations; the actuarial survival of recipients is greater than 80% at one year post transplant and approximately 67% at five years post transplant.[2,3] Functional status is also excellent for recipients, with studies suggesting that more than 80% of patients return to New York Heart Association Class I.[3] Factors contributing to the current clinical success of heart transplantation include improved donor management, better perioperative care, advances in immunosuppression (including especially the introduction of cyclosporine) and the development of endomyocardial biopsy for diagnosis of rejection.

Despite these significant advances, numerous problems remain unsolved in clinical cardiac transplantation. Medically, the most challenging problem is that of achieving optimal immunosuppression. Immunologic complications, or the complications of their treatment, are the most important causes of morbidity and mortality in the transplant population.[2,4] Among the most common causes of death early after transplantation are rejection (due to insufficient immunosuppression) and infection (due to excessive, or too nonspecific, immunosuppression). Late causes of death include neoplasia (also a consequence of immunosuppression) and graft atherosclerosis (which appears to be due to immunologic attack on the vasculature of the graft). Finally, some of the most troublesome nonfatal complications of transplantation are related to immunosuppression: renal failure (a side effect of cyclosporine), hypertension (due to both cyclosporine and prednisone), glucose intolerance (due to prednisone), and osteoporosis (due to prednisone). All of these complications have a serious impact on the likelihood that a heart transplant patient will return to a healthy, active life after receiving a new heart. Furthermore, even if no complications actually occur, a schedule of frequent clinical follow-up is essential for the patient to remain in good health. Frequent office visits, blood tests and endomyocardial biopsies are necessary, as is annual cardiac catheterization to monitor for the development of coronary disease. All of this routine care greatly increases the expense and inconvenience of maintaining a transplant recipient. For these reasons, improvements in the immunologic management of heart (and other organ) transplant recipients are sought eagerly. Improved immunotherapy for transplant patients could have a very great impact on patient survival and well-being and possibly also on the cost of care.

Most of the advances in the pharmacotherapy of transplant patients have occurred with only a limited understanding of the underlying immunobiology. Ideally, new and better immunosuppressive agents should be developed by proceeding from clear knowledge of immune mechanisms to the identification of treatments designed to influence known pathways of the immune response. Unfortunately, the immune system is sufficiently complex that it is not yet possible to construct a complete model of the process of allograft rejection. To some extent, the design of optimal immunosuppressives awaits a more thorough knowledge of the normal physiology of the immune system. However, as parts of the immune response become better understood, they reveal new avenues for therapeutic intervention. This chapter will discuss the contributions of molecular immunology to the development of new techniques for treating allograft rejection.

Cyclosporine, FK-506, and rapamycin

Cyclosporine is a cyclic peptide derived from the soil fungus *Tolypocladium inflatum* (see Figure 14.1). Discovered in 1972, it quickly became of potential clinical interest when it was found to suppress immune responsiveness in several animal models. Bone-marrow suppression, a typical feature of most previously known immunosuppressive agents, was not seen with cyclosporine, suggesting a more specific mechanism of action on the immune system than that of other drugs.[5] It was introduced in clinical renal transplantation in 1978 and quickly led to conspicuously better survival of grafts and patients.[6] Largely as a result of these studies, interest in the transplantation of other organs, including the heart, increased. The advent of cyclosporine use, more than any other innovation, has made cardiac transplantation clinically feasible.

Although cyclosporine was developed (as noted above) without knowledge of its molecular mechanism of action, studies of the drug since then have revealed important details of the workings of the immune system. Cyclosporine has therefore been described as a 'pharmacologic probe' for the study of immunobiology;[7] this work has led to the recognition of new potential targets for intervention in the immune response to allografts.

Cyclosporine's effects, when cataloged, seem complex, but some clear themes have been recognized. *In vitro*, it influences primarily T-cell function, especially T-cell activation by various stimuli. T cells can ordinarily be stimulated in culture by several means, such as the addition of monoclonal antibodies to the T-cell receptor,

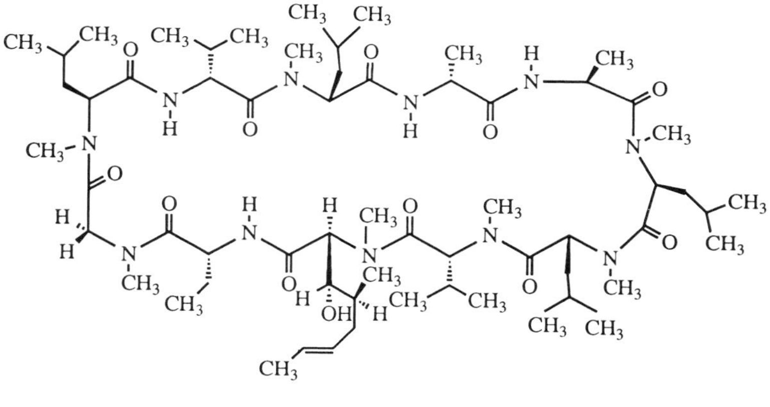

Cyclosporin A

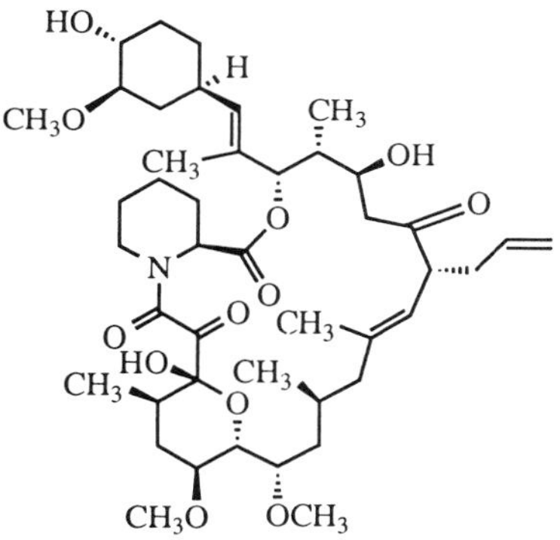

FK-506

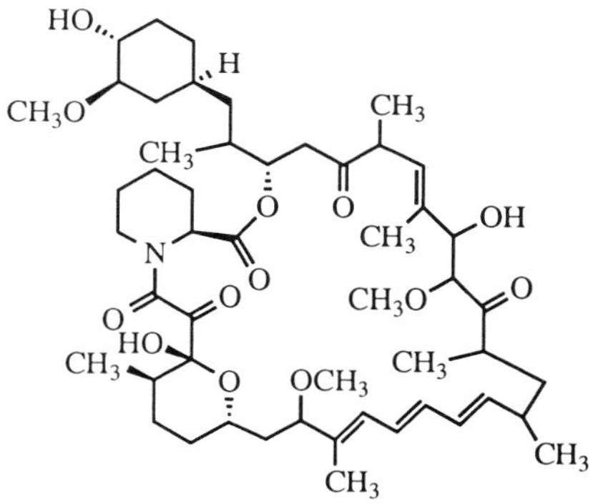

Rapamycin

Figure 14.1 The structures of cyclosporine A, FK-506 and rapamycin. (With permission from Sigal, N. H. and Dumont, F. J. (1992) Cyclosporin A, FK-506, and rapamycin: pharmacologic probes of lymphocyte signal transduction. *Annu. Rev. Immunol.*, **10**, 519–560.)

which cross-link adjacent receptors and in so doing activate the cells. T cells can also be stimulated by plant lectins (a group of polymeric proteins) or by a combination of the calcium ionophore ionomycin and the phorbol ester PMA (phorbol myristate acetate), which activates protein kinase C. Responses to all of these stimuli are blocked by cyclosporine.[7] However, in another model, T cells may be stimulated by the combination of antibodies to the T-cell surface molecule CD28 and PMA. This pathway is cyclosporine-resistant.[8] These findings are revealing because the cyclosporine-sensitive T-cell stimuli are all associated with an increase in the intracellular calcium concentration, while cyclosporine-resistant stimuli are not.[9]

When stimulated, T cells also release a variety of soluble products which can be measured in the culture medium. These include the lymphokines IL-2, IL-3, IL-4, interferon-γ (IFN-γ) and tumor necrosis factor (TNF). Production of all of these factors is prevented by cyclosporine, a blockade which takes place at the level of gene transcription.[10,11] If T cells are stimulated in the presence of cyclosporine, activation and proliferation do not occur; however, if exogenous IL-2 is added to the culture, the blockade is reversed.[9,12] Taken together, these data indicate that cyclosporine interferes with T-cell activation by blocking a calcium-dependent pathway which leads to IL-2 gene transcription.

In 1987, the immunosuppressive agent FK-506 was isolated from cultures of an actinomycete also found in the soil.[13] FK-506 is a macrolide compound chemically unrelated to cyclosporine (see Figure 14.1). However, it soon became apparent that the biologic actions of FK-506 are strikingly similar to those of cyclosporine, despite the chemical dissimilarity. Like cyclosporine, FK-506 acts primarily on T cells. Like cyclosporine, FK-506 blocks calcium-dependent pathways of activation exclusively.[9] Like cyclosporine, FK-506 interferes with the production of IL-2, IL-3 and IL-4, as well as IFN-γ and TNF, all at the transcriptional level.[14] FK-506 is an effective immunosuppressant in the same animal models of transplantation, autoimmunity and inflammation as cyclosporine. The only significant difference is that FK-506 is 10- to 100-fold more potent.[15]

Rapamycin is another macrolide which was discovered before either cyclosporine or FK-506, but which was realized to have immunosuppressive potential only after FK-506 was discovered. Then the structures of these two agents were compared and were found to be very similar (see Figure 14.1). Despite its structural similarity to FK-506, the immunosuppressive actions of rapamycin were actually found to differ significantly from its sister compound. Rapamycin is an effective immunosuppressant in animal models of allograft rejection;[16] like cyclosporine and FK-506, it inhibits T-cell activation specifically.[17] However, the effects of rapamycin are not limited to calcium-dependent activation pathways; it effectively blocks CD28-dependent stimulation *in vitro*.[18] The production of cytokines is not inhibited by rapamycin[19] and the blockade of T-cell activation by rapamycin cannot be reversed by exogenous IL-2.[19]

Understanding of the molecular basis of action of these drugs began in 1984 with the isolation of cyclophilin, a small cytosolic protein which binds to cyclosporine with very high affinity.[20] Cyclophilin A, the first of these binding proteins to be identified, is actually a member of a family of cyclophilins, of which four species (cyclophilins A to D) are found in humans.[21] These cyclosporine-binding proteins are found in great abundance in all cell types and may constitute as much as 0.4% of the total cytosolic protein.[22] In addition, cyclophilins have been found in a wide range of species.[21,22] These observations suggest that cyclophilins serve a fundamental and essential cellular function. In 1989, the analogous target for FK-506 was identified[23,24] and called simply FKBP (FK-506 binding protein). It, too, is a small cytosolic protein which is both abundant and widely distributed. It is perhaps not surprising, given the dissimilarity of their structures, that cyclosporine and FK-506 do not bind to each other's ligands. However, rapamycin binds to FKBP with high affinity.[25]

FKBP and cyclophilin have a common enzymatic activity: they are both able to catalyze the *cis–trans* isomerization of proline residues in peptides.[26,27] They are therefore described as peptidylprolyl isomerases, or as rotamases, because isomerization leads to a rotational change about the proline amide bond. Rotamase activity is thought to play an important role in the folding of proteins, which is necessary for them to attain the correct tertiary structure. Cyclosporine inhibits the rotamase activity of cyclophilin;[21,26] FK-506 and rapamycin both inhibit the rotamase activity of FKBP.[27] It was therefore proposed that the two rotamases are necessary for the folding of cellular proteins required for T-cell activation, and that when either of these enzymes is bound by its ligand, proper protein folding cannot occur and T-cell activation is prevented.

There are several problems with this model, however. First, it does not explain why the effects of cyclosporine and FK-506 are so similar, and why they differ from that of rapamycin. Given that FK-506 and rapamycin bind the same ligand, one might expect that cyclosporine would be the agent to differ in action from the other two. Second, cyclophilin and FKBP are present in all cell types,[21] yet the effects of their ligands are confined to T cells (and to those cell types implicated in the side effects of the drugs). Third, cyclophilin and FKBP are present in high concentration in the cell; large amounts of cyclosporine, FK-506 or rapamycin are needed to inhibit cellular rotamase activity – much larger amounts than are actually necessary to produce immunosuppression.[21,28] Finally, analogs of cyclosporine and FK-506 have been synthesized which block rotamase activity but which are not themselves immunosuppressants.[28,29] These observations effectively exclude a simple blockade of immunophilin activity as the mechanism of action of these drugs.

The search for a clearer understanding of this confusing picture led in 1991 to the demonstration that the cyclosporine–cyclophilin complex and the FK-506–FKBP complex both bind to, and inhibit, a protein phosphatase called calcineurin.[30] Neither drug alone blocks calcineurin, nor do the binding proteins alone. Furthermore, the complex of FKBP with rapamycin does not inhibit calcineurin.[30] A synthetic analog of FK-506 called 506BD, which binds to FKBP but is not immuno-suppressive, is also unable to block calcineurin when complexed to FKBP.[30] In short, the behavior of these drugs and their binding proteins in blocking the action of calcineurin reproduces the known pattern of their immunosuppressive interactions. Further studies with analogs of FK-506 and cyclosporine have demonstrated that the immunosuppressive potency of a given synthetic analog correlates very well with its ability to block calcineurin, but not with its ability to block rotamase activity.[31]

Calcineurin is an enzyme which dephosphorylates proteins on serine and threo-nine residues.[32] This activity thus seems to be the true target of the immunosuppressive action of cyclosporine and FK-506, but not of rapamycin. Since (as noted above) transcription of the gene encoding IL-2 is an important effect of these drugs, analysis of IL-2 promoter activity has been undertaken to explain the role of calcineurin.[33] Enhancer sites within the IL-2 promoter region have been identified that bind several transcription factors, including NFAT (nuclear factor of activated T cells).[34] It has been established that NFAT is actually a complex consisting of $NFAT_n$, a nuclear component, and $NFAT_p$, a cytoplasmic component.[35,36] The cytoplasmic component must be dephosphorylated and migrate to the nucleus to form the active complex. The cytoplasmic component has now been shown to be a substrate of calcineurin, and cyclosporine and FK-506 have been shown to inhibit translocation of this component to the nucleus.[37]

It therefore appears that the action of cyclosporine and related drugs can now be explained on a molecular level. Cyclosporine binds to cyclophilin; the complex of cyclosporine and cyclophilin then binds to, and blocks, the action of calcineurin. Blockade of calcineurin results in an inability to dephosphorylate $NFAT_p$ (and probably other transcription factors as well), preventing it from moving into the nucleus to activate the IL-2 promoter. Hence IL-2 transcription in response to T-cell stimulation is inhibited. FK-506 binds to FKBP, and the complex of FK-506 and FKBP likewise inhibits calcineurin. Rapamycin binds to FKBP, but the complex of rapamycin and FKBP has a different configuration from that of FK-506–FKBP; the rapamycin–FKBP complex apparently blocks a different, and later, step in T-cell activation and proliferation.

Deciphering the mechanism of action of cyclosporine has given much new insight into the mechanism of T-cell activation, and in so doing has suggested directions for the development of new and better immunosuppressive agents. Drugs which bind to the immunophilins cyclophilin and FKBP are not without toxic side effects; these effects are probably also due to inhibition of calcineurin, which is found in other tissues outside of the immune system. The transcription factor NFAT, however, is found only in lymphoid cells. Drugs designed to inhibit NFAT might be much more specific immunosuppressives than cyclosporine or FK-506. As other sites of calcineurin action are identified, they may reveal additional targets for new drug development.

Antilymphocyte antibodies

The use of antibodies against lymphocytes to prevent tissue graft rejection was first demonstrated by Woodruff and Anderson in 1963.[38] They used a crude antilymphocyte serum, prepared in rabbits, against rat thoracic duct lymphocytes, and were able to show prolongation of the survival of skin homografts derived from a second strain of rats. Subsequent studies showed the ability of antilymphocyte serum to protect solid organ grafts, first in animals[39,40] and then, in 1967, in human kidney transplants.[40] Early clinical studies suggested that antilymphocyte preparations made at several different institutions were able to improve graft function and reduce the incidence of rejection,[41–43] although they were not able to show prolongation of either graft or patient survival.[44] A reduction in rejection frequency was also seen in heart transplant recipients by the Stanford group.[45]

Initial experience in humans was marked by the occurrence of frequent side effects, including significant allergic reactions (fever, urticaria, skin rashes, anaphylaxis[41–43]), anemia and thrombocytopenia (due to antibodies against other blood components in the crude sera[43]) and glomerulonephritis (due to antibodies cross-reacting with glomerular basement membrane[43]). Attempts were therefore made to refine the preparations to generate reagents of maximal potency with minimal toxicity. Comparisons were made between sera derived from horses, rabbits, goats and cows.[43] Attempts were made to remove contaminating erythrocytes, platelets and proteins from the inocula, and antibodies generated to these other targets were removed by adsorption.[41] The gamma-globulin fraction, separated from the other serum proteins, made a purer preparation ('antilymphocyte globulin' or ALG) with a reduced incidence of serum sickness.[41] Peripheral blood lymphocytes, thoracic duct lymphocytes, lymph-node suspensions, spleen cells, and thymocytes (hence ATG, for 'antithymocyte globulin') were all explored as sources of antigen.[43] Even with more refined preparations, however, side effects, especially allergic reactions, were frequent, especially if the agent was given for longer than two-to-three weeks.

Given the drawbacks associated with this form of therapy, there was considerable debate about the best use of ALG in transplant patients. Eventually two discrete settings were defined in which ALG or ATG were thought to be useful: as initial therapy immediately following transplantation ('induction') and for treatment of steroid-resistant rejection.

When ALG or ATG is used for initial control of post-transplant rejection it is usually given for a period of from three days to two weeks, starting either immediately before or as many as three days after surgery.[46–49] In this setting, antilymphocyte therapy has been shown to be useful for two reasons. First, it significantly reduces the occurrence of rejection in the early post-transplant period, when surgical recovery is still occurring and rejection is particularly dangerous.[46,47] Second, it makes it possible to reduce the use of the other drugs in the immunosuppressive regimen. This feature has been particularly important since the advent of cyclosporine use. Because cyclosporine is nephrotoxic, its use at full doses immediately after transplant may sometimes delay the recovery of postoperative renal function.[50] In this setting, antilymphocyte 'induction' with low-dose cyclosporine (or even no cyclosporine initially) may allow the kidneys to recover.[51] Studies of the longer-term benefit of such therapy have had conflicting results, with some institutions reporting improved graft and patient survival, and others finding no such difference.[52] Interpretation of these data has been hampered by the fact that different studies have used different antilymphocyte preparations.

When used for treatment of acute episodes of rejection, ALG is more potent than the standard intervention of steroid pulse therapy. It reverses a greater percentage of rejection episodes on the first attempt than does methylprednisolone, and may reduce the frequency of recurrent rejection.[53,54] However, repeated administration of ALG for subsequent episodes of rejection is problematic. Since all antilymphocyte preparations are made in other species (especially horse and rabbit), they are foreign proteins not previously encountered by the recipient. If ALG is used frequently, an immune response to the antibody preparation develops, which may interfere with efficacy.[54] For this reason, ALG is not typically used as the agent of first choice for rejection. Instead, it is reserved for specific situations, such as steroid-resistant rejection or particularly severe rejection. If a patient has repeated episodes of severe or intractable rejection, it may be necessary to switch from one ALG preparation to another.

Despite the observation that ALG can be a very effective immunosuppressant in all types of organ transplants, controversy persists about the best way to use antilymphocyte therapy. In particular, there is doubt about its utility in the initial post-transplant period. This form of treatment has been labeled 'induction' because of the expectation by some investigators that the use of antilymphocyte therapy to eliminate mature lymphocytes at the same time as engraftment would 'induce' a state of true tolerance to the new organ.[55] It quickly became evident that tolerance was not being created with ALG, but the term has persisted because it is convenient, if inaccurate. Some authors have preferred to use the term 'prophylaxis' to describe the use of ALG initially at the time of transplant.[47,48] In any event, no adequate prospective multicenter-controlled trial of 'induction' versus 'noninduction' has ever been performed. Individual institutions have reviewed their own patient experience and drawn their own conclusions, but the variations in patient management from center to center make it difficult to generalize from these findings.

With the advent of monoclonal antibody technology, it became possible to distinguish lymphocyte subsets precisely based on their expression of specific cell surface antigens. OKT3, a murine monoclonal antibody directed against a human antigen present on all T cells (but not on B cells or nonlymphoid cells), quickly attracted the attention of transplant physicians. It was found to reverse acute renal allograft rejection within seven days when used alone.[56] A large multicenter randomized study of its use in renal transplants proved that it was significantly more effective than steroids in reversing a first episode of allograft rejection, and that long-term graft survival was significantly improved.[57] The use of OKT3 for prophylaxis has also been studied; it is clear that, in this setting, OKT3 delays the first rejection episode[58] and in some reports long-term graft survival is improved as well.[59]

OKT3 was expected to be superior to ATG because of its defined specificity, which would presumably eliminate side effects related to cross-reactions with other cell types and increase the immunosuppressive potency of the reagent. In addition, a monoclonal antibody, because of its uniformity, should eliminate the problem of unpredictable batch-to-batch variability seen with polyclonal preparations. Several prospective studies were undertaken to compare ATG with OKT3 for prophylaxis in heart transplant recipients.[60–68] None of these single-center trials was able to show a difference between the two agents in terms of one-year or two-year survival. Some of the studies seemed to confirm that the onset of a first rejection episode was delayed with OKT3,[63,64,66] although one center found much more rejection with OKT3 than with ATG.[62] This issue, like that of the role of prophylaxis itself, has yet to be settled by a prospective multicenter trial.

A more significant aspect of OKT3 was that it represented the first therapeutic agent in the transplant armamentarium designed with some specific knowledge of its biologic target. OKT3 was one of several monoclonal antibodies specifically generated against T cells, and selected because it recognized all peripheral T cells but no other cell types.[69] At the time of the first use of OKT3 the function of the target molecule was unknown, although it was soon demonstrated to play a role in antigen recognition.[70,71] With the development of a system of nomenclature for antibody-defined leukocyte cell-surface molecules, this target molecule became known as CD3. The CD3 molecule is now known to be a multimeric structure which is a component of the T-cell receptor complex[72,73] (see Figure 14.2).

The mechanism of action of OKT3 is still only partly understood. T cells are abruptly depleted from the circulation soon after administration of OKT3;[57,74] this process is probably a consequence of opsonization of the target cells for phagocytosis.[75] The murine antibody does not bind human complement well and hence

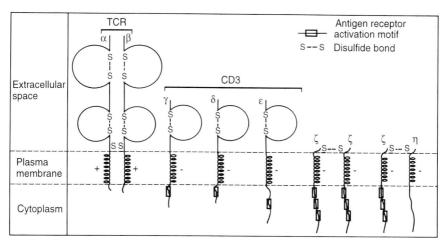

Figure 14.2 The T-cell receptor complex. The α and β chains confer specificity for antigen/MHC. The γ, δ, and ε chains are collectively referred to as the CD3 proteins, and are recognized by the monoclonal antibody OKT3. The ζ and η chains are found either as $\zeta\zeta$ or $\zeta\eta$ dimers. The CD3 proteins and the ζ and η chains are necessary for signal transduction by the T-cell receptor, and are also required for cell-surface expression of the entire complex. (With permission from Abbas, A. K., Lichtman, A. H. and Pober, J. S. (1994) Molecular basis of T cell antigen recognition and activation. In: *Cellular and Molecular Immunology*, 2nd edn, p. 145. Philadelphia: W.B. Saunders.

probably does not cause complement-mediated cell lysis.[54] However, attention has also focused on the fact that, when T cells reappear in the circulation, they no longer express CD3 on their surfaces. This phenomenon is referred to as 'modulation' of the target molecule, and is associated with a loss of immunologic competence by these cells.[76,77] Furthermore, OKT3 possesses the ability to activate T cells *in vivo* prior to removing them from the circulation.[78] As a result, cytokines such as tumor necrosis factor, interferon-γ, and IL-2 are released into the circulation, resulting in a variety of clinical side effects including fever, vomiting, diarrhea, aseptic meningitis, and pulmonary edema. This phenomenon is referred to as the 'cytokine release syndrome', and can occasionally be life-threatening.[79,80]

The clinical utility of OKT3, and the power of monoclonal antibody development for the specific targeting of immunosuppressive therapy, have led to intensive investigation of antibodies against leukocyte cell-surface molecules. An increasing number of such antibodies have been developed, with research focused in two directions: (1) identification of new, potentially useful antibodies against previously untargeted structures; and (2) modification of available antibodies to improve their potency or reduce their toxicity.

Several antibodies have been developed which have similar specificity to that of OKT3. These include BMA031,[81] WT32[82] and T10B9,[83] all of which are also directed against the T-cell receptor/CD3 complex. None of these antibodies has been found to be more effective than OKT3 itself, although they may all cause the cytokine release syndrome less frequently. Another antibody, anti-T12, is directed against the CD6 antigen, a molecule of unknown function found on most T cells and some B cells.[84] The antibody CAMPATH-1 is directed against CD52, an antigen found on all lymphocytes; it has been used to induce remission in patients with lymphoid malignancies[85] and there is limited experience with it in transplantation as well.[86] It has also proven to be no more effective than OKT3.

The antibodies above were developed to target large populations of lymphocytes generally. However, antibodies of increasing functional sophistication have also been designed to block specific lymphocyte functions. An early achievement of monoclonal antibody studies of lymphocytes was the distinction of 'helper', CD4+ T cells from 'cytotoxic', CD8+ T cells. These two groups of T cells have been shown, with some exceptions, to subserve separate roles in the immune response. They also interact differently with foreign antigens; CD4+ T cells recognize antigen only when bound to class II MHC (major histocompatibility complex, see below) molecules, while CD8+ T cells recognize antigen only when bound to class I MHC molecules.[87] Because CD4+ T cells are mostly of the 'helper' phenotype, that is, they provide signals necessary for most other effector functions of both T and B cells, they are an attractive target for immunosuppression.[88] Antibodies directed against CD4 have been studied in primate[89] and rodent[90] transplant models and have been shown to prolong allograft survival and, in rats, to induce long-term allograft tolerance.[91] The mechanism of action of these antibodies is also not precisely defined. Some such antibodies are 'lytic' or 'depleting' and act, at least in part, by eliminating CD4+ T cells.[90] Others, which are nonlytic, may act either by interfering with the T-cell receptor interaction with antigen-presenting cells or by blocking some necessary secondary signal (delivered through the CD4 molecule) during antigen recognition.[92] In other studies, antibodies against CD4 have been combined with antibodies against CD8, also conferring tolerance in mice.[93]

In designing a specific immunosuppressive antibody, it would be desirable to target only those lymphocytes which are actually activated by interaction with the graft, in such a way as to inhibit their activation and proliferation. The binding of the cytokine IL-2 to its receptor is a crucial early step in T-cell activation, which is required for clonal expansion (as noted earlier in the discussion of cyclosporine). The IL-2 receptor is therefore an attractive target for monoclonal antibody therapy. Monoclonal antibodies developed against the IL-2 receptor have been tested in a variety of animal models.[94,95] In rodents, these antibodies have been able to produce graft tolerance.[96] In human studies, tolerance has not been demonstrated. Nonetheless, effective immunosuppression has been achieved with IL-2 receptor antibodies in humans. In one randomized study comparing IL-2 targeted antibody therapy with ATG in renal transplant recipients, the two groups of patients had similar rejection rates, with fewer side effects in the IL-2 group.[97]

In addition to CD4 and CD8, several other cell surface molecules have been discovered which appear to play an accessory role in T-cell activation. These accessory molecules serve to promote attachment of cells to one another and to the intercellular substrate; some of them belong to the integrin superfamily of adhesion molecules.[98] They may serve more than a simply adhesive role, however; intracellular signalling through these accessory molecules may play an important role in activation of the T cell.[99] They are therefore sometimes referred to as 'costimulatory' molecules. An important pair of such molecules are LFA-1 (for leukocyte function-associated antigen-1), which is expressed on most T cells, B cells, monocytes and granulocytes[100] and ICAM-1 (for intercellular adhesion molecule-1), which is expressed on T cells, B cells, fibroblasts and endothelial cells.[101] LFA-1 and ICAM-1 are a complementary pair of ligands which bind to each other,[102] promoting attachment of T cells to antigen-presenting cells and delivering a costimulatory signal. This interaction has been shown to be necessary for optimal T-cell activation.[103] Monoclonal antibodies against ICAM-1 and LFA-1, when administered together to mice, have been shown to induce donor-specific graft tolerance.[104] This finding is of particular interest since it has been shown that engagement of the T-cell receptor in the absence of costimulatory signaling can cause T-cell inactivation.[105] Hence, the strategy of blocking costimulation may point the way to methods of tolerance induction.

Modification of antibodies to improve their effectiveness as therapeutic agents is also an area of active investigation. An important drawback of classical monoclonals is that, because they are murine antihuman antibodies, they constitute a foreign protein not previously encountered by the human recipient. As such, they are capable of inducing an immune response directed against themselves, with formation of 'anti-idiotypic antibodies'.[80,106] Efforts have been made to reduce the antigenicity of monoclonals by modifying the genes encoding them. Hybrid immunoglobulin genes have been designed in which the constant regions (and even some parts of the variable regions) are derived from human antibodies, with the hypervariable, antigen-binding regions (sometimes referred to as 'complementarity-determining regions') encoded by murine sequences. Such hybrid genes can then be introduced into cell lines capable of translating the genetic information into their protein product. These 'humanized' antibodies retain their antigenic specificity while losing some of their own antigenicity.[107] *In vitro* studies of humanized OKT3 have shown it to bind to T cells, compete for binding with murine OKT3, modulate the T-cell receptor, induce expression of the IL-2 receptor, and inhibit cytotoxic T-cell lysis of target cells.[108] All of these properties indicate that the new, humanized molecule has retained its effectiveness as both a T-cell activator and inhibitor. There is very limited experience with such antibodies in humans; the published data do suggest, however, that the humanized agents may be less immunogenic.[109]

Attempts are currently underway to make the production of humanized antibodies simpler. Using the technique of gene targeting, Zou *et al.* have replaced the constant region of the mouse kappa light chain (a structural component of the immunoglobulin molecule) with the equivalent human constant region. Such mice, when immunized against foreign antigens, produce chimeric antibodies which contain the human kappa light chain.[110] A similar approach can be used to replace the murine heavy-chain constant region with its human equivalent. Therefore, it should soon be possible to make humanized antibodies by immunization of chimeric mice, avoiding the difficult process of designing each antibody individually.

Another modification of immunosuppressive antibodies which has been proposed is the removal of the constant region of the antibody molecule, which is responsible for the binding of the antibody to Fc receptors on leukocytes during the antibody-mediated limb of the immune response. Without its constant region, the antibody, consisting of only its F(ab')$_2$ portion, becomes a 'coating protein', capable of binding to its target and inhibiting it without activating the host immune system.

Such antibodies, when administered to mice, have been shown to retain their immunosuppressive properties without causing the cytokine-release syndrome described above.[111]

A third approach to antibody modification is that of linking the immunoglobulin to a biologic toxin. Such antibody–toxin conjugates should work, not by blocking or downmodulating the target molecule, but by selectively poisoning the target cell. Several toxins have been studied for use in this setting including diphtheria toxin, *Pseudomonas* exotoxin A and ricin A chain.[112,113] These toxins, when they gain access to a cell interior, interfere with mRNA translation, thus bringing the protein synthesis of the cell to a halt. Because the process of 'modulation' of the target molecule involves internalization, linkage to an antibody is an effective way to bring the toxin molecule into the cell. Unfortunately, it has proven difficult to modify toxins for antibody conjugation in such a way as to avoid nonspecific side effects and yet maintain potency. An 'immunotoxin' consisting of anti-CD5 monoclonal antibody linked to a ricin A chain has been tested clinically in bone-marrow transplantation to prevent graft-versus-host disease.[114] In a related approach, some investigators are currently studying the use of toxins linked, not to antibodies, but to the natural ligand of the targeted cell-surface receptor. One such agent, consisting of diphtheria toxin linked to IL-2, has been tested in a variety of hematologic malignancies, with response rates as high as 44%.[115]

As our understanding of the biology of T cells continues to improve, more and more cell-surface molecules are identified which become attractive targets for antibody therapy. Regardless of their structure, antibodies will probably never be suitable for long-term use because they will ultimately provoke an immune response themselves and because they must be given intravenously. They are therefore likely to find their place in the transplant regimen as agents for treatment of acute rejection episodes, rather than as agents for prophylaxis. In such a role, however, they have already been shown to be extremely effective. In conjunction with appropriate maintenance drugs, such as cyclosporine, they play an essential part in the clinical success of cardiac transplantation.

Antigen presentation and tolerance induction

Patients with end-stage renal disease typically develop anemia as their kidneys fail, as a result of the loss of erythropoietin production. Exogenous erythropoietin is now available to manage such patients. Previously, frequent blood transfusions were performed to help maintain a stable hematocrit. For this reason, most patients coming to renal transplantation in the 1950s and 1960s had had many blood transfusions; it was not uncommon for the typical kidney patient to have received transfusions on ten or more occasions. In the late 1960s, however, it was demonstrated that transfusion recipients become sensitized to the HLA (human leukocytes antigen) types present on donor white blood cells, and that such sensitization may result in hyperacute rejection of a renal allograft.[116] As a result, pretransplant crossmatching was introduced: recipient serum was tested against potential donor leukocytes for evidence of a cytotoxic response prior to acceptance for transplantation. In addition, an attempt was made to minimize blood transfusion in patients with renal failure, to prevent sensitization.[117]

The doctrine of minimizing pretransplant transfusions persisted until 1973, when Opelz *et al.*[118] found the graft survival rate in patients receiving blood transfusions to be better, in general, than the rate in patients who have not been transfused. Furthermore, they were able to show that the more transfusions a patient received before transplant, the better their graft survival was likely to be, as long as prospective cross-matching was performed.[118] In 1980 this discovery was extended further by Salvatierra *et al.*[119] They showed that, for living-related donors matched for one HLA haplotype but not the other ('one haplotype matched'), if blood transfusions from the organ donor preceded the transplant, then graft survival was similar to that of an HLA-identical transplant.[119]

These findings led to renewed enthusiasm for planned blood transfusion before transplant. However, with the introduction of cyclosporine, graft survival improved significantly and interest in blood transfusion waned.[120] It was anticipated that cyclosporine would confer the same benefit as blood transfusion without the risks of sensitization and transmission of viral infection.

Interest in the role of blood transfusion before transplant was revived by a study by Lagaaij *et al.* reported in 1989.[121] This study examined both heart and kidney transplant recipients prospectively as well as a group of kidney transplant recipients retrospectively. Heart transplant candidates were transfused with a single unit of blood which was either completely mismatched for HLA-DR, or which was mismatched at one HLA-DR antigen and matched at the other, followed subsequently by transplantation. Recipients who had had a single DR-matched transfusion had fewer episodes of rejection than those who had received fully DR-mismatched blood. The renal transplant patients studied prospectively were tested for cytotoxic antibodies before and after transfusion of blood with either one or zero DR matches. The one DR-matched recipients had a much lower incidence of sensitization. Finally, a group of renal transplant recipients were evaluated retrospectively for graft survival according to the DR matching of prior transfusions. Patients receiving one DR-matched blood had significantly better graft survival than those who had received DR-mismatched blood or who had not been transfused.[121] This study suggested that the important variable in the transfusion effect is not the degree of matching between the blood donor and the organ donor, but the degree of matching between the blood donor and the recipient. In a related study, Lazda *et al.* showed that fully HLA-compatible transfusions did not reduce the incidence of allograft rejection, while single DR mismatches did.[122]

The study of Lagaaij *et al.*[121] suggests that, clinically at least, the transfusion effect is a broadly immunosuppressive one, reducing rejection regardless of the HLA type of the transplanted organ. Studies of unmatched (or 'third-party') transfusions seem to confirm that the suppressive effect encompasses other HLA types. However, a more recent study has shown that T-cell mediated cytotoxicity is reduced only for the HLA type of the transfused blood itself, with third-party cytotoxicity being unaffected.[123] This distinction is of particular importance in cardiac transplantation, where is it not possible to 'choose' the HLA type of the donor heart. Unfortunately, the clinical data to date are contradictory on this point.

The mechanism of the blood transfusion effect remains unknown. Several possible mechanisms have been suggested for the observed immunosuppression, including clonal deletion (the elimination of T cells specific for the graft[124,125]), clonal anergy (the inactivation, but not deletion, of graft-reactive T cells[126,127]), the generation of T suppressor cells (that is, antigen-specific T cells which actively block the immune response[128,129]), and the formation of anti-idiotype antibodies (antibodies which bind the antigen-specific regions of the T-cell receptor and thereby block antigen recognition[130,131]), Data from various studies provide provisional but not conclusive support for each of these hypotheses.

In the absence of definitive information about the mechanism of the transfusion effect, investigators have taken a variety of approaches to try to produce the same effect by other means. Doing so has depended on a steadily growing knowledge of the role of the HLA molecules themselves in the process of antigen presentation. Most of what is known about this process comes from studies in mice.

Antigen presentation to the immune system requires the cell-surface molecules of the HLA system. Because it has been shown that human HLA molecules (which are analogous to the H-2 system in mice) are the principal barriers to allogeneic tissue transplantation, they are collectively referred to as major histocompatibility complex (MHC) molecules.[132] MHC class I molecules, which are expressed on virtually all cell types, consist of an α-chain polypeptide which contains all of the polymorphic variability of the class I molecule, and an invariant β-chain polypeptide called β_2-microglobulin.[132,133] Class I molecules are designed chiefly to present endogenous antigen (foreign antigen manufactured within the host cell, such as a viral protein[134]). The endogenous protein is 'processed' by being broken down into small peptides within the cell; these peptides are then complexed to newly synthesized class I molecules as they are produced inside the cell. The class I molecule is so constructed that it has a distinct 'cleft' into which a short polypeptide (8–10 amino acids long) will fit.[135] The class I molecule, bearing the fragment of processed antigen, is then transferred to the cell surface and stably inserted in the cell membrane, with the antigen cleft containing the foreign polypeptide on the extracellular side of the membrane (see Figure 14.3A). When a CD8$^+$ T cell subsequently interacts with this class I-expressing cell, it will do so by means of its T-cell receptor; the T-cell receptor will actually recognize, and bind to, the complex of class I molecule and antigen together.[136]

MHC class II molecules are expressed on only a few cell types, which are sometimes referred to as 'professional antigen-presenting cells'; these include B lymphocytes, macrophages, dendritic cells and endothelial cells.[132,134] Class II molecules, like class I molecules, consist of two polypeptide chains designated α and β. However, unlike the β-chains of class I molecules, both chains of the class II molecule are polymorphic.[137] Class II molecules are designed to present exogenous antigen (that is, antigen which is endocytosed from outside the antigen-presenting cell, such as bacteria phagocytosed by a macrophage). As with class I-mediated antigen presentation, the exogenous antigen is broken down into smaller peptides for binding to the antigen-presenting cleft of the class II molecule. Peptides presented by class II molecules may be larger than class I-presented peptides, ranging from 12 to 24 amino acids in length.[138] As in class I antigen presentation, the

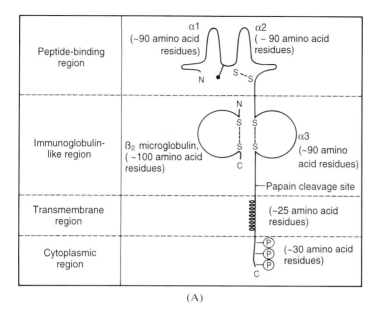

(A)

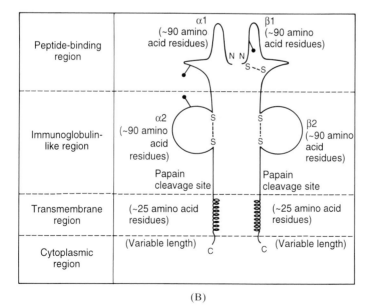

(B)

Figure 14.3 The MHC molecules. (A) The class I MHC molecule. (B) The class II MHC molecule. The amino and carboxy termini of the polypeptides are designated N and C, respectively. Intrachain disulfide bonds are designated S--S. Phosphorylation sites are designated –Ⓟ. Carbohydrate ligands are designated –●. (With permission from Abbas, A. K., Lichtman, A. H. and Pober, J. S. (1994) The major histocompatibility complex. In: *Cellular and Molecular Immunology*, 2nd edn, pp. 103 and 106. Philadelphia: W.B. Saunders.)

antigenic peptide is complexed to the class II molecule in its cleft before the complex is expressed on the cell surface (see Figure 14.3B). A CD4$^+$ T cell will bind to the class II molecule bearing the foreign antigen via its T-cell receptor. The subsequent activation of both CD4$^+$ and CD8$^+$ T cells, including proliferation, cytokine production and cell-mediated cytotoxicity, is dependent on this recognition event.[136]

The human genome contains DNA sequences sufficient to encode 10^{10} to 10^{15} distinct T-cell receptors, each capable of recognizing a different combination of antigen and MHC molecule.[139] This immense repertoire of T cells makes an effective response to a wide variety of antigens feasible. However, the initial repertoire includes T cells with receptors which would be capable of recognizing self-antigens bound to MHC molecules, and also receptors which would not require that the host's own MHC be a component of the recognized complex. These cells must be eliminated from the pool of T-cell clones to prevent autoimmune disease and to ensure that all responses are MHC-restricted (that is, that such responses only occur in conjunction with host MHC). The process whereby certain T-cell clones are removed from the repertoire and others are preserved is called 'selection', and it occurs in the thymus. The purpose of thymic selection is to limit the final pool of T-cell clones to those that recognize host MHC, but only in conjunction with foreign (nonhost) antigens.[140–142]

T-cell recognition of an allograft is essentially a cross-reaction between a T-cell receptor designed to recognize a host HLA molecule bearing a foreign peptide and a foreign HLA molecule (bearing either a host or a foreign peptide[143,144]). Recognition of transplanted tissue usually causes a vigorous reaction involving many T-cell clones because the variety of target molecules presented by a transplanted organ (including multiple foreign HLA molecules bearing a variety of either host or foreign peptides) is much greater than the variety of foreign peptides presented as targets during a viral or bacterial infection.

It was first demonstrated by Medawar that tolerance to foreign antigens can be induced by exposing the recipient to the antigen *in utero* or during the neonatal period. If mice are inoculated with lymphocytes from a second, nonidentical strain early after birth, they will not reject a subsequent skin graft from the second strain. However, their ability to reject a skin graft from a third unrelated strain is not diminished.[145] The immature lymphopoietic system of the neonatal mouse, exposed to a foreign antigen, accepts the antigen as 'self' and deletes T-cell clones which react with that antigen. Although tolerance is less easily induced in the mature lymphopoietic system, under some conditions exposure to antigens may lead to tolerance rather than activation in adult mice. For example, inoculation with antigen by subcutaneous injection typically stimulates an immune response,[146] while intravenous[147] or oral[148] administration of antigen may induce tolerance. The reason for this difference is unknown.

Several modifications to the blood-transfusion approach for allograft tolerance have now been studied in animals. In one approach, lymphocytes from the intended organ donor have been heated to 60°C prior to reinfusion. These heat-treated cells continue to express MHC antigens on their surface, but fail to activate allogeneic cells in a mixed-lymphocyte response *in vitro*.[149] The survival of a subsequent allograft after the infusion of heat-treated cells is prolonged.[150] It has been hypothesized that heat treatment prevents the cell from delivering a costimulatory signal (such as the ICAM-1/LFA-1 interaction described previously).

In another approach, first described in 1988, cells from the proposed organ recipient were cultured *in vitro* and then transfected with MHC class I genes from the organ donor. The transfected cells, which expressed the transfected MHC antigens on their surface, were then infused back into the organ recipient before transplantation of a graft which was both class I and class II mismatched. Graft survival was prolonged by this technique.[151] In 1993, a further elaboration of this approach was reported, in which the transfected cells of the recipient were bone-marrow cells.[152] The technique resulted in only a low level of expression of the transfected class I antigen at the cell surface. Nonetheless, survival of the subsequent skin grafts was prolonged, though not indefinitely.[152] Since the isolation and subsequent reinfusion of bone marrow are already established methods in clinical medicine, the potential of this approach for application in humans is clear.

Because T-cell selection takes place in the thymus, investigators have proposed that the introduction of donor alloantigens directly into the thymic tissue of the recipient should be an effective way to induce tolerance.[153] If T cells maturing in the thymus could be brought into contact with the donor antigens, presumably those antigens should be recognized as 'self' and the clones reacting with those antigens should be deleted. This approach was first attempted by Posselt *et al.* using pancreatic islet tissue.[154] In their study, inoculation of pancreatic islet cells into the thymus of diabetic rats protected the islet tissue from rejection. The islet grafts also induced donor-specific tolerance to subsequent extrathymic allografts from the same strain. Further work by the same group and by others showed that the same effect can be obtained by intrathymic injection of lymphoid cells; indefinite ($>$300 days) cardiac allograft survival in rats has been achieved by this means.[155] Variants of this approach have included intrathymic inoculation with bone-marrow cells[156] and, in one kidney allograft model, glomeruli.[157] Knechtle *et al.* have combined intrathymic inoculation with the class I MHC transfection method described above; in their study, recipient myoblasts and myotubes were transfected with donor MHC class I antigen, then injected into the thymus. The recipient animals were tolerant of subsequent liver and cardiac allografts, but not tolerant of third-party grafts.[158] Finally, Oluwole *et al.* have demonstrated that even soluble antigens extracted from class I-bearing donor cells, when inoculated into the thymus, lead to indefinite allograft survival in rats.[159]

It was mentioned above that oral administration of an antigen may induce tolerance in murine models. There has been considerable interest recently in the potential of this approach for the control of autoimmune disease. Animal studies which show the potential of this technique have included such examples as feeding Lewis rats myelin basic protein to prevent experimental autoimmune encephalomyelitis[160] and feeding type II collagen to prevent adjuvant arthritis.[161] The same method has now been applied to MHC antigens. Sayegh *et al.* developed a model of rejection in which a skin graft, transplanted between rat strains, activated the immune response and led to rejection of a subsequent cardiac graft. If the recipient was fed allogeneic MHC peptides at the time of the skin graft, the survival of the subsequent cardiac graft was prolonged.[162]

In some of the models described above, the tolerant state which is induced is long-lasting, and persists beyond the expected survival of peripheral leukocytes. Indeed, the human clinical model of blood transfusion is one such example; the beneficial effect has been documented in patients who were transplanted more than two years after the transfusion.[121] Since new T cells continue to be made and to mature throughout the life of a patient, persistent tolerance implies the persistent presence of the alloantigen. Presumably the only way that exogenous HLA antigens can persist in the recipient is by the establishment of allogeneic stem cells from the donor in the host – a state referred to as chimerism.[163] In transfused peripheral blood there are probably small numbers of hematopoietic precursors – perhaps enough to maintain the production of the allogeneic line in small quantity.[164]

Larger numbers of stem cells are present in harvested bone marrow, and it has long been recognized that bone-marrow transplantation would provide a means of guaranteeing allograft survival. In early models of this approach, recipients were prepared for transplantation by whole-body irradiation to destroy the host hemato-poietic system, followed by bone-marrow infusion from the organ donor.[165] Although this approach is effective in prolonging allograft survival, the recipient animals become nonspecifically immunosuppressed. Sachs[164] theorizes that this is due to the fact that the new, donor-derived T cells are selected in the thymus for recognition of antigen associated with recipient MHC (on the host's thymic epi-thelium) but then face exogenous antigen challenges (as during infection) in association with donor MHC (on the new, donor-derived antigen-presenting cells).

Sachs and his colleagues have therefore developed a murine model of 'mixed chimerism', in which bone-marrow infusion given after irradiation consists of a mixture of host and donor marrow.[166] Both the host and donor marrow are depleted of mature T cells before being infused into the recipient. The recipients of such marrow transplants form hematopoietic cell lineages from both the host and the donor. They accept allografts from the same strain as the donor marrow, but will reject third-party grafts. Since they have T cells, thymic epithelium and antigen-presenting cells all derived from the host, they exhibit normal immunocompetence toward foreign antigens.[167] A similar approach involves using a preparative regimen which does not completely ablate the host bone marrow, followed by donor marrow transplantation. The host marrow will subsequently recover, producing mixed chimerism without requiring total host marrow ablation.[168] Such an approach may be feasible clinically for the transplantation of some organs. The time interval between marrow recovery and the subsequent solid-organ transplant poses prob-lems for cardiac transplantation, since the donor heart cannot be preserved intact while the marrow is engrafted.

Sachs and his colleagues have taken the concept of mixed chimerism a step further, into the realm of xenotransplantation. Xenografting (the transplantation of organs from another species) has been a subject of longstanding interest in organ transplantation, because it represents a potential solution to the problem of donor availability. The immunologic barriers between species are even more formidable than those within a species. Two types of xenotransplantation barriers exist. Between similar species (such as chimpanzee and man) the antigenic differences are qualitatively similar to, though wider than, those seen within a species. Such species combinations are referred to as 'concordant'. More distant species (such as pig and man) are separated by an additional barrier. With such 'discordant' species combinations, preformed antibodies are found in the putative recipient (man) which react against the donor (pig) tissue, producing hyperacute rejection with rapid antibody-mediated necrosis of the graft.[169–171] These xenotransplantation barriers are not effectively breached by standard immunosuppression with agents like cyclosporine. However, they appear to be surmountable using the mixed chimerism approach. In studies of rat organ transplantation into mouse recipients (a concordant model), mixed chimerism has been achieved and led to host acceptance of the subsequent xenograft.[172] Discordant grafting using mixed chimerism is currently under investigation.

Xenografting presents the opportunity to use even more powerful approaches to alter antigen presentation. Recently, methods have been developed to manipulate the structure of genes in animals using a technique known as homologous recombination, or gene targeting. In this approach, cells derived from an animal embryo ('embryonic stem cells') are cultured *in vitro* under conditions which preserve their pluripotential character.[173] The gene of interest is cloned and modified (or disrupted) and then introduced into the cultured embryonic stem cells. A small but finite proportion of the cultured cells will execute a precise exchange of the new DNA for the native sequence ('homologous recombination'[174]). If the new DNA contains a selectable marker (such as the sequence for neomycin resistance), then the progeny colonies of stem cells may be screened for recombinants. Ultimately, each potential colony must be screened by DNA analysis to verify that the desired alteration has been achieved. Colonies which have been successfully modified may then be injected into developing blastocysts of the same species. Some proportion of the tissues of the progeny animals will be derived from the cultured cells and will carry the altered gene. If the tissues so derived include the germ line of the animal, then the mutation may be propagated from generation to generation.[175]

The animals used as sources of xenograft organs are potential targets for this new technology. In theory, the cell-surface molecules of a donor animal could be modified by homologous recombination so as to make the organs less antigenic. Considerable interest has focused on the use of gene targeting to overcome the hyperacute rejection seen with discordant xenografting. The pig in particular seems to be a suitable species for gene targeting in cardiac transplantation, because the porcine heart is anatomically similar to the human heart and because enough pigs could readily be bred to supply the recipient need.[176] The preformed antibodies against porcine tissue (which probably result from a cross-reaction of antibodies directed against resident bacterial flora in the human gastrointestinal tract) have come under recent study. Many of these antibodies appear to be directed against sugar residues complexed to various cell-surface proteins.[177] It has thus been proposed that targeted disruption of the glycosyltransferases which catalyze the glycosylation of porcine peptides might enable the resulting grafted organs to escape hyperacute rejection.[178]

Manipulation of antigen presentation to transplant recipients appears to be the most promising route to true graft tolerance. The ideal technique, which may combine more than one of the approaches described above, would be one which makes continued pharmacologic immunosuppression unnecessary. Such a technique would enable the organ recipient to accept the donor tissue as 'self' without compromising the immunocompetence of the host in any way. If this goal can be achieved, an important barrier to the increased use of cardiac transplantation (and the transplantation of other organs) will have been overcome. Patients transplanted by such means will lead healthier lives with fewer complications, and perhaps longer lives as well.

Summary

Modern molecular biology has made possible important advances in organ transplantation, most notably in the development of new approaches to immunosuppression. Cyclosporine, FK-506 and rapamycin are in current clinical use or in clinical trials. The mechanisms of their immunosuppressive actions continue to be studied. Each of the three agents binds to an intracellular ligand. In the case of cyclosporine and FK-506, the drug–ligand complex then binds to a protein phosphatase called calcineurin. Calcineurin binding inactivates the phosphatase; this inhibition prevents an important transcription factor ($NFAT_p$) from moving to the nucleus from the cytoplasm. $NFAT_p$ is part of a complex required for the transcription of IL-2, the main cytokine responsible for T-cell activation. Rapamycin, though it binds to the same intracellular ligand as FK506, has a different mechanism of action; its target has not yet been identified.

Antilymphocyte antibodies are also an important part of the therapeutic armamentarium in transplantation, and are used mainly to treat serious episodes of rejection. Antibodies of increasing specificity and sophistication have gradually been developed. Some target particular lymphocyte subsets (such as $CD3^+$ or $CD4^+$ cells). Some target cell surface molecules known to play a specific role in immune activation (such as the IL-2 receptor or costimulatory adhesion molecules). The antibodies themselves have been modified to reduce their own antigenicity or to link them to toxins to increase their efficacy.

Methods to alter the immune response by manipulating antigen presentation are the subject of intensive research. It has been shown that blood transfusions before organ transplantation can reduce rejection and improve graft survival. Studies of this phenomenon suggest that the mode of introducing foreign HLA antigens to a host may have a significant impact on whether immune activation or tolerance is the result. In animal models, recipient lymphoid cells transfected with donor antigens can induce tolerance, as can donor-cell injection into the thymus. Even cell-free peptides derived from HLA antigens may induce tolerance when injected into the thymus or administered orally. Long-term tolerance, which requires the persistence of the foreign antigen, can be induced by introduction of donor hematopoietic stem cells (bone-marrow transplantation). Such marrow grafts lead to a state of chimerism in which the host produces donor-derived T cells. The recipient's marrow may be ablated with chemo- and radiotherapy, but some studies suggest that it is desirable to ensure that some host marrow persists ('mixed chimerism'). Xenografting may offer an even wider range of possibilities for tolerance induction. Mixed chimeras may be created across species lines. Animal xenograft donors are also being genetically modified using gene targeting to reduce the antigenicity of their organs, making them more suitable for transplantation into a foreign host. The ideal approach to true graft tolerance has not yet been identified, but the many methods now under study will likely lead to improved clinical immunologic management in the near future.

References

1. *1993 Annual Report of the U.S. Scientific Registry for Transplant Recipients and the Organ Procurement and Transplantation Network – Transplant Data: 1988–1991.* UNOS, Richmond, VA, and the Division of Organ Transplantation, Bureau of Health Resources Development, Health Resources and Services Administration, U.S. Department of Health and Human Services, Bethesda, MD.
2. 24th Bethesda Conference: Cardiac Transplantation (1993). *J. Am. Coll. Cardiol.*, **22**, 1–64.
3. The Registry of the International Society for Heart and Lung Transplantation: Tenth Official Report (1993). *J. Heart Lung Transplant.*, **12**, 541–62.
4. Reitz, B. (1992) Heart and heart–lung transplantation. In: Braunwald, E. (ed.) *Heart Disease: A Textbook of Cardiovascular Medicine*, 4th edn, pp. 520–34. Philadelphia: W. B. Saunders.
5. Borel, J. F., Feurer, C., Gubler, H. U. and Stahelin, H. (1976) Biological effects of cyclosporin A: a new antilymphocyte agent. *Agents Actions*, **6**, 468–75.
6. Kahan, B. D. (1989) Drug therapy: cyclosporine. *N. Engl. J. Med.*, **321**, 1725–38.
7. Sigal, N. H. and Dumont, F. J. (1992) Cyclosporin A, FK-506, and rapamycin: pharmacologic probes of lymphocyte signal transduction. *Annu. Rev. Immunol.*, **10**, 519–60.
8. June, C. H., Ledbetter, J. A., Gillespie, M. M., *et al.* (1987) T-cell proliferation involving the CD28 pathway is associated with cyclosporin-resistant interleukin 2 gene expression. *Mol. Cell. Biol.*, **7**, 4472–81.
9. Lin, C. S., Boltz, R. C., Siekierka, J. J. and Sigal, N. H. (1991) FK-506 and cyclosporin A inhibit highly similar signal transduction pathways in human T lymphocytes. *Cell. Immunol.*, **133**, 269–84.
10. Kronke, M., Leonard, W. J., Depper, J. M. *et al.* (1984) Cyclosporin A inhibits T-cell growth factor gene expression at the level of mRNA transcription. *Proc. Natl Acad. Sci. USA*, **81**, 5214–18.
11. Herold, K. C., Lancki, D. W., Moldwin, R. L. and Fitch, F. W. (1986) Immunosuppressive effects of cyclosporin A on cloned T cells. *J. Immunol.*, **136**, 1315–21.
12. Hess, A. D. (1985) Effect of interleukin 2 on the action of cyclosporin. *Transplantation*, **39**, 62–8.
13. Kino, T., Hatanaka, H., Hashimoto, M. *et al.* (1987) FK-506, a novel immunosuppressant isolated from a *Streptomyces*. I. Fermentation, isolation, physico-chemical and biological characteristics. *J. Antibiot.*, **40**, 1249–55.
14. Tocci, M. J., Matkovich, D. A., Collier, K. A. *et al.* (1989) The immunosuppressant FK506 selectively inhibits expression of early T cell activation genes. *J. Immunol.*, **143**, 718–26.
15. Johansson, A. and Moller, E. (1990) Evidence that the immunosuppressive effects of FK506 and cyclosporine are identical. *Transplantation*, **50**, 1001–7.
16. Calne, R. Y., Lim, S., Samaan, A. *et al.* (1989) Rapamycin for immunosuppression in organ allografting. *Lancet*, **ii**, 227.
17. Morris, R. E. (1992) Rapamycins: antifungal, antitumor, antiproliferative, and immunosuppressive macrolides. *Transplant. Rev.*, **6**, 39–87.
18. Kay, J. E., Kromwel, L., Doe, S. E. A. and Denyer, M. (1991) Inhibition of T and B lymphocyte proliferation by rapamycin. *Immunology*, **72**, 544–9.

19. Dumont, F. J., Staruch, M. J., Koprak, S. L. *et al.* (1990) Distinct mechanisms of suppression of murine T cell activation by the related macrolides FK-506 and rapamycin. *J. Immunol.*, **144**, 251–8.
20. Handschumacher, R. E., Harding, M. W., Rice, J. *et al.* (1984) Cyclophilin. A specific cytosolic binding protein for cyclosporin A. *Science*, **226**, 544–7.
21. Walsh, C. T., Zydowsky, L. D. and McKeon, F. D. (1992) Cyclosporin A, the cyclophilin class of peptidylprolyl isomerases, and blockade of T cell signal transduction. *J. Biol. Chem.*, **267**, 13115–18.
22. Wiederrecht, G., Lam, E., Hung, S. *et al.* (1993) The mechanism of action of FK-506 and cyclosporin A. In: Allison, A. C., Lafferty, K. J. and Fliri, H. (eds) Immunosuppressive and Antiinflammatory Drugs. *Ann. NY Acad. Sci.*, **696**, pp. 9–19. New York: New York Academy of Sciences.
23. Siekierka, J. J., Hung, S. H., Poe, M. *et al.* (1989) A cytosolic binding protein for the immunosuppressant FK506 has peptidyl-prolyl isomerase activity but is distinct from cyclophilin. *Nature*, **341**, 755–7.
24. Harding, M. W., Galat, A., Uehling, D. E. and Schreiber, S. L. (1989) A receptor for the immunosuppressant FK506 is a *cis–trans* peptidyl-prolyl isomerase. *Nature*, **341**, 758–60.
25. Bierer, B. E., Mattila, P. S., Standaert, R. F. *et al.* (1990) Two distinct signal transmission pathways in T lymphocytes are inhibited by complexes formed between an immunophilin and either FK-506 or rapamycin. *Proc. Natl Acad. Sci. USA*, **87**, 9231–5.
26. Fischer, G., Wittman-Liebold, B., Lang, K. *et al.* (1989) Cyclophilin and peptidyl-prolyl *cis–trans* isomerase are probably identical proteins. *Nature*, **337**, 476–8.
27. Harding, M. W., Galat, A., Uehling, D. E. and Schreiber, S. L. (1989) A receptor for the immunosuppressant FK506 is a *cis–trans* peptidyl-prolyl isomerase. *Nature*, **341**, 758–60.
28. Bierer, B. E., Hollander, G., Fruman, D. and Burakoff, S. J. (1992) Cyclosporin A and FK506: molecular mechanisms of immunosuppression and probes for transplantation biology. *Curr. Opin. Immunol.*, **5**, 763–73.
29. Bierer, B. E., Somers, P. K., Wandless, R. J. *et al.* (1990) Probing immunosuppressant action with a nonnatural immunophilin ligand. *Science*, **250**, 556–8.
30. Liu, J., Farmer, J. D. J., Lane, W. S. *et al.* (1991) Calcineurin is a common target of cyclophilin–cyclosporin A and FKBP–FK506 complexes. *Cell*, **66**, 807–15.
31. Liu, J., Albers, M. W., Wandless, T. J. *et al.* (1992) Inhibition of T cell signalling by immunophilin–ligand complexes correlates with loss of calcineurin phosphatase activity. *Biochemistry*, **31**, 3896–901.
32. Clipstone, N. A. and Crabtree, G. R. (1992) Identification of calcineurin as a key signalling enzyme in T-lymphocyte activation. *Nature*, **357**, 695–7.
33. O'Keefe, S. J., Tamura, J., Kincaid, R. L. *et al.* (1992) FK-506- and CsA-sensitive activation of the interleukin-2 promoter by calcineurin. *Nature*, **357**, 692–4.
34. Ullman, K. S., Northrop, J. P., Verweij, C. L. and Crabtree, G. R. (1990) Transmission of signals from the T lymphocyte antigen receptor to the genes responsible for cell proliferation and immune function: the missing link. *Annu. Rev. Immunol.*, **8**, 421–52.
35. Flanagan, W. M., Corthesy, B., Bram, R. J. and Crabtree, G. R. (1991) Nuclear association of a T-cell transcription factor blocked by FK-506 and cyclosporine A. *Nature*, **352**, 803–7.
36. Jain, J., McCaffrey, P. G., Valge-Arthur, V. E. and Rao, A. (1992) Nuclear factor of activated T-cells contains *fos* and *jun*. *Nature*, **356**, 801–4.
37. McCaffrey, P. G., Perrino, B. A., Soderling, T. R. and Rao, A. (1993) NF-ATp, a T lymphocyte DNA-binding protein that is a target for calcineurin and immunosuppressive drugs. *J. Biol. Chem.*, **268**, 3747–52.
38. Woodruff, M. F. A. and Anderson, N. A. (1963) Effect of lymphocyte depletion by thoracic duct fistula and administration of anti-lymphocyte serum on survival of skin homografts in rats. *Nature*, **200**, 702.
39. Monaco, A..P., Abbott, W. M., Othersen, H. B. *et al.* (1966) Antiserum to lymphocytes: prolonged survival of canine renal allografts. *Science*, **153**, 1264–7.

40. Starzl, T. E., Marchioro, T. L., Porter, K. A. *et al.* (1967) The use of heterologous antilymphoid agents in canine renal and liver homotransplantation and in human renal homotransplantation. *Surg. Gynecol. Obstet.*, **124**, 301–8.
41. Starzl, T. E. (1968) Current concepts. Heterologous antilymphocyte globulin. *N. Engl. J. Med.*, **279**, 700–3.
42. Sheil, A. G. R., Kelly, G. E., Storey, B. G. *et al.* (1971) Controlled clinical trial of antilymphocyte globulin in patients with renal allografts from cadaver donors. *Lancet*, **ii**, 359–63.
43. Najarian, J. S. and Simmons, R. L. (1971) The clinical use of antilymphocyte globulin. *N. Engl. J. Med.*, **285**, 158–66.
44. Monaco, A. P. and Codish, S. D. (1976) Survey of the current status of the clinical use of antilymphocyte serum. *Surg. Gynecol. Obstet.*, **142**, 417–26.
45. Griepp, R. B., Stinson, E. B., Bieber, C. P. *et al.* (1977) Increasing patient survival following heart transplantation. *Transplant. Proc.*, **9**, 197–201.
46. Najarian, J. S., Simmons, R. L., Condie, R. M. *et al.* (1976) Seven years' experience with antilymphoblast globulin for renal transplantation from cadaver donors. *Ann. Surg.*, **184**, 352–68.
47. Kawaguchi, A., Szentpetery, S., Mohanakumar, T. *et al.* (1987) Effects of prophylactic rabbit antithymocyte globulin in cardiac allograft recipients treated with cyclosporine. *J. Heart Transplant.*, **6**, 214–17.
48. Kormos, R. L., Herlan, D. B., Armitage, J. M. *et al.* (1990) Monoclonal versus polyclonal antibody therapy for prophylaxis against rejection after heart transplantation. *J. Heart Transplant.*, **9**, 1–10.
49. Copeland, J. G., Icenogle, T. B., Williams, R. J. *et al.* (1990) Rabbit antithymocyte globulin. A 10-year experience in cardiac transplantation. *J. Thorac. Cardiovasc. Surg.*, **99**, 852–60.
50. McGiffin, D. C., Kirklin, J. K. and Naftel, D. C. (1985) Acute renal failure after heart transplantation and cyclosporine therapy. *J. Heart Transplant.*, **4**, 396–9.
51. Deeb, G. M., Kolff, J., McClurken, J. B. *et al.* (1987) Antithymocyte gamma globulin, low-dosage cyclosporine, and tapering steroids as an immunosuppressive regimen to avoid early kidney failure in heart transplantation. *J. Heart Transplant.*, **6**, 79–83.
52. Carey, J. A. and Frist, W. H. (1990) Use of polyclonal antilymphocytic preparations for prophylaxis in heart transplantation. *J. Heart Transplant.*, **9**, 297–300.
53. Shield, C. F., Cosimi, A. B., Tolkoff- Rubin, N. *et al.* (1979) Use of antithymocyte globulin for reversal of acute allograft rejection. *Transplantation*, **28**, 461–4.
54. Norman, D. J. (1992) Antilymphocyte antibodies in the treatment of allograft rejection: targets, mechanisms of action, monitoring, and efficacy. *Semin. Nephrol.*, **12**, 315–24.
55. Lance, E. M. and Medawar, P. B. (1970) Antilymphocyte serum and the induction of tolerance to transplantation antigens. *Fed. Proc.*, **29**, 151–2.
56. Cosimi, A. B., Burton, R. C., Colvin, R. B. *et al.* (1981) Treatment of acute renal allograft rejection with OKT3 monoclonal antibody. *Transplantation*, **32**, 535–9.
57. Ortho Multicenter Transplant Study Group (1985) A randomized clinical trial of OKT3 monoclonal antibody for acute rejection of cadaveric renal transplants. *N. Engl. J. Med.*, **313**, 337–42.
58. Chatenoud, L. and Bach, J-F. (1992) Selective immunosuppression with anti-T cell monoclonal antibodies. *Clin. Nephrol.*, **38** (Supp. 1), S53–S60.
59. Norman, D. J. (1993) Rationale for OKT3 monoclonal antibody treatment in transplant patients. *Transplant. Proc.*, **25** (Suppl 1), 1–3.
60. Renlund, D. G., O'Connell, J. B., Gilbert, E. M. *et al.* (1989) A prospective comparison of murine monoclonal CD-3 (OKT3) antibody-based and equine antithymocyte globulin-based rejection prophylaxis in cardiac transplantation. *Transplantation*, **47**, 599–605.
61. Laufer, G., Laczkowics, A., Wollenek, G. *et al.* (1989) Impacts of low-dose steroids and prophylactic monoclonal versus polyclonal antibodies on acute rejection in

cyclosporine- and azathioprine-immunosuppressed cardiac allografts. *J. Heart Transplant.*, **8**, 253–61.

62. Griffith, B. P., Kormos, R. L., Armitage, J. M. *et al.* (1990) Comparative trial of immunoprophylaxis with RATG versus OKT3. *J. Heart Transplant.*, **9**, 301–5.

63. Costanzo-Nordin, M. R., O'Sullivan, E. J., Johnson, M. R. *et al.* (1990) Prospective randomized trial of OKT3- versus horse antithymocyte globulin-based immunosuppressive prophylaxis in heart transplantation. *J. Heart Transplant.*, **9**, 306–15.

64. Frist, W. H., Merrill, W. H., Eastburn, T. E. *et al.* (1990) Unique antithymocyte serum versus OKT3 for induction immunotherapy after heart transplantation. *J. Heart Transplant.*, **9**, 489–94.

65. Kirklin, J. K., Bourge, R. C., White-Williams, C. *et al.* (1990) Prophylactic therapy for rejection after cardiac transplantation. A comparison of rabbit antithymocyte globulin and OKT3. *J. Thorac. Cardiovasc. Surg.*, **99**, 716–24.

66. Laske, A., Gallino, A., Schneider, J. *et al.* (1992) Prophylactic cytolytic therapy in heart transplantation: monoclonal versus polyclonal antibody therapy. *J. Heart Lung Transplant.*, **11**, 557–63.

67. Menkis, A. H., Powell, A.-M., Novick, R. J. *et al.* (1992) A prospective randomized controlled trial of initial immunosuppression with ALG versus OKT3 in recipients of cardiac allografts. *J. Heart Lung Transplant.*, **11**, 569–76.

68. Ladowski, J. S., Dillon, T., Schatzlein, M. H. *et al.* (1993) Prophylaxis of heart transplant rejection with either antithymocyte globulin-, Minnesota antilymphocyte globulin- or an OKT3-based protocol. *J. Cardiovasc. Surg.*, **34**, 135–140.

69. Kung, P. C., Goldstein, G., Reinherz, E. L. and Schlossman, S. F. (1979) Monoclonal antibodies defining distinctive human T cell surface antigens. *Science*, **206**, 347–9.

70. Chang, T. W., Kung, P. C., Gingras, S. P. and Goldstein, G. (1981) Does OKT3 monoclonal antibody react with an antigen-recognition structure on human T cells? *Proc. Natl Acad. Sci. USA*, **78**, 1805–8.

71. Reinherz, E. L., Meuer, S., Fitzgerald, K. A. *et al.* (1982) Antigen recognition by human T lymphocytes is linked to surface expression of the T3 molecular complex. *Cell*, **30**, 735–43.

72. Abbas, A. K., Lichtman, A. H. and Pober, J. S. (1994) Molecular basis of T cell antigen recognition and activation. In: *Cellular and Molecular Immunology*, 2nd edn, pp. 136–65. Philadelphia: W.B. Saunders.

73. Marrack, P. and Kappler, J. W. (1986) The antigen-specific, major histocompatibility complex-restricted receptor on T cells. *Adv. Immunol.*, **38**, 1–30.

74. Cosimi, A. B., Colvin, R. B., Burton, R. C. *et al.* (1981) Use of monoclonal antibodies to T-cell subsets for immunologic monitoring and treatment in recipients of renal allografts. *N. Engl. J. Med.*, **305**, 308–14.

75. Descamps-Latscha, B., Golub, R. M., Nguyen, A. T. and Feuillet-Fieux, M. N. (1983) Monoclonal antibodies against T cell differentiation antigens initiate stimulation of monocyte/macrophage oxidative metabolism. *J. Immunol.*, **131**, 2500–7.

76. Chatenoud, L., Baudrihaye, M. F., Kreis, H. *et al.* (1982) Human *in vivo* antigenic modulation induced by the anti-T cell OKT3 monoclonal antibody. *Eur. J. Immunol.*, **12**, 979–82.

77. Hirsch, R., Eckhaus, M., Auchincloss, H. *et al.* (1988) Effects of *in vivo* administration of anti-T3 monoclonal antibody on T cell function in mice. I. Immunosuppression of transplantation responses. *J. Immunol.*, **140**, 3766–72.

78. Van Wauwe, J. P., De May, J. R. and Goossens, J. G. (1980) OKT3: a monoclonal anti-human T lymphocyte antibody with potent mitogenic properties. *J. Immunol.*, **124**, 2708–13.

79. Chatenoud, L., Ferran, C., Reuter, A. *et al.* (1989) Systemic reaction to the monoclonal antibody OKT3 in relation to serum levels of tumor necrosis factor and interferon-γ. *N. Engl. J. Med.*, **320**, 1420–6.

80. Norman, D. J., Chatenoud, L., Cohen, D. *et al.* (1993) Consensus statement regarding OKT3-induced cytokine-release syndrome and human antimouse antibodies. *Transplant. Proc.*, **25** (Supp. 1), 89–92.

81. Land, W., Hillebrand, G., Illner, W. D. *et al.* (1988) First clinical experience with a new TCR/CD3-monoclonal antibody (BMA 031) in kidney transplant patients. *Transplant. Int.*, **1**, 116–17.

82. Frenken, L. A. M., Hoitsma, A. J., Tax, W. J. and Koene, R. A. (1991) Prophylactic use of anti-CD3 monoclonal antibody WT32 in kidney transplantation. *Transplant. Proc.*, **23**, 1072–3.

83. Waid, T. H., Lucas, B. A., Thompson, J. S. *et al.* (1992) Treatment of acute cellular rejection with T10B9.1A-31 or OKT3 in renal allograft recipients. *Transplantation*, **53**, 80–6.

84. Kirkman, R. L., Araujo, J. L., Busch, G. J. *et al.* (1983) Treatment of acute renal allograft rejection with monoclonal anti-T12 antibody. *Transplantation*, **36**, 620–6.

85. Dyer, M. J., Hale, G., Hayhoe, F. G. and Waldmann, H. (1989) Effects of CAMPATH-1 antibodies *in vivo* in patients with lymphoid malignancies: influence of antibody isotype. *Blood*, **73**, 1431–9.

86. Hale, G., Waldmann, H., Friend, P. and Calne, R. (1986) Pilot study of CAMPATH-1, a rat monoclonal antibody that fixes human complement, as an immunosuppressant in organ transplantation. *Transplantation*, **42**, 308–11.

87. Reinherz, E. L. and Schlossmann, S. F. (1980) The differentiation and function of human T lymphocytes. *Cell*, **19**, 821–9.

88. Shizuru, J. A., Alters, S. E. and Fathman, C. G. (1992) Anti-CD4 monoclonal antibodies in therapy: creation of nonclassical tolerance in the adult. *Immunol. Rev.*, **129**, 105–30.

89. Cosimu, A. B., Delmonico, F. L., Wright, J. K. *et al.* (1990) Prolonged survival of nonhuman primate renal allograft recipients treated only with anti-CD4 monoclonal antibody. *Surgery*, **108**, 406–14.

90. Shizuru, J. A., Seydel, K. B., Flavin, T. F. *et al.* (1990) Pre-transplant anti-CD4 monoclonal antibody therapy induces donor unresponsiveness to cardiac allografts in rat. *Transplantation*, **50**, 366–74.

91. Herbert, J. and Roser, B. (1988) Strategies of monoclonal antibody therapy that induce permanent tolerance of organ transplants. *Transplantation*, **46**, 128S–134S.

92. Carteron, N. L., Wofsy, D. and Seaman, W. E. (1988) Induction of immune tolerance during administration of monoclonal antibody to L3T4 does not depend on depletion of L3T4 cells. *J. Immunol.*, **140**, 713–16.

93. Chen, Z., Cobbold, S., Metcalfe, S. and Waldmann, H. (1992) Tolerance in the mouse to major histocompatibility complex-mismatched heart grafts, and to rat heart xenografts, using monoclonal antibodies to CD4 and CD8. *Eur. J. Immunol.*, **22**, 805–10.

94. Granstein, R. D., Goulston, C. and Gaulton, G. N. (1986) Prolongation of murine skin allograft survival by immunologic manipulation with anti-interleukin 2 receptor antibody. *J. Immunol.*, **136**, 898–902.

95. Reed, M. H., Shapiro, M. E., Strom, T. B. *et al.* (1988) Prolongation of primate renal allografts with anti-Tac monoclonal antibody. *Curr. Surg.*, **45**, 28–30.

96. Strom, T. B., Kelley, V. R., Murphy, J. R. *et al.* (1993) Interleukin-2 receptor-directed therapies: antibody- or cytokine-based targeting molecules. *Annu. Rev. Med.*, **44**, 343–53.

97. Soulillou, J-P., Cantarovich, D., Le Mauff, B. *et al.* (1990) Randomized controlled trial of a monoclonal antibody against the interleukin-2 receptor (33B3.1) as compared with rabbit antithymocyte globulin for prophylaxis against rejection of renal allografts. *N. Engl. J. Med.*, **322**, 1175–82.

98. Hynes, R. O. (1992) Integrins: versatility, modulation, and signalling in cell adhesion. *Cell*, **69**, 11–25.

99. Springer, T. A. (1990) Adhesion receptors of the immune system. *Nature*, **346**, 425–34.

100. Springer, T. A., Dustin, M. L., Kishimoto, T. K. and Marlin, S. D. (1987) The lymphocyte function associated LFA-1, CD2, and LFA-3 molecules: cell adhesion receptors of the immune system. *Annu. Rev. Immunol.*, **5**, 223–52.

101. Dustin, M. L., Rothlein, R., Bhan, A. K. *et al.* (1986) Induction by IL-1 and interferon-γ: tissue distribution, biochemistry, and function of a natural adherence molecule (ICAM-1). *J. Immunol.*, **137**, 245–54.

102. Marlin, S. D. and Springer, T. A. (1987) Purified intercellular adhesion molecule-1 (ICAM-1) is a ligand for lymphocyte function-associated antigen 1 (LFA-1). *Cell*, **51**, 813–19.

103. van Seventer, G. A., Shimizu, Y., Horgan, K. J. and Shaw, S. (1990) The LFA-1 ligand ICAM-1 provides an important costimulatory signal for T cell receptor-mediated activation of resting T cells. *J. Immunol.*, **144**, 4579–86.

104. Isobe, M., Yagita, H., Okumura, K. and Ihara, A. (1992) Specific acceptance of cardiac allograft after treatment with antibodies to ICAM-1 and LFA-1. *Science*, **255**, 1125–7.

105. Mueller, D. J., Jenkins, M. K. and Schwartz, R. H. (1989) Clonal expansion versus functional inactivation. *Annu. Rev. Immunol.*, **7**, 445–80.

106. Jaffers, G. J., Fuller, T. C., Cosimi, A. B. *et al.* (1986) Monoclonal antibody therapy: anti-idiotypic and non-anti-idiotypic antibodies to OKT3 arising despite intense immunosuppression. *Transplantation*, **41**, 572–5.

107. Bruggemann, M., Winter, G., Waldmann, H. and Neuberger, M. S. (1989) The immunogenicity of chimeric antibodies. *J. Exptl Med.*, **170**, 2153.

108. Woodle, E. S., Thistlethwaite, J. R., Jolliffe, L. K. *et al.* (1992) Humanized OKT3 antibodies: successful transfer of immune modulating properties and idiotype expression. *J. Immunol.*, **148**, 2756–63.

109. LoBuglio, A. F., Wheeler, R. H., Trang, J. *et al.* (1989) Mouse/human chimeric monoclonal antibody in man: kinetics and immune response. *Proc. Natl Acad. Sci. USA*, **86**, 4220–3.

110. Zou, Y. R., Gu, H. and Rajewsky, K. (1993) Generation of a mouse strain that produces immunoglobulin kappa chains with human constant regions. *Science*, **262**, 1271–4.

111. Ferran, C., Sheehan, C., Dy, M. *et al.* (1990) Cytokine related syndrome following injection of anti-CD3 monoclonal antibody: further evidence for transient *in vivo* T cell activation. *Eur. J. Immunol.*, **20**, 509–15.

112. Pastan, I., Willingham, M. C. and Fitzgerald, D. S. P. (1986) Immunotoxins. *Cell*, **47**, 641–8.

113. Olsnes, S., Sandrig, K., Petersen, O. W. and VanDews, B. (1989) Immunotoxins – entry into cells and mechanisms of action. *Immunol. Today*, **10**, 291–5.

114. Henslee, P. J., Byers, V. S., Jennings, C. D. *et al.* (1989) A new approach to the prevention of graft-versus-host disease using XomaZyme-H65 following histo-incompatible partially T-depleted marrow grafts. *Transplant. Proc.*, **21**, 3004–7.

115. LeMaistre, C. F., Meneghetti, C., Rosenblum, M. *et al.* (1992) Phase I trial of an interleukin-2 (IL-2) fusion toxin (DAB$_{486}$IL-2) in hematologic malignancies expressing the IL-2 receptor. *Blood*, **79**, 2547–54.

116. Kissmeyer-Nielsen, F., Olsen, S., Petersen, V. P. and Fjeldborg, O. (1966) Hyperacute rejection of kidney allografts, associated with pre-existing humoral antibodies against donor cells. *Lancet*, **ii**, 662–5.

117. Williams, G. M., Hume, D. M., Hudson, R. P. *et al.* (1968) 'Hyperacute' renal-homograft rejection in man. *N. Engl. J. Med.*, **279**, 611–18.

118. Opelz, G., Sengar, D. P. S., Mickey, M. R. and Terasaki, P. I. (1973) Effect of blood transfusions on subsequent kidney transplants. *Transplant. Proc.*, **5**, 253–9.

119. Salvatierra, O., Vincenti, F., Amend, W. *et al.* (1980) Deliberate donor-specific blood transfusions prior to living related renal transplantation: a new approach. *Ann. Surg.*, **192**, 543–52.

120. Opelz, G. (1987) Improved kidney graft survival in nontransfused recipients. *Transplant. Proc.*, **19**, 149–52.

121. Lagaaij, E. L., Hennemann, P. H., Ruigrok, M. *et al.* (1989) Effect of one-HLA-DR-antigen-matched and completely HLA-DR-mismatched blood transfusions on survival of heart and kidney allografts. *N. Engl. J. Med.*, **321**, 701–5.

122. Lazda, V. A., Pollak, R., Mozes, M. R. *et al* (1990) Evidence that HLA class II disparity is required for the induction of renal allograft enhancement by donor-specific blood transfusions in man. *Transplantation*, **49**, 1084–7.

123. van Twuyver, E., Mooijaart, R. J. D., ten Berge, I. J. M. *et al.* (1991) Pretransplantation blood transfusion revisited. *N. Engl. J. Med.*, **325**, 1210–13.

124. Takiff, H., Novak, M., Yin, L. *et al.* (1987) Examination of the clonal deletion hypothesis following transfusions in rat cardiac transplants. *Transplantation*, **43**, 145–51.

125. Wood, M. L. and Monaco, A. P. (1984) Induction of unresponsiveness to skin allografts in adult mice disparate at defined regions of the H-2 complex. *Transplantation*, **37**, 39–42.

126. Kast, W. M., van Twuyver, E., Mooijaart, R. J. D. *et al.* (1988) Mechanism of skin allograft enhancement across an H-2 class I mutant difference. Evidence for involvement of veto cells. *Eur. J. Immunol.*, **18**, 2105–8.

127. Heeg, K. and Wagner, H. (1990) Induction of peripheral tolerance to class I major histocompatibility complex (MHC) alloantigens in adult mice: transfused class I MHC-incompatible splenocytes veto clonal responses of antigen-reactive Lyt-2$^+$ T cells. *J. Exptl Med.*, **172**, 719–28.

128. Hutchinson, I. V. (1986) Suppressor T cells in allogeneic models. *Transplantation*, **41**, 547–55.

129. Shelby, J., Marushack, M. M. and Nelson, E. W. (1987) Prostaglandin production and suppressor cell induction in transfusion-induced immune suppression. *Transplantation*, **43**, 113–16.

130. Singal, D. P., Ludwin, D., Joseph, S. *et al.* (1986) Induction of anti-idiotypic antibodies by blood transfusions. *Transplantation*, **42**, 632–5.

131. Reed, E., Hardy, M., Benvenisty, A. *et al.* (1987) Effect of anti-idiotypic antibodies to HLA on graft survival in renal allograft recipients. *N. Engl. J. Med.*, **316**, 1450–5.

132. Abbas, A. K., Lichtman, A. H. and Pober, J. S. (1994) The major histocompatibility complex. In: *Cellular and Molecular Immunology*, 2nd edn, pp. 96–114. Philadelphia: W.B. Saunders.

133. Ploegh, H. L., Orr, H. T. and Strominger, J. L. (1981) Major histocompatibility antigens: the human (HLA-A, -B, -C) and murine (H-2K, H-2D) class I molecules. *Cell*, **24**, 287–99.

134. Germain, R. N. (1994) MHC-dependent antigen processing and peptide presentation: providing ligands for T lymphocyte activation. *Cell*, **76**, 287–99.

135. Falk, K., Rotzschke, O., Stevanovic, S. *et al.* (1991) Allele-specific motifs revealed by sequencing of self-peptides eluted from MHC molecules. *Nature*, **351**, 290–6.

136. Germain, R. N. (1986) The ins and outs of antigen processing and presentation. *Nature*, **322**, 687–9.

137. Kaufman, J. F., Auffray, C., Korman, A. J. *et al.* (1984) The class II molecules of the human and murine major histocompatibility complex. *Cell*, **36**, 1–13.

138. Rudensky, A., Preston, H. P., Hong, S. C. *et al.* (1991) Sequence analysis of peptides bound to MHC class II molecules. *Nature*, **353**, 622–7.

139. Davis, M. M. and Bjorkman, P. J. (1988) T-cell receptor antigen genes and T-cell recognition. *Nature*, 334, 395–402.

140. Blackman, M., Kappler, J. and Marrack, P. (1990) The role of the T cell receptor in positive and negative selection of developing T cells. *Science*, **248**, 1335–41.

141. von Boehmer, H. (1994) Positive selection of lymphocytes. *Cell*, **76**, 219–28.

142. Nossal, G. J. V. (1994) Negative selection of lymphocytes. *Cell*, **76**, 229–39.

143. Krensky, A. M., Weiss, A., Crabtree, G. *et al.* (1990) T-lymphocyte–antigen interactions in transplant rejection. *N. Engl. J. Med.*, **322**, 510–17.

144. Sherman, L. A. and Chattopadhyay, S. (1993) The molecular basis of allorecognition. *Annu. Rev. Immunol.*, **11**, 385–402.

145. Billingham, R. E., Brent, L. and Medawar, P. B. (1953) Actively acquired tolerance of foreign cells. *Nature*, **172**, 603–6.

146. Ptak, W., Rozycka, D., Askenase, P. W. and Gershon, R. K. (1980) Role of antigen-presenting cells in the development and persistence of contact hypersensitivity. *J. Exptl Med.*, **151**, 362–75.

147. Dixon, F. J. and Maurer, P. H. (1955) Immunologic unresponsiveness induced by protein antigens. *J. Exptl Med.*, **101**, 245–57.

148. Thomas, H. C. and Parrott, D. M. V. (1974) The induction of tolerance to a soluble protein antigen by oral administration. *Immunology*, **27**, 631–9.

149. Baird, M. A., Enosawa, S. and Heslop, B. F. (1992) Evidence that changes in expression of major histocompatibility complex antigens may underlie the immunosuppressive effect of heat-treated cells *in vivo* and *in vitro*. *Transplantation*, **53**, 1329–33.
150. Baird, M. A., Bradley, M. P. and Heslop, B. F. (1986) Prolonged survival of cardiac allografts in rats following administration of heat-treated donor lymphocytes. *Transplantation*, **42**, 1–7.
151. Madsen, J. C., Superina, R. A., Wood, K. J. and Morris, P. J. (1988) Immunological unresponsiveness induced by recipient cells transfected with donor MHC genes. *Nature*, **332**, 161–4.
152. Sykes, M., Sachs, D. H., Nienhuis, A. W. *et al.* (1993) Specific prolongation of skin graft survival following retroviral transduction of bone marrow with an allogeneic major histocompatibility complex gene. *Transplantation*, **55**, 197–202.
153. Jenkinson, E. J., Jhittay, P., Kingston, R. and Owen, J. J. T. (1985) Studies of the role of the thymic environment in the induction of tolerance to MHC antigens. *Transplantation*, **39**, 331–3.
154. Posselt, A. M., Barker, C. F., Tomaszewski, J. E. *et al* (1990) Induction of donor-specific unresponsiveness by intrathymic islet transplantation. *Science*, **249**, 1293–5.
155. Oluwole, S. F., Chowdhury, N. C. and Fawwaz, R. A. (1993) Induction of donor-specific unresponsiveness to rat cardiac allografts by intrathymic injection of UV-B-irradiated donor spleen cells. *Transplantation*, **55**, 1389–95.
156. Posselt, A. M., Odorico, J. S., Barker, C. F. and Naji, A. (1992) Promotion of pancreatic islet allograft survival by intrathymic transplantation of bone marrow. *Diabetes*, **41**, 771–5.
157. Remuzzi, G., Rossini, M., Imberti, O. and Perico, N. (1991) Kidney graft survival in rats without immunosuppressants after intrathymic glomerular transplantation. *Lancet*, **337**, 750–2.
158. Knechtle, S., Wang, J., Jiao, S. *et al.* (1994) Induction of specific tolerance by intrathymic injection of recipient muscle cells transfected with donor class I major histocompatibility complex. *Transplantation*, **57**, 990–6.
159. Oluwole, S. F., Chowdhury, N. C., Jin, M-X. and Hardy, M. A. (1993) Induction of transplantation tolerance to rat cardiac allografts by intrathymic inoculation of allogeneic soluble peptides. *Transplantation*, **56**, 1523–7.
160. Higgins, P. and Weiner, H. (1988) Suppression of experimental autoimmune encephalomyelitis by oral administration of myelin basic protein and its fragments. *J. Immunol.*, **140**, 440–5.
161. Zhang, Z. J., Lee, C. S. Y., Lider, O. and Weiner, H. L. (1990) Suppression of adjuvant arthritis in Lewis rats by oral administration of type II collagen. *J. Immunol.*, **145**, 2489–93.
162. Sayegh, M. H., Zhang, Z. J., Hancock, W. W. *et al.* (1992) Downregulation of the immune response to histocompatibility antigens and prevention of sensitization by skin allografts by orally administered alloantigen. *Transplantation*, **53**, 163–6.
163. McDaniel, D. O., Naftilan, J., Hulvey, K. *et al.* (1994) Peripheral blood chimerism in renal allograft recipients transfused with donor bone marrow. *Transplantation*, **57**, 852–6.
164. Sachs, D. H. (1991) Specific transplantation tolerance. *N. Engl. J. Med.*, **325**, 1240–2.
165. Rayfield, L. S. and Brent, L. (1983) Tolerance, immunocompetence, and secondary disease in fully allogeneic radiation chimeras. *Transplantation*, **36**, 183–9.
166. Ildstad, S. T. and Sachs, D. H. (1984) Reconstitution with syngeneic plus allogeneic or xenogeneic bone marrow leads to specific acceptance of allografts or xenografts. *Nature*, **307**, 168–70.
167. Sykes, M. and Sachs, D. H. (1988) Mixed allogeneic chimerism as an approach to transplantation tolerance. *Immunol. Today*, **9**, 23–7.
168. Sharabi, Y. and Sachs, D. H. (1989) Mixed chimerism and permanent specific transplantation tolerance induced by a nonlethal preparative regimen. *J. Exptl Med.*, **169**, 493–502.
169. Calne, R. Y. (1970) Organ transplantation between widely disparate species. *Transplant. Proc.*, **2**, 550–6.
170. Auchincloss, H. Jr. (1988) Xenogeneic transplantation: a review. *Transplantation*, **46**, 1–20.

171. Miyagawa, S., Hirose, H., Shirakura, R. *et al.* (1988) The mechanism of discordant xenograft rejection. *Transplantation*, **46**, 825–30.
172. Sharabi, Y., Aksentijevich, I., Sundt, T. M. *et al.* (1990) Specific tolerance induction across a xenogeneic barrier: production of mixed rat/mouse lymphohematopoietic chimeras using a nonlethal preparative regimen. *J. Exptl Med.*, **172**, 195–202.
173. Thomas, K. R. and Capecchi, M. R. (1987) Site-directed mutagenesis by gene targeting in mouse embryo-derived stem cells. *Cell*, **51**, 503–12.
174. Capecchi, M. R. (1989) Altering the genome by homologous recombination. *Science*, **244**, 1288–92.
175. Koller, B. H. and Smithies, O. (1992) Altering genes in animals by gene targeting. *Annu. Rev. Immunol.*, **10**, 785–807.
176. Sachs, D. H. (1994) The pig as a xenograft donor. *Pathol. Biol.*, **42**, 217–19.
177. Oriol, R., Ye, Y., Koren, E. and Cooper, D. K. (1993) Carbohydrate antigens of pig tissues reacting with human natural antibodies as potential targets for hyperacute vascular rejection in pig-to-man organ xenotransplantation. *Transplantation*, **56**, 1433–42.
178. Sandrin, M. S., Vaughan, H. A., Dabkowski, P. L. and McKenzie, I. F. (1993) Anti-pig IgM antibodies in human serum react predominantly with Gal(α 1–3) epitopes. *Proc. Natl Acad. Sci. USA*, **90**, 11391–5.

15

Gene and Cell-based Therapies for Myocardial Dysfunction

Mark W. Chang
Jeffrey M. Leiden

Introduction

Chronic congestive heart failure (CHF) remains a leading cause of cardiovascular morbidity and mortality in the United States. The disorder affects approximately four million Americans, is diagnosed in 10% of the population by the age of 75 years and is the leading cause of hospitalization in patients over the age of 65 years.[1] While recent studies have demonstrated that several newer pharmacologic agents, particularly the angiotensin-converting enzyme (ACE) inhibitors, can improve survival in this disease,[2–5] CHF continues to cause significant mortality. For example, in the CONSENSUS trial in which patients with severe (NYHA class IV) CHF were treated with either placebo or the ACE inhibitor, enalapril, patients who received enalapril had improved survival rates as compared to those who received placebo. However, the one-year mortality in the enalapril group was still almost 50%.[2] Similarly, patients with mild-to-moderate heart failure (NYHA functional classes I to III) and ejection fractions of <35% who received enalapril in the treatment arm of the Studies of Left Ventricular Dysfunction (SOLVD) trial fared better than those who received placebo, but still had a two-year mortality of nearly 20%.[4] It is also worth emphasizing that although a large number of inherited and acquired cardiovascular diseases can cause CHF, the poor prognosis associated with this syndrome has been consistently demonstrated in multiple trials and appears to be independent of its etiology.

   In recent years, major advances have been made in elucidating the cellular and molecular bases of a number of cardiovascular diseases, including CHF. Taken together, these advances have suggested several novel approaches to the treatment of myocardial dysfunction. Included among these are somatic gene therapy, the ability to introduce and express recombinant genes into nongerm-line cells of a recipient organism *in vivo*, and cellular cardiocyte transplantation, the implantation of normal or genetically modified myocytes into the myocardium *in vivo*. This review will summarize the recent progress in cardiovascular gene therapy and cellular transplantation with an emphasis on assessing the feasibility of these approaches for the treatment of CHF. We will first describe the recent methodologic advances concerning *in vivo* gene transfer into the heart. We will then discuss specific candidate genes that could be used for the prevention and treatment of CHF. These include: the dystrophin gene for the treatment of the cardiomyopathy associated with Duchenne muscular dystrophy; angiogenesis factor genes to program the growth of coronary collaterals in patients with chronic ischemic heart disease; the skeletal troponin C gene to reduce the sensitivity of cardiac myocytes to acute ischemic insults; and the β_2-adrenergic receptor to modify myocardial contractility. Finally, we will discuss the potential of cardiomyocyte transplantation as a novel cell-based therapy for CHF. The reader is referred to several recent reviews for additional discussions of gene therapy for cardiovascular disease.[6-9]

In vivo gene transfer into the heart – vector and delivery systems

The ability to introduce recombinant genes into cardiac myocytes *in vivo* is critically dependent upon the unique biologic features of these cells. Human cardiomyocytes are terminally differentiated cells which lack the ability to proliferate *in vivo* or *in vitro*.[10,11] Thus, *ex vivo* gene-transfer approaches that involve the removal of cardiac myocytes from the organism followed by *in vitro* gene transfer and reimplantation into the host are not feasible for cardiac gene transfer. Similarly, recombinant retroviruses cannot be used for *in vitro* or *in vivo* gene transfer into cardiac myocytes because these vectors require cell proliferation for successful gene transduction. Thus, the development of successful somatic gene therapy approaches involving cardiomyocytes must be used on *in vivo* gene-transfer technologies using vector and delivery systems capable of transducing nonproliferating cells. Two such approaches have been described in the last five years: direct DNA injection into the myocardium and the use of replication-defective adenovirus vectors, delivered either by direct intramyocardial injection or by catheter-mediated intracoronary artery infusion. The advantages and limitations of these two methods are discussed in detail below.

Direct injection of plasmid DNA into the myocardium

The direct injection of naked plasmid DNA into the myocardium represents a technically straightforward method for introducing recombinant genes into cardiac myocytes *in vivo*.[12] Wolff and Felgner were the first to demonstrate the feasibility of *in vivo* gene transfer into skeletal myocytes by direct DNA injection. Their initial work showed that intramuscular injection of plasmid DNA resulted in the uptake and expression of the recombinant DNA by a small percentage of myocytes immediately surrounding the injection site.[13] Subsequent studies demonstrated that cardiac myocytes are also capable of expressing a variety of reporter genes directly injected into myocardium, and that the efficiency of expression in cardiac muscle following direct injection is even greater than that of skeletal myofibers.[14–16] Successful gene transfer into cardiac myocytes using direct DNA injection has now been demonstrated in a number of species, including rats,[14–16] rabbits and pigs.[17]

Direct DNA injection has several advantages as a method of *in vivo* gene transfer into the heart. It is technically simple and utilizes noninfectious, plasmid-based eukaryotic expression vectors which can be easily prepared in large quantities. The delivery system itself limits gene expression to the myocyte. No recombinant gene expression has been observed in nonmyocytic cells in the heart or elsewhere in the organism following direct DNA injection into the heart. In addition, recombinant gene expression following direct DNA injection is relatively long-lived. Although levels of recombinant gene expression reach a peak 7–20 days after injection, persistent gene expression has been observed for as long as eight months after DNA injection in the rat heart.[12] Finally, the injected DNA is maintained as a circular episome. Thus, there is little risk of insertional mutagenesis.

Despite these advantages, the use of direct DNA injection for human therapy has thus far been limited by two important problems. First, the efficiency of *in vivo* gene transfer following direct DNA injection is quite low. Less than 1% of the cardiomyocytes adjacent to the injection site take up and express the injected DNA. Second, DNA injection is associated with a mild-to-moderate mononuclear cell inflammatory response, which in some cases leads to myocyte necrosis and myocardial fibrosis in the area of injection.[12] Although this inflammatory response can be limited by the careful preparation of the plasmid DNA, the arrhythmogenic potential of this response must be carefully assessed prior to human therapy.

Little is known about the mechanism of uptake of the injected DNA by cardiac myocytes. The ability to take up and express recombinant genes following the direct injection of plasmid DNA is limited to skeletal and cardiac muscle,[15] suggesting that striated muscle cells have unique features that may be important for DNA uptake and expression *in vivo*. Current hypotheses include a role for muscle-specific transport systems such as the T-tubules or a unique capacity of these cells to survive transient sarcolemmal disruption during plasmid DNA injection. It will be particularly important to better understand the mechanism of DNA uptake and to improve the efficiency of gene transfer following direct DNA injection in order to extend the feasibility of this approach for the treatment of human myocardial dysfunction.

In addition to its potential usefulness for somatic gene therapy, the direct injection of plasmid DNA is a useful method for studying cardiac gene transcription *in vivo*. For example, Leinwand and coworkers demonstrated that transcriptional regulatory elements injected directly into the heart are regulated in a tissue-specific fashion, and respond appropriately to thyroid hormone *in vivo*.[16] Leiden and coworkers[18] used the technique to define the *cis*-acting sequences regulating cardiac-specific expression of the slow/cardiac troponin C gene (*cTnC*). Thus, direct DNA injection may be particularly useful for studies of altered gene expression during the development and progression of CHF. For example, it should be possible to determine the changes in cardiac-specific transcription that occur in response to specific physiologic manipulations (e.g. pressure or volume overload) during the development of hypertrophy and subsequent systolic dysfunction by directly injecting transcriptional reporter constructs into animal hearts prior to specific physiologic manipulations. This method is much simpler, more economical, and less time consuming than the generation of transgenic animals. It is also more physiologically relevant than transient transfections of cultured fetal or neonatal cardiac myocytes which are known to lose their differentiated phenotypes when cultured *in vitro*.

Replication-defective adenoviruses for *in vivo* gene transfer into cardiac myocytes

Recent studies have shown that replication-defective adenoviruses represent a useful vector system for programming therapeutic levels of recombinant proteins in the myocardium. Adenoviruses are double-stranded linear DNA viruses which cause respiratory tract infections in humans. The adenovirus genome is a 36 kD DNA molecule which is divided evenly into 100 map units (mu). Adenoviruses are particularly well suited for cardiomyocyte gene transfer because, unlike retroviruses, they efficiently infect nonreplicating cells such as cardiac myocytes both *in vitro* and *in vivo*. Moreover, unlike retroviruses, which can be produced at titers of 10^5–10^6 pfu ml^{-1}, replication-defective adenovirus vectors can be produced in titers of 10^{10}–10^{11} pfu ml^{-1}. Thus, efficient *in vivo* gene transfer can be effected by the administration of relatively small volumes of virus. Replication-defective adenovirus vectors also have the advantage of being able to accommodate cDNA or genome inserts of at least to 7–9 kb. Finally, adenovirus vectors display a relatively favorable safety profile; they do not integrate into the host genome and have not been associated with human malignancies. Moreover, wild-type adenoviruses have been used safely to vaccinate large numbers of military recruits.

The majority of the adenovirus vectors used for *in vivo* gene transfer experiments have been derived from adenovirus serotypes 2 (Ad2) and 5 (Ad5), both of which are minimally pathogenic for humans.[19] These viruses have been made replication-defective by deletion of the E1 region (mu 1–9), which encodes two early transcriptional regulatory proteins (E1A and E1B) that are required for the induction of the viral lytic cycle and for the capacity of adenoviruses to transform cells *in vitro*. In addition to the E1 deletion, many of the first-generation adenovirus vectors contain a deletion of the nonessential E3 region of the viral genome (mu 78.5–84.7) in order to allow for the incorporation of larger cDNA or genomic inserts.[20] Because they are rendered replication-defective, these adenoviruses can only be propagated by infection of a permissive cell line such as 293 human embryonic kidney cells which stably express the adenovirus E1 proteins in *trans*. Following *in vivo* administration, these viruses are able to efficiently infect a wide variety of rodent and human cells. However, because these normal cells lack the E1 gene products, they are nonpermissive for replication of the E1-deleted adenovirus vectors thus preventing either persistent or generalized infections of the host.

Recent studies from several groups have demonstrated that replication-defective adenoviruses can be used to efficiently program recombinant gene expression in cardiac myocytes from a variety of mammalian species. Stratford-Perricaudet and coworkers[21] reported that simple intravenous injection of replication defective adenovirus into neonatal mice resulted in stable, low efficiency (1–2%) recombinant gene expression in cardiac myocytes. More recently, Leinwand and colleagues have reported efficient *in vivo* gene transfer into cardiac myocytes in rats following direct intramyocardial injection of virus. Recombinant gene expression was seen in up to 15% of the cardiomyocytes adjacent to the area of injection in these experiments.[22] Leiden and coworkers reported that a single intracoronary infusion of 10^{10} pfu of replication-defective adenovirus in adult rabbits results in recombinant gene expression in 30–60% of cardiac myocytes in the area of distribution of the infused coronary artery.[23] This result is important from a therapeutic perspective, because it suggests that it will be possible to use catheter-mediated adenovirus infusions to program efficient recombinant gene expression in large, but localized areas of myocardium.

Despite the relatively high efficiency of *in vivo* gene transfer into the myocardium observed with replication-defective adenovirus vectors, the feasibility of using these vectors for the somatic gene therapy of human myocardial dysfunction is currently limited by two important biological problems. First, adenovirus-mediated recombinant gene expression in the heart (and most other organs) is short lived in adult immunocompetent animals.[21,23] Leiden and coworkers showed that recombinant gene expression in cardiac myocytes declines rapidly two weeks after viral administration and is undetectable in the majority of animals two months after intracoronary adenovirus infusion. Similar transient recombinant gene expression has been observed by a number of groups in liver, skeletal muscle, and joint following *in vivo* administration of the first generation of adenovirus vectors.[21–28] Recent studies have suggested that the transient nature of recombinant gene expression seen after adenovirus-mediated *in vivo* gene transfer in adult immunocompetent animals is due to a CD8[+] cytotoxic T-cell response directed against late viral proteins produced by the adenovirus infected cells *in vivo*. The strongest evidence in support of this model is the observation that in contrast to the transient recombinant gene expression seen in immunocompetent hosts, the first generation adenoviruses produce stable recombinant gene expression in a variety of organs in immunocompromised SCID, nude, and class I MHC-deficient and RAG-2-deficient mice, each of which lack a normal CD8[+] CTL response.[25,29] This finding is important because it suggests that adenovirus vectors will be capable of producing stable recombinant gene expression *in vivo* if it is possible to circumvent the host immune response. Current studies are focused on developing a new generation of vectors and/or immunosuppressive regimens that will decrease the immunogenicity of the adenovirus vectors *in vivo*, and thereby allow long-term recombinant gene expression in the heart and other organs.

The use of replication-defective adenovirus vectors for the treatment of human myocardial diseases is also currently limited by our ability to restrict recombinant gene expression to the heart. Intravenous or intracoronary artery infusions of virus result in the infection of many organs including liver, spleen, kidney, lung, brain and testis in addition to the heart. There are at least two approaches which could be used to localize recombinant gene expression to the heart following the intracoronary administration of these vectors. First, it may be possible to develop a local delivery system which prevents the spread of virus into the systemic circulation. Secondly, cardiac-specific transcriptional regulatory elements could be used to control the expression of the recombinant gene in the adenovirus vector, thereby restricting recombinant gene expression to the heart following intracoronary virus infusions.

In summary, replication-defective adenovirus vectors display two important advantages as compared to direct DNA injection for the somatic gene therapy of myocardial dysfunction: (1) they program 50–100-fold more efficient *in vivo* gene transfer into cardiac myocytes; and (2) they can be delivered to relatively large areas of the myocardium by intracoronary infusion, thereby avoiding the need for multiple intramyocardial injections. However, before these vectors can be used for the therapy of human myocardial disease, it will be necessary to construct a new generation of vectors (or immunosuppressive regimens) which will produce stable recombinant gene expression *in vivo* and to develop novel delivery systems or transcriptional regulatory elements which will restrict recombinant gene expression to the heart following intravascular virus infusions.

Candidate genes for the therapy of CHF

The feasibility of developing somatic gene therapies for CHF depends both upon an efficient *in vivo* delivery system and upon the availability of appropriate candidate genes to prevent the onset of CHF or to treat the systolic or diastolic dysfunction associated with most of the inherited or acquired cardiomyopathies. In considering candidate genes for the somatic gene therapy of CHF, it is useful to divide the cardiomyopathies into several distinct groups. First, there are the relatively rare inherited recessive disorders in which the mutation or deletion of a single gene leads directly or indirectly to myocardial dysfunction. In these diseases, the ultimate goal of gene therapy would be to correct the genetic defect by the introduction of a normal gene into a significant fraction of diseased cardiomyocytes. The cardiomyo-pathy associated with Duchenne muscular dystrophy is an example of such a single-gene disorder that is discussed below.

The second, and much more common group of cardiomyopathies are acquired or multigenic. Of these, approximately half are due to chronic ischemic heart disease. In a significant proportion of patients with nonischemic etiologies, termed 'idio-pathic', the specific cause is unknown. In the remainder of cases, underlying structural abnormalities such as valvular heart disease or direct toxic damage to the myocardium, such as that resulting from alcohol, nutritional deficiencies or viral infections are identified as the cause. Somatic gene therapy for the acquired forms of CHF can be approached in two ways. Ideally, the therapeutic gene or genes would be delivered sufficiently early to alter the natural course of the underlying disease and to thereby prevent myocardial damage and/or the progression to a dilated cardiomyopathy. In the remainder of patients in whom myocardial damage has already occurred, gene therapy would be directed toward improving the contractile function of the failing myocardium. Specific examples of each of these two ap-proaches are discussed below. It should be emphasized that these examples are by no means comprehensive, and, instead were chosen to illustrate a number of possible approaches to the gene therapy of CHF. Rapid progress in understanding the molecular and cellular biology of normal and abnormal cardiac function should lead to the identification of novel candidate genes and approaches to this problem.

Gene therapy for the cardiomyopathy of Duchenne muscular dystrophy

Duchenne muscular dystrophy (DMD) is an example of a single-gene inherited cardiomyopathy that might be amenable to somatic gene therapy. DMD is an X-linked, progressive, and fatal myopathy that affects approximately 1 in 3500 newborn males. While symptoms of proximal skeletal weakness dominate the clinical picture early in life, the disease progresses to affect distal muscles, then respiratory muscles with inevitable respiratory failure and death by the third decade of life.[30] DMD is also characterized by a cardiomyopathy that represents a significant cause of morbidity and mortality in these patients.[31] Evidence of cardiac involvement in the early stages of the disease is limited to changes on the surface electrocardiogram, but sinus tachycardia, conduction abnormalities and atrial arrhythmias can develop later in the course of the disease. Rapidly progressive congestive heart failure and severe ventricular arrhythmias may develop and lead to sudden death in some patients.[32] Histologically, DMD is characterized by active myocyte degeneration. In the heart, degenerative fibers can be seen in both the atria and ventricles,[31,32] but the His–Purkinje cells appear to be particularly affected.[33]

Duchenne muscular dystrophy is caused by mutations and deletions in the dystrophin gene located at Xp21.[34] This gene encodes a 427-kD protein that is expressed in skeletal, cardiac and smooth muscle and in the central nervous system. The function of dystrophin remains unknown. However, it has been suggested that dystrophin in association with a membrane-spanning glycoprotein complex may reinforce the sarcolemma during mechanical stresses such as contraction. Alternatively, it has been postulated that the dystrophin–glycoprotein complex is involved in the maintenance of the transmembrane Ca^{2+} gradient and that the increased susceptibility of dystrophic myocytes to rupture from mechanical stress may be due to abnormally functioning Ca^{2+} channels.

Recent transgenic studies in the murine *mdx* model of DMD have suggested that both the skeletal and cardiac myopathies of DMD can be effectively treated by expression of dystrophin in skeletal and cardiac myocytes *in vivo*. Thus, *mdx* mice overexpressing a dystrophin transgene under the control of the murine muscle creatine kinase promoter/enhancer showed no clinical or histologic evidence of myopathy.[35] Importantly, it was shown that levels of dystrophin 50-fold higher than those found in normal mice had no adverse effects *in vivo*. Several groups have reported that it is possible to express dystrophin in murine skeletal myocytes *in vivo* following either direct DNA injection of plasmid expression vectors containing a dystrophin cDNA or intramuscular injection of replication-defective adenovirus vectors encoding a dystrophin minigene. Acsadi *et al.*[36] used direct intramuscular injection of plasmid DNA encoding the full-length dystrophin cDNA in *mdx* mouse muscle and demonstrated expression of dystrophin in approximately 1% of the skeletal myofibers in the area of injection. Stratford-Perricaudet and coworkers[37] reported that intramuscular injection of 2.5×10^9 pfu of a recombinant, replication-defective adenovirus containing a dystrophin minigene under the control of the Rous sarcoma virus (RSV) long terminal repeat (LTR) into neonatal *mdx* mice resulted in recombinant dystrophin gene expression in 6–50% of skeletal myocytes in the area of injection for periods of up to three months. Although promising, the feasibility of both of these local approaches for the treatment of DMD is limited by the fact that they cannot be used to program dystrophin expression in the large number of skeletal and cardiac muscles *in vivo*. In addition, the efficiency of *in vivo* gene transfer associated with direct DNA injections is too low to allow even effective local therapy. Thus, the ability to successfully treat both the skeletal and cardiac myopathies of DMD will almost certainly depend on the development of gene-delivery systems that will allow efficient dystrophin gene transfer into large areas of skeletal and cardiac muscle following intravascular delivery. In this regard, the recent studies of Leiden and coworkers demonstrating efficient *in vivo* gene transfer into large areas of rabbit myocardium following intracoronary infusions of replication-defective adenoviruses suggest that catheter-mediated intracoronary delivery of replication-defective adenoviruses encoding dystrophin may represent a feasible approach for the treatment of the cardiomyopathy associated with DMD. Studies to assess the feasibility of intra-arterial delivery of adenovirus vectors to skeletal muscle are ongoing in a number of laboratories.

Gene therapy of ischemic cardiomyopathies

Coronary artery disease (CAD) is an etiologic factor in 40–75% of patients presenting with signs and symptoms of CHF.[38] CAD precipitates CHF either by causing sufficient myocyte necrosis to impair left-ventricular contractile function, or by causing the contractile dysfunction of viable myocytes due to chronic ischemia, a disorder termed 'ischemic cardiomyopathy'. Below, we will discuss two specific gene-therapy approaches for the prevention of CHF due to ischemic heart disease.

Myocardial angiogenesis

Numerous studies in animals and humans have demonstrated that an effective coronary collateral circulation can preserve myocardial structure and function, and even prevent myocardial infarction following the occlusion of a large epicardial coronary artery.[39] Clinical studies have shown that the presence of collateral vessels is associated with greater viability of the myocardium in the setting of acute infarction,[40] preservation of overall ejection fraction postinfarction[41] and reduction in the incidence of left-ventricular aneurysm formation following acute infarction and failed thrombolysis.[42] These studies suggest that the ability to promote collateralization in regions of ischemic myocardium could prove useful for the treatment of patients with severe CAD.

Genes encoding a large number of diffusible angiogenic factors have now been identified and cloned.[43] Furthermore, recent studies have demonstrated that intravascular and intracoronary infusions of two angiogenesis factors, basic fibroblast growth factor[44,45] and vascular endothelial growth factor,[46] result in increased collateral blood flow to ischemic myocardium. The availability of these cloned angiogenesis factors and their demonstrated angiogenic potential have suggested the possibility of using *in vivo* gene transfer to overexpress angiogenesis factors to program neovascularization in ischemic myocardium. Leiden and coworkers examined the feasibility of this approach in a recent series of experiments. Plasmid DNA encoding the secreted angiogenesis factor, fibroblast growth factor-5 (FGF-5),[47] was injected into the left ventricle of Sprague–Dawley rats resulting in a 30–40% increase in capillary density three weeks after injection. While these preliminary results demonstrate the potential of programming myocardial angiogenesis *in vivo*, a number of important questions must be addressed prior to considering this approach for human therapy. For example, the optimum timing of gene delivery and the stability of neovascularization following gene transfer will need to be studied. From a safety perspective, the potential for widespread neovascularization is a concern. Thus, it will be critical to restrict expression of these genes to regions of ischemic myocardium. Furthermore, many of the angiogenesis factors are proto-oncogenes and others are associated with inflammatory responses in a number of organ systems. Thus, it will be important to carefully assess the systemic effects of *in vivo* delivery of these genes independent of myocardial neovascularization.

Altering myocyte dysfunction in response to hypoxia and acidosis

A second approach to the prevention of ischemic cardiomyopathy involves modifying specific properties of cardiomyocytes in the setting of acute or chronic ischemia. Prerequisites for this strategy include the need to identify and characterize molecular pathways that are important in maintaining normal cardiac function during ischemia, and that could be manipulated by the introduction of a single recombinant gene. For example, ischemia and the resultant intracellular acidosis markedly impairs myocardial contractile force.[48] In a recent study, Metzger *et al.*[49] ectopically expressed the skeletal isoform of the troponin C gene (*sTnC*) in cardiac myocytes, which normally express only the cardiac isoform of troponin C. Cardiac myocytes from the transgenic mice were shown to be significantly more resistant to the negative inotropic effects of intracellular acidosis as compared to myocytes from control mice. These results suggest that overexpression of *sTnC* using *in vivo* gene transfer could be effective in maintaining ventricular function during acute ischemic insults. The feasibility and efficacy of such an approach for the prevention of ischemic cardiomyopathy are currently under investigation.

Gene therapy for the modification of myocardial contractility

Direct enhancement of the contractile function of the failing myocardium represents another potential application of somatic gene therapy in the treatment of chronic CHF. The β-adrenergic receptor (β-AR) system is the most powerful endogenous mediator of inotropic support in normal myocardium[50,51] and derangements in the β-AR system contribute significantly to impaired myocardial contractility in CHF. Failing myocardium contains 50% fewer β-ARs than normal myocardium, and inotropic responses to β-agonists are markedly reduced, probably as a result of the focal β-AR deficits.[52] Thus, somatic gene therapy directed toward restoring β-AR number and function in the failing myocardium could restore myocardial contractility either through improved responsiveness to endogenous or exogenously administered β-agonists, or through agonist-independent mechanisms. To test this hypothesis, Lefkowitz and coworkers produced a transgenic mouse which overexpressed the β_2-AR under the control of the cardiac α-myosin heavy chain promoter.[53] These mice were shown to express nearly 200-fold increased levels of β-AR. Studies of myocardial function of these transgenic mice revealed increases in contractility and heart rate as well as high levels of intracellular adenylyl cyclase activity. All of these changes were equivalent to those seen with maximal isoproterenol stimulation and occurred in the absence of agonist. In addition, the authors reported no serious adverse effects of high levels of β_2-AR expression in these animals.[53]

The transgenic mouse models described above demonstrate that overexpression or ectopic expression of cell-surface receptors or contractile proteins by *in vivo* gene-transfer methods may prove useful in enhancing myocardial function in patients with CHF. It is important to note, however, that both reports involved studies of recombinant gene expression in normal myocytes. Whether such approaches can be used to modify the contractile function of diseased myocytes is currently unknown. Also, because chronic administration of several positive inotropic drugs has been associated with increased mortality in CHF,[54,55] it will be particularly important to demonstrate a decrease in morbidity and mortality using these gene-therapy approaches.

Myocyte transplantation for the therapy of CHF

As discussed above, the adult cardiac myocyte is a terminally differentiated nonproliferating cell. Thus, the myocardium has no regenerative capacity following myocyte damage or loss. Organ transplantation remains the only therapeutic option currently available for the treatment of end-stage, refractory CHF. Recently, Field and coworkers demonstrated the ability of transplanted fetal cardiomyocytes from transgenic mice to form stable grafts in the host myocardium.[56] In this study, single-cell suspensions were prepared from the myocardium of 15-day embryos of these transgenic animals and transplanted by direct injection into the left-ventricular free wall of syngeneic nontransgenic mice. Transmission electron microscopy demonstrated the presence of intercalated disks between the injected and recipient cells, suggesting the transplanted cells had become functionally coupled to the host myocardium. Importantly, the grafted myocytes remained stably incorporated into the host myocardium for at least two months. Furthermore, histological analyses revealed no significant inflammation at or near the graft site and the surface electrograms of the graft-bearing mice were identical to those of control mice.[56]

There are two important implications of these findings with regard to gene and cell-based therapies for chronic CHF. First, this study raised the possibility of transplanting normal, unaltered cardiomyocytes into the failing myocardium in order to directly enhance myocardial function by increasing the number of normally contracting cells. Also, because the authors transplanted genetically modified myocytes which stably expressed the *LacZ* reporter gene, this study raised the possibility of utilizing fetal cardiomyocyte transplantation as a novel delivery system for introducing specific recombinant gene products into the myocardium. Important questions to be addressed include whether cardiomyocyte transplantation would yield similar results in the diseased heart. For example, it is currently unknown whether intercellular coupling is possible between transplanted and diseased myocytes, or whether stable recombinant gene expression would occur in the setting of the failing myocardium following myocyte implantation. In addition, the ability of cell transplantation to enhance myocardial contractility will almost certainly require the development of a novel delivery system that will allow safe and efficient transplantation of large numbers of cardiomyocytes.

Summary and future directions

Gene and cell-based therapies represent a novel approach to the treatment of inherited and acquired forms of chronic CHF, and may provide significant advantages over currently available pharmacologic therapies. The feasibility of therapeutic gene transfer in the heart utilizing direct DNA injection and replication-defective adenovirus has now been established in a number of animal models. Recent studies which have identified mutant genes responsible for inherited cardiomyopathies and have delineated the *in vivo* effects of overexpressing specific genes in the myocardium and have suggested novel gene therapy approaches for the treatment of inherited and acquired forms of CHF. While these early results are promising, several major issues must be addressed prior to the use of somatic gene therapy for the treatment of human CHF. These include:

1. Further refinement and modification of the currently available gene delivery systems. It will be particularly important to develop strategies that restrict expression of recombinant genes to the myocardium and that increase the duration of expression of therapeutic genes in the heart.
2. The development of relevant animal models with which to test the efficacy and safety of specific candidate genes in the treatment of myocardial dysfunction.
3. Once efficacy and safety are established in such animal models, large-scale clinical trials must be performed to carefully delineate the relative benefits and risks of gene and cell-based approaches as compared to standard pharmacologic therapy for CHF.

Studies designed to address these issues and to further elucidate the mutant genes responsible for inherited forms of CHF, as well as to study the effects of overexpression of specific genes on cardiac function, promise to yield important new cell and gene therapy approaches for the prevention and treatment of CHF.

References

1. Massie, B. M. and Packer, M. (1990) Congestive heart failure: Current controversies and future prospects. *Am. J. Cardiol.*, **66**, 429–30.

2. The CONSENSUS Trial Group (1987) Effects of enalapril on mortality in severe congestive heart failure: Results of the Cooperative North Scandinavian Enalapril Survival Study. *N. Engl. J. Med.*, **316**, 1429–35.
3. Cohn, J. N., Archibald, D. G., Ziesche, S. *et al.* (1986) Effect of vasodilator therapy on mortality in chronic congestive heart failure: Results of a Veterans Administration Cooperative Study (V-HeFT). *N. Engl. J. Med.*, **314**, 1547–52.
4. SOLVD Investigators (1991) Effect of enalapril on survival in patients with reduced left ventricular ejection fractions and congestive heart failure. *N. Engl. J. Med.*, **325**, 293–302.
5. Pfeffer, M. A., Braunwald, E., Moye, L. A. *et al.* (1992) Effect of captopril on mortality and morbidity in patients with left ventricular dysfunction after myocardial infarction. Results of the survival and ventricular enlargement trial. *N. Engl. J. Med.*, **327**, 725–7.
6. Wolf, J. A. (1994) *Gene Therapeutics: Methods and Applications of Direct Gene Transfer.* Boston: Birkhauser.
7. Swain, J. L (1989) Gene therapy: A new approach to the treatment of cardiovascular disease. *Circulation*, **80**, 1495–6.
8. Nabel, E. G., Plautz, G. and Nabel, G. J. (1991) Gene transfer into vascular cells. *J. Am. Coll. Cardiol.*, **17**, 189B–94B.
9. Leinwand, L. A. and Leiden, J. M. (1991) Gene transfer into cardiac myocytes *in vivo. Trends Cardiovasc. Med.*, **1**, 271–6.
10. Zak, R. (1974) Development and proliferation capacity of cardiac muscle cells. *Circ. Res.*, **34–35** (Supp. 2), II-17.
11. Wantanabe, A. M., Green, F. J. and Farmer, B. B. (1986) Preparation and use of cardiac myocytes in experimental cardiology. In: Fozzard, H. A., Haber, E., Jennings, R. B. *et al.* (eds) *The Heart and Cardiovascular System.* New York: Raven Press.
12. Leiden, J. M. and Barr, E. (1994) *In vivo* gene transfer into the heart. In: Wolff, J. A. (ed.) *Gene Therapeutics: Methods and Applications of Direct Gene Transfer*, pp. 363–81. Boston: Birkhauser.
13. Wolff, J. A., Malone, R. W., Williams, P. *et al.* (1990) Direct gene transfer into mouse muscle *in vivo. Science*, **247**, 1465–8.
14. Lin, H., Parmacek, M. S., Morle, G. *et al.* (1990) Expression of recombinant genes in myocardium *in vivo* after direct injection of DNA. *Circulation*, **82**, 2217–21.
15. Acsadi, G., Jiao, S., Jani, A. *et al* (1991) Direct gene transfer and expression into rat heart *in vivo. New Biology*, **3**, 71–81.
16. Kitsis, R., Buttrick, P., McNally, E. *et al.* (1991) Hormonal modulation of a gene injected into rat heart *in vivo. Proc. Natl Acad. Sci. USA*, **88**, 4138–42.
17. Gal, E., Weir, L., LeClerc, G. *et al.* (1993) Direct myocardial transfection in two animal models. Evaluation of parameters affecting gene expression and percutaneous gene delivery. *Lab. Invest.*, **68**, 18–25.
18. Parmacek, M. S., Vora, A. J., Shen, T. *et al.* (1992) Identification and characterization of a cardiac-specific transcriptional regulatory element in the slow/cardiac troponin C gene. *Mol. Cell. Biol.*, **12**, 1967–76.
19. Horwitz, M. S. (1990) The adenoviruses. In: Fields, B. N. and Knipe, D. M. (eds) *Virology.* New York: Raven Press.
20. Berkner, K. L. (1988) Development of adenovirus vectors for the expression of heterologous genes. *Biotechniques*, **6**, 616–29.
21. Stratford-Perricaudet, L. D., Makeh, I., Perricaudet, M. and Briand, P. (1992) Widespread long-term gene transfer to mouse skeletal muscles and heart. *J. Clin. Invest.*, **90**, 626–30.
22. Eisler, A., Falck-Pedersen, E., Alvira, M. *et al.* (1993) Quantitative determination of adenovirus-mediated gene delivery to rat cardiac myocytes *in vitro* and *in vivo. Proc. Natl Acad. Sci. USA*, **90**, 11498–502.
23. Barr, E., Carroll, J., Tripathy, S. K. *et al.* (1994) Efficient catheter-mediated gene transfer into the heart using replication-defective adenovirus. *Gene Therapy*, **1**, 51–8.
24. Kass-Eisler, A., Falk-Pedersen, E., Elfenbein, D. *et al.* (1994) The impact of developmental stage, route of administration and the immune system on adenovirus-mediated gene transfer. *Gene Therapy*, **1**, 395–402.

25. Engelhardt, J. F., Ye, X., Doranz, B. and Wilson, J. M. (1994) Ablation of E2a in recombinant adenovirus improves transgene persistence and decreases immune response in mouse liver. *Proc. Natl Acad. Sci. USA*, **91**, 6196–6200.
26. Engelhardt, J. F. (1993) Adenovirus-mediated transfer of the CFTR gene to lung of non-human primates: biological efficacy study. *Human Gene Therapy*, **4**, 759–69.
27. Zabner, J., Petersen, D. M., Puga, A. P. *et al.* (1994) Safety and efficacy of repetitive adenovirus-mediated transfer of CFTR cDNA to airway epithelia of primates and cotton rats. *Nature-Genetics*, **6**, 75–83.
28. Zabner, J., Couture, L. A., Gregory, R. J. *et al.* (1993) Adenovirus-mediated gene transfer transiently corrects chloride transport defect in nasal epithelia of patients with cystic fibrosis. *Cell*, **75**, 207–16.
29. Tripathy, S. K., Goldwasser, E., Barr, E., Leiden, J. M. (1994) Stable delivery of physiologic levels of recombinant erythropoietin to the systemic circulation by intramuscular injection of replication-defective adenovirus. *Proc. Natl Acad. Sci. USA*, **91**, 11557–61.
30. Miller, G. and Wessle, H. B. (1993) Diagnosis of dystrophinopathies: review for the clinician. *Ped. Neurol.*, **9**, 3–9.
31. Perloff, J. K. (1992) Neurologic disorders and heart disease. In: Braunwald, E. (ed.) *Heart Disease*, pp. 1810–13. Philadelphia: W.B. Saunders.
32. Moser, H. (1984) Duchenne muscular dystrophy: pathogenetic aspect and genetic prevention. *Human Genetics*, **66**, 17–40.
33. Bies, R. D., Friedman, D., Roberts, R. *et al.* (1992) Expression and localization of dystrophin in human cardiac Purkinje fibers. *Circulation*, **86**, 147–53.
34. Anderson, M. S. and Kunkel, L. M. (1992) The molecular and biochemical basis of Duchenne muscular dystrophy. *Trends Biochem. Sci.*, **17**, 289–92.
35. Cox, G. A., Cole, N. M., Matsumura, K. *et al.* (1993) Overexpression of dystrophin in transgenic *mdx* mice eliminates dystrophic symptoms without toxicity. *Nature*, **364**, 725–9.
36. Acsadi, G., Dickson, G., Love, D. R. *et al.* (1991) Human dystrophin expression in *mdx* mice after intramuscular injection of DNA constructs. *Nature*, **352**, 815–18.
37. LeGal-LaSalle, G., Robert, J. J., Berrard, R. S. *et al.* (1993) An adenovirus vector for gene transfer into neurons and glia in the brain. *Science*, **259**, 988–90.
38. Franciosa, J. A., Wilen, M., Ziesche, S. *et al.* (1983) Survival in men with severe chronic left ventricular failure due to either coronary heart disease or idiopathic dilated cardiomyopathy. *Am. J. Cardiol.*, **51**, 831–6.
39. Sasayama, S. and Fujita, M. (1992) Recent insights into coronary collateral circulation. *Circulation*, **85**, 1197–204.
40. Sabia, P. J., Powers, E. R., Ragosta, M. *et al.* (1992) An association between collateral blood flow and myocardial viability in patients with recent myocardial infarction. *N. Engl. J. Med.*, **327**, 1825–31.
41. Habib, G. B., Heibig, J., Forman, S. A. *et al.* and the TIMI Investigators (1991) Influence of coronary collateral vessels on myocardial infarct size in humans: Results of phase I Thrombolysis in Myocardial Infarction (TIMI) Trial. *Circulation*, **83**, 739–46.
42. Hirai, T., Fujita, M., Nakajima, H. *et al.* (1989) Importance of collateral circulation for prevention of left ventricular aneurysm formation in acute myocardial infarction. *Circulation*, **79**, 791–6.
43. Folkman, J. and Klagsbrun, M. (1987) Angiogenic factors. *Science*, **235**, 442–7.
44. Yanagisawa-Miwa, A., Uchida, Y., Nakamura, F. *et al.* (1992) Salvage of infarcted myocardium by angiogenic action of basic fibroblast growth factor. *Science*, **257**, 1401–3.
45. Battler, A., Scheinowitz, M., Bor, A. *et al.* (1933) Intracoronary injection of basic fibroblast growth factor enhances angiogenesis in infarcted swine myocardium. *J. Am. Coll. Cardiol.*, **22**, 2001–6.
46. Banai, S., Jaklitsch, M. T., Shou, M. *et al.* (1994) Angiogenic-induced enhancement of collateral blood flow to ischemic myocardium by vascular endothelial growth factor in dogs. *Circulation*, **89**, 1–7.
47. Zhan, X., Bates, B., Hu, X., Goldfarb, M. (1988) The human *FGF-5* oncogene encodes a novel protein related to fibroblast growth factors. *Mol. Cell. Biol.*, **8**, 3487–95.

48. Lee, J. A., Allen, D. G. (1991) Mechanisms of acute ischemic contractile failure of the heart. Role of intracellular calcium. *J. Clin. Invest.*, **88**, 361–7.
49. Metzger, J. M., Parmacek, M. S., Barr, E. *et al.* (1993) Skeletal troponin C confers contractile sensitivity to acidosis in cardiac myocytes from transgenic mice. *Proc. Natl Acad. Sci. USA*, **90**, 9036–40.
50. Bristow, M. R., Kantrowitz, N. E., Ginsburg, R. and Fowler, M. B. (1985) β-adrenergic function in heart muscle disease and heart failure. *J. Mol. Cell. Cardiol.*, **17** (Supp. 2), 41–52.
51. Bristow, M. R., Hershberger, R. E., Port, J. D. *et al.* (1990) β-adrenergic pathways in nonfailing and failing human ventricular myocardium. *Circulation*, **82** (Supp. 1), I-12–I-25.
52. Bristow, M. R., Ginsburg, R., Minobe, W. *et al.* (1982) Decreased catecholamine sensitivity and β-adrenergic-receptor density in failing human hearts. *N. Engl. J. Med.*, **307**, 205–11.
53. Milano, C. A., Allen, L. F., Rockman, H. A. *et al.* (1994) Enhanced myocardial function in transgenic mice overexpressing the β_2-adrenergic receptor. *Science*, **264**, 582–6.
54. Packer, M., Carver, J. R., Rodeheffer, R. J. *et al.* and the PROMISE Study Research Group (1991) Effect of oral milrinone on mortality in severe chronic heart failure. *N. Engl. J. Med.*, **325**, 1468–75.
55. Lerer, C. V. (1992) Current status of non-digitalis positive inotropic drugs. *Am. J. Cardiol.* **69**, 120G–8G.
56. Soonpaa, M. H., Koh, G. Y., Klug, M. G. and Field, L. J. (1994) Formation of nascent intercalated disks between grafted fetal cardiomyocytes and host myocardium. *Science*, **264**, 98–101.

16

Electrophysiologic Disorders

John Kenneth Gibson
Robert J. Levy

Introduction

Although the thrust of this section will be local drug delivery and the use of devices to treat cardiac arrhythmias, this chapter will focus on 'traditional' antiarrhythmic therapy. That is the use of oral and/or intravenous agents to treat cardiac arrhythmias. Whereas substantial progress has been made in the use of implanted devices and/or ablation procedures to treat cardiac arrhythmias, a recent survey of electrophysiologists who treat cardiac arrhythmias showed they still use antiarrhythmic agents even when internal cardioversion devices are implanted.[1] While the goal is to reduce the number of times the device must discharge to maintain the patient in normal rhythm, recent studies have suggested that newer antiarrhythmic agents also may increase the efficacy of defibrillation and lower the energy necessary for cardioversion. Thus, this chapter will briefly address the electrophysiologic basis of cardiac arrhythmias, review the classification of antiarrhythmic agents and the recent clinical trials which have addressed the use of these antiarrhythmic agents. The final sections will briefly present the preclinical models that are used to identify new antiarrhythmic agents and discuss some of the newer agents being developed for the treatment of cardiac arrhythmias. This chapter also will consider the electrophysiologic and pharmacologic basis for local drug-delivery strategies for the treatment of cardiac arrhythmias. This therapeutic approach has been used only in experimental studies thus far, but published results have raised a number of important issues and considerations with respect to efficacy, device testing and relevance of preclinical models of cardiac rhythm disorders.

The genesis of cardiac arrhythmias

It is not the intent of this chapter to present a comprehensive review of re-entrant cardiac conduction and the role of antiarrhythmic agents in treating these cardiac arrhythmias. However a brief review demonstrates these basic concepts have been explored in the laboratory for almost a century and outlines how we have reached our current target of novel, class III antiarrhythmic agents for the treatment of serious cardiac arrhythmias.

It is generally accepted that cardiac arrhythmias result from disorders in the initiation of a cardiac impulse, abnormal conduction of the cardiac impulse or simultaneous abnormalities of impulse initiation and conduction.[2] The recent interest in the development of new class III antiarrhythmic agents has been fueled in part by the hypothesis that both atrial and ventricular tachyarrhythmias result from abnormalities in cardiac conduction which produce a re-entrant conduction pathway or circus movement of the cardiac electrical impulse. It has been thought that intrinsic or induced structural abnormalities in the cardiac ion channels which are responsible for cardiac conduction and repolarization create abnormalities in the conduction of the cardiac impulse. However, a recent hypothesis is that the discontinuous nature or anisotropic properties of the myocardium provide a unique mechanism for functionally different conduction pathways to allow re-entrant cardiac conduction to occur in the heart.[3]

While Mayer is credited with making the first key observations on re-entry in jellyfish rings,[4] critical observations on cardiac re-entry were reported by Mines[5] when he observed the importance of slow cardiac conduction and short refractory periods to produce re-entrant cardiac conduction or a circulating excitation as he described it. Likewise Garrey[6] observed the importance of transient conduction block producing multiple re-entrant or 'circus contractions' which were manifest as ventricular fibrillation. Weiner and Rosenblueth[7] proposed a mathematical model of a re-entrant circuit for a continuous, isotropic two-dimensional sheet in which they demonstrated the 'wavelength' of a re-entrant circuit. While their work suggests that they considered a fixed anatomic block to be essential for re-entry, the 'wavelength' equation (wavelength equals the conduction velocity multiplied by the refractory period) is still used today and has been applied to generate re-entrant cardiac arrhythmias in the presence of fixed anatomic or functional obstacles to cardiac conduction. Computer modeling was first evident in 1964, when Moe *et al.* presented a computer model of atrial fibrillation based upon a two-dimensional sheet of atrial cells with repolarization abnormalities.[8] While Garrey had reported '... ringlike circuits of shifting locations ...' as the cause of fibrillation, the Moe model which did not require a fixed anatomical block produced '... numerous vortices, shifting in position and direction like eddies in a turbulent pool ...'. Since this initial report, we have seen three decades of computer modeling and mapping of re-entrant cardiac conduction and arrhythmogenesis.

At the same time this work was being conducted on re-entrant cardiac conduction and its role in cardiac arrhythmias, simultaneous work was underway in a number of laboratories on the role of ventricular repolarization and its role in the genesis and pharmacologic treatment of cardiac arrhythmias. Quinidine was introduced in 1918 for the treatment of arrhythmias such as atrial fibrillation. The ability of this agent to increase the effective refractory period of the heart was recognized by Sir Thomas Lewis in 1926 as the mechanism of this agent's therapeutic action.[9] While it was known that quinidine was able to increase the duration of the QT interval and also increase the duration of the QRS interval, the latter action initially was viewed as a sign of potential toxicity. However, the use of intracellular microelectrode recording techniques demonstrated the ability of agents such as quinidine to block sodium currents in atrial and ventricular muscle, reduce the maximum rate of depolarization of the cardiac action potential and consequently slow cardiac conduction. While both electrophysiologic actions of quinidine could prevent cardiac arrhythmias, both also are able to cause cardiac arrhythmias.

'Quinidine syncope' was recognized as a paroxysmal ventricular fibrillation associated with prolongation of the QT interval by quinidine.[10] The characteristic electrocardiographic features of this proarrhythmic response were eventually included in the original description of torsades de pointes described by Dessertenne.[11] Sudden cardiac death associated with quinidine-induced prolongation of the QT interval clearly overwhelmed the issue of prolonging the QT interval to achieve an antiarrhythmic effect. Consequently, blockade of the inward sodium current in cardiac muscle was viewed as the significant way to achieve control of malignant cardiac arrhythmias. A number of quinidine-like drugs such as procainamide, disopyramide, and orally effective analogs of lidocaine were evaluated as antiarrhythmic agents. Indeed, even more potent agents that inhibit the inward cardiac sodium current were synthesized and developed for their ability to suppress the frequent premature ventricular beats that were recognized as markers of an increased risk of ventricular fibrillation. However, as discussed below, the CAST trial has placed serious doubts on the role of agents that selectively suppress the inward sodium current for the prevention of cardiac arrhythmias including sudden cardiac death. A further discussion of this large clinical trial is included below.

In discussing the repolarization of the cardiac action potential, the QT interval is used as a noninvasive surrogate. Indeed, it is often corrected for variations in heart rate to provide a correction for the natural decrease in the QT interval that is seen with faster heart rates. In many preclinical and clinical papers, the Bazett formula is used to provide this correction, generating the 'QTc interval'.[12] The Bazett formula was derived to determine the duration of electrical (ventricular) systole or K as a function of pulse rate. It was not intended to correct the QT interval of the electrocardiogram as it is now used by many authors. Indeed, it was not until 1947, that Taran and Szilagyi,[13] defined the term 'QTc'.

Despite its wide spread application to normalize or 'correct' the QT interval for pulse rate, the Bazett formula has been reviewed and/or criticized by many authors.[14–17] A major inadequacy of the Bazett formula is its overcorrection at fast heart rates. This is demonstrated in a clinical study by Ahnve and Vallin[18] in which application of the Bazett formula produced an apparent inversion of the effect of propranolol and atropine on the QT interval. Likewise, in a preclinical study using rats, Nattel,[19] showed that use of the Bazett formula overcorrected for fast heart rates, i.e. 200–250 beats per minute. In a preclinical study using dogs, Sarma *et al.*[20] suggested that over a wide range of heart rates the relation between the QT interval and the heart rate is best expressed as an exponential formula.

In summary, while the Bazett formula has been criticized and praised since it was first described, it continues to be used by many and we must be careful in its use and interpretation particularly when a fast heart rate is a consequence of the experimental protocol. In most electrophysiologic studies, parameters of agents that prolong cardiac repolarization such as the QT interval, duration of the monophasic action potential duration or refractory period are measured during pacing at constant heart rate to eliminate rate dependent changes in these parameters.

Classification of antiarrhythmic agents

Vaughan Williams classification

In 1970, Singh and Vaughan Williams[21] proposed a classification of antiarrhythmic agents based upon the drug's ability to produce clearly definable electrophysiologic actions (Table 16.1). He originally described four groups: class I agents or membrane-stabilizing agents that block the fast, inward Na^+ currents; class II drugs consisted of beta-adrenergic blocking agents; class III compounds increased the duration of the cardiac action potential by delaying the repolarization of the cardiac action potential; and class IV agents were calcium channel antagonists that blocked Ca^{2+} channels. Later, class I drugs were subdivided (into class IA, IB and IC based on the kinetics of blockade). This system has been very useful and has provided a simple way to group a variety of compounds, particularly new compounds as they are first studied.[22]

It has become clear, however, that almost all drugs possess multiple actions (e.g. amiodarone blocks Na^+ channels,[23] K^+ channels,[24,25] Ca^{2+} channels[26] and causes beta-adrenoceptor blockade). In addition, the Vaughan Williams classification system has been based on the drug's acute actions on normal tissue, which is electrophysiologically different from cardiac tissue that is acutely or chronically stressed by conditions such as ischemia or disease.[27,28] For example in a recent study, Furukawa et al.[29] demonstrated the enhanced susceptibility of myocytes from hypertrophied feline hearts to reperfusion arrhythmias resulted from a significant reduction of outward potassium current(I_K) over the action potential plateau range. Thus, although the hypertrophied myocytes demonstrated a prolonged action potential when compared to control cells at baseline, reperfusion further increased the duration of the action potential and produced repolarization arrhythmias. Likewise, age-related increases and decreases in K^+-channel density have been reported.[30] Also, as newer agents such as adenosine are developed for the treatment of cardiac arrhythmias are developed, they may not 'fit' within the confines of this

Table 16.1 Vaughan Williams Classification of antiarrhythmic agents

Class	Examples
Class I: Membrane-stabilizing agents	
IA: Block Na^+ channel, increase action potential duration	Quinidine, disopyramide procainamide
IB: Block Na^+ channel, shorten action potential duration	Lidocaine, mexiletine
IC: Block Na^+ channel	Encainide, flecainide, propafenone
Class II: Beta-adrenergic blocking agents	Propanolol, nadolol, metroprolol, atenolol
Class III: Increase action-potential duration	Amiodarone, sotalol,* clofilium, dofetilide, ibutilide
Class IV: Calcium antagonists	Verapamil, diltiazem

*While *d,l*-sotalol is a racemic mixture, the *l*-isomer possesses beta-adrenergic blocking properties and class III actions, the *d*-isomer possesses class III actions.

classification system. Therefore, it was suggested that a revised classification system was needed.

The Sicilian gambit

In 1991 the Task Force of the Working Group on Arrhythmias of the European Society of Cardiology published 'The Sicilian Gambit. A New Approach to the Classifiction of Antiarrhythmic Drugs based on their Actions on Arrhythmogenic Mechanisms'.[31] The authors were dissatisfied with existing classification systems and hoped to provide a new framework for antiarrhythmic drugs that would be flexible to accommodate and encourage new advances in antiarrhythmic drug research. The Sicilian Gambit classifies antiarrhythmic agents on the basis of their targets of action such as channels, pumps and receptors with intensity/potency of action also included. The article also reviewed the effects of antiarrhythmic drugs in relation to the mechanisms responsible for cardiac arrhythmias and the application of these agents to clinical therapy. The major advantage of this classification system is its ability to assimilate new knowledge about drugs and cardiac electrophysiology as it becomes available.

Clinical trials and antiarrhythmic agents

The results of recent clinical trials have raised a number of concerns about the pharmacologic basis of many of the antiarrhythmic pharmaceuticals currently being considered for human use, and has even effected the use of a number of already approved agents. These clinical trials also have stimulated a redistribution of research activities concerning the development of new antiarrhythmic agents, as well as increased interest in the use of device-related therapies for cardiac arrhythmias. Furthermore, the failures and side effects observed in a number of clinical trials also have served to emphasize the potential importance of regional cardiac drug delivery strategies to avoid the untoward side effects of conventional antiarrhythmic drug administration.

Class I agents – the CAST and CAST II study

Frequent ventricular premature depolarizations and left-ventricular dysfunction are independent predictors for cardiac death after myocardial infarction. Specifically, several studies have shown an independent association between the presence of ventricular premature complexes and increased risk of arrhythmic death following mycardial infarction.[32,33] The hypothesis of the CAST study (Cardiac Arrhythmia Suppression Trial) was that pharmacologic suppression of asymptomatic or mildly asymptomatic ventricular premature beats in survivors of acute myocardial infarction would reduce arrhythmic death.[34] Based upon an earlier CAPS (Cardiac

Arrhythmia Pilot Study) trial, the agents used in the CAST trial included encainide, flecainide and moricizine.

After ten months of followup, interim analysis of data established an excess of deaths from arrhythmia in patients treated with encainide or flecainide. The potential causes of this enhanced mortality remain uncertain. It has been hypothesized that a proarrhythmic action of these agents, i.e. creation of a stable re-entrant circuit, was enhanced in the presene of myocardial ischemia. It also has been suggested that the negative inotropic effects of these agents resulted in a reduced cardiac oxygen supply in the face of increased oxygen demand exacerbating ischemia and increasing mortality. Finally, it also has been observed that a low incidence of mortality was observed in the placebo group and this may have effected the analysis.[35,36]

The investigators of the CAST trial concluded that although asymptomatic or mildly asymptomatic patients with ventricular premature beats or nonsustained ventricular tachycardia after a myocardial infarction may have an increased risk of mortality, these patients do not benefit from the use of encainide or flecainide to treat these arrhythmias. Subsequently, it has been recommended that these conclusions apply to all class IC drugs.

Despite their disappointment with the interim analysis, the CAST investigators made significant changes in the design of the trial and the CAST II trial was continued with moricizine. They lowered the left-ventricular ejection fraction for acceptance into the trial and reduced the entry window to 90 days after infarction. In consequence, patients with more severe disease and a higher event rate now were enrolled in the study. In August 1991, however, CAST II was stopped upon recommendation from the CAST II data and safety monitoring board to the CAST II executive committee.[37] While in April 1989, only four patients receiving moricizine had died compared to 11 receiving placebo, a July review of the mortality data showed that of the 1346 CAST II patients, 74 patients in the placebo group had died versus 97 patients in the moricizine treated group. Although this was not statistically significant, the safety board felt the trial should not continue with this trend of increased mortality in patients treated with moricizine.

Both CAST and CAST II had a major impact on many groups including patients, physicians, the pharmaceutical industry and regulatory agencies.[38] It was reported that patients refused treatment with antiarrhythmic agents and arrhythmic death ensued in some who discontinued their treatment. The decision of when and how to treat patients with potentially life-threatening arrhythmias has been problematic. Indeed, the medical community has become somewhat reluctant to use any antiarrhythmic agent, even when there may be legitimate medical reasons for its use to prevent serious supraventricular or ventricular arrhythmias. The pharmaceutical industry has re-evaluated new drug development in this area in the face of a shrinking market, substantially reducing the number of new drugs being developed for what remains an unmet medical need. Finally, in the face of the uncertainties observed in these groups, regulatory agencies now have a major responsibility to provide new guidelines for the approval of antiarrhythmic agents and restore confidence that this process is based upon the best possible scientific evaluation. This is particularly true if the newer agents presented in this review are to be carefully studied in the clinic.

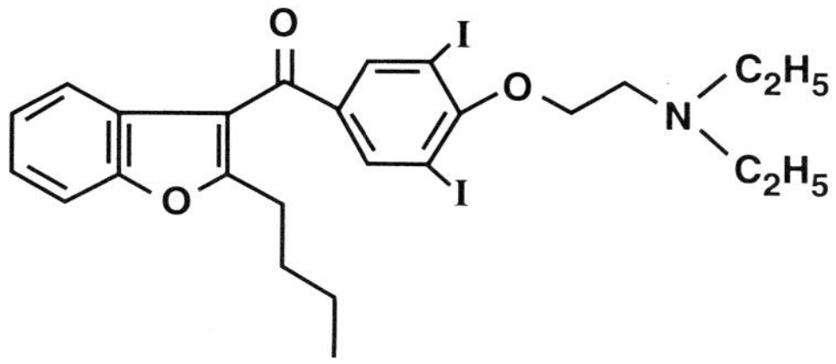

Figure 16.1   Chemical structure of amiodarone.

Class III agents – amiodarone and sotalol

Amiodarone

A number of major clinical trials, SAVE, Consensus II and SOLVD have demonstrated that converting enzyme inhibitors such as captopril and enalapril do not prevent sudden cardiac death in the first year after myocardial infarction.[39] Their beneficial effects to prevent sudden cardiac death appear in the second and subsequent years after myocardial infarction. Earlier clinical trials, BASIS and CASCADE, have shown the ability of amiodarone (Figure 16.1) to reduce postinfarction ventricular fibrillation and sudden cardiac death. Three large-scale prospective trials are underway to determine the ability of amiodarone to prevent ventricular fibrillation and prevent sudden cardiac death.

The Cardiac Arrest in Seattle: Conventional Versus Amiodarone Drug Evaluation (CASCADE) study evaluated antiarrhythmic drug therapy in survivors of out-of-hospital cardiac arrest.[40] To be enrolled in this study, patients had to have been resuscitated from out-of-hospital ventricular fibrillation and not demonstrate a Q-wave myocardial infarction at the time of ventricular fibrillation. The patients also had to demonstrate at least 10 ventricular complexes per hour on Holter recording or an inducible, sustained ventricular tachycardia or fibrillation at baseline electrophysiologic study. The primary endpoints were cardiac mortality, resuscitated cardiac arrest due to ventricular fibrillation or complete syncope followed by a shock from an automatic defibrillator. Although patients with a more severe depression of left-ventricular function had a poorer outcome, baseline clinical variables were similar in the two treatment groups. After randomization, the amiodarone group consisted of 113 patients and the conventional antiarrhythmic therapy group consisted of 115 patients. Patients in the conventional antiarrhythmic therapy arm were treated with the class I antiarrhythmic agents procainamide, quinidine, disopyramide, tocainide, mexilitine, encainide, flecainide, propafenone, moricizine or combination therapy. Although larger loading doses of amiodarone were administered, maintenance doses of amiodarone were reduced to avoid adverse side effects; the mean amiodarone maintenance dose was $185 \, \text{mg day}^{-1}$ at 36 months of treatment. Cardiac survival, free of the primary endpoints, was substantially greater ($P = 0.007$) in patients treated with amiodarone; at six years, 53% amiodarone versus 40% conventional therapy. This success with amiodarone occurred despite the higher, cumulative incidence of side effects observed with the relatively low maintenance doses of amiodarone. These side effects included pulmonary toxicity, neurotoxicity, hepatotoxicity and thyroid dysfunction and at six years, 41% of the patients receiving amiodarone had stopped their assigned therapy. During the study, the investigators began to implant internal defibrillators in all patients in whom surgery was not contraindicated. An unexpected finding was that patients treated with amiodarone had fewer syncopal shocks ($P = 0.032$) and indeed amiodarone treated patients had fewer total shocks from their devices ($P = 0.014$). The investigators concluded that future studies should compare amiodarone to placebo inpatients with an implanted cardioverter/defibrillator. They also suggested that newer class III antiarrhythmic agents should be tested in light of the side effects observed with amiodarone in this study. They acknowledged that the small number of enrolled patients prevented detailed subgroup analyses.

The BASIS study (Basel Antiarrhythmic Study and Infarct Survival) evaluated the effects of prophylactic antiarrhythmic treatment in patients with persisting asymptomatic complex ventricular arrhythmias two weeks after myocardial infarction.[41] The patients were consecutively screened and randomized to individualized antiarrhythmic treatment with quinidine or mexiletine (group 1), low-dose amiodarone treatment (group 2, 200 mg day^{-1}) or placebo. In the one year followup, survival was greater ($P < 0.05$) and arrhythmic events were reduced ($P < 0.01$) in the patients given amiodarone. In a followup study (55–125 months, 72-month mean), this reduction in mortality remained lower in the amiodarone-treated patients apparently due to a first-year reduction in cardiac death.[42]

The CASCADE and the BASIS studies have led to the initiation of the European Myocardial Infarct Amiodarone Trial (EMIAT).[43] Since these earlier trials suggested a beneficial action of amiodarone to reduce mortality in a relatively small number of postinfarction patients, EMIAT was designed to test the efficacy of amiodarone on the mortality of patients with depressed cardiac function after acute myocardial infarction. In addition to enrolling a larger number of patients, unlike the earlier trials, EMIAT will stratify the patients by cardiac ejection fraction. The patients are enrolled between 5 and 21 days after infarction if their ejection fraction is ≤40%. This is a double-blind randomized study in which the patients will receive amiodarone or placebo. It is anticipated that >700 patients will be enrolled in 13 European countries and the trial will be completed in 1995.

While EMIAT is evaluating postinfarction patients with reduced left-ventricular function, the Canadian Amiodarone Myocardial Infarction Arrhythmia Trial (CAMIAT) is enrolling patients with frequent of repetitive ventricular premature depolarization 6–45 days after myocardial infarction.[44] It is anticipated that 1200 patients will be randomized and treated for 16 months with amiodarone or placebo treatment. The principal outcome is presumed arrhythmic death or resuscitated ventricular fibrillation.

The VA320 study will enroll 700 patients with dilated cardiomyopathy, ejection fraction ≤45% and more than 10 premature ventricular beats per hour.

Sotalol

While several studies have or are currently investigating the effects of antiarrhythmic therapy with amiodarone on various patient populations, the Electrophysiologic

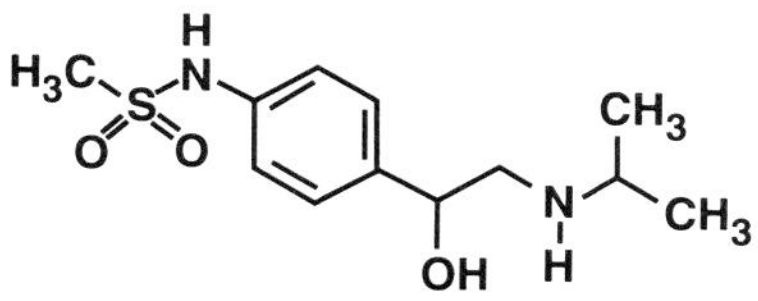

Figure 16.2   Chemical structure of sotalol.

Study Versus Electrocardiographic Monitoring study (EVESM) examined the relative efficacy of various antiarrhythmic drugs in the treatment of ventricular tachyarrhythmias. In this study patients with documented ventricular tachyarrhythmias that were inducible during electrophysiologic testing and demonstrated ten or more premature ventricular beats per hour during Holter monitoring were randomly assigned to serial testing of antiarrhythmic drug efficacy by Holter monitoring or electrophysiologic testing. The patients received long-term treatment with the first antiarrhythmic drug predicted to be effective on the basis of Holter monitoring or electrophysiologic testing. The agents used included the class I agents: imipramine, mexiletine, pirmenol, procainamide, propafenone, quinidine and the class III agent sotalol (Figure 16.2). Arrhythmia recurrence, death from any causee, death from arrhythmia and adverse drug effects were significantly lower for sotalol than any of the other agents in the four-year followup.

Surgical and interventional approaches to treat cardiac arrhythmias have been increasingly used and clinical results have been received with enthusiasm. The initial surgical resections and open operative ablations of re-entry pathways and regions of pre-excitation have been replaced by catheter-based ablation procedures of the same regions of interest. Various forms of energy including microwave and radiofrequency are now used to successfully carry out catheter ablation. Device-mediated therapies have been used increasingly in the past five years or so and also have demonstrated excellent efficacy. Device-related therapies have included the use of antitachycardia pacemakers and implantable countershock defibrillators. All of these developments plus the undesirable results noted in the clinical trials cited above have led to an increased interest on the part of clinical cardiologists for device-related therapies and interventional ablations as the treatment of choice wherever possible for life-threatening cardiac arrhythmias.

Preclinical models used to study antiarrhythmic agents

In vitro electrophysiologic models of cellular impulse conduction, as well as animal models of cardiac arrhythmias, leave a great deal to be desired in terms of their ability to predict drug efficacy and untoward effects in clinical use. Nevertheless, these particular preclinical models represent the best means currently available for testing drugs and optimizing their use. It has been difficult to standardize animal model use in particular because of species variation in the dog, the principal animal used in most of these studies. In addition, the use of acute ischemia and infarction models (chiefly canine models) of cardiac arrhythmias results in large numbers of control

Table 16.2 *In vitro* models used to study antiarrhythmic agents

Preparation	Species	Reference
Isolated cells	Cultured cells and cloned channels	Sakuta et al.;[45] Yanagishi et al.[46]
	Guinea pig	Jurkiewicz and Sanguinetti[47]
	Rabbit	Velkamp et al.[48]
	Ferret	Campbell et al.[49,50]
	Cat	Spinelli et al.[51]
Intact tissues	Guinea pig	Yang et al.[52]
	Rabbit	Abrahamsson et al.[53]
	Ferret	Baskin et al.[54]
	Dog	Butera et al.[55]
Intact organs	Guinea pig	Flores and Sheridan[56]
	Rabbit	Chi et al.[57]

and drug-treated animals and, in general, the experimental methods tend to be individualized for each laboratory performing these types of experiments.

In vitro models

A variety of *in vitro* methods are used to study the electrophysiologic actions of antiarrhythmic agents. Although Table 16.2 lists representative model systems and tissues used in these studies it should be emphasized that this is not a complete listing nor is it a listing of the preferred systems. It also should be noted that ion channels cloned from a variety of species including man are used with increasing frequency to characterize the electrophysiologic actions of antiarrhythmic agents. The rat is not listed in Table 16.2 since I_{to} is the major current responsible for the repolarization of its ventricular action potential and I_{to} does not appear to be a major current of cardiac repolarization in other species including man.

In vivo models of cardiac arrhythmias

A variety of *in vivo* methods also are used to study the electrophysiologic and antiarrhythmic actions of antiarrhythmic agents. Although Table 16.3 lists representative model systems used in these studies it should be emphasized that this is not a

Table 16.3 *In vivo* models used to study antiarrhythmic agents

Preparation	Species	Reference
Atrial arrhythmias		
flutter-Y incision, intercaval crush	Dog	Inoue et al.[58]
flutter-pericarditis	Dog	Shimizu et al.[59]
fibrillation	Dog	Nabih et al.[60]
Ventricular arrhythmias		
ischemia	Rat, dog, rabbit	Curtis et al.;[61] Sano et al.[62]
reperfusion	Rat, dog, rabbit	Bril et al.[63]
infarction	Dog, rabbit	Lynch et al.;[64] Kohdoh et al.[65]
Torsades de pointes	Rabbit, dog	Carlsson et al.;[66] Ben-David and Zipes[67]
Cardiac electrophysiology	Dog	Wallace et al.[68]
Ventricular defibrillation	Dog	Dorian et al.[69]

complete listing nor is it a listing of the preferred models. A particular concern is that when using smaller species such as the rat or guinea pig, the physically small size of the heart predisposes these animals to spontaneous cardioversion of many arrhythmias to normal sinus rhythm.

In vivo experiments to test antiarrhythmic drugs often lack uniformity and the methods used to produce the arrhythmias and their pharmacologic treatment are often inconsistently reported. In 1987 a group of scientists assembled the Lambeth Conventions[70] in an effort to overcome 'the paralyzing influence of the dead hand of tradition' for the study of cardiac arrhythmias in myocardial ischemia and reperfusion. Although these conventions are primarily applicable to animal studies, it was hoped that they also would be useful for clinical trials. While the first eleven conventions address experimental design, the remaining nine describe the classification, quantification and analysis of cardiac arrhythmias. Although these statements may seem obvious, it has been the experience of the authors that many times these simple conventions are not considered in the development of antiarrhythmic agents and therapies.

The Lambeth conventions as listed in Table 16.4 are relatively simple and perhaps obvious to all investigators. We would like to provide a few additional comments. While dose–response studies are useful in preclinical studies they may not be ethical in clinical trials. The background details should be reported since arrhythmias may be influenced by the sex, strain, species, housing conditions and perhaps even the diet of the animals being used. While untreated controls may be used, when testing drugs it may be necessary to use a drug vehicle control group. In addition, when an

Table 16.4 The Lambeth conventions

Experimental design	Classification of arrhythmias
1. Treatment randomization and blind administration of agents is mandatory	1. Ventricular premature beats (VPBs) are discrete, premature QRS complexes
2. Dose–response designs should be used for drug studies	2. Two or three VPBs constitute a salvo. Four or more consecutive VPBs are defined as ventricular tachycardia
3. Pilot studies while useful are reported only in the methods	3. Ventricular fibrillation (VF) is manifest when individual QRS complexes cannot be observed and rate can no longer be measured
4. All species and models have limitations	4. VPBs, bigeminy, salvos, VT and VF describe ventricular arrhythmias
5. Report background information on animals – source, sex, weight, etc.	5 The incidence of the arrhythmias described above must be analyzed separately
6. Exclusion criteria are clearly stated and are consistently applied at the start of each experiment	6. Quantification of other variables depends upon their frequency characteristics
7. Contemporary controls should be used	7. Arrhythmia scores must be used with caution
8. Ischemia, infarction and/or reperfusion must be validated in every experiment	8. The statistical procedures and group sizes must be determined prior to the start of the experiments
9. The effects of anesthetics on hemodynamics and blood gases must be monitored	9. Loss of experimental animals during the experiment should be reported and analyzed
10. Variables other than arrhythmia count should be measured	
11. Arrhythmias must be determined from ECG or electrogram recordings	

agent has more than one pharmacologic mechanism of action such as beta-adrenergic blockade and class III actions, it may be necessary to add an additional control treatment group such as a beta-adrenergic blocker alone. When using a preparation as its own control in arrhythmic research one must be careful that the arrhythmic response does not undergo time-dependent or procedure-dependent changes. Coronary collateral circulation is species dependent, while cats and dogs often have an extensive collateral circulation, rats, rabbits and pigs generally do not. Therefore, while coronary flow is controlled by the investigator in global models of ischemia and reperfusion, in models of regional coronary occlusion coronary flow must be measured to ensure that consistent levels of ischemia have been achieved. While some antiarrhythmic agents may have direct antiarrhythmic actions, the indirect actions of an anesthetic such as hypotension, fast heart rate, may influence the initiation of cardiac arrhythmias and these actions should be considered, particularly since these agents will primarily be used in unanesthetized patients. Although the authors of the Lambeth conventions stated that a single ECG lead is sufficient to monitor cardiac arrhythmias, their major concern was that ancillary parameters such as mean arterial blood pressure or heart rate alone should not be used for the detection and classification of arrhythmias.

A major concern of the authors of the Lambeth conventions was the lack of consistency in the reporting of ventricular arrhythmias. The distinction of ventricular premature beats, salvos and ventricular tachycardia was not based upon consistent, objective criteria. In the first four conventions on the classification of arrhythmias they addressed these issues. They developed a model independent classification based solely upon ECG patterns. Ventricular premature beats must be premature in relation to the P wave of the ECG and hence a defined P wave is necessary. Since ventricular tachycardia was not defined in terms of its rate, this definition is species and model-independent. Since asystole was defined as a flatline ECG record with no rate, it clearly differs from ventricular fibrillation which also has no rate and consists of QRS deflections which can no longer be distinguished from each other.

Torsades de pointes

Torsades de pointes is a potentially life-threatening arrhythmia which has become of increasing concern with respect to the use of a number of drugs. Torsades de pointes is a polymorphic ventricular tachycardia with a progressive twisting of the QRS complex around the isoelectric baseline with a change in amplitude every 10–15 ventricular beats. The prolonged ventricular repolarization observed with torsades de pointes may be idiopathic or acquired but it produces a prolonged QT interval. Acquired prolongation of the QT interval is observed following treatment with a variety of drugs, particularly agents that delay cardiac repolarization, and has also been associated with electrolyte abnormalities. While a slow heart rate favors the onset of torsades de pointes, a unique conduction sequence, the long–short–long cycle length appears to precede the onset of torsades de pointes.[71]

Several hypotheses have been proposed to explain the electrophysiologic causes of torsades de pointes. One hypothesis suggests that heterogeneous prolongation of the cardiac action potential duration produces a dispersion of refractory periods and cardiac conduction block. This provides the substrate for re-entrant cardiac conduction to produce torsades de pointes. However, this substrate generally presents a stable substrate for abnormal cardiac conduction and would tend to produce a monomorphic ventricular tachycardia which torsades de pointes is not. In addition, this type of re-entrant cardiac substrate should allow initiation of the arrhythmia by premature stimuli delivered during repolarization. Again, induction of torsades de pointes in this manner is not observed in patients with QT prolongation. Lazzara and coworkers have suggested that early afterdepolarizations produce a form of abnormal automaticity or triggered activity that initiates torsades de pointes.[72,73] These early afterdepolarizations occur during repolarization of the cardiac action potential and their amplitude is enhanced at slow heart rates.[74] When these afterdepolarizations reach the activation threshold a new action potential is initiated and the tachycardia ensues.

Monophasic action potential recording techniques allow us to measure the duration of the cardiac action potential *in vivo*.[75] In addition, they have shown that acquired torsaides de pointes occurs in patients with a marked dispersion of repolarization and the presence of early afterdepolarizations.[76] This suggests that acquired or drug-induced torsades de pointes may actually be a combination of these two hypotheses. Early afterdepolarizations may serve as the 'trigger foci' while the heterogeneous electrical substrate may be necessary to sustain this abnormal tachycardia.

Removal of the agent responsible for acquired torsades de pointes and/or correction of electrolyte imbalance is obviously the first therapeutic choice in the management of this arrhythmia. If this does not control the arrhythmia, temporary pacing or intravenous administration of 1–2 g of magnesium sulfate is the treatment of choice. The pharmacologic mechanisms by which magnesium suppresses torsades de pointes are not clear, but its calcium blocking properties[77] may depress the early afterdepolarizations responsible for torsades de pointes.[78]

Newer class III antiarrhythmic agents

E-4031

The sotalol derivative E-4031 (Figure 16.3), produced dose-dependent increases in the effective refractory period of isolated rabbit papillary muscle.[79] In these *in vitro* studies E-4031 also produced dose-dependent increases in contractility. Intravenous

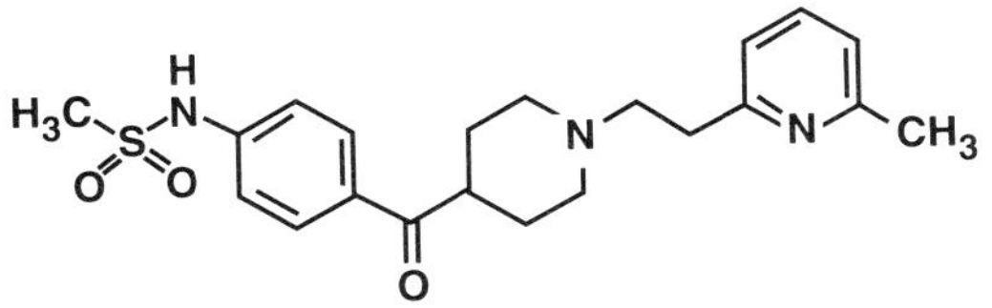

Figure 16.3 Chemical structure of E-4031.

administration of E-4031 in anesthetized dogs prolonged the cardiac action potential and produced positive inotropic effects.[79] E-4031 terminated atrial flutter in a canine model by increasing the refractory period of the atria while causing a minimal slowing of conduction.[80] Following myocardial infarction E-4031 increased the refractory periods in noninfarcted and infarcted myocardium and prevented ventricular fibrillation in a canine model.[81] The electrophysiologic effects of E-4031 were evaluated in 15 patients with supraventricular tachyarrhythmias. Intravenous administration (loading infusion $5\,\mu g\,kg^{-1}$ for 5 min plus maintenance infusion $0.15\,\mu g\,kg^{-1}\,min^{-1}$) significantly increased the QT and QTc intervals, and effective refractory periods of the atria and ventricle while having no effect on RR interval, PR interval, QRS duration, or AH or HV intervals. While blood pressure did not change and this dose of E-4031 produced no undesirable side effects, it prevented repetitive atrial arrhythmias in only 1 of 3 patients with inducible atrial firing and could not prevent induction of AV re-entrant tachycardia in patients with an inducible AV re-entrant arrhythmia.[82]

Dofetilide

In single myocytes from rabbits and guinea pigs, dofetilide (UK-68,798, Figure 16.4) blocked I_{Kr}, the rapid component of the delayed rectifier.[83] This block was voltage- and time-dependent, was greater at more depolarized membrane potentials and exhibited a slow recovery at hyperpolarized membrane potentials. This inhibition of repolarizing potassium currents by dofetilide prolonged action-potential duration and effective refractory period in isolated guinea-pig papillary muscle, canine ventricular muscle and Purkinje fiber.[84,85] Concentrations as high as 10–5 M had no effect on rat papillary muscle or atria demonstrating the absence of I_K in rat myocardium. While dofetilide prevented the initiation of ventricular arrhythmias in a canine model of myocardial infarction, it also substantially reduced the incidence of sudden death in these animals following formation of an occlusion thrombus in the circumflex coronary artery.[86] In a rabbit model of torsades de pointes (polymorphic ventricular tachycardia), administration of dofetilide increased the QT_c 38%, and produced early afterdepolarizations and proarrhythmia in 73% of the treated animals.[87]

   In phase I clinical trials, dofetilide produced significant dose-dependent increases in the QT_c interval after intravenous or oral administration. In these patients no significant changes in the PR interval, QRS width, heart rate or blood pressure were

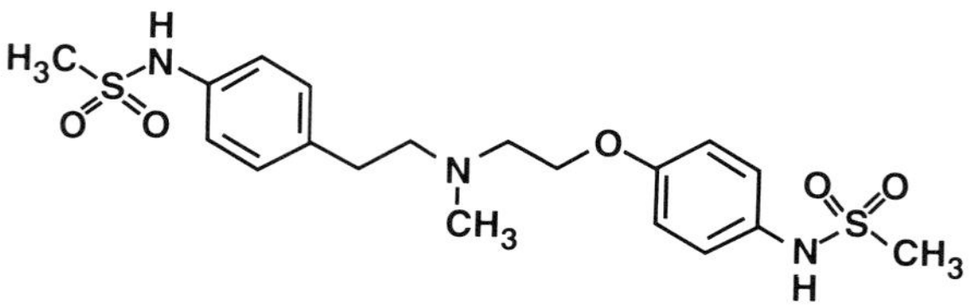

Figure 16.4   Chemical structure of dofetilide (UK-68,798).

observed following administration of dofetilide.[88] However, in one subject, intravenous administration of dofetilide increased the QT_c interval from 415 to 808 ms and an asymptomatic run of polymorphic ventricular tachycardia and multifocal ventricular ectopic beats was transiently observed. In patients with coronary artery disease, intravenous dofetilide prolonged the effective and functional refractory periods of the atria and the ventricles while not affecting the PA, AH, HV, PR or QRS intervals or heart rate.[89] In a similar patient population, intravenous dofetilide increased the duration of the monophasic action potentials and refractory periods recorded from the right ventricular apex or the right ventricular outflow tract. These increases in action potential duration and refractory period showed little use or reverse-use dependence and were remarkably similar between the two electrode sites.[90] In an open-label, dose-ranging study, intravenous dofetilide converted 53% of the patients with atrial fibrillation and 80% of the patients with atrial flutter to normal sinus rhythm.[91] While dose-related efficacy was not seen in the small number of patients (19 in atrial fibrillation, 5 in atrial flutter) treated in this study, the QRS duration and blood pressure remained unchanged, while the QT_c interval showed an overall increase of 77 ms following dofetilide treatment.

NE-10064

While it has been reported that these newer class III agents exert their electrophysiologic actions by inhibiting the I_{Kr}, the rapid component of the delayed rectifier, a recent report has suggested that NE-10064 (azimilide, Figure 16.5) selectively inhibits I_{Ks}, the slow component of the delayed rectifier[92] in isolated guinea-pig myocytes with an IC_{50} of 2 μM. However, while other investigators also using guinea pig myocytes have demonstrated that NE-10064 inhibits I_{Na}, the fast inward sodium current, with an IC_{50} of 100 μM, they also have reported that NE-10064 is not selective for I_{Ks} over I_{Kr}, with respective IC_{50} values of 2 μM and 0.2 μM, respectively.[93,94] An *in vitro* study using sheep Purkinje fibers has shown that NE-10064 increases the duration of the action potential by delaying the terminal phase of repolarization without affecting the plateau phase.[95] In these studies, the potency of NE-10064 to increase the cardiac action potential was E-4031 > NE-10064 > sotalol; increases in APD_{90} of 20 ± 6, 27 ± 6 and 33 ± 9 ms were reported for 1 μM E-4031, 3 μM NE-10064, 300 μM sotalol, respectively.

NE-10064 has shown *in vivo* efficacy against a variety of ventricular arrhythmias in animal models. It suppresses ischemia/reperfusion arrhythmias in the rat[96] and programmed stimulation induced arrhythmias in the postinfarction anesthetized

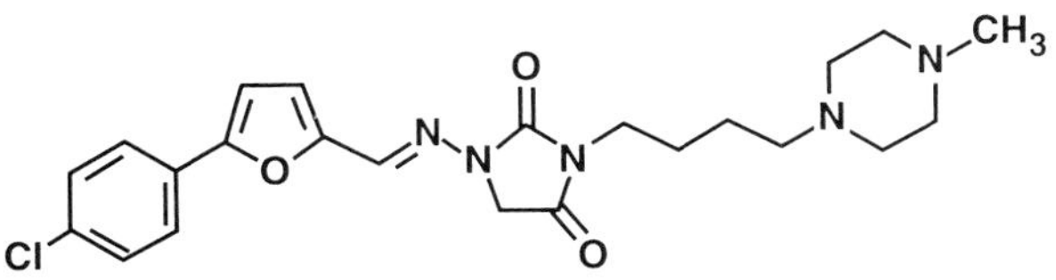

Figure 16.5   Chemical structure of NE-10064.

dog.[97] In both these models, NE-10064 was well tolerated hemodynamically after intravenous administration of up to 30 mg kg^{-1}. In addition to its intravenous activity, NE-10064 is effective after oral administration.[98] When 10 mg kg^{-1} NE-10064 was administered intravenously to postinfarction conscious dogs, it significantly reduced the incidence of sudden cardiac death following acute ischemia at a site distant to the infarcted tissue.[99] NE-10064 (average dose 6.5 ± 3.2 mg kg^{-1} i.v.) also has been shown to be effective in converting atrial flutter in a canine model of stable atrial flutter subsequent to creation of a Y-shaped lesion in the right atria of the dog.[100]

Ibutilide

It has been reported that ibutilide (Figure 16.6) prolongs the action potential duration of guinea-pig myocytes by a unique ionic mechanism.[101] At low concentrations such as 10^{-9} to 10^{-8} M, ibutilide appears to increase a slow inward sodium current, I_{Na-s}, and prolongs the duration of the action potential. A subsequent comparison to other class III agents such as sotalol, E-4031, sematilide or dofetilide showed these agents do not appear to increase this slow inward sodium current but prolong the duration of the cardiac action potential by inhibiting the outward repolarization potassium current I_K.[102] Additional *in vitro* studies have shown that ibutilide significantly increases the effective refractory period of isolated rabbit papillary muscles when they are externally paced at rates of 1 and 3 Hz.[103] These studies also demonstrated that ibutilide does not exert positive or negative inotropic actions while high concentrations, i.e. 10^{-5} M, do depress cardiac conduction when the tissues are paced at a rate of 3 Hz.

The antiarrhythmic actions of ibutilide have been demonstrated in models of atrial and ventricular arrhythmias. Nabih *et al.*[104] used a closed-chest canine model of acute left-ventricular dysfunction to generate sustained atrial fibrillation. Intravenous ibutilide prolonged the QT$_c$ interval by 27% and converted all seven dogs to normal sinus rhythm with a median conversion time of 3 min in this study. In this study there were no significant hemodynamic changes after ibutilide or placebo. Creation of a Y-shaped incision in the right atria of relatively large dogs facilitates the initiation of a sustained atrial flutter. In this model, administration of ibutilide significantly increases the effective refractory period of the atria and terminates the atrial flutter.[105] In addition to its class III actions in these preclinical models of atrial arrhythmias, ibutilide also has been shown to suppress ventricular tachyarrhythmias and fibrillation.[106] An interesting property of class III agents such as ibutilide is their ability to lower the energy necessary to defibrillate a fibrillating

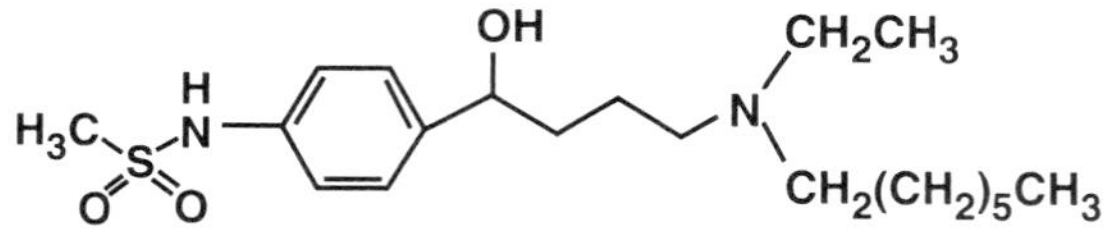

Figure 16.6   Chemical structure of ibutilide (U-70226E).

heart.[107] This is in direct contrast to class I agents such as lidocaine that actually increase the energy necessary to defibrillate an arrested heart.[108] As discussed at the beginning of this chapter, torsades de pointes is a concern with any agent that prolongs the QT interval of the electrocardiogram. While several preclinical models have been proposed to study this specific type of arrhythmia, none has been shown to be uniquely predictive of the clinical situation. In a rabbit model of polymorphic ventricular tachycardia or torsades de pointes, ibutilide has been shown to have lower proarrhythmic potential than *d*-sotalol, clofilium, E-4031 or dofetilide.[109] However, whether this preclinical observation is true in clinical practice remains to be seen, particularly in patients with ventricular tachyarrhythmias, since at present ibutilide is being developed for the treatment of atrial tachyarrhythmias. In a recent clinical trial, Stambler *et al.* demonstrated that intravenous ibutilide converted 42% of the patients with atrial fibrillation and 47% of the patients with atrial flutter to normal sinus rhythm.[110] In contrast, intravenous procainamide converted only 9% of the patients with atrial fibrillation to normal sinus rhythm. While these antiarrhythmic actions of ibutilide were associated with an increase in the duration of the atrial action potential and a decrease in the excitable gap of the re-entrant circuit, procainamide produced an increase in the excitable gap.

Local application of antiarrhythmic agents

While bioavailability considerations can be overcome with specific chemical synthesis programs, bioavailability considerations as well as systemic toxicity problems also can be overcome through the use of cardiac implantable drug-delivery systems. Cardiac-controlled release of antiarrhythmic agents through the direct cardiac implantation of drug–polymer composites, known as 'controlled release matrices', has been studied experimentally with a number of different arrhythmia models, and other experimental designs considering relevant electrophysiologic situations. Initial work in this area demonstrated efficacy of lidocaine containing polyurethane matrices for the conversion of ouabain-induced ventricular tachycardia in dogs.[111,112] Subsequent studies demonstrated efficacy for the prevention of ischemia-induced ventricular tachycardia through epicardial administration of conventional antiarrhythmic agents in class I,[113] III[114] and IV[115] but not beta-adrenergic antagonists (class II).[116]

Recent polymer matrix investigations with class III agents have demonstrated efficacy for preventing ischemia-induced ventricular tachycardia with *d*-sotalol,[111] as well as prolongation of refractoriness and conduction time with polymeric administration of racemic sotalol using polyurethane matrices.[117] Furthermore, enhanced myocardial accumulation of antiarrhythmic agents has been demonstrated with silicone rubber implants used for up to two months in dog studies, as well as pericardial infusions of biodegradable microspheres containing racemic sotalol.[114]

The obvious advantage of cardiac implantable polymeric drug-delivery systems has to do with the very high regional concentrations of antiarrhythmic agents, with sustained release, and minimization of the possibility of systemic side effects.

Interestingly, for several of the agents investigated thus far with controlled cardiac release, lidocaine and verapamil, sonomicrometry studies for ventricular function have demonstrated no adverse effects of regional administration of these agents to the myocardium on cardiac function as measured by sonomicrometry.[109,112]

Ibutilide, a class III antiarrhythmic agent, is of particular interest with respect to local drug delivery, since its bioavailability limitations and pharmacokinetic parameters limit its routine conventional use.[110] Because of a high first-pass elimination, ibutilide has only a 2% bioavailability after oral administration. Furthermore, its plasma half-life is 1.25 hours because of its rapid liver metabolism. However, ibutilide administration directly to the heart using a polymeric controlled-release matrix bypasses these limitations and results in a significant therapeutic advantage for the use of this compound, which is effective at doses of $\leqslant 1\ \mu g\ kg^{-1}$.[118] Very recent studies using ibutilide controlled-release matrices have demonstrated not only effective prolongation of refractoriness with epicardial ibutilide–polyurethane implants in dog, but reduction of the ventricular defibrillation energy threshold as well. The defibrillation threshold reduction is of particular importance, since this particular drug effect could result in favorable design improvements for implantable defibrillators in terms of lessened requirements for use, as well as diminished power needs. Both considerations could result in significant reduction in overall size of the device.

Structure–activity relationships for class III antiarrhythmic agents

Based upon a review of traditional and the newer class III antiarrhythmic agents in clinical use, questions arise concerning drug design and development for optimal antiarrhythmic efficacy as parenteral agents or in combination with local delivery systems. In regard to structure–activity relationships in the newer class III agents, Colatsky has suggested a basic pharmacophore that is required for class III activity.[119] The importance of a methanesulfonamide group in the *para* position on the aryl ring has been reported by several authors.[120–122] Substitution within the methanesulfonamide side chain at the carbon or the nitrogen reduces the class III activity. While changes can occur in the linker group between the aryl ring and the basic amine, the overall spacing between these sites is critical.[123] Connector groups with class III activity include alcohols (sotalol, ibutilide), ethers (UK-68,798), carbonyls (E-4031) separated from the basic amine by 1–3 methylene groups. Although class III activity is observed with secondary or tertiary amines, a variety of side chains and modification of the basic amine still retain class III activity. However, the individual ionic currents that an agent acts upon to produce its class III actions may depend upon specific modifications of this basic amine.

Whereas bioavailability considerations can be overcome with the use of specific tools such as cardiac implantable drug delivery systems, directed chemical synthesis programs also can overcome limitations in bioavailability. For example, L-691,121 (Figure 16.7), was the initial compound tested by Merck Research Laboratories as a class III antiarrhythmic agent. Subsequent modification to increase the metabolic stability created L-702,958, a new active candidate.[124] However, it was found that the oxygen at the 4-position in this second candidate was metabolized to an alcohol at

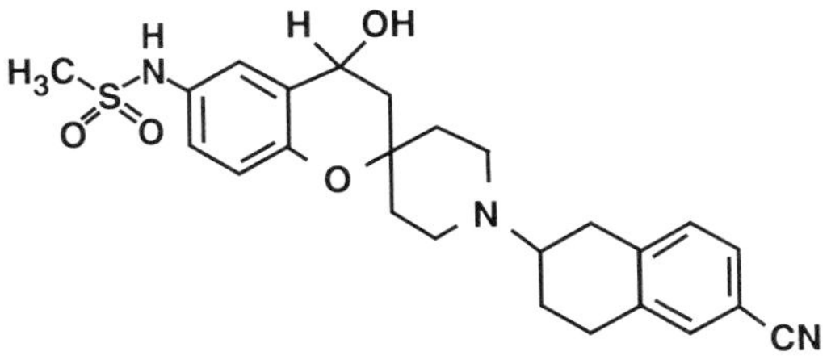

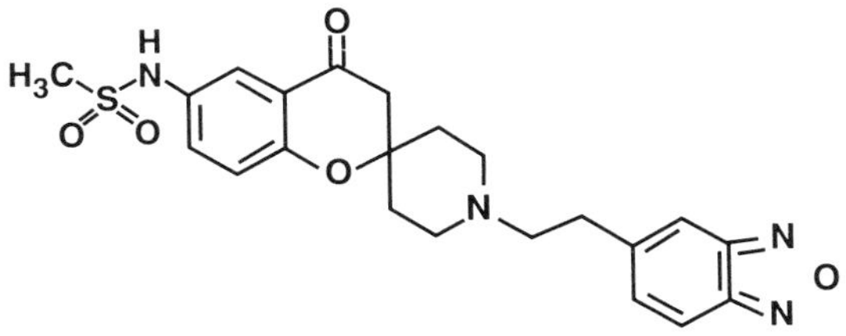

Figure 16.7 Chemical structure of L-691,121 and L-706,000 (MK-499).

this 4-position creating an active metabolite that is now the current clinical candidate L-706,000 (Figure 16.7).[125]

Conclusion

Clearly, the present classification of antiarrhythmic agents began with the initial Vaughan Williams classification published in 1970. The use of new class III antiar-rhythmic agents is the current focus of drug therapy for the treatment of atrial and ventricular tachyarrhythmias. Indeed, this classification system described these class III agents at a time where there were few examples available. The current interest in the use of class III agents is in contrast to the emphasis on the use of class I agents in the 1970s and 1980s. Since the CAST trials have shown the liabilities of these agents that directly depress cardiac conduction, the concepts of cardiac refractoriness and re-entry first proposed at the beginning of this century have taken on new significance. While we now can electrically 'map' the path of a cardiac arrhythmia in both preclinical and clinical situations, it is interesting to note that the concept of re-entrant, wave fronts of conduction has been a constant hypothesis in this field. While beta-blockers, class II agents, have shown their value in reducing postinfarction mortality, not all patients can tolerate these agents and a variety of serious arrhythmias do not necessarily follow acute myocardial infarction.

A new concept is that these class III agents decrease the energy necessary to defibrillate a fibrillating heart in contrast to the increase in energy observed with class I agents. This suggests the concurrent use of class III agents as adjuncts to implanted cardiac defibrillators. This application leads to a new concept of local drug delivery in conjunction with devices or perhaps as a 'stand-alone' application to treat severe cardiac arrhythmias while minimizing the systemic actions of directly-acting antiarrhythmic agents. These are concepts that will need to be developed further in the preclinical laboratory before they can undergo clinical testing.

References

1. Antiarrhythmic Agents – Part 2: Survey, Drug Markets, Devices (1994) *Drug Market Development*, 10 March, **4**, 243–54.
2. Waldo, A. L. and Wit, A. L. (1993) Mechanisms of cardiac arrhythmias. *Lancet*, **341**, 1189–93.
3. Spach, M. S. and Josephson, M. E. (1994) Initiating reentry: the role of nonuniform anisotropy in small circuits. *J. Cardiovasc. Electrophysiol.*, **5**, 182–209.
4. Mayer, A. G. (1908) VII. Rhythmical pulsations in Scyphomedusae. II. Papers from the Tortugas Laboratory of the Carnegie Institution of Washington. Carnegie Institute of Washington, Publication 102, Part VII, **1**, 113–31.
5. Mines, G. R. (1913) On dynamic equilibrium in the heart. *J. Physiol.*, **46**, 349–83.
6. Garrey, W. E. (1914) The nature of fibrillatory contraction of the heart. Its relation to tissue mass and form. *Am. J. Physiol.*, **33**, 397–414.
7. Wiener, N. and Rosenblueth, A. (1946) The mathematical formulation of the problem of conduction impulses in a network of connected excitable elements, specifically in cardiac muscle. *Arch. Inst. Cardiol. Mexico*, **16**, 205–65.
8. Moe, G. K., Rheinboldt, W. C. and Abildskov, J. V. (1964) A computer model of atrial fibrillation. *Am. Heart J.*, **67**, 200–20.
9. Lewis, T. and Drury, A. N. (1926) Revised views of refractory period, in relation to drugs reputed to prolong it, and in relation to circus movement. *Heart*, **13**, 95–100.
10. Selzer, A. and Wray, H. W. (1964) Quinidine syncope and paroxysmal ventricular fibrillation occurring during treatment of chronic atrial arrhythmias. *Circulation*, **30**, 17–26.
11. Dessertenne, F. (1966) Un chapitre nouveau d'electrocardiographie: les variations progressives de l'amplitude de l'electrocardiogramme. *Actualites Cardiologiques et Angiologique Internationale*, **15**, 241–58.
12. Bazett, H. C. (1920) An analysis of the time-relations of electrocardiograms. *Heart*, **7**, 353–70.
13. Taran, L. M. and Szilagyi, N. (1947) Duration of electrical systole (Q-T) in acute rheumatic carditis in children. *Am. Heart J.*, **33**, 14–26.
14. Sarma, J. S., Sarma, R. J., Blitich, M. *et al.* (1984) An exponential formula for heart rate. Dependence of QT interval during exercise and cardiac pacing in human: reevaluation of Bazett's formula. *Am. J. Cardiol.*, **54**, 103–8.
15. Ahnve, S. (1985) Correction of the QT interval for heart rate: review of different formulas and the use of Bazett's formula in myocardial infarction. *Am. Heart J.*, **109**, 568–74.
16. Kovacs, S. J. (1985) The duration of the QT interval as a function of heart rate: a derivation based on physical principles and a comparison to measured values. *Am. Heart J.*, **110**, 872–8.
17. Sagie, A., Larson, M. G., Goldberg, R. J. *et al.* (1992) An improved method for adjusting the QT interval for heart rate (the Framingham Heart Study). *Am. J. Cardiol.*, **70**, 797–801.
18. Ahnve, S. and Vallin, H. (1982) Influence of heart rate and inhibition of autonomic tone on the QT interval. *Circulation*, **65**, 435–9.
19. Nattel, S. (1986) Pharmacodynamic studies of amiodarone and its active *N*-desethyl metabolite. *J. Cardiovas. Pharm.*, **8**, 771–7.

20. Sarma, J. S. M., Bilitich, M. and Melinte, S. G. (1983) Ventricular refractory periods in relation to rate and test-site VT intervals in anesthetized and conscious dogs: a canine model for conscious state measurements. *PACE. Pacing Clin. Electrophysiol.*, **6**, 735–45.
21. Singh, B. N. and Vaughan Williams, E. M. (1970) Classification of antiarrhythmic drugs. In: Sandoe, E., Flentsed-Jensen, E. and Olesen, K. H. (eds) *Symposium on Cardiac Arrhythmias*. Sodertalje: AB Astra.
22. Vaughan Williams, E. M. (1984) A classification of antiarrhythmic drugs reassessed after a decade of new drugs. *J. Clin. Pharmacol.*, **24**, 129–47.
23. Follmer, C. H., Aomine, M., Yeh, J. Z. and Singer, D. H. (1987) Amiodarone-induced block of sodium current in isolated cardiac cells. *J. Pharmacol. Exptl Therapeut.*, **243**, 187–94.
24. Balser, J. R., Bennett, P. B., Hondeghem, L. M. and Roden, D. M. (1991) Suppression of time-dependent outward current in guinea-pig ventricular myocytes. Actions of quinidine and amiodarone. *Circ. Res.*, **69**, 519–29.
25. Sato, R., Koumi, S-I., Singer, D. H. *et al.* (1994) Amiodarone blocks the inward rectifier potassium channel in isolated guinea pig ventricular cells. *J. Pharmacol. Exptl Therapeut.*, **269**, 1213–19.
26. Nishimura, M., Follmer, C. H. and Singer, D. H. (1989) Amiodarone blocks calcium current in single guinea-pig ventricular myocytes. *J. Pharmacol. Exptl Therapeut.*, **251**, 650–9.
27. Morgan, H. E. and Baker, K. M. (1991) Cardiac hypertrophy. Mechanical, neural, and endocrine dependence. *Circulation*, **83**, 13–25.
28. Lynch, J. J., Sanguinette, M. C., Kimura, S. and Bassett, A. L. (1992) Therapeutic potential of modulating potassium current in the diseased myocardium. *FASEB J.*, **6**, 2952–60.
29. Furukawa, T., Bassett, A. L., Furukawa, N. *et al.* (1991) The ionic mechanism of reperfusion-induced early afterdepolarizations in feline left ventricular hypertrophy. *J. Clin. Invest.*, **91**, 1521–31.
30. Huynh, T. V., Chen, F., Wetzel, G. T. *et al.* (1992) Developmental changes in membrane Ca^{2+} and K^+ currents in fetal, neonatal, and adult rabbit ventricular myocytes. *Circ. Res.*, **70**, 508–15.
31. Task Force of the Working Group on Arrhythmias of the European Society of Cardiology (1991) The Sicilian Gambit. A new approach to the classification of antiarrhythmic drugs based on their actions on arrhythmogenic mechanisms. *Circulation*, **84**, 1831–51.
32. Bigger, J. T., Fleiss, J. L., Klieger, R. *et al.* and The Multicenter Post-Infarction Research Group (1984) The relationships among ventricular arrhythmias, left ventricular dysfunction, and mortality in the 2 years after myocardial infarction. *Circulation*, **69**, 250–8.
33. Mukharji, C. J., Rude, R. E., Poole, W. K. *et al.* (1984) Risk factors for sudden death after acute myocardial infarction: two-year follow-up. *Am. J. Cardiol.*, **54**, 31–6.
34. Echt, D. S., Liebson, P. R., Mitchell, L. B. *et al.* and the CAST Investigators (1991) Mortality and morbidity in patients receiving encainide, flecainide, or placebo. The Cardiac Arrhythmia Suppression Trial. *N. Engl. J. Med.*, **324**, 781–8.
35. Epstein, A. E., Bigger, J. T. Jr, Wyse, D. G. *et al.* (1991) Events in the Cardiac Arrhythmia Suppression Trial (CAST): mortality in the entire population enrolled. *J. Am. Coll. Cardiol.*, **18**, 14–19.
36. Pratt, C. M. and Moye, L. A. (1990) The Cardiac Arrhythmic Suppression Trial: background, interim results and implications. *Am. J. Cardiol.*, **65**, 20B–9B.
37. The Cardiac Arrhythmia Suppression Trial II Investigators (1992) Effect of the antiarrhythmic agent moricizine on survival after myocardial infarction. *N. Eng. J. Med.*, **327**, 227–33.
38. Kowey, P. R., Marinchak, R. A. and Rials, S. J. (1990) The cardiac arrhythmia suppression trial: how has it impacted on contemporary arrhythmia management? *J. Cardiovasc. Electrophysiol.*, **1**, 457–63.
39. Nademanee, K., Singh, B. N., Stevenson, W. G. and Weiss, J. N. (1993) Amiodarone and post-MI patients. *Circulation*, **88**, 764–74.

40. The CASCADE Investigators (1993) Randomized Antiarrhythmic Drug Therapy in Survivors of Cardiac Arrest (the CASCADE Study). *Am. J. Cardiol.*, **72**, 280–7.

41. Burkart, F., Pfisterer, M., Kiowski, W. *et al.* (1990) Effect of antiarrhythmic therapy on mortality in survivors of myocardial infarction with asymptomatic complex ventricular arrhythmias: Basel Antiarrhythmic Study of Infarct Survival (BASIS). *J. Am. Coll. Cardiol.*, **16**, 1719–921.

42. Kiowski, W., Pfisterer, M., Brunner, H. *et al.* (1992) Long-term effect of one year amiodarone treatment for persistent complex ventricular arrhythmias after myocarcial infarction. *Circulation*, **86**, I-534.

43. Camm, A. J., Julian, D., Janse, G. *et al.* (1993) The European Myocardial Infarct Amiodarone Trial (EMIAT). *Am. J. Cardiol.*, **72**, 95F–8F.

44. Cairns, J. A., Connolly, S. J., Roberts, R. and Gent, M. (1993) Canadian Amiodarone Myocardial Infarction Arrhythmia Trial (CAMIAT): rationale and protocol. *Am. J. Cardiol.*, **72**, 87F–94F.

45. Sakuta, H., Okamoto, K. and Watanabe, Y. (1993) Antiarrhythmic drugs, clofilium and cibenozoline are potent inhibitors of glibenclamide-sensitive K^+ currents in *Xenopus* oocytes. *Br. J. Pharmacol.*, **109**, 866–72.

46. Yanagishi, T., Ishii, K. and Taira, N. (1993) Absence of effects of class III antiarrhythmic agents on cloned cardiac K^+ channels. *Jap. J. Pharmacol.*, **61**, 371–3.

47. Jurkiewicz, N. K. and Sanguinetti, M. C. (1993) Rate-dependent prolongation of cardiac action potentials by a methanesulfonanilide class III antiarrhythmic agent. Specific block of rapidly activating delayed rectifier K^+ current by dofetilide. *Circ. Res.*, **72**, 75–83.

48. Velkamp, M. W., van-Ginneken, A. C. and Bouman, L. N. (1993) Single delayed rectifier channels in the membrane of rabbit ventricular myocytes. *Circ. Res.*, **72**, 865–78.

49. Campbell, D. L., Rasmusson, R. L., Qu, Y. and Strauss, H. C. (1993) The calcium-independent transient outward potassium current in isolated ferret right ventricular myocytes. I. Basic characterization and kinetic analysis. *J. Gen. Physiol.*, **101**, 571–601.

50. Campbell, D. L., Qu, Y., Rasmusson, R. L. and Strauss, H. C. (1993) The calcium-independent transient outward potassium current in isolated ferret right ventricular myocytes. II. Closed state reverse use-dependent block by 4-aminopyridine. *J. Gen. Physiol.*, **101**, 603–26.

51. Spinelli, W., Moubarak, I. F., Parsons, R. W. and Colatsky, T. J. (1993) Cellular electrophysiology of WAY-123,398, a new class III antiarrhythmic agent: specificity of I_K block and lack of reverse use dependence in cat ventricular myocytes. *Cardiovasc. Res.*, **27**, 1580–91.

52. Yang, T., Tande, P. M., Lathrop, D. A. and Refsum, H. (1992) Class III antiarrhythmic action by potassium channel blockade: dofetilide attenuates hypoxia induced electromechanical changes. *Cardiovasc. Res.*, **26**, 1109–15.

53. Abrahamsson, C., Duker, G., Lundberg, C. and Carlsson, L. (1993) Electrophysiological and inotropic effects of H234/09 (almokalant) *in vitro*: a comparison with two other novel I_K blocking drugs, UK-68,798 (dofetilide) and E-4031. *Cardiovasc. Res.*, **27**, 861–7.

54. Baskin, E. P., Serik, C. M., Wallace, A. A. *et al.* (1991) Effects of new and potent methanesulfonanilide class III antiarrhythmic agents on myocardial refractoriness and contractility in isolated cardiac muscle. *J. Cardiovasc. Pharmacol.*, **18**, 406–14.

55. Butera, J. A., Spinelli, W., Anantharaman, V. *et al.* (1991) Synthesis and selective class III antiarrhythmic activity of novel N-heteroaralkyl-substituted 1-(aryloxy)-2-propanolamine and related propylamine derivatives. *J. Med. Chem.*, **43**, 3212–28.

56. Flores, N. A. and Sheridan, D. J. (1989) Electrophysiological and antiarrhythmic effects of UK 52,046-27 during ischaemia and reperfusion in the guinea pig heart. *Br. J. Pharmacol.*, **96**, 670–4.

57. Chi, L., Black, S. C., Kuo, P. I. *et al.* (1993) Actions of pinacidil at a reduced potassium concentration: a direct cardiac effect possibly involving the ATP-dependent potassium channel. *J. Cardiovasc. Pharmacol.*, **21**, 179–90.

58. Inoue, H., Yamashita, T., Nozaki, A. and Sugimoto, T. (1991) Effects of antiarrhythmic drugs on canine atrial flutter due to reentry: role of prolongation of refractory period and depression of conduction to excitable gap. *J. Am. Coll. Cardiol.*, **18**, 1098–104.
59. Shimizu, A., Kaibara, M., Centurion, O. A. *et al.* (1993) Electrophysiologic effects of a new class III antiarrhythmic agent, E-4031, on atrial flutter, atrial refractoriness, and conduction delay in a canine sterile pericarditis model. *J. Cardiovasc. Pharmacol.*, **21**, 656–62.
60. Nabih, M. A., Prcevski, P, Fromm, B. S. *et al.* (1993) Effect of ibutilide, a new class III agent, on sustained atrial fibrillation in a canine model of acute ischemia and myocardial dysfunction induced by microembolization. *PACE. Pacing Clin. Electrophysiol.* **16**, 1975–83.
61. Curtis, M. J., Macleod, B. A. and Walker, M. J. A. (1987) Models for the study of arrhythmias in myocardial ischaemia and infarction: the use of the rat. *J. Mol. Cell. Cardiol.*, **19**, 399–419.
62. Sano, T., Sugiyama, S., Taki, K. *et al.* (1990) Effects of antiarrhythmic agents classified as class III group on ischaemia-induced myocardial damage in canine hearts. *Br. J. Pharmacol.*, **99**, 577–81.
63. Bril, A., Landais, L. and Gout, B. (1993) Actions and interactions of E-4031 and tedisamil on reperfusion-induced arrhythmias and QT interval in rat *in vivo. Cardiovasc. Drugs Therapy*, **7**, 233–40.
64. Lynch, J. J., Heaney, L. A., Wallace, A. A. *et al.* (1990) Suppression of lethal ischemic ventricular arrhythmias by the class III agent E-4031 in a canine model of previous myocardial infarction. *J. Cardiovasc. Pharmacol.*, **15**, 764–75.
65. Kohdoh, K., Hashimoto, H., Nishiyama, H. *et al.* (1994) Effects of MS-551, a new class III antiarrhythmic drug, on programmed stimulation-induced ventricular arrhythmias, electrophysiology, and hemodynamics in a canine myocardial infarction model. *J. Cardiovasc. Pharmacol.*, **23**, 674–80.
66. Carlsson, L., Abrahamsson, C., Drews, L. and Duker, G. (1992) Antiarrhythmic effects of potassium in rhythm abnormalities related to delayed repolarization. *Circulation*, **85**, 1491–500.
67. Ben-David, J. and Zipes, D. P. (1988) Differential response to right and left ansae subclaviae stimulation of early afterdepolarizations and ventricular tachycardia induced by cesium in dogs. *Circulation*, **78**, 1241–50.
68. Wallace, A. A., Stupienski, R. F., Brookes, L. M. *et al.* (1991) Cardiac electrophysiologic and inotropic actions of new and potent methanesulfonanilide class III antiarrhythmic agents in anesthetized dogs. *J. Cardiovasc. Physiol.*, **18**, 687–95.
69. Dorian, P., Wang, M., David, I. and Fiendel, C. (1991) Oral clofilium produces sustained lowering of defibrillation energy requirements in a canine model. *Circulation*, **83**, 614–21.
70. Walker, M. J. A., Curtis, M. J., Hearse, D. J. *et al.* (1988) The Lambeth Convention. Guidelines for the study of arrhythmias in ischaemia, infarction and reperfusion. *Cardiovasc. Res.*, **22**, 447–55.
71. Roden, D. M., Woosley, R. L. and Primm, R. K. (1986) Incidence and clinical features of the quinidine associated long QT syndrome: implications for patient care. *Am. Heart J.*, **111**, 1088–94.
72. Brachmann, J., Scherlag, B. J., Rosenshtraukh, L. V. and Lazzara, R. (1983) Bradycardia-dependent triggered activity: relevance to drug-induced multiform ventricular tachycardia. *Circulation*, **68**, 846–56.
73. Jackman, W. M., Friday, K. J., Anderson, J. L. *et al.* (1988) The long QT syndromes: a critical review, new clinical observations and unifying hypothesis. *Progr. Cardiovasc. Dis.*, **31**, 115–72.
74. Wit, A. L. and Rosen, M. R. (1986) After depolarizations and triggered activity. In: Fozzard, H. A. (ed.) *The Heart and the Cardiovascular System*, pp. 1449–89. New York: Raven Press.
75. Franz, M. R., Burkhoff, D., Spurgeon, H. *et al.* (1986) *In vitro* validation of a new catheter technique for recording monophasic action potentials. *Eur. Heart J.*, **7**, 34–41.
76. Habbab, M. A. and El-Sherif, N. (1990) Drug-induced torsades de pointes: role of early afterdepolarizations and dispersion of repolarization. *Am. J. Med.*, **89**, 241–6.

77. Carlsson, L., Almgren, O. and Duker, G. (1990) QTU-prolongation and torsades de pointes induced by putative class III antiarrhythmic agents in the rabbit: etiology and interventions. *J. Cardiovasc. Pharmacol.*, **16**, 276–85.
78. Bailie, D. S., Inoue, H., Kaseda, S. *et al.* (1988) Magnesium suppression of early afterdepolarizations and ventricular tachyarrhythmias induced by cesium in dogs. *Circulation*, **77**, 1395–402.
79. Cingolani, H. E., Wiedmann, R. T., Lynch, J. J. *et al.* (1991) Myocardial contractile behavior of a new sotalol derivative. *J. Cardiovasc. Pharmacol.*, **17**, 83–9.
80. Inoue, H., Yamashita, T., Usui, M. *et al.* (1991) Effects of pentisomide and E-4031 on canine atrial flutter due to reentry: a comparative study with disopyramide. *J. Cardiovasc. Pharmacol.*, **18**, 137–43.
81. Chi, L., Mu, D-X. and Lucchesi, B. R. (1991) Electrophysiology and antiarrhythmic actions of E-4031 in the experimental animal model of sudden coronary death. *J. Cardiovasc. Pharmacol.*, **17**, 285–95.
82. Fujiki, A., Tani, M., Mizumaki, K. *et al.* (1994) Electrophysiologic effects of intravenous E-4031, a novel class III antiarrhythmic agent, in patients with supraventricular arrhythmias. *J. Cardiovasc. Pharmacol.*, **23**, 374–8.
83. Carmeliet, E. (1992) Voltage- and time-dependent block of the delayed K^+ current in cardiac myocytes by dofetilide. *J. Pharmacol. Exptl Therapeut.*, **262**, 809–17.
84. Yang, T., Tande, P. M., Lathrop, D. A. and Refsum, H. (1992) Class III antiarrhythmic action by potassium channel blockade: dofetilide attenuates hypoxia induced electromechanical changes. *Cardiovasc. Res.*, **26**, 1109–15.
85. Gwilt, M., Arrowsmith, J. E., Blackburn, R. A. *et al.* (1991) UK-68,798 is a novel, potent and highly selective class III antiarrhythmic agent which blocks potassium channels in cardiac membranes. *J. Pharmacol. Exptl Therapeut.*, **256**, 318–24.
86. Blackburn, S. C., Chi, L., Mu, D.-X. and Lucchesi, B. R. (1991) The antifibrillatory actions of UK-68,798, a class III antiarrhythmic agent. *J. Pharmacol. Exptl Therapeut.*, **258**, 416–23.
87. Buchanan, L. V., Kabell, G., Brunden, M. N. and Gibson, J. K. (1993) Comparative assessment of ibutilide, *d*-sotalol, clofilium, E-4031, and UK-68,798 in a rabbit model of proarrhythmia. *J. Cardiovasc. Pharmacol.*, **220**, 540–9.
88. Tham, T. C., Maclennan, B. A., Burke, M. T. and Harron, D. W. (1993) Pharmacodynamics and pharmacokinetics of the class III antiarrhythmic agent dofetilide (UK-68,798) in humans. *J. Cardiovasc. Pharmacol.*, **21**, 507–12.
89. Sedgwick, M. L., Rasmussen, H. S. and Cobbe, S. M. (1992) Clinical and electrophysiologic effects of intravenous dofetilide (UK-68,798), a new class III antiarrhythmic drug, in patients with angina pectoris. *Am. J. Cardiol.*, **69**, 513–17.
90. Sedgwick, M. L., Rasmussen, H. S. and Cobbe, S. M. (1992) Effects of the class III antiarrhythmic drug dofetilide on ventricular monophasic action potential duration and QT interval dispersion in stable angina pectoris. *Am. J. Cardiol.*, **70**, 1432–7.
91. Suttorp, M. J., Polak, P. E., van't Hof, A. *et al.* (1992) Efficacy and safety of a new selective class III antiarrhythmic agent dofetilide in paroxysmal atrial fibrillation or atrial flutter. *Am. J. Cardiol.*, **69**, 417–19.
92. Busch, A. E., Malloy, K. J., Varnum, M. D. *et al.* (1993) A slowly activating potassium current I_{Ks} is the target for the class III antiarrhythmic drug NE-10064. *Circulation*, **88**, I-231.
93. Conder, M. L., Hess, T. A., Smith, M. A. *et al.* (1994) The effects of NE-10064 on cardiac sodium channels. *FASEB J.*, **8**, A609.
94. Conder, M. L., Smith, M. A., Atwal, K. S. and McCullough, J. R. (1994) Effects of NE-10064 on K^+ currents in cardiac cells. *Biophysics J.*, **66**, A326.
95. Mcintosh, M. A., Tanira, M., Pacini, D. and Kane, K. A. (1994) Comparison of the cardiac electrophysiologic effects of NE-10064 with sotalol and E-4031 and their modification by simulated ischemia. *J. Cardiovasc. Pharmacol.*, **23**, 653–7.
96. Brooks, R. R., Carpenter, J. F., Maynard, A. E. and Decker, G. E. (1993) Efficacy of a novel class III antiarrhythmic agent NE-10064 against ischemia/reperfusion arrhythmias in rats. *FASEB J.*, **7**, A97.

97. Drexler, A. P., Micklas, J. M. and Brooks, R. R. (1993) Effects of intravenously administered NE-10064 on programmed electrical stimulation (PES)-induced ventricular arrhythmias in anesthetized infarcted dogs. *FASEB J.*, **7**, A97.
98. Brandt, M. A. and Maynard, A. E. (1994) NE-10064 inhibits class III antiarrhythmic effects after intravenous or oral activity in conscious dogs. *FASEB J.*, **8**, A7.
99. Black, S. C., Butterfield, J. L. and Lucchesi, B. R. (1993) Protection against programmed electrical stimulation-induced ventricular tachycardia and sudden cardiac death by NE-10064, a class III antiarrhythmic drug. *J. Cardiovasc. Pharmacol.*, **22**, 810–18.
100. Pinto, J., Boyden, P., Wit, A. and Brooks, R. (1994) The effects of a class III antiarrhythmic agent NE-10064 which blocks the slowly activating delayed rectifier current (I_{Ks}) on canine atrial flutter. *PACE*, **17**, 777.
101. Lee, K. S. (1992) Ibutilide, a new compound with potent class III antiarrhythmic activity, activates a slow inward Na^+ current in guinea pig ventricular cells. *J. Pharmacol. Exptl Therapeut.*, **262**, 99–108.
102. Lee, K. S., Tsai, T. D. and Lee, E. W. (1993) Membrane activity of class III antiarrhythmic compounds; a comparison between ibutilide, *d*-sotalol, E-4031, sematilide and dofetilide. *Eur. J. Pharmacol.*, **234**, 43–53.
103. Cimini, M. G., Brunden, M. N. and Gibson, J. K. (1992) Effects of ibutilide fumarate, a novel antiarrhythmic agent, and its enantiomers on isolated rabbit myocardium. *Eur. J. Pharmacol.*, **222**, 93–8.
104. Nabih, M. A., Prcevski, P., Fromm, B. S. *et al.* (1993) Effect of ibutilide, a new class III agent, on sustained atrial fibrillation in a canine model of acute ischemia and myocardial dysfunction induced by microembolization. *PACE. Pacing Clin. Electrophysiol.*, **16**, 1975–83.
105. Buchanan, L. V., Turcotte, U. M., Kabell, G. G. and Gibson, J. K. (1993) Antiarrhythmic and electrophysiologic effects of ibutilide in a chronic canine model of atrial flutter. *J. Cardiovasc. Pharmacol.*, **33**, 10–14.
106. Buchanan, L. V., Kabell, G., Turcotte, U. M. *et al.* (1992) Effects of ibutilide on spontaneous and induced ventricular arrhythmias in 24-hour canine myocardial infarction: a comparative study with sotalol and encainide. *J. Cardiovasc. Pharmacol.*, **19**, 256–63.
107. Wesley, R. C., Farkhani, F., Morgan, D. and Zimmerman, D. (1993) Ibutilide: enhanced defibrillation via plateau sodium current activation. *Am. J. Physiol.*, **264**, H1269–H74.
108. Dorian, P., Fain, E. S., Davy, J. M. and Winkle, R. A. (1968) Lidocaine causes a reversible, concentration-dependent increase in defibrillation energy requirements. *J. Am. Coll. Cardiol.*, **8**, 327–32.
109. Buchanan, L. V., Kabell, G., Brunden, M. N. and Gibson, J. K. (1993) Comparative assessment of ibutilide, *d*-sotalol, clofilium, E-4031, and UK-68,798 in a rabbit model of proarrhythmia. *J. Cardiovasc. Pharmacol.*, **220**, 540–9.
110. Stambler, B. S., Wood, M. A., Belz, M. K. *et al.* (1993) Electrophysiologic determinants of pharmacologic conversion of human atrial fibrillation and flutter: enhanced efficacy of ibutilide a new class III antiarrhythmic drug. *Circulation*, **88**, I-445.
111. Sintov, A., Scott, W., Dick, M. and Levy, R. J. (1988) Cardiac controlled release for arrhythmia therapy: lidocaine–polyurethane matrix studies. *J. Controlled Release*, **8**, 157–65.
112. Sintov, A., Scott, W. A., Gallagher, K. P. and Levy, R. J. (1990) Conversion of ouabain-induced ventricular tachycardia in dogs with epicardial lidocaine: pharmacodynamics and function effects. *Pharmaceut. Res.*, **7**, 28–33.
113. Levy, R. J., Golomb, S. F., Siden, R. *et al.* (1991) Polymeric controlled release of cardiovascular drugs. In: Gebelein, C. (ed.) *Cosmetic and Pharmaceutical Applications of Polymers*, pp. 231–8. Edgewater, FL: Lionfire.
114. Labhasetwar, V., Kadish, A., Underwood, T. *et al.* (1993) The efficacy of controlled release *d*-sotalol–polyurethane epicardial implants for ventricular arrhythmias due to acute ischemia in dogs. *J. Controlled Release*, **23**, 75–86.
115. Siden, R., Kadish, A., Flowers, W. *et al.* (1992) Epicardial controlled release verapamil prevents ventricular tachycardia episodes induced by acute ischemia in a canine model. *J. Cardiovasc. Pharmacol.*, **19**, 798–809.

116. Siden, R., Flowers, W. and Levy, R. J. (1992) Epicardial propranolol administration for ventricular arrhythmias in dogs: matrix formulation and characterization. *Biomaterials*, **13**, 764–70.
117. Labhasetwar, V., Underwood, T., Gallagher, M. *et al.* (1994) Sotalol controlled-release systems for arrhythmias: *in vitro* characterization, *in vivo* drug disposition, and electrophysiologic effects. *J. Pharmaceut. Sci.*, **83**, 157–64.
118. Labhasetwar, V., Underwood, T., Hell, R. W. *et al.* (1994) Epicardial administration of ibutilide from polyurethane matrices: effects on defibrillation threshold and electrophysiologic parameters. *J. Cardiovasc. Pharmacol.*, **24**, 826–40.
119. Colatsky, T. J. (1993) Potassium channel blockers: synthetic agents and their antiarrhythmic potential. In: Weston, A. H. and Hamilton, T. C. (eds) *Potassium Channel Modulators*, pp. 304–40. London: Blackwell Scientific Publications.
120. Lumma, W. C. Jr., Wohl, R. A., Davey, D. D. *et al.* (1987) Rational design of 4-[(methylsulfonyl)amino]benzamides as class III antiarrhythmic agents. *J. Med. Chem.*, **30**, 755–8.
121. Elliot, J. M., Selnick, H. G., Claremon, D. A. *et al.* (1992) 4-Oxospiro[benzopyran-2,4'-piperidines] as class III antiarrhythmic agents. Pharmacological studies on 3,4-dihydro-1'-[2-(benzofurazan-5-yl)-ethyl]-6-methanesulfonamidospiro[(2H)-1-benzopyran-2,4'-piperidin]-4-one (L-691,121). *J. Med. Chem.*, **35**, 3973–6.
122. Oinuma, H., Miyake, K., Yamanaka, M. *et al.* (1990) 4'[(4-piperidyl)carbonyl]-methanesulfonamides as potent, selective bioavailable class III antiarrhythmic agents. *J. Med. Chem.*, **33**, 903–5.
123. Hester, J. B., Gibson, J. K., Cimini, M. G. *et al.* (1991) N-[ω-amino-1-hydroxyalkyl)phenyl]methanesulfonamide derivatives with class III antiarrhythmic activity. *J. Med. Chem.*, **34**, 308–15.
124. Piquet, V., Appenzeller, M., Buclin, T. *et al.* (1993) L-702,958, a novel class III antiarrhythmic agent in healthy volunteers. *Clin. Pharmacol. Therapeut.*, **53**, 138.
125. Singh, B. N., Ellenbogen, K. A., Zoble, R. G. *et al.* (1994) Electrocardiographic effects of oral MK-499, a new class III antiarrhythmic agent in patients with coronary artery disease. *J. Am. Coll. Cardiol.*, **23**, 92A.

17

The Molecular Biology of the Long QT Syndrome

Mark W. Russell
Lawrence C. Brody

Introduction

Traditionally, disease genes have been identified through characterization of the biochemical defect. The knowledge of the protein's functions were then used to identify and isolate the protein and, from the amino acid sequence, to determine the gene responsible. However, for many inherited diseases, the pathophysiologic processes are too complex to unravel by examining the intact system or through experimental models. For these diseases, an alternative approach termed 'positional cloning' has been devised. Positional cloning identifies the disease gene by its physical location in the genome, and uses the gene's sequence and structure to trace its expression and function (see Figure 17.1).[1]

Congenital abnormalities of myocardial repolarization, such as the Romano–Ward and Jervell–Lange–Nielsen long QT syndromes, have been difficult to characterize and treat due to the complex interaction of physiologic factors which influence repolarization. Experimental models of the long QT syndrome have been able to represent some, but not all, of the pathophysiologic defects present in affected individuals.[2–8] Therefore, positional cloning techniques are currently being used to determine the genes responsible.[9] The identification of one genetic locus responsible for the Romano–Ward long QT syndrome closely linked to the Harvey-*ras*-1 (H-*ras*-1) oncogene locus on chromosome 11p15.5 marked the first step of the positional cloning effort.[9] The region around the H-*ras*-1 locus is currently being searched for this gene. Identification and characterization of the genes responsible for the long QT syndromes offers an exciting opportunity to determine how these genes affect myocardial repolarization and how they function in normal and disease states. Ultimately, understanding the genes that influence myocardial repolarization should aid not only the diagnosis and treatment of individuals with congenital repolarization abnormalities but should improve the understanding and treatment of other ventricular arrhythmias.

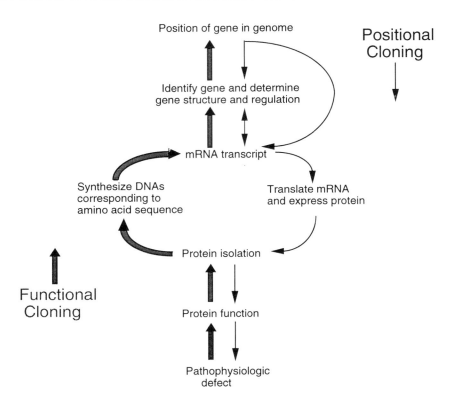

Figure 17.1 Comparison of positional versus functional cloning approach to disease characterization.

Long QT syndromes

History

The QT interval is an electrocardiographic measurement which reflects the time course of ventricular depolarization and repolarization (Figure 17.2). Long QT syndrome patients have abnormalities of myocardial repolarization which cause lengthening of the QT interval. There are three forms of congenital prolongation of the QT interval: (1) the Romano–Ward syndrome[10,11] which is inherited as an autosomal dominant disorder; (2) the Jervell–Lange–Nielsen syndrome[12] which is autosomal recessive and associated with congenital sensorineural deafness; and (3) the sporadic or idiopathic form. To date, >1500 patients have been diagnosed with the long QT syndrome.[13] Over 90% have normal hearing and 75–80% have a positive family history.[13] Of the long QT syndromes, the Romano–Ward syndrome, being the most prevalent and best suited for positional cloning, has attracted the most attention.

The Romano–Ward long QT syndrome was first described in 1963 and is typified by prolongation of the QT interval with syncope and sudden death secondary to torsades de pointes[10,11] (Figure 17.3). The symptoms usually begin during late

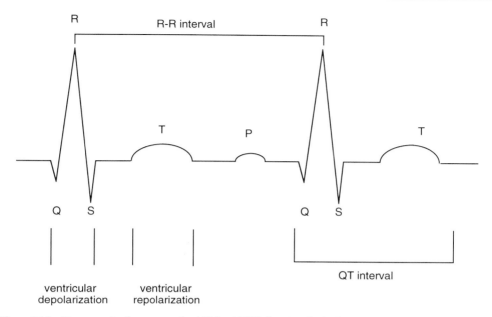

Figure 17.2   One complex from a standard 12-lead ECG showing the P, Q, R, S, and T waves as well as the QT interval.

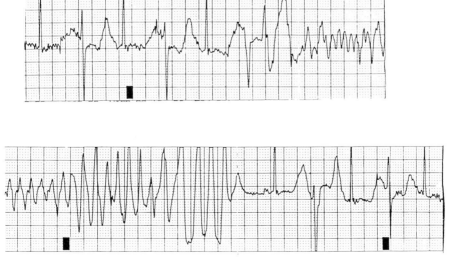

Figure 17.3   Episode of torsades de pointes in a pediatric patient with Romano–Ward long QT syndrome. The tracing is from lead II of a standard 12-lead ECG recorded at a paper speed of 25 mm s^{-1} (tracing courtesy of M. Dick II).

Table 17.1 Clinical diagnostic criteria for the long QT syndromes. After Schwartz *et al.*[19]

Parameter		Points
*ECG findings**		
A.	QT_c†	
	≥480 ms$^{\frac{1}{2}}$	3
	460–470 ms$^{\frac{1}{2}}$	2
	450 ms$^{\frac{1}{2}}$ (in males)	1
B.	Torsade de pointes‡	2
C.	T-wave alternans	1
D.	Notched T wave in three leads	1
E.	Low heart rate for age§	0.5
Clinical history		
A.	Syncope‡	
	With stress	2
	Without stress	1
B.	Congenital deafness	0.5
Family history‖		
A.	Family members with definite LQTS#	1
B.	Unexplained sudden cardiac death below age 30 among immediate family members	0.5

LQTS, long QT syndrome.
*In the absence of medications or disorders known to affect these electrocardiographic features.
†QT_c calculated by Bazett's formula, where $QT_c = QT/\sqrt{RR}$.
‡Mutually exclusive.
§Resting heart rate below the second percentile for age.
‖The same family member cannot be counted in A and B.
#Definite LQTS is defined by an LQTS score ≥4.
Scoring: ≤1 point, low probability of LQTS; 2–3 points, intermediate probability of LQTS; ≥4 points, high probability of LQTS.

childhood and occur during periods of heightened sympathetic tone. In general, these episodes occur during episodes of neural sympathetic responses, elicited by emotion, as opposed to hormonal sympathetic responses, such as during exercise.[14] Typically, a patient with long QT syndrome will have episodes of syncope associated with excitement or anger. Estimates on mortality have varied from 70% by the age of 15 years in untreated patients[15] to 5–7% in patients treated with β-blockade or left cardiac sympathetic ganglionectomy (-LCSG).[16–18]

Accurate identification of affected individuals has been difficult, particularly during childhood. Unfortunately, the diagnosis is often not made until symptoms such as syncope or sudden death occur. The diagnosis of long QT syndrome is based on prolongation of the corrected QT interval which is often accompanied by T-wave abnormalities such as notching or T-wave alternans, abnormally slow sinus heart rate for age, and syncopal attacks which usually occur with excitement. While traditionally the diagnosis has been based almost entirely on the length of the corrected QT interval and symptoms, recently Schwartz *et al.*[19] outlined a scoring system for the diagnosis of the long QT syndrome (see Table 17.1) which includes weighted scores for each of the characteristic abnormalities found in patients with the long QT syndrome. The scoring system is largely empirical, based on the clinical experience of the authors, and further study will be required to determine if this scoring system aids in the identification of affected individuals and reduces the number of incorrectly diagnosed patients.

Pathophysiology

The prolonged QT interval in these patients represents an abnormality of myocardial repolarization. The exact nature of the abnormality is unknown. Due to the exacerbation of symptoms during increased sympathetic tone, the role of the sympathetic nervous system in the long QT syndrome has been widely investigated.

The ability of the central nervous system to influence the electrocardiogram, and the QTU interval in particular, was first documented by Burch *et al.*[20] They noted large T waves, prominent U waves and prolongation of the QT interval in patients with cerebrovascular accidents. Manning and Cotton[21] demonstrated the induction of ventricular arrhythmias by the central nervous system, eliciting ectopic ventricular beats and idioventricular rhythms upon stimulation of the midbrain reticular formation and posterior hypothalamus in the anesthetized cat. Furthermore, this ectopy was eliminated by pharmacologic or surgical vagotomy and by bilateral stellate ganglionectomy.

The differential influence of the right and left stellate ganglia on the QT interval and on the functional refractory periods (FRP) of the ventricles was delineated by Yanowitz *et al.*[22] This study determined that left stellate stimulation and right stellate blockade prolonged the QT interval while left or bilateral stellate blockade had little effect on the QT interval length. Left and right stellate blockade were demonstrated to increase the FRP of the posterior and anterior left ventricle (LV), respectively. These findings led to the first LCSG for the treatment of the long QT syndrome by Moss and McDonald in 1971.[23]

Based on these studies and work in his own laboratory, Schwartz *et al.*[24] postulated that a congenital defect in the balance of sympathetic innervation to the heart from the right and left stellate ganglia, resulting in exaggerated left stellate or diminished right stellate activity, was responsible for the long QT syndrome. In a series of animal studies, Schwartz demonstrated that manipulations of sympathetic tone could reproduce many, if not all, of the clinical features of the long QT syndrome.[2,25–28] He and others found stimulation of the left stellate ganglion transiently prolonged the ventricular refractory period,[31] could produce T-wave alternans,[27] decrease the ventricular fibrillation threshold,[25] exaggerate early[29] and induce delayed afterdepolarizations[26] and transiently lengthen the QT interval.[22] Stimulation of the right stellate ganglia transiently increased the ventricular refractory period but decreased the ventricular fibrillation threshold. Right stellate blockade produced sinus bradycardia, decreased the ventricular fibrillation threshold during coronary artery occlusion,[25] and prolonged the QT interval.[22,30] Proponents of the sympathetic imbalance theory interpret these findings as indicating the following relationships between asymmetric alteration of cardiac sympathetic tone and myocardial repolarization.[16,46] Briefly, right and left stellate stimulation increases sympathetic tone resulting in QT prolongation; right stellate blockade causes a reflex increase in left stellate activity, increasing the right–left asymmetry, and causing prolongation of the QT interval through greater dispersion of ventricular recovery forces. Left stellate blockade, likewise, causes reflex increase in right sympathetic activity but to a degree insufficient to compensate for the loss of left-sided sympathetic activity, thereby causing a net decrease in sympathetic activity and a reversal of the sympathetic asymmetry.

Supportive animal studies include demonstration of QT prolongation and myocardial sympathetic denervation after nerve growth factor antiserum injection into neonatal rats[32] and QT prolongation in the chick embryo after placode, or sympathetic efferent, node ablation.[33] Pathologic case reports have demonstrated inflammation[34] and inflammatory degeneration[35] of the stellate ganglion. However, in another study by Schwartz et al.,[24] the myocardium was normal. Attempts have been made to demonstrate asymmetric myocardial sympathetic neurotransmitter uptake using positron emission tomography (PET) imaging with MIBG (metaiodobenzyl-guanidine) in patients with the long QT syndrome. Results of the MIBG scanning have been mixed with some studies reporting symmetric MIBG uptake[3,36] while others have demonstrated decreased uptake in the inferior and inferior-septal portions of the left ventricle which would be consistent with a right-sided sympathetic dysinnervation.[37,38] Recently, a genetic model which supports the possibility of inherited, asymmetric sympathetic innervation was described by Lee et al.[39] who demonstrated that a defect in the neurotrophin receptor p75 in mice affected the development of a specific population of sympathetic neurons resulting in the absence of innervation of specific tissues including the pineal and sweat glands. A defect in a related neurotrophin receptor might account for abnormal cardiac sympathetic innervation.

However, several investigators have proposed that an intrinsic myocardial repolarization defect could be responsible for the long QT syndrome and that manipulations of sympathetic tone may be exerting effects through the complex second-messenger system which controls ion-channel conductance.[2–8] The predominant ion currents involved in myocardial repolarization include the outward delayed rectifier potassium current and I_{to}, a potassium current that rapidly activates and then inactivates after depolarization.[16] Factors which influence potassium flux, such as hypokalemia, cesium chloride blockade of potassium channels, hypocalcemia, hypomagnesemia, acidosis and class IA and class III antiarrhythmic therapy prolong the QT interval and cause exaggerated early afterdepolarizations which can generate ventricular arrhythmias.[40–43] In patients, alteration of potassium-channel conductance by one of these methods causes pause-dependent ventricular arrhythmias. A prolonged ventricular cycle length causes exaggerated early afterdepolarizations which, if sufficient in amplitude, can cause triggered activity and ventricular extrasystoles.[40] The long–short–long cycle length of ventricular bigeminy can increase U-wave amplitude and cause more severe ventricular arrhythmias such as ventricular tachycardia or torsades de pointes.[42] With pause-dependent prolongation of the QT interval, β-adrenergic stimulation mildly decreases the incidence of ventricular arrhythmias[40] by decreasing the the cycle length and the frequency of sinus pauses. In contrast, in Romano–Ward, Jervell–Lange–Nielsen and most sporadic congenital long QT syndrome patients as well as patients with QT prolongation secondary to CNS disturbances, ventricular arrhythmias are

Table 17.2   Long QT syndromes

I. Congenital (>1500 patients)

A.   Romano–Ward syndrome (75–80%)
      autosomal dominant
      adrenergic-dependent ventricular arrhythmias
      two types:
            1. linked to H-*ras*-1 locus (LQT1)
            2. not linked to H-*ras*-1
B.   Jervell–Lange–Neilsen syndrome (<10%)
      autosomal recessive
      sensorineural deafness
      adrenergic-dependent ventricular arrhythmias
C.   Sporadic (10–15%)
      no family history
      several types:
            1. adrenergic-dependent ventricular arrhythmias
            2. pause-dependent ventricular arrhythmias
            3. mixed adrenergic- and pause-dependent

II. Acquired

A.   CNS disturbance – excluding subarachnoid hemorrhage, stroke adrenergic-dependent
B.   Electrolyte abnormalities
      hypokalemia, hypocalcemia, hypomagnesemia
      pause-dependent
C.   Drug-induced
      class IA and class III antiarrhythmics, phenothiazines, tricyclic antidepressants, erythromycin,
            sotalol
      pause-dependent

---

adrenergic-dependent, occurring with increased sympathetic tone and decreasing with β-blockade.[40] Only rarely do patients with sporadic congenital long QT syndrome demonstrate pause-dependent or mixed pause- and adrenergic-dependent ventricular arrhythmias[40] (see Table 17.2).

However, electrolyte abnormalities such as hypokalemia and hypomagnesemia can exacerbate symptoms in all patients with a congenital long QT syndrome[40] and left stellate stimulation can exacerbate cesium-induced ventricular arrhythmias.[29] Furthermore, both pause- and adrenergic-dependent arrhythmias may be due to exaggerated early afterdepolarizations.[40,44,45] It has even been proposed that pause-, mixed- and adrenergic-dependent arrhythmias may represent a spectrum of a single repolarization defect in ion-channel conductance with the adrenergic-dependent LQTS being the most severe manifestation.[40] Therefore, an intrinsic defect in myocardial repolarization may account for the long QT syndrome and, if so, may involve the signal transduction from the sympathetic nervous system to the ion channels which effect repolarization.

Therapy

Due to the adrenergic-dependent nature of the ventricular arrhythmias, β-blockade[11] with or without LCSG[23] was the initial treatment for the long QT syndromes. Beta-blockade alone has been reported to be effective in preventing

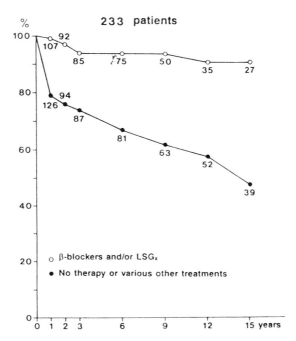

Figure 17.4 The effect of therapy, after the first syncopal episode, on the survival of 233 long QT syndrome patients. Therapy with β-blockade or LCSG markedly decreased mortality. (After Schwartz.[67])

syncope and sudden death in 75–80% of the patients with long QT syndrome.[16,40,46,47] Patients who continued to have symptoms despite β-blockade were considered for LCSG. Although only 11% of the patients were reported to have permanent shortening of the QT interval in response to LCSG,[47] there was a reduction in number of patients with symptoms and nonfatal cardiac arrests, from 99% to 45% and from 60% to 15%, respectively. The absolute effectiveness of this therapy is clouded by the variety of surgical techniques and the heterogeneity of the population which included Romano–Ward syndrome (most likely both types, linked and not linked to H-*ras*-1), Jervell–Lange–Nielsen and sporadic long QT syndrome patients. However, these studies do demonstrate that therapies directed at modifying the myocardial sympathetic response by LCSG or peripheral β-blockade have successfully decreased the mortality in patients with all types of congenital long QT syndrome (Figure 17.4).

Currently, long QT syndrome patients are most commonly treated with 2.5–4 mg kg^{-1} day^{-1} propranolol. The use of other β-blocking agents such as nadolol has been reported[17,49] with equivalent efficacy in the amerlioration of symptoms and prevention of ventricular arrhythmias in pediatric patients.[17] However, atenolol use in the treatment of the long QT syndrome has declined due to concerns over its efficacy in preventing episodes of torsades de pointes and sudden death (M. Dick II, pers. commun.). For those patients who continue to have symptoms despite adequate β-blockade, concurrent administration of phenytoin or mexilitene has been tried but, used alone, each agent has been less successful than the β-blockers.[17] Furthermore, multiple-drug regimens have not generally proven to be successful when single-drug therapy has failed.[17] As a consequence, patients with symptoms despite therapy have had LCSG[47] or atrial pacing[49–52] with successful treatment of symptoms. For severe, refractory cases, implantable defibrillators have been placed, and have been effective in some patients.[17] However, despite all therapy, mortality from fatal arrhythmia continues to be 5–8% for patients with the long QT syndromes[16,17] and may be higher in some families.

Defining the phenotype

In order to perform linkage studies in preparation for positional cloning, a very strict definition of the affected phenotype is required. Misclassification of an unaffected individual as affected or vice versa can have profound implications when defining the region of interest for the gene responsible. Several difficulties have complicated the identification of individuals affected with the long QT syndrome. First, the precise termination of the T wave can be difficult to define, particularly with a gradually sloped T wave or superimposition of a prominent U wave. Determination of a patient's QT interval may vary by as much as 0.04 s between observers.[53] Furthermore, the QT varies with the time of day, and can be affected by serum electrolyte concentrations, and certain drugs such as class IA antiarrhythmics. Females have slightly longer corrected QT intervals than males (0.421 ± 0.018 and 0.409 ± 0.014 s, respectively)[54] and the corrected QT interval tends to decrease from early childhood to early adulthood in males.[55–57]

Furthermore, the most accurate method of correcting the QT interval for heart rate in patients with the long QT syndrome has been debated.[58] Traditionally, investigators have used Bazett's correction for heart rate [$QT/(R–R \text{ interval})^{1/2}$] of the QT interval measured in lead II or V5 of a standard 12 lead electrocardiogram. Linear[58,60] and exponential models[61] as well as JT interval measurement[62] have been suggested as more accurate corrections and are currently being evaluated in patients with the long QT syndrome to determine if affected patients will be more readily distinguished from unaffected individuals.[53] At this time, most investigators continue to use Bazett's formula to correct the QT interval for heart rate.[53]

The precise identification of patients affected with the long QT syndrome is further complicated by the range of corrected QT intervals in affected individuals regardless of the method. In a retrospective study in which 'affected' individuals were determined by linkage to the H-*ras*-1 allele which cosegregated with the affected phenotype (see Figure 17.5), there was a significant overlap in the corrected QT interval in affected and unaffected individuals ranging from 0.41 to 0.59 s and from 0.39 to 0.47 s, respectively.[63] Therefore, diagnosis of the long QT syndrome, for the purpose of linkage analysis, has been defined as a QTc of ⩾0.47 s or ⩾0.45 s in patients with a history of syncope during excitement or torsades de pointes with an onset of symptoms during childhood or early adulthood.[64] Unaffected individuals are defined by a QTc ⩽ 0.41 s. Individuals not categorized as affected or unaffected by these criteria are designated 'indeterminate' and are not used for linkage analysis.

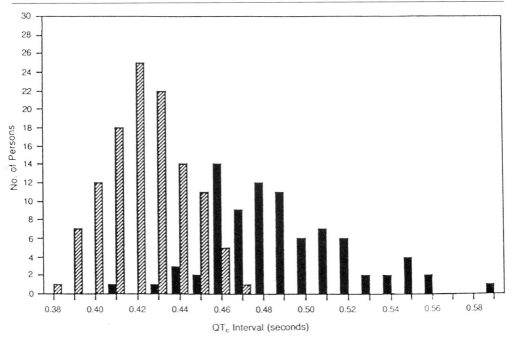

Figure 17.5 Distribution of QTc measurements among carriers (solid bars) and noncarriers (hatched bars) of the long QT syndrome. Carriers of the Romano–Ward long-QT gene were identified by presence of the H-*ras*-1 allele which cosegregated with the long QT syndrome in each family studied. (After Vincent et al.[63])

These criteria allow the identification of the maximum number of affected individuals while not miscategorizing patients. Note that these criteria are much stricter than in the clinical setting where it is critical to identify all potentially affected individuals.

Once the genes responsible for the long QT syndrome are determined, genetic testing may be beneficial to identify affected individuals with an indeterminant phenotype, since QT interval length has not consistently correlated with the risk of sudden death in patients with the syndrome. Although two studies found that children with an extremely prolonged QT interval, $\geqslant$0.55–0.60 ms,[17,65] have an increased risk of sudden death, the risk of sudden death in patients with an altered gene but a normal QT interval remains to be determined. The clinical observation of excitement-induced torsades de pointes and sudden death despite a normal or borderline QT interval attests to the lethality of this syndrome even when the QT interval is not prolonged.[16,17,66]

Molecular biology of the long QT syndromes

Linkage analysis

Recently, a positional cloning effort has sought to identify the genes responsible for the Romano–Ward syndromes. The first phase of positional cloning is the identification of the chromosomal region which is near the disease gene. If a chromosomal rearrangement is present in patients with the disease, then the search can be focused on the affected region(s). Unfortunately, no chromosomal anomalies have been detected in patients with Romano–Ward syndrome 1 (LQT1)[64] (M. Russell, unpubl. observ.).

If no chromosomal abnormalities are detected then the genome will need to be 'searched' using linkage analysis. This process relies on minor differences in the DNA sequences between individuals. The genomic DNA differences that can be utilized in this process include microsatellite repeats, variable number of tandem repeats (VNTRs) and restriction fragment-length polymorphisms (RFLPs) (Figure 17.6). Many of these differences, called polymorphic markers, have been well characterized and can be used to distinguish DNA segments from different individuals. The sequence variations that can be detected for any polymorphic marker are termed 'alleles'. The polymerase chain reaction has made the detection of microsatellite marker alleles possible through the specific amplification of the DNA segment containing the polymorphic repeat (Figure 17.7).

During meiosis, crossover or recombination occurs between an individual's two homologous chromosomes (Figure 17.8). The further apart two markers are, the greater the likelihood that a recombination event will occur between them. The frequency of recombination between two markers will determine the genetic distance between them. The genetic distance is measured in centimorgans (cM) where 1 cM approximates 1% recombination for distances <30 cM. Markers that are very far apart ($\geqslant$50 cM) on the same chromosome will segregate independently as if they were on separate chromosomes. The genetic distance between markers correlates with the physical distance, measured in basepairs (bp). On average, 1 cM or 1% recombination corresponds to a physical distance of 1×10^6 bp (1 megabase or 1 Mb)[68] but can be severalfold greater or less than that depending on the recombination characteristics in that region.

To determine linkage of an autosomal disease to a specific marker, markers distributed throughout the 22 autosomal chromosomes are traced through a large, affected family to determine the frequency with which the disease cosegregates with a specific allele for that marker. From the frequency of recombination between the disease phenotype and the marker, a statistic reflecting the odds that the markers and the disease are linked, referred to as a LOD score or logarithm (base 10) of the odds, can be calculated. A LOD score of $\geqslant$3 indicates linkage of the disease gene to that marker with a likelihood of 1000:1.[69]

Using this approach, Keating *et al.*[9,70] found that the Romano–Ward long QT phenotype was closely linked to the H-*ras*-1 locus on the short arm of chromosome 11 in seven families. The LOD score for linkage of the long QT syndrome to the H-*ras*-1 locus was 16.44 in the largest family. However, in several recently described pedigrees, the long QT phenotype was shown not to be linked to the H-*ras*-1 locus,[71–74] indicating that a different locus is responsible in those families. Using the pedigrees not linked to the H-*ras*-1 locus, a search for a marker linked to the other gene(s) responsible for the Romano–Ward long QT phenotype is in progress, but, to date, no alternative locus has been identified (J. A. Towbin, pers. commun.).

Therefore, at least two separate genetic loci can cause the Romano–Ward long QT syndrome phenotype. This genetic heterogeneity currently prevents genetic

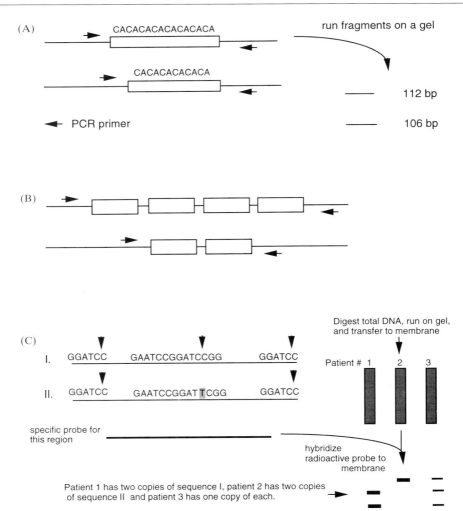

(A)

CACACACACACACACA

run fragments on a gel

CACACACACA

← PCR primer

—— 112 bp

—— 106 bp

(B)

(C)

I. GGATCC   GAATCCGGATCCGG   GGATCC

II. GGATCC   GAATCCGGAT T CGG   GGATCC

specific probe for
this region

Digest total DNA, run on gel,
and transfer to membrane

Patient # 1   2   3

hybridize
radioactive probe to
membrane

Patient 1 has two copies of sequence I, patient 2 has two copies
of sequence II and patient 3 has one copy of each.

Figure 17.6 Polymorphic markers. The major categories of polymorphic markers are the following: **A**. Microsatellite – A very short segment of DNA, usually 2–4 basepairs, is tandemly repeated and can be detected by polymerase chain reaction (PCR). **B**. VNTR – A variable number of tandem repeats are longer segments of repeated DNA sequence which can be detected by PCR or a complementary segment of DNA called a probe. **C**. RFLP – A restriction fragment-length polymorphism is a change in DNA sequence that results in the gain or loss of a restriction endonuclease (an enzyme which cuts the DNA at specific sequences) site.

diagnosis of the Romano–Ward syndrome in small families where there are not enough affected individuals and their first-degree relatives to generate a LOD score ⩾3. With smaller families, apparent linkage to the H-*ras*-1 locus, i.e. cosegregation of the Romano–Ward phenotype with the H-*ras*-1 marker, may occur by chance, even in families where the syndrome is not linked to that locus. Therefore, genetic counseling based on linkage of the syndrome must necessarily be delayed in smaller families until the genes have been found. In larger families with definite linkage to

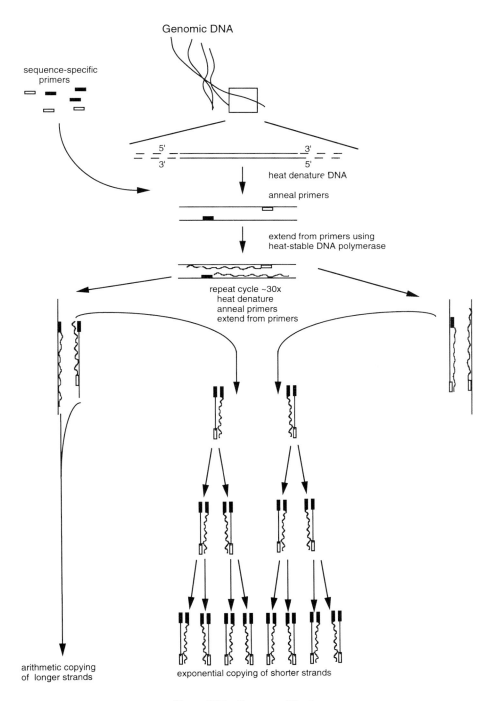

Figure 17.7 Gene amplification.

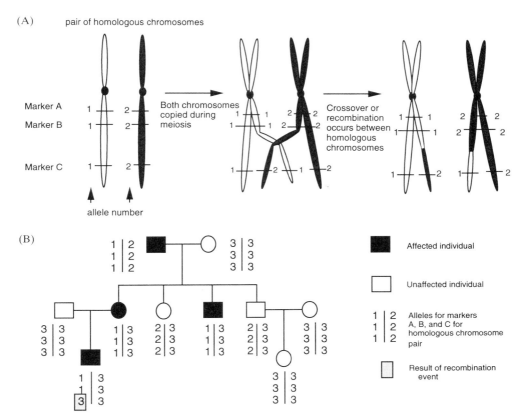

Figure 17.8 Recombination. **A**. Polymorphic markers can be used to trace the inheritance of chromosomes through a pedigree. The closer two polymorphic markers are to each other, the more likely they are to travel through the pedigree together. **B**. Recombination analysis. These markers can be followed through the family and the recombination events identified. The frequency of recombination between a marker and the long QT phenotype indicates the genetic distance between that marker and the affected gene. Therefore, the gene affected in this syndrome is close to markers A and B, since the phenotype cosegregates with these markers, and distant from marker C. By examining additional markers around markers A and B for evidence of recombination with the syndrome phenotype in a large number of families, the interval of the chromosome that must contain the affected gene may be identified.

the H-*ras*-1 locus based on a LOD score of ⩾3, genetic diagnosis of the long QT syndrome can be considered since it offers the potential of identifying affected individuals before they become symptomatic. Since the gene responsible for the LQT1 is within 10 cM of the H-*ras*-1 locus,[75] using linkage to the H-*ras*-1 locus to identify affected individuals will correctly identify >90% of affected and unaffected individuals, even when the clinical diagnosis is indeterminate.

There is no published information concerning positional cloning efforts to find the gene for the Jervell–Lange–Nielsen syndrome. Because it is an autosomal recessive disorder, linkage analysis may rely on tracing a marker that is homozygous in an affected patient back to the parents' common ancestor, called 'homozygosity mapping'.

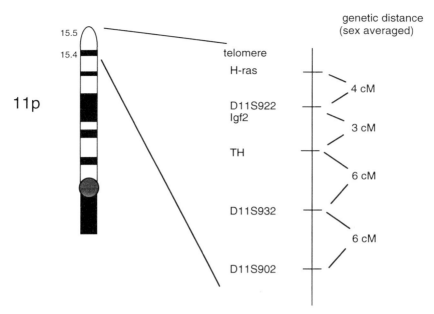

Figure 17.9 H-*ras*-1 region. (After Litt *et al.*[83] and Weissenbach *et al.*[84])

Positional cloning

Genetic mapping

After linkage to the H-*ras*-1 locus was established in several large families, the markers near H-*ras*-1 were examined for recombination with the LQT1 phenotype. Although no published information concerning recombination between LQT1 and the flanking markers is currently available, the region of interest for the gene responsible has been described as within 3–5 cM of the H-*ras*-1 locus on chromosome 11p15.5 (see Figure 17.9).[64] A recent reanalysis of the largest published pedigree[9] by Wymore *et al.*[75] determined that the candidate gene for LQT1 may be as far as 10 cM from the H-*ras*-1 locus.

Unfortunately, even a 6 cM interval presents a daunting problem for positional cloning efforts. A 6 cM interval corresponds to approximately 6×10^6 bp (6 Mb). Since there are an estimated 1×10^5 genes in the human genome coded within approximately 3×10^9 bp,[91] a 6 Mb interval may contain 200 genes which would need to be identified, fully characterized and analyzed for evidence of mutation in affected individuals. Additional families are currently being studies in an effort to reduce this interval as much as possible and to minimize the number of genes that will need to be characterized. However, due to the genetic heterogeneity, relatively large pedigrees capable of generating LOD scores of ⩾3 are required to yield useful recombination information.

Candidate genes

Faced with such a sizeable interval, the region has been examined for suitable candidate genes which might account for the pathophysiology of the LQT1. The 'candidate-gene' approach has proved successful for several other disease genes,[76,77] such as the gene for Marfan's syndrome.[78] For the Marfan's syndrome, the disease phenotype was mapped to the long arm of chromosome 15 based on linkage analysis. The region of interest included the fibrillin gene which encodes a connective-tissue protein that proved to be consistently abnormal in Marfan's syndrome patients, making fibrillin an excellent candidate gene. Demonstration of a fibrillin genetic abnormality in Marfan's syndrome patients identified the fibrillin gene as the responsible gene, thereby bypassing the remainder of the positional cloning process.[79]

The first candidate gene to be evaluated for LQT1 was the H-*ras*-1 gene which had been used for the linkage studies. Given that there was no evidence of recombination between the H-*ras*-1 locus and the Romano–Ward long QT phenotype in several large pedigrees, the H-*ras*-1 gene was extensively investigated for evidence of mutation in patients with the Romano–Ward syndrome. A member of the G-protein family which can effect signal transduction through the binding and hydrolysis of GTP, the H-*ras*-1 gene product is a 21-kDa protein involved in cell growth and differentiation. The rationale for the H-*ras*-1 gene being responsible for the long QT syndrome was based on the role of related G proteins in the regulation of atrial potassium channels.[80] A similar role for H-*ras*-1 in the regulation of ventricular potassium channels was postulated.[5] To date, no evidence of alteration of the H-*ras*-1 gene has been found in LQT1 patients.[64] However, since the genome occasionally has related genes in close physical proximity to each other, it is possible that there is another member of the family of G proteins that is closely linked to the H-*ras*-1 locus and may be responsible for LQT1.[4]

The region was searched for other candidate genes and the mapping of a delayed rectifier potassium channel, ngk2-kv4, to 11p15 using fluorescent *in situ* hybridization[81] attracted particular attention (Figure 17.10). Delayed rectifier potassium channel activity is thought to have an important role in myocardinal repolarization and therefore, on the length of the QT interval.[16,40,82] However, ngk-kv4 has recently been mapped in the mouse very near to MyoD.[75] This region is relatively well conserved between the mouse and the human genome and in the human maps to chromosome 11p14.3–15.2.[75] If ngk-kv4 proves to map to this region in the human, then it will no longer be considered a candidate gene for the LQT1, since this region is at least 25 cM from the H-*ras*-1 locus.[75,83]

Other genes which have been previously described and are within the region of interest include: DRD4, a dopamine receptor; insulin and insulin growth factor II; cathespin D; and mucin 2.[83] To date, limited studies have not revealed mutations in any of these genes in patients with long QT syndrome, none of which seems to be a strong biologic candidate.

Human Chromosome 11p

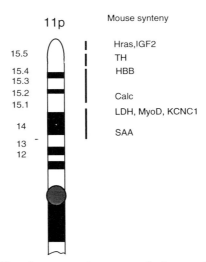

Figure 17.10   KCNC1 and mouse synteny groups for human chromosome 11p15.

Physical mapping

Once the flanking markers for the region of interest have been determined through recombination analysis, a physical map of the region is constructed. To estimate the length of the region, genomic DNA is digested with infrequently-cutting restriction endonucleases, which recognize specific 8 bp sequences and therefore 'cut' DNA approximately every 50 000–100 000 bp. These large DNA fragments are separated by pulsed field gel electrophoresis (PFGE) and transferred to a nylon membrane in a process called a Southern blot. The membrane is then probed with markers from the region of interest to determine the physical distance between the markers. Next, the markers from the region are used to isolate large segments of human DNA cloned into vectors such as yeast artificial chromosomes (YACs), cosmids, P1 clones, and bacterial artificial chromosomes (BACs). The average size of the human genomic DNA insert for each vector is 400, 40, 100 and 200 kb for the YAC, cosmid, P1 and BAC, respectively. Probes can be made from the end of each isolated clone and used to identify additional clones which contain the DNA segments between the markers. Each of the probes derived from YACs in this manner needs to be carefully mapped back to the region of interest by fluorescent *in situ* hybridization (FISH) or other methods since approximately 40–50% of YACs contain DNA from more than one human chromosome.[85] This approach, termed 'chromosome walking', is continued until all the DNA between the flanking markers is covered by DNA within the isolated vectors, as demonstrated in Figure 17.11. The coverage of the region of interest by this cloned DNA is termed a 'contig', referring to the contiguous coverage of the interval.

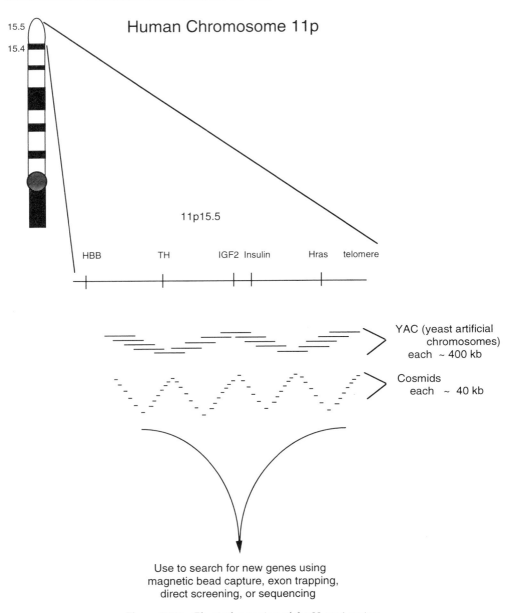

Figure 17.11   Physical mapping of the H-*ras*-1 region.

Once identified and precisely mapped, these genomic clones can be searched for new polymorphic markers, which can be subjected to recombination analysis in an effort to further restrict the region of interest. Furthermore, as will be described in the next section, these clones can be used to identify and characterize all of the genes in the region of interest.

Physical and genetic mapping efforts for LQT1 are currently in progress. Since there are no published markers between H-*ras*-1 and the telomere,[83] the region is being mapped from the centromeric boundary, as determined by recombination analysis, to the telomere. However, there is also no published information about recombination events which would define the centromeric boundary. Based on the analyses of Keating *et al.*[64] and Wymore *et al.*,[75] this centromeric boundary may be 3–10 cM from the H-*ras*-1 locus.

Finding new genes

Novel genes are identified by isolation of the mRNA message that it encodes or by utilizing one of the characteristics of gene structure to separate transcribed from non-transcribed DNA. Figure 17.12 reviews the aspects of gene structure, transcription, and message modification that are utilized to find new genes.

Many methods for finding new genes have been described. Currently, four of the most prevalent include (1) exon amplification, (2) magnetic bead capture (direct selection), (3) direct screening, and (4) genomic sequencing. Figure 17.13 outlines the basic concepts of the first two methods. The *exon trapping procedure* utilizes a shuttle vector with strong splice donor and acceptor sites.[86–88] In this procedure, genomic DNA in the region of interest is obtained from YAC, cosmids, or P1 genomic clones and subcloned into a specialized plasmid which contains a splice donor site. The resulting plasmid DNA is isolated and is transfected into a cell line such as mammalian COS cells. The transfected DNA is transcribed *in vivo* and if the inserted genomic sequence contains an exon with splice donor and acceptor sites, it should be spliced into the vector's splice donor and acceptor sites during RNA processing. The RNA from the cell line is isolated and reverse transcribed to double-stranded cDNA. The resultant cDNAs are amplified by the polymerase chain reaction and directionally cloned into a different plasmid vector. DNA sequencing using a primer from the original vector will identify an exon from a potential novel gene.

In the *magnetic bead capture technique*, cDNAs, which are derived from mRNA and represent the message-encoding DNA sequences, are hybridized to digested YAC and cosmid DNA from the region of interest to which a paramagnetic bead has been attached. The cDNA sequences which hybridize to the YAC or cosmid DNA are removed from solution by a small magnet. They are then amplified and subjected to a repeat hybridization step.[89,90] Only those cDNAs that hybridize to the genomic clones from the region are retained and amplified. With this procedure and with direct screening, the choice of cDNA libraries is critical and is based on an understanding of the disease pathophysiology. If the affected gene is not expressed in the tissue from which the cDNA library has been constructed, then the direct screening and magnetic bead capture techniques will not aid the search for the affected gene. For the long QT syndromes the tissue of primary interest is the myocardium. However, as demonstrated by the sympathetic imbalance model, the peripheral or central nervous system may be the affected tissue. Furthermore, some genes are only expressed at certain times during development, potentially necessitating the screening of fetal and adult cDNA libraries for each tissue of interest.

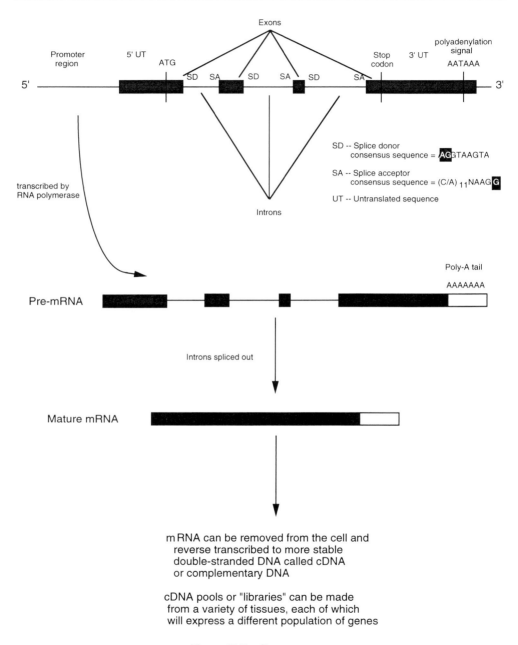

SD -- Splice donor
  consensus sequence = AG|GTAAGTA

SA -- Splice acceptor
  consensus sequence = (C/A) $_{11}$NAAG|G

UT -- Untranslated sequence

mRNA can be removed from the cell and
reverse transcribed to more stable
double-stranded DNA called cDNA
or complementary DNA

cDNA pools or "libraries" can be made
from a variety of tissues, each of which
will express a different population of genes

Figure 17.12   Gene structure.

Direct screening of cDNA libraries and sequencing are, conceptually, the most
straightforward of the methods. Direct screening involves radioactively labeling
large regions of cloned genomic DNA (40–200 kb) and using it to probe cDNA
libraries. In theory, this method should isolate all transcripts from the region that are

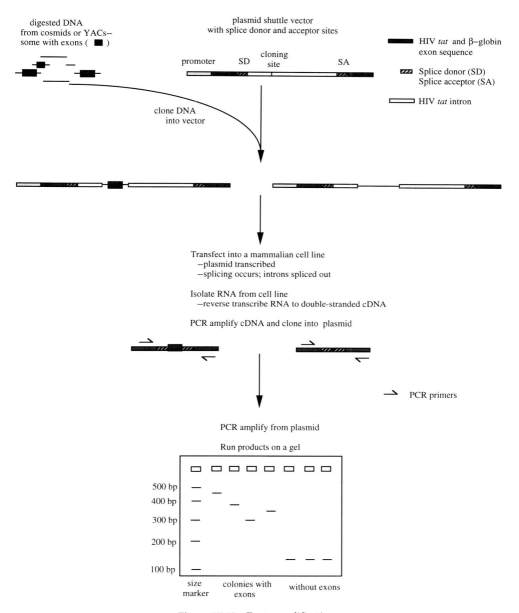

Figure 17.13 Exon amplification.

expressed in the tissues of interest. However, the detection of the matches between the genomic clones and the cDNAs is hindered by the abundance of nontranscribed intergenic DNA, intronic and high copy repetitive DNA (e.g. SINE and LINE elements) which compromise over 90% of the human genome.[91] To eliminate hybridization to transcribed repetitive sequences which would mask the unique or single copy transcribed sequences, the probes are preannealed to a vast excess of unlabeled human genomic DNA. The preannealing conditions are chosen such that any highly repetitive sequences are bound to the cold competitor DNA and therefore not available to hybridize with the filter-bound cDNAs.[92]

Sequencing strategies, although better suited to smaller candidate regions than currently exists for the LQT1, have been receiving more attention and may be of use in searching a region of 1–2 Mb. For this method, the cloned genomic DNA from the region of interest is isolated, digested and subcloned into a smaller phage vector which is used for sequencing. The sequence from these subclones is aligned by computer analysis and searched using sensor algorithms.[93] The sensor information, which is based on DNA-sequence characteristics of coding and noncoding DNA, is evaluated by a neural network to localize the coding regions. The sequencing method can identify an estimated 90% of exons $\geqslant 100$ bp and 50% of exons < 100 bp.[93] Although effective, the time and effort required for large-scale sequencing at this time is too great to be feasible for intervals >2 Mb.

Each of these methods will miss a significant number of the genes in any given region. Therefore, a combination of two or more of these methods, in addition to other methods not described in this chapter, are often utilized in the search for new genes. Furthermore, each of these methods will yield only fragments of genes. The reconstruction of the entire gene requires a combination of these methods as well as the rescreening of cDNA libraries with specific probes from the known part of the gene. Once the coding sequence for each new gene has been determined, it is subjected to mutation analysis.

Identifying mutations

Occasionally, mutations which cause clinical disease involve gross chromosomal insertions, deletions, or rearrangements which can be identified microscopically using cytogenetic techniques. However, as previously mentioned, the chromosomes of patients with the long QT syndrome have been extensively evaluated without evidence of gross chromosomal rearrangement. Therefore, each candidate or novel gene that is identified in the region of interest will need to be examined for evidence of mutation in individuals affected with the long QT syndrome.

Mutations are changes in a patient's DNA sequence which significantly alter the formation of the gene's product. If a stable RNA product is made then it can be examined for either gross or minute alterations. Gross alterations, such as large insertions, deletions or truncations of the coding sequence are detected by electrophoresing the patient's and unaffected individual's RNA, extracted from a variety of tissues, on a sizing gel and transferring it to a nylon membrane (Northern blot). The membrane can be hybridized with probes from each novel gene to determine if there is any difference in the size or amount of the mRNA products between affected and unaffected individuals.

However, if no stable mRNA product is made by the abnormal gene, the genomic DNA coding sequence is examined for differences between affected and unaffected individuals. First, DNA from affected and unaffected individuals is digested with several different restriction endonucleases, electrophoresed and transferred to a nylon membrane (Southern blot). Again the membrane is hybridized with probes from each novel gene. However, only large insertions or deletions, and single nucleotide changes which alter a restriction endonuclease 'cutting' site will be detected.

If the mutation cannot be detected by Northern or Southern blot analysis, then large segments of the patient's DNA or RNA will need to be scanned for subtle mutations of that gene. RNA analysis does not require precise knowledge of the genomic structure but is dependent upon a stable nRNA product of the defective gene and expression of the gene in an accessible tissue. For instance, RNA is easily obtained from a patient's leukocytes and skin fibroblasts but difficult to obtain from the less-accessible myocardium. Therefore, genes only expressed in myocardium will be more difficult to evaluate. Conversely, DNA analysis is not dependent on the production of a stable transcript or on tissue specificity. However, it usually requires a precise knowledge of the genomic structure for each gene including the location and surrounding sequence of each intron/exon boundary.

For RNA or DNA analysis, the methods currently employed to find single basepair changes or microinsertions or deletions include single-strand conformational polymorphism (SSCP), denaturing gradient gel electrophoresis (DGGE) and chemical mismatch cleavage (CMC).[94–97] Each method amplifies short overlapping segments (100–400 bp) of the gene's coding sequence from either genomic DNA or cDNA (derived from tissue mRNA) and can identify single basepair differences between individuals. Each method has an 80–90% success rate for identifying most single basepair changes so a combination of methods is often used to ensure that no mutations are missed. All identified differences between affected and unaffected individuals, which cosegregate with the disease phenotype, are verified by sequencing and compared to determine whether or not the alteration is likely to significantly affect the protein. Although beyond the scope of this chapter, the identification and characterization of disease-causing mutations is a complex process and represents the culmination of the positional cloning effort. For an overview of these techniques, please see the review by Grompe.[98]

Future applications

Once the gene responsible for the Romano–Ward long QT syndrome is identified, it will be characterized and its role in myocardial repolarization defined. The integrity of the gene in patients with the Jervell–Lange–Nielsen and sporadic congenital long QT syndromes will be examined to determine if that gene is also responsible for the phenotype in some or all of these patients.

The ultimate goal will be to utilize the knowledge gained about the gene product(s) to improve diagnosis and management of the long QT syndromes. Understanding the genes responsible for each of the long QT syndromes will enable the tailoring of therapy to best treat the physiologic defect responsible for each. Treatment advances may include more specific pharmacologic therapy or gene therapy directed at correcting or ameliorating the genetic defect. For the autosomal dominant syndromes this may entail ceasing or decreasing the production of an

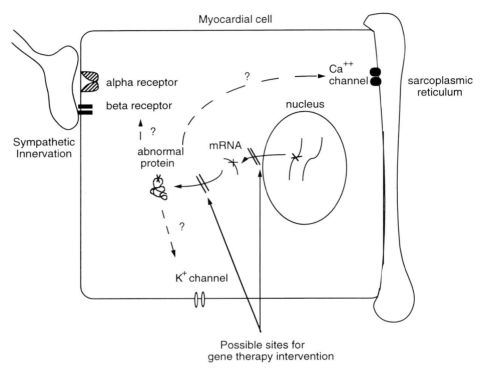

Figure 17.14   Diagram of the myocardial cell in a patient with Romano–Ward syndrome. Included in the diagram are the possible sites for intervention with gene therapy and several of the proteins involved in myocardial repolarization which might be targets for pharmacotherapy.

abnormal protein, either at the transcriptional or translational level or through functional inactivation of the abnormal protein. However, for some of the autosomal dominant syndromes and for the autosomal recessive Jervell–Lange–Nielsen syndrome, the genetic defect may be corrected through introduction of the normal gene (Figure 17.14). In the future, it may be possible to correct the genetic defect of the long QT syndrome before the patient can exhibit the phenotypic manifestations of cardiac arrest and sudden death. Eventually, the increased understanding of myocardial repolarization gained by the investigation of the genes responsible for the long QT syndrome may improve the treatment of many other ventricular arrhythmias.

Acknowledgments

The authors would like to thank Dr. Francis Collins and Dr. Macdonald Dick II for their thoughtful review of this manuscript. Dr. Russell is a Kenneth Rosen Fellow supported by the North American Society for Pacing and Electrophysiology.

References

1. Collins, F. S. (1992) Positional cloning: Let's not call it reverse anymore. *Nature-Genetics*, **1**, 3–6.
2. Schwartz, P. J. (1986) Prevention of arrhythmias in the long QT syndrome. In: Kulbertus, H. E. (ed.) *Medical Management of Cardiac Arrhythmias*, pp. 153–62. Edinburgh: Churchill Livingstone.
3. Moss, A. J. (1992) Molecular genetics and ventricular arrhythmias. *N. Engl. J. Med.*, **327**, 885–7.
4. Moss, A. J. (1986) Prolonged QT interval syndrome. *JAMA*, **256**, 2985–7.
5. Vincent, G. M. (1992) Hypothesis for the molecular physiology of the Romano–Ward long QT syndrome. *J. Am. Coll. Cardiol.*, **20**, 500–3.
6. Abildiskov, J. A. (1991) The sympathetic imbalance hypothesis of QT interval prolongation. *J. Cardiovasc. Electrophysiol.*, **2**, 355–9.
7. Manoach, M., Fein, A., Hecht, Z. and Varon, D. (1992) A cellular basis for the prolonged QT interval in mammals. *Ann. NY Acad. Sci.*, **644**, 84–92.
8. Zipes, D. P. (1991) The long QT interval syndrome. A Rosetta stone for sympathetic related ventricular tachyarrhythmias. *Circulation*, **84**, 1414–19.
9. Keating, M., Atkinson, D., Dunn, C. *et al.* (1991) Linkage of a cardiac arrhythmia, the long QT syndrome, and the Harvey *ras*-1 gene. *Science*, **252**(5006), 704–6.
10. Romano, C., Gemme, G. and Pongiglione, R. (1963) Aritmie cardiache rare dell'eta pediatria. *Clin. Pediatr.*, **45**, 658–83.
11. Ward, O. C. (1964) New familial cardiac syndrome in children. *J. Irish Med. Assoc.*, **54**, 103–6.
12. Jervell, A. and Lange-Nielsen, F. (1957) Congenital deaf-mutism, functional heart diseases, with prolongation of the QT interval and sudden death. *Am. Heart J.*, **54**, 59–68.
13. Moss, A. J. (1992) Molecular genetics and ventricular arrhythmias. *N. Engl. J. Med.*, **327**, 885–7.
14. Coumel, P. (1990) Early afterdepolarizations and triggered activity in clinical arrhythmias. In: Rosen, M. R., Janse, M. J. and Wit, A. L. (eds) *Cardiac Electrophysiology*, pp. 387–411. Mount Kisko. (NY): Futura.
15. Moss, A. J. and Schwartz, P. J. (1982) Delayed repolarization (QT or QTU prolongation) and malignant ventricular arrhythmias. *Mod. Concepts Cardiovasc. Dis.*, **51**, 85–90.
16. Schwartz, P. J., Bonazzi, Q., Locati, E. *et al.* (1992) Pathogenesis and therapy of the idiopathic long QT syndrome. *Ann. NY Acad. Sci.*, **644**, 112–41.
17. Garson, A. Jr., Dick, M. II, Fournier, A. *et al.* (1993) The long QT syndrome in children. An international study of 287 patients. *Circulation*, **87**, 1866–72.
18. Moss, A. J., Schwartz, P. J., Crampton, R. S. *et al.* (1991) The long QT syndrome. Prospective longitudinal study of 328 families. *Circulation*, **84**, 1136–44.
19. Schwartz, P. J., Moss, A. J., Vincent, G. M. and Crampton, R. S. (1993) Diagnostic criteria for the long QT syndrome. An update. *Circulation*, **88**, 782–4.
20. Burch, G. E., Meyers, R. and Abildskov, J. A. (1954) A new electrocardiographic pattern observed in cerebrovascular accidents. *Circulation*, **9**, 719–23.
21. Manning, J. W. and Cotton, M. (1962) Mechanism of cardiac arrhythmias induced by diencephalic stimulation. *Am. J. Physiol.*, **203**, 1120–32.
22. Yanowitz, F., Preston, J. B. and Abildskov, J. A. (1966) Functional distribution of the right and left stellate innervation to the ventricles. Production of neurogenic electrocardiographic changes by unilateral alteration of sympathetic tone. *Circ. Res.*, **18**, 416–38.
23. Moss, A. J. and McDonald, J. (1971) Unilateral cervicothoracic sympathetic ganglionectomy for the treatment of the long QT syndrome. *N. Engl. J. Med.*, **285**, 903–4.
24. Schwartz, P. J., Periti, M. and Malliani, A. (1975) The long QT syndrome. *Am. Heart J.*, **89**, 378–90.

25. Schwartz, P. J., Snebold, N. G. and Brown, A. M. (1976) Effects of unilateral cardiac sympathetic denervation on the ventricular fibrillation threshold. *Am. J. Cardiol.*, **37**, 1034–40.
26. Priori, S. G., Mantica, M. and Schwartz, P. J. (1988) Delayed afterdepolarizations elicited *in vivo* by left stellate ganglion stimulation. *Circulation*, **78**, 178–85.
27. Schwartz, P. J. and Malliani, A. (1975) Electrical alternation of the T wave. Clinical and experimental evidence of its relationship with the sympathetic nervous system and with the long QT syndrome. *Am. Heart J.*, **89**, 45–50.
28. Schwartz, P. J. and Stone, H. L. (1978) Unilateral stellatectomy and sudden death. In: Schwartz, P. J., Brown, A. M., Malliani, A. and Zanchetti, A. (eds) *Neural Mechanisms in Cardiac Arrhythmias*, pp. 107–22. New York: Raven Press.
29. Ben-David, J. and Zipes, D. P. (1988) Differential response to right and left ansae subclaviae stimulation of early afterdepolarizations and ventricular tachycardia induced by cesium in dogs. *Circulation*, **78**, 1241–50.
30. Austoni, P., Rosati, R., Gregorini, L. *et al.* (1979) Stellatectomy and exercise in man. *Am. J. Cardiol.*, **43**, 399.
31. Schwartz, P. J., Verrier, R. L. and Lown, B. (1977) Effect of stellatectomy and vagotomy on ventricular refractoriness. *Circ. Res.*, **40**, 536–40.
32. Malfatto, G., Steinberg, S. F., Rosen, T. S. *et al.* Experimental QT interval prolongation. *Ann. NY Acad. Sci.*, **644**, 74–83.
33. Christiansen, J. L., Stadt, H. A., Mulroy, M. J. and Kirby, M. L. (1989) Electrocardiographic QT prolongation after ablation of the nodose placode in the chick embryo: a development model of the idopathic long QT syndrome. *Pediatr. Res.*, **26**, 11–15.
34. James, T. N., Froggatt, P., Atkinson, W. J. *et al.* (1978) De subitaneis morbitus. XXX. Observations on the pathophysiology of the long QT syndromes with special reference to the neuropathology of the heart. *Circulation*, **57**, 1221–31.
35. Pfeiffer, D., Fiehring, H., Henkel, H. G. *et al.* (1989) Long QT syndrome associated with inflammatory degeneration of the stellate ganglia. *Clin. Cardiol.*, **12**, 222–4.
36. Calkins, H., Lehmann, M. H., Allman, K. *et al.* (1993) Scintigraphic pattern of regional cardiac sympathetic innervation in patients with familial long QT syndrome using positron emission tomography. *Circulation*, **87**, 1616–21.
37. Gohl, K., Feistel, H., Weikl, A. *et al.* (1991) Congenital myocardial sympathetic dysinnervation (CMSD) – a structural defect of idiopathic long QT syndrome. *Pacing Clin. Electrophysiol.*, **14**, 544–53.
38. Muller, K. D., Jakob, H., Neuzner, J. *et al.* (1993) ^{123}I-metaiodobenzylgluanidine scintigraphy in the detection of irregular regional sympathetic innervation in long QT syndrome. *Eur. Heart J.*, **14**, 316–25.
39. Lee, K.-F., Bachman, K., Landis, S. and Jaenisch, R. (1994) Dependence on p75 for innervation of some sympathetic targets. *Science*, **263**, 1447–9.
40. Jackman, W. M., Friday, K. J., Anderson, J. L. *et al.* (1988) The long QT syndromes: a critical review, new clinical observations and a unifying hypothesis. *Prog. Cardiovasc. Dis.*, **31**, 115–72.
41. Ejvinsson, G. and Ornius, E. (1980) Prodromal ventricular premature beats preceded by a diastolic wave. *Acta Med. Scand.*, **208**, 445–50.
42. Kay, G. N., Plumb, V. J., Arciniegas, J. G. *et al.* (1983) Torsades de Pointes: the long–short initiating sequence and other clinical features: observations in 32 patients. *J. Am. Coll. Cardiol.*, **2**, 806–17.
43. Bissett, J. K., Watson, J. W., Scovil, J. A. *et al.* (1980) Sudden death in cardiomyopathy: role of bradycardia dependent repolarization changes. *Am. Heart J.*, **99**, 625–9.
44. Zhou. J. T., Zheng, L. R. and Liu, W. Y. (1992) Role of early afterdepolarization in familial long QTU syndrome and torsade de pointes. *Pacing Clin. Electrophysiol.*, **15**, 164–8.
45. Shimizu, W., Ohe, T., Kurita, T. *et al.* (1991) Early afterdepolarizations induced by isoproterenol in patients with congenital long QT syndrome. *Circulation*, **84**, 1915–23.
46. Schwartz, P. J. (1985) The idiopathic long QT syndrome: Progress and questions. *Am. Heart J.*, **109**, 399–411.

47. Schwartz, P. J., Locati, E. H., Moss, A. J. *et al.* (1991) Left cardiac sympathetic denervation in the therapy of congenital long QT syndrome. A worldwide report. *Circulation*, **84**, 503–11.
48. Chien, W. W., Foster, E., Phillips, B. *et al.* (1991) Pacemaker syndrome in a patient with DDD pacemaker for long QT syndrome. *Pacing Clin. Electrophysiol.*, **14**, 1209–12.
49. Eldar, M., Griffin, J. C., Van Hare, G. F. *et al.* (1992) Combined use of beta-adrenergic blocking agents and long-term cardiac pacing for patients with the long QT syndrome. *J. Am. Coll. Cardiol.*, **20**, 830–7.
50. Eldar, M., Griffin, J. Y., Abbott, J. A. *et al.* (1987) Permanent cardiac pacing in patients with the long QT syndrome. *J. Am. Coll. Cardiol.*, **10**, 600–7.
51. Moss, A. J., Liu, J. E., Gottlieb, S. *et al.* (1991) Efficacy of permanent pacing in the management of high-risk patients with long QT syndrome. *Circulation*, **84**, 1524–9.
52. Pfeiffer, D., Fiehring, H., Warnke, H. *et al.* (1992) Treatment of tachyarrhythmias in a patient with the long QT syndrome by autotransplantation of the heart and sinus node-triggered atrial pacing. *J. Thorac. Cardiovasc. Surg.*, **104**, 491–4.
53. Vincent, G. M. (1993) The long-QT syndrome. *N. Engl. J. Med.*, **328**, 287.
54. Merri, M., Benhorin, J., Alberti, M. *et al.* (1989) Electrocardiographic quantitation of ventricular repolarization. *Circulation*, **80**, 1301–8.
55. Moss, A. J. (1993) Measurement of the QT interval and the risk associated with QTc interval prolongation: a review. *Am. J. Cardiol.*, **72**, 23B–5B.
56. Hashiba, K. (1992) Sex differences in phenotypic manifestation and gene transmission in the Romano–Ward syndrome. *Ann. NY Acad. Sci.*, **644**, 142–56.
57. Moss, A. J. and Robinson, J. L. (1992) The long-QT syndrome: genetic considerations. *Trends Cardiovasc. Med.*, **2**, 81–3.
58. Spodick, D. H. (1993) The long-QT syndrome (Letter). *N. Engl. J. Med.*, **328**, 287.
59. Bazett, H. C. (1988) An analysis of the time relations of electrocardiograms. *Heart*, **7**, 353–70.
60. Sagie, A., Larson, M. G., Goldberg, R. J. *et al.* (1992) An improved method for adjusting the QT interval for heart rate (the Framingham Heart Study). *Am. J. Cardiol.*, **70**, 797–801.
61. Yoshinaga, M., Tomari, T., Aihoshi, S. *et al.* (1993) Exponential correction of QT interval to minimize the effect of the heart rate in children. *Jpn. Circ. J.*, **57**, 102–8.
62. Spodick, D. H. (1992) Reduction of QT-interval imprecision and variance by measuring the JT interval. *Am. J. Cardiol*, **70**, 103.
63. Vincent, G. M., Timothy, K., Leppert, M. and Keating, M. (1992) The spectrum of symptoms and QT intervals in carriers of the gene for the long-QT syndrome. *N. Engl. J. Med.*, **327**, 846–52.
64. Keating, M. (1992) Linkage analysis and the long QT syndrome: using genetics to study cardiovascular disease. *Circulation*, **85**, 1973–86.
65. Timothy, K., Fox, J. and Vincent, G. M. (1992) QTc duration correlates with symptom severity in long QT syndrome patients. *Circulation*, (Supp. 1), **86**, I-391.
66. Schwartz, P. J. (1980) The long QT syndrome. In: Kulbertus, H. E. and Wellens, H. J. J. (eds) *Sudden Death*, pp. 153–61. London: Martinus Nijhoff.
67. Schwartz, P. J. (1990) Long QT syndrome. In: Horowitz, L. N. (ed.) *Current Management of Arrhythmias*, pp. 194–8. Philadelphia: W. B. Saunders.
68. Gelehrter, T. D. and Collins, F. S. (1990) Anatomy of the human genome: gene mapping and linkage. In: Gardner, J. N. (ed.) *Principles of Medical Genetics*, pp. 193–227. Baltimore, MD: Williams and Wilkins.
69. Ott, J. (1992) *Analysis of Human Genetic Linkage*, 302 pp. Baltimore, MD: Johns Hopkins University Press.
70. Keating, M., Dunn, C., Atkinson, D. *et al.* (1991) Consistent linkage of the long QT syndrome to the Harvey *ras*-1 locus on chromosome 11. *Am. J. Hum. Genet.*, **49**, 1335–9.
71. Towbin, J. A., Pagotto, L., Siu, B. *et al.* (1992) Romano–Ward long QT syndrome (RWLQTS): evidence of genetic heterogeneity. *Pediatr. Res.*, **31**, 22A (Abstract).
72. Satler, C., Walsh, E., Korf, B. *et al.* (1992) Linkage Analysis with H-*ras*-1 probe identifies genetic heterogeneity of the long QT syndrome. *Circulation*, (Supp.), **86**, I-348.

73. Benhorin, J., Kalman, Y. M., Medina, A. *et al.* (1993) Evidence of genetic heterogeneity in the long QT syndrome. *Science*, **260**, 1960–1.
74. Curran, M., Atkinson, D., Timothy, K. *et al.* (1993) Locus heterogeneity of autosomal dominant long QT syndrome. *J. Clin. Invest.*, *92*, 799–803.
75. Wymore, R. S., Korenberg, J. R., Kinoshita, K. D. *et al.* (1994) Genomic organization, nucleotide sequence, biophysical properties, and localization of the voltage-gated K^+ channel gene KCNA/4Kv 1.4 to mouse chromosome 2/human 11p14 and mapping of KCNC1/Kv 3.1 to mouse 7/human 11p14.3-p15.2 and KCNA1/Kv1.1 to human 12p13. *Genomics*, **20**, 191–202.
76. Geisterfer-Lowrance, A. A. T., Kass, S., Tanigawa, G. *et al.* (1990) A molecular basis for familial hypertrophic cardiomyopathy: a β-cardiac myosin heavy chain gene missense mutation. *Cell*, **62**, 999–1006.
77. Goate, A., Chartier-Harlin, M. C., Mullan, M. *et al.* (1991) Segregation of a missense mutation in the amyloid precursor protein gene with familial Alzheimer's disease. *Nature*, **349**, 704–6.
78. Dietz, H. C., Cutting, G. R., Pyeritz, R. E. *et al.* (1991) Marfan syndrome caused by a recurrent *de novo* missense mutation in the fibrillin gene. *Nature*, **352**, 337–9.
79. Dietz, H. C. and Pyeritz, R. E. (1994) Molecular biology – to the heart of the matter. *N. Engl. J. Med.*, **330**, 930–2.
80. Yatani, A., Okabe, K., Codina, J. *et al.* (1990) Heart rate regulation by G proteins acting on the cardiac pacemaker channel. *Science*, **249**, 1163–6.
81. Ried, T., Rudy, B., Vega-Saenz de Miera, E. *et al.* (1993) Localization of a highly conserved human potassium channel gene (NGK2-KV4, KCNC1) to chromosome 11p15. *Genomics*, **15**, 405–11.
82. Pressler, M. L. and Hathaway, D. R. (1992) The long QT syndrome: A G or not a G? *J. Am. Coll. Cardiol.*, **20**, 504–5.
83. Litt, M., Kramer, P., Hauge, X. Y. *et al.* (1993) A microsatellite-based index map of human chromosome 11. *Hum. Mol. Genet.*, **2**, 909–13.
84. Weissenbach, J., Gyapay, G., Dib, C. *et al.* (1992) A second-generation linkage map of the human genome. *Nature*, **59**, 794–801.
85. Bronson, S. K., Pei, J., Taillon-Miller, P. *et al.* (1991) Isolation and characterization of yeast artificial chromosome clones linking the HLA-B and HLA-C loci. *Proc. Natl Acad. Sci. USA*, **88**, 1676–80.
86. Buckler, A. J., Chang, D. D., Graw, S. L. *et al.* (1991) Exon amplification: a strategy to isolate mammalian genes based on RNA splicing. *Proc. Natl Acad. Sci. USA*, **88**, 4005–9.
87. Duyk, G. M., Kim, S., Myers, R. M. and Cox, D. R. (1990) Exon trapping: a genetic screen to identify candidate transcribed sequences in cloned mammalian genomic DNA. *Proc. Natl Acad. Sci. USA*, **87**, 8995–9.
88. Church, D. M., Stolter, C. J., Rutter, J. L. *et al.* (1994) Isolation of genes from complex sources of mammalian genomic DNA using exon amplification. *Nature-Genetics*, **6**, 98–105.
89. Lovett, M., Kere, J. and Hinton, L. M. (1991) Direct selection: a method for the isolation of cDNAs encoded by large genomic regions. *Proc. Natl Acad. Sci. USA*, **88**, 9628–32.
90. Tagle, D. A., Swaroop, M., Lovett, M. and Collins, F. S. (1993) Magnetic bead capture of expressed sequences encoded within large genomic segments. *Nature*, **361**, 751–3.
91. Schmid, C. W. and Deininger, P. L. (1975) Sequence organization of the human genome. *Cell*, **6**, 345–58.
92. Wallace, M. R., Marchuk, D. A., Andersen, L. B. *et al.* (1990) Type 1 neurofibromatosis gene: identification of a large transcript disrupted in three NF1 patients. *Science*, **249**, 181–6.
93. Uberbacher, E. C. and Mural, R. J. (1991) Locating protein-coding regions in human DNA sequences by a multiple sensor-neural network approach. *Proc. Natl Acad. Sci. USA*, **88**, 11261–5.
94. Michaud, J., Brody, L. C., Steel, G. *et al.* (1992) Strand-separating conformational polymorphism analysis: efficacy of detection of point mutations in the human ornithine ∂-aminotransferase gene. *Genomics*, **13**, 389–94.

95. Orita, M., Suzuki, Y., Sekiya, T. and Hayashi, K. (1989) Rapid and sensitive detection of point mutations and DNA polymorphisms using the polymerase chain reaction. *Genomics*, **5**, 874–9.
96. Myers, R. M., Lumelsky, N., Lerman, L. and Maniatis, T. (1985) Detection of single base substitutions in total genomic DNA. *Nature*, **313**, 495–8.
97. Cotton, R. G. H., Rodriquez, N. R. and Campbell, R. D. (1988) Reaction of cytosine and thymidine in single base pair mismatches with hydroxylamine and osmium tetroxide and its application to the study of mutations. *Proc. Natl Acad. Sci. USA*, **85**, 4397–401.
98. Grompe, M. (1993) The rapid detection of unknown mutations in nucleic acids. *Nature-Genetics*, **5**, 111–17.

18

Iontophoresis for Modulating Cardiac Delivery of Antiarrhythmic Agents

Vinod Labhasetwar
Steven P. Schwendeman
Tam Nguyen
Thomas Underwood
Robert J. Levy

Introduction

Cardiovascular controlled release has been successfully used in a limited number of clinical applications, and in a growing number of experimental studies for optimal cardiac and blood vessel-related disease states for site-specific delivery of therapeutic agents.[1-7] The general rationale involved in cardiovascular controlled release hypothesizes that regional drug delivery of therapeutic agents of interest using polymer composites results in optimal local drug levels, while minimizing the possibilities for systemic side effects. Furthermore, this rationale also makes possible the use of therapeutic agents which have bioavailability limitations because of rapid metabolic inactivation or poor oral absorption.[8] Thus far, the most successful clinical example of cardiovascular controlled release is the use of a dexamethasone-releasing cardiac pacing catheter.[9-11] In this particular device design, the tip of the pacemaker catheter electrode, which makes contact with the endocardium, contains a dexamethasone–silicone rubber matrix. The purpose of this drug-delivery system is to reduce the extent of scar-tissue formation around the lead contact point so that increased electrical resistance (resulting from excessive scar tissue) will not take place. This innovation has been highly successful and has resulted in the subsequent development of the smallest and most energy-efficient cardiac pacemaker to date.

Experimental cardiovascular controlled-release systems, such as the dexamethasone system just described, have consisted of controlled-release drug–polymer composites implanted in direct contact with the heart or with blood vessels, where they can locally release drugs of interest to prevent or treat local disease processes. Successful local controlled-release experimental studies thus far have been carried out for preventing bioprosthetic heart valve calcification,[4] ventricular arrhythmias,[12–17] heart transplant rejection,[3] arterial restenosis[1,18] and cardiac valve prosthesis infection.[19] In each of these examples, local drug delivery has been efficacious with dosages typically orders of magnitude below those effective systemically. Furthermore, no local or systemic side effects with site-specific drug delivery administered by these means have been noted.

All of the drug-delivery systems for cardiovascular diseases just described, however, have involved sustained drug-release kinetics which are predetermined by the formulation and fabrication characteristics of the drug–polymer composites. Thus such systems have the limitation of altering drug-release kinetics depending upon disease activity which is most desirable in an ideal setting.[20] For example, feedback modulation of drug-delivery rates would be advantageous for increasing or decreasing dosages depending on disease activity or side effects. Modulation has been possible in experimental controlled-release systems using a number of different energy sources including electromagnetism,[21] ultrasound,[3,22] implantable mechanical drug pumps,[23] and iontophoresis.[24–28]

Iontophoresis offers a more energy-efficient possibility for modulated controlled release, compared to the other modulated systems investigated. Iontophoresis may be defined as the transport of charged molecules under an applied electrical field which can theoretically be calculated from the Nernst–Planck equation and the Laws of Conservation of Mass and Charge. In the present chapter, we will review the general principles of iontophoresis and consider how this technique can be applied in modulating drug delivery for cardiovascular disease, specifically for cardiac arrhythmias. Thus, we will address the following issues:

1. The theoretical basis for iontophoretic modulation of drug-release kinetics including equations for predicting iontophoretic delivery of antiarrhythmic agents through heterogeneous cation-exchange membranes.
2. A review of other drug delivery iontophoresis applications.
3. The development of rate-limiting heterogeneous cation-exchange membranes for use in cardiac implants.
4. The fabrication of cardiac iontophoretic drug-delivery devices and their characterization *in vitro*.
5. The examination of short-term and long-term antiarrhythmic therapy with an iontophoretic cardiac device that has been implanted in dogs and the critical issues involved in cardiac iontophoresis.

Heterogeneous cation-exchange membranes (HCMs)

Iontophoretic drug delivery and HCM development

Iontophoretic drug delivery involves controling the movement of drugs (usually ions) by externally modulating the electrical driving force across the rate-limiting medium(s) of the transported drug. An essential aspect in developing an iontophoretic device is to identify the rate-limiting barrier(s) to transport and to prepare a membrane for the iontophoretic device that provides such a barrier. Barriers to transport typically consist of implanted polymeric materials, biological tissues, and unstirred aqueous boundary layers that develop adjacent to polymeric or biological membranes. A second important consideration is membrane selectivity for the drug. Ion-exchange membranes offer the most basic type of selectivity that is based on charge of the ion. According to Donnan equilibrium, cation exchangers exclude anions (prevent transport in) and anion exchangers exclude cations.

However, not all ion-exchange membranes are rate-limiting in the absence of an electrolytic current under diffusion conditions. Membranes used in electrodialysis, Nafion[29] for example, are highly conductive and diffusion to and from the membrane in the unstirred boundary layers most often will control transport under zero-current conditions as the boundary layer resistance exceeds that of the membrane. One simple way to control the membrane resistance is to formulate a heterogeneous membrane consisting of conductive microparticles embedded in an inert non-conductive matrix. Control may then be accomplished by adjusting particle size, particle content and membrane thickness.

The above two fundamental design criteria led us to the development of hetero-geneous cation-exchange membranes that consist of common laboratory Dowex 50W cation-exchange resin embedded in a flexible and biocompatible silicone rubber matrix. These colloidian-type ion-exchange membranes were prepared as early as the 1950s[30] using wax and other inert materials as the nonconductive matrix.

Transport of ions and transport through HCMs

General transport equations

To evaluate the transport of ions, a law that governs the rate of movement of each ion within the rate-limiting medium must first be considered. The most basic of these rate laws is the Nernst–Planck equation, which is based on the proportionality between ion flux (rate of ion movement divided by area normal to transport) and the gradient of electrochemical potential written in one-dimensional form:

$$j_i = -D_i[\partial c_i/\partial x + (z_i F/RT)c_i(\partial \phi/\partial x)] \tag{1}$$

where D_i, j_i, c_i, z_i, are the self-diffusion coefficient, unidirectional mass flux, concentration and charge of species i, respectively; ϕ and x are the electric potential and position coordinate; F, R and T are Faraday's constant, the universal gas constant and absolute temperature, respectively. We note here that both flux of i (j_i) and position coordinate (x) are technically vectors and thus, have both magnitude and direction. The most critical requirements for the above equation to be completely valid are the absence of convective mass transport (e.g. water movement due to electro-osmosis) and the independence of the logarithm of the activity coefficients with respect to concentration (and thus, position coordinate). The inclusion of these latter two phenomena in equation (1) is discussed more completely elsewhere.[31] The first term in the Nernst–Planck equation (containing $\partial c_i/\partial x$) is representative of transport due to the chemical driving force and the second term (containing $\partial \phi/\partial x$) is representative of transport due to the electrical driving force. As the electric field strength, $|\partial \phi/\partial x|$, is increased by an external source of electromotive force (i.e. a power supply), diffusing ions begin to migrate at a terminal velocity in the direction dictated by the electric field and the charge of the ion.

In order to assemble a general partial differential equation (PDE) for each ion in the rate-limiting medium, the above flux expression must be inserted into the continuity equation (based on the conservation of mass) written as follows (no chemical reaction in the medium of interest):

$$\partial c_i / \partial \theta = -\partial j_i / \partial x \tag{2}$$

where θ is time. We also note that while equation (1) requires assumptions as described above, equation (2) is an exact relationship.

In ion transport, constraints based on the conservation of charge (the medium is electrically neutral) are required:

$$\sum_i z_i c_i + \omega X = 0, \tag{3}$$

and

$$I/A = F \sum_i z_i j_i, \tag{4}$$

where X is the concentration of fixed or physically trapped charge (if present) having charge ω; I and A are current (also a vector) and area normal to transport, respectively. The equations (3) and (4) require that the electric permittivity of the medium be low such that any accumulation of charge is negligible.

From equations (1)–(4), the general spatial and time-dependent transport behavior of the one-dimensional problem is fixed. What is necessary to solve the above system of PDEs are boundary conditions (at the boundary of the medium) and an initial condition (condition of the entire medium at time 0). A specific example of this transport analysis will be given in the next section.

Steady-state bi-ionic transport through HCMs

We describe the solution to the above equations (1)–(4) for the specific case of interest, a drug cation (such as an antiarrhythmic drug) is delivered through a rate-limiting cation-exchange membrane into a Na^+-containing release medium after some long time following any current adjustment (at steady state, no time dependence). We assume perfect Donnan exclusion of co-ions so equation (2) need be considered for cations only. Thus, equations (1)–(4) may be rewritten using reduced variables (no dimensions) and as ordinary differential equations (ODEs) in the absence of any time dependence as follows:

$$j_1^* = -dc_1^*/d\xi + c_1^* s \tag{5}$$
$$j_2^* = -\gamma(dc_2^*/d\xi - c_2^* s)$$

$$dj_i^*/d\xi = 0; \quad i = 1, 2 \tag{6}$$

$$c_1^* + c_2^* = 1 \tag{7}$$

$$I^* = j_1^* + j_2^* \tag{8}$$

where subscripts 1 and 2 denote Na^+ and the drug cation, respectively, and the reduced variables γ, j_i^*, c_i^*, ξ, I^* and s are related to their dimensional counterparts D_i, j_i, c_i, x, I and $d\phi/dx$ by:

$$\xi \equiv x/L \tag{9}$$

$$s \equiv -d\phi/dx[RT/(FL)] \tag{10}$$

$$c_i^* \equiv c_i/X; \qquad i = 1.2 \tag{11}$$

$$I^* \equiv I/(D_1 XAF/L) = I/[RT/(FR_{s1})] \tag{12}$$

$$j_i^* \equiv j_i/(D_1 X/L) = (j_i A)/[RT/(F^2 R_{s1})]; \quad i = 1, 2 \tag{13}$$

$$\gamma \equiv D_2 //D_1 = R_{s1}/R_{s2} \tag{14}$$

where R_{s1} and R_{s2} are the observed electrical resistance of the membrane in the presence of species 1 (Na^+) and 2 (drug cation), respectively; L is the membrane thickness and s is reduced electric field (a vector). Equations (12)–(14) utilize the relationship between D_i and R_{s_i}:

$$R_{s_i} = (RT/F)[L/(D_i XAF)]; \quad i = 1, 2 \tag{15}$$

and assume the swollen state of the cation-exchange membrane is not altered when changing between drug and Na^+ forms (form refers to the ion that neutralizes the fixed charge groups of the exchanger).

In the bi-ionic system of interest the drug cation would reside within the implant and Na^+ (the physiologically relevant cation) would be outside. Therefore, the boundary conditions state that the drug cation and Na^+ each neutralize the fixed charges within the cation exchanger on opposing sides of the membrane as follows:

$$\xi = 0; \qquad c_1^* = 0, \quad c_2^* = 1 \quad \text{(inside)} \tag{16}$$

$$\xi = 1; \qquad c_1^* = 1, \quad c_2^* = 0 \quad \text{(outside)} \tag{17}$$

The above system of equations (5)–(8) with boundary conditions as per equations (16) and (17) has been solved analytically and is given as:[32]

$$I^*(s) = s(\gamma e^s - 1)/(e^s - 1) \tag{18}$$

$$j_2^*(s) = \gamma s e^s/(e^s - 1) \tag{19}$$

$$c_2^*(s, \xi) = (e^s - e^{sx})/(e^s - 1) \tag{20}$$

$$\eta_m(s) = s + \ln K_1^2 \tag{21}$$

$$t_2(s) = \gamma e^s/(\gamma e^s - 1) \tag{22}$$

where η_m is the observed membrane potential divided by RT/F (26.7 mv at 37°C) and K_1^2 is the drug–Na^+ selectivity coefficient, which describes the competition of the two cations for neutralizing a fixed charge site. The variable t_2 is the transference number of the drug cation. In addition, the electric field(s) is not spatially dependent in this steady-state solution (constant electric field).

Hence, all variables of interest: current (I^*), drug-delivery rate (j_2^*), concentration of drug as a function of position within the membrane (c_2^*), membrane potential (η_m) and drug transference number (t_2) are written in terms of electric field (s). The variable s can be calculated from equation (18), if the current is controlled by a constant current source and the resistances (R_{s1} and R_{s2}) are measured. All other variables then can be evaluated explicitly from equations (19)–(22). Calculation of the dimensional values is also straight forward with this information from equations (9)–(14).

Design equations

Two of the most important variables for design are the 'on' and 'off' drug-delivery rates corresponding to when the power to the iontophoretic implant is turned 'on' and 'off'. From equations (12), (13), (18) and (19), these are easily shown to be:

$$j_2 A = I/F \qquad\qquad\qquad \text{(on)} \qquad\qquad (23)$$

$$j_2 A = [\gamma \ln \gamma/(\gamma - 1)][RT/(F^2 R_{s1})] \quad \text{(off)} \qquad\qquad (24)$$

Typically, it is found that these relationships are correct to within 20% for very small cations (e.g. a molecular weight of about 150).[26,32] However, for slightly larger antiarrhythmic drugs, factors of 0.75 and 2 are found to work well when inserted on the right-hand sides of equations (23) and (24), respectively. The deviation of equation (23) is considered due to small penetration of Cl^- in between the exchanger beads and the silicone rubber, and the deviation of equation (24) is considered to be primarily due to nonvalidity of the independence of counterion form assumption described above. We also note for equation (23) to be valid $I/F \gg [\gamma \ln \gamma/(\gamma - 1)][RT/(F^2 R_{s1})]$, otherwise the current is too small and will simply serve to perturb the electrodiffusion in the membrane.

Electro-osmotic considerations

It has been extremely well documented that water transport (electro-osmosis) will accompany the passage of electrolytic current through membranes containing fixed charges (e.g. ion-exchange membranes).[31] This is relevant, for several reasons, to implantable iontophoresis of charged drugs (e.g. antiarrhythmic drugs) through ion-exchange membranes. If appreciable water moves out of the implant (the water movement will be in the direction of counterion flow), a decrease in pressure inside would result, which will potentially damage the implant. Likewise, water movement through HCMs may potentially dislodge the resin beads from their position in the cluster of beads, which make up the transport path through the membrane to cause a loss of control of the release rate.

Another potential difficulty is an alteration of drug-release rate because of a convective term in the flux expression (equation 1). In the bi-ionic system where the drug cation resides in the implant and Na^+ is outside, the delivery rate during migrating current is predicted to be I/F if perfect Donnan exclusion of co-ions (anions in our case) holds. It is therefore impossible for electro-osmosis to increase the flux of the drug during constant current iontophoresis, since this would increase the flux of the charge (or current density) above that which is externally regulated by the external power source. At zero current, there is negligible water movement. Thus, the design rates, equations (23) and (24), are valid whether or not conditions in our system are favorable for electro-osmosis. The membrane potential, given by equation (21), will be affected by electro-osmosis. We have observed a nonlinear voltage–current behavior in the presence of dilute salt solutions (e.g., 0.01 M NaCl)[32] which we expect to be due to electro-osmosis. This becomes important as the device potential would increase from the energy required to move the solvent.

The mechanism responsible for water movement has classically been described in terms of counterions which are moving at a terminal velocity in the diffuse side of the electric double layer within the membrane (electro-osmosis).[33] These ions form a moving boundary adjacent to the solvent and impart momentum to the solvent, which in turn, moves in the same direction. Another mechanism has been proposed that suggests that water movement also occurs because of an induced osmotic pressure difference on either side of the membrane due to concentration polarization.[34,35] In the former mechanism, the solvent flow is favored as ionic strength of external media is reduced (and the electric double layer thickness is increased) and as membrane water content is increased (and pore size is increased).

Drug delivery and iontophoresis

Over the past 10–15 years, iontophoretic drug delivery has been investigated mainly for transdermal iontophoresis where the rate-limiting membrane is the skin. An electrical circuit is formed by placing two electrodes in their respective solutions on the epidermis and connecting a source of electromotive force. The current travels beginning from the power supply and reaching in the anodal reservoir via the anode, through the skin into the blood circulation, back through the skin into the cathodal reservoir, and reaching once again to the supply via the cathode. If the positively charged drug is placed in the anodal reservoir, or a negatively charged drug in the cathodal reservoir, a portion of the current is carried by the drug and the component reaches the blood circulation. Delivery of neutral therapeutic agents has also been shown to be enhanced during iontophoresis. Transdermal administration has been used with a number of drugs in an effort to lower dosage requirements and also to reduce the frequency of drug administration by providing sustained and constant drug levels by continuous drug input. Several therapeutic agents such as sotalol, phenylethylamine, lignocaine and cyclosporine have been studied for transdermal ionotophoresis. A number of drugs with a large molecular size, such as insulin, thyrotropin releasing hormone and leuprolide acetate have also been investigated by transdermal iontophoresis.[36] Transdermal iontophoresis has also been useful for treating localized disease process such as the delivery of dexamethasone sodium phosphate for the treatment of localized tissue inflammation.[24] Conventional direct current (d.c.) iontophoresis uses a constant current density of the magnitude of 0.5 mA cm^{-2} to enhance the movement of charged drugs through the skin. However, d.c. constant-current iontophoresis inevitably causes a skin polarization potential to develop, irritating the skin. The pulsed d.c. mode constant-current or alternating current (a.c.) have been reported to increase the efficiency of iontophoretic transdermal drug delivery by minimizing skin irritation.[37,38]

Cardiovascular iontophoresis with transtissue current flow has been investigated by several groups. In a study by Avitall,[27] transmyocardial iontophoretic delivery of procainamide using a dialysis membrane as a part of defibrillator electrode system was examined. The delivery of high amounts of procainamide directly into infarct myocardium using pulsed current iontophoresis was shown to be feasible and effective. Fuster's group studied catheter-based transarterial iontophoresis demonstrating higher localized levels of hirudin in the arterial wall using iontophoresis after balloon angioplasty to prevent restenosis. Anionic hirudin was transported into the wall of the artery with an Ag|AgCl cathode in a specially designed delivery balloon positioned inside the lumen of the artery and an adhesive electrode patch placed on the skin served as the anode. Vascular levels of hirudin after active iontophoresis ($4\,mA\,cm^{-2}$, 5 min) were 80-fold greater than those achieved by passive diffusion (without electricity). The autoradiography studies revealed distribution of hirudin throughout the entire circumference of the arterial wall within the intima, media and adventitia. Iontophoresis-mediated vessel wall trauma was reported as <10% endothelial denudation and medial smooth-muscle damage.[28]

Conceptualization of HCMs for cardiac iontophoresis

The principles of iontophoresis have not been explored substantially to develop systems beyond the transdermal applications, to treat other disease conditions where modulated release of the drug could be more effective. Our laboratory has been investigating the principle of iontophoresis in the epicardial and endocardial delivery of antiarrhythmic agents in acute and chronic studies using cation-selective HCMs. Conventional therapy for treating ventricular arrhythmias is complicated by inadequate myocardial drug levels when given at clinically tolerable doses by conventional routes, and adverse systemic effects associated with these drugs. In our earlier studies, epicardial administration of antiarrhythmic agents from drug-loaded controlled release polymer matrices has been shown to be an effective alternative to deliver antiarrhythmic drugs. The drug levels due to epicardial implants in the coronary circulation are usually 10–20-fold higher than in the peripheral circulation, thus optimizing the drug effect at the location of the disease. Furthermore, the drug effect is observed with a dose 20–30-fold lower than that which is effective intravenously.[12,17] However, such systems can deliver the drug only at a fixed predetermined rate. An additional feature in such systems of modulating the release rates depending upon the state of the disease condition or other pharmacologic considerations will have significant importance in several clinical settings for an effective treatment of cardiac arrhythmias. The possibility of electrocardiogram monitoring techniques such as those used in the automatic implantable defibrillators would provide an optimal online arrhythmia-detection system to trigger the drug release from the modulatable drug implant. Such modulatable systems eventually will optimize the drug effect by delivering it only when it is most required. Such a feedback system is explained in detail in Chapter 19.

Formulation and characterization of HCMs

In our studies we have typically formulated HCMs as rate-limiting membranes for drug-delivery reservoir implants, regulatable with iontophoresis. We have characterized these HCMs for cation permselectivity under *in vitro* conditions using cationic drugs including antiarrhythmic agents.

Conditioning of the cation-exchange resin

Cation-exchange resin (Dowex 50W-200X, Sigma) is initially conditioned to remove impurities by repeated washing with alternate cycles of 1 N NaOH and 1 N HCl. The cycle is repeated six times followed by six washes of 1 M NaCl in order to convert the resin into the sodium form. The resin is then rinsed with distilled water repeatedly until the pH of the filtrate is the same as distilled water. The wet resin is freeze-dried overnight and stored under reduced pressure in the presence of silica gel.

Formulation of heterogeneous cation-exchange membranes (HCMs)

HCMs are usually prepared by mixing the dry conditioned resin processed as above at 42–52% w/w loading (53–75 μm size resin fraction) with the prevulcanized form of the Silastic (Dow Corning, Midland, MI) Q-7 4840 (Part A and B mixture in 1:1 ratio) in an aluminum mold. A circular disk of 0.2 cm^2 cut through HCM is further vulcanized with silicone as previously described so that HCM forms an ion-conducting port in the matrix of insulated silicone membrane.[32] The HCM thus prepared was either used in diffusion cells to study release characteristics or to fabricate cardiac iontophoretic devices.

Iontophoretic cardiac drug implant design

The HCM prepared as above is sealed to the silicone reservoir (2 cc capacity) with a Ag|AgCl anode inside and a cathode outside the HCM. The cathode is separated from the HCM by a silicone gasket for HCM swelling and covered with a low protein-binding blood-biocompatible Millipore® membrane (pore size 5 μm, filter type SV) (Figure 18.1).

Swelling and conditioning of HCM to drug form

The iontophoresis device is typically filled with a 0.15 M NaCl solution and is left in a beaker of the same ionic strength NaCl solution for 48 hours at 37°C for equilibrium swelling of the HCM. Next, the HCM, which is originally in sodium form, is converted to the drug form by replacing the inside and outside sodium chloride solutions with drug solution. A current of 150 μA is passed until a steady membrane potential (~8 hours) is noted. The HCMs for *in vitro* characterization are first put in a

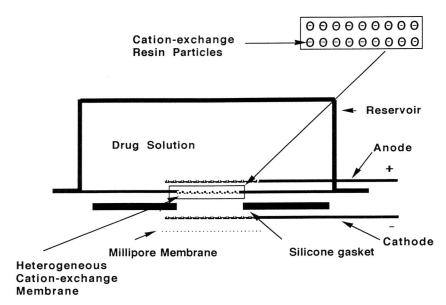

Figure 18.1 Schematic representation of a cardiac iontophoretic device design.

NaCl solution in a beaker for equilibrium swelling and then conditioned to drug form in double diffusion cell (Crown Glass Co., Somerville, NJ).

In vitro iontophoretic modulation of antiarrhythmic drugs

In vitro iontophoretic modulation of antiarrhythmic agents was carried out in a double diffusion cell after converting the HCM into the drug form. Modulation studies were carried out with various current protocols depending upon the drug used. Sotalol as a model class III antiarrhythmic agent was used to study iontophoretic modulation using the HCM. The HCM-reservoir device filled with fresh 0.15 M sotalol hydrochloride, and the HCM previously conditioned to sotalol form, was initially evaluated *in vitro* for modulated release of the drug at 'off' and 450 μA currents for two off/on cycles with each phase lasting for 60 min. The *in vitro* study was performed in a double-jacketed beaker with water circulation at 37°C in Sörenson's buffer of pH 7.3. The drug was analyzed spectrophotometrically at 227 nm.

In vivo cardiac iontophoretic implant study

The iontophoretic device previously conditioned to the sotalol form (as above) was evaluated *in vivo* in acute and chronic dog studies. The implant is typically placed over the left epicardium and the electrical leads are connected to power unit to run the off/on current protocol. The blood from the coronary vein proximal to the device, and the cephalic vein were collected to quantitate sotalol levels by high-performance liquid chromatography. In chronic studies, the device was implanted under sterile conditions. The electrical leads from the device were placed below the skin in the ventrodorsal region. The leads were exposed briefly to run a $900\,\mu A$ current protocol for 30 minutes on the day of implantation, and again after two weeks and four weeks postimplantation. Blood samples were collected from the cephalic vein before and after the current was passed.

HCM-facilitated iontophoresis: drug transport and disposition

The iontophoretic modulation in a double diffusion cell was studied using antiarrhythmic drugs *d*-sotalol, lidocaine and acebutolol. Figure 18.2 typically demonstrates the release rates of *d*-sotalol modulated between ~ 1000 and $400\,\mu g\,h^{-1}$ for two on/off cycles. The 'on' current phase was adjusted to reduce the lag phase that is usually observed after the current is turned on. The negative currents were also used to halt the drug release. The *in vitro* iontophoretic modulation of *d,l*-sotalol from the cardiac implant device at 'off'/450 μA current was carried out in a double jacketed beaker at 37°C. The steady-state release rate at 'off' current was $0.363\,mg\,h^{-1}$ whereas at $450\,\mu A$ it was $3.88\,mg\,h^{-1}$ (Figure 18.3). The anticipated dosing rate, calculated from the *in vitro* release characteristics, is $0.015\,mg\,kg^{-1}\,h^{-1}$ during 'off' current phase and $0.155\,mg\,kg^{-1}\,h^{-1}$ during $450\,\mu A$ current phase in a 25 kg dog. The steady-state device potential measured simultaneously at $450\,\mu A$ was $6.04 \pm 0.8\,V$. *In vitro* release rates and device potential at a $450\,\mu A$ of current were used as parameters for each device before *in vivo* implantation.

In an example of an acute iontophoretic drug-implant study in the dog, the sotalol release-rate modulation was achieved at 'off' and 'on' current cycles with an 'on'

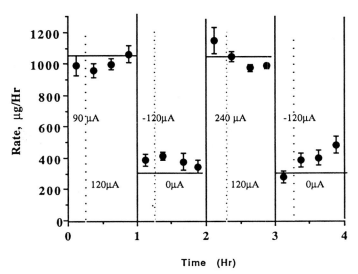

Figure 18.2 *In vitro* modulation of the release of *d*-sotalol through HCM for two on/off current cycles from 0.01 M sotalol hydrochloride into 0.01 M NaCl in a double diffusion cell at 37°C. Resin (74–89 μm size) loading 52% w/w in HCM. Symbols represent the mean ($n = 3$) $\pm$ SEM; (———), the expected steady-state values based on equations (23) and (24) and empirical factors of 0.75 and 2. (Reproduced with permission from *Macromolecules*.)

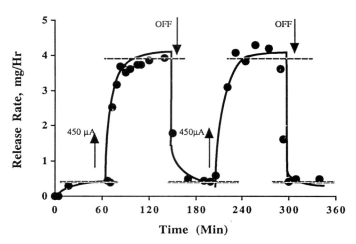

Figure 18.3 *In vitro* modulation of the release of *d,l*-sotalol hydrochloride from an iontophoretic device for two 'off'/450 mA current cycles from 0.15 M drug solution into Sörenson's buffer at 37°C. Resin (53–75 μm size) loading 42% w/w in HCM. Each point is a mean of three readings; (– – – –), the expected steady-state values based on equations (23) and (24) and empirical factors of 0.75 and 2.

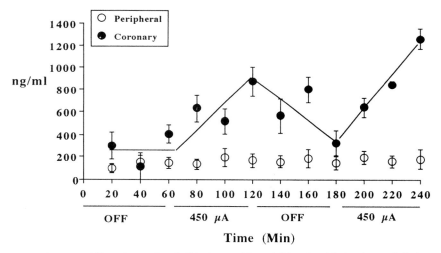

Figure 18.4 Coronary (●) and peripheral (○) plasma *d,l*-sotalol levels with *in vivo* modulation of drug release from iontophoretic device at two 'off'/450 μA current cycles. Iontophoretic reservoir contained 0.15 M *d,l*-sotalol hydrochloride solution. The anticipated dosing rate, calculated from the *in vitro* release characteristics is 0.015 mg kg^{-1} h^{-1} during 'off' current phase and 0.155 mg kg^{-1} h^{-1} during 450 μA current phase in a 25-kg dog. Each symbol represents mean ($n = 3$) ± SEM.

current phase of either 100 μA, 450 μA or 900 μA in three different protocols studied. Figure 18.4 represents *in vivo* modulation of drug with off/450 μA/off/450 μA current protocol with each 'off' or 'on' phase lasting for 60 minutes. As shown (Figure 18.4), coronary venous sotalol levels demonstrated phasic changes with off/on current cycles. The peripheral sotalol levels measured during the same period display

Table 18.1 Chronic cardiac iontophoretic implant results

Parameter	Time postimplant		
	Same day	2 weeks	4 weeks
Zero-current baseline sotalol peripheral levels (ng ml^{-1})	101.8 ± 13.2	86.1 ± 7.9	79.1 ± 8.1
Post-900 μA current sotalol peripheral levels (ng ml^{-1})	227.2 ± 38.8	185.5 ± 25.4	132.4 ± 8.2
Percentage increase in sotalol levels post-900 μA current	123.2	115.4	67.3
Device potential at 900 μA current (volts)	12.1 ± 1.7	9.8 ± 1.5	11.8 ± 1.8

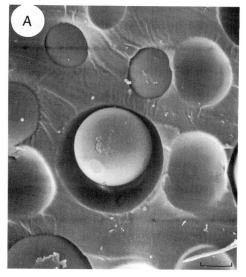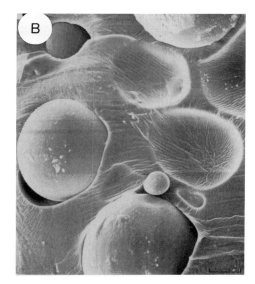

Figure 18.5 Scanning electron micrograph (400×) of the surface of the HCM from nonimplanted (A) and 30-day implanted (B) iontophoretic device. Bar represents 30 μm.

relatively less effect of 'off' or 'on' current cycles. The peak coronary levels attained with the 'on' current phase in different protocols were linear with the current density (113.5 ng/100 μA, $r^2 = 0.996$). This study demonstrated a current responsive characteristics of the iontophoretic implant for efficient modulation of drug release *in vivo*.

In our chronic 30-day dog-implant study, the effect of current modulation was observed with 'off' and 900 μA current for 30 minutes on peripheral sotalol levels at the time of implantation, two weeks and four weeks postdevice implantation. The data in the Table 18.1 indicate the effect of 900 μA current on peripheral sotalol levels compared to baseline drug levels at various time points. The rise in the peripheral plasma sotalol levels with the $900\,\mu A$ current is indicative of device responsiveness even after 30-day implantation. The overall decrease in the drug plasma levels was due to depletion of the drug ($52.8\% \pm 4.8$ in a 30-day period) from the device because of diffusion through HCM. In addition, the device potential measured at each time point was almost unchanged (12.1 ± 1.7, 9.8 ± 1.5 and $11.8 \pm 1,8$ V at $900\,\mu A$, on the day of implant, two weeks and four weeks postimplantation, respectively) indicating stable electrical properties of the HCM. Furthermore, scanning electron microscopy of the HCM of pre- and postimplanted device indicates no apparent changes in the resin particles such as pores and cracks (Figure 18.5).

Our studies demonstrate a successful epicardial iontophoretic cardiac implant device design for iontophoretic modulation of antiarrhythmic agents. Furthermore, the modulation of the release rate could be achieved at microampere current densities. Other iontophoretic studies have used non-ion-selective membranes as rate-limiting membranes such as polyhydroxymethacrylate to modulate drug release. However such membranes have distinct disadvantages as compared to the system described in our study. The modulation of the drug release with nonselective membranes can only be achieved at very high current density. The membrane system described in our study uses a cationic exchange material (resin particles) which is ideally permselective for cations. Therefore, the modulation of drug release can be achieved with high efficiency with microampere current densities.[39,40] In addition, with the iontophoretic device design proposed in our study, current is confined across the HCM and does not pass through the myocardium. Thus the possibility of myocardial injury due to d.c. current-induced tissue polarization or its effect on normal heart electrophysiologic function is minimized. The drug once released from the device can diffuse passively throughout the heart because of the perfused nature of the myocardium.

Future perspectives

Cardiac iontophoretic drug systems can be best used in conjunction with an arrhythmia detection system in a feedback loop so the antiarrhythmic agent is released at a desired time and rate. Such a feedback system is very successful in an automatic implantable defibrillator. Iontophoretic systems that contain more potent drugs such as ibutilide and that can be refilled through a subcutaneous access device will be useful for long-term applications.[27] However, some critical factors, such as scar-tissue buildup around the device and its effect on long-term release rates, drug stability in solution, etc. require consideration for its effective applications in the clinical setting.

References

1. Edelman, E. R., Adams, D. H. and Karnovsky, M. J. (1990) Effect of controlled adventitial heparin delivery on smooth muscle cell proliferation following endothelial injury. *Proc. Natl Acad. Sci. USA*, **87**, 3773–7.

2. Golomb, G., Dixon, M., Smith, M. S. *et al.* (1987) Controlled-release drug delivery of diphosphonates to inhibit bioprosthetic heart valve calcification: release rate modulation with silicone matrices via drug solubility and membrane coating. *J. Pharm. Sci.*, **76**, 271–6.

3. Gorecki, D., Kruszewski, A., Jakobisiak, M. and Lasek, W. (1989/90) Local administration of cyclosporin allows reduction of the dose prolonging survival of heart tissue allografts. *Immunol. Lett.*, **23**, 247–50.

4. Levy, R. J., Wolfrum, J., Schoen, F. J. *et al.* (1985) Inhibition of calcification of bioprosthetic heart valves by local controlled-release diphosphonate. *Science*, **228**, 190–2.

5. Labhasetwar, V. and Levy, R. J. (1992) Polymer systems for cardiovascular drug delivery. *Polymer News*, **17**, 336–42.

6. Wilensky, R. L., March, K. L. and Hathaway, D. R. (1991) Direct intraarterial wall injection of microparticles via a catheter: a potential drug delivery strategy following angioplasty. *Am. Heart J.*, **122**, 1136–40.

7. Wilensky, R. L., March, K. L., Gradus-Pizlo, I. *et al.* (1993) Methods and devices for local drug delivery in coronary and peripheral arteries. *Trends Cardiovasc. Med.*, **3**, 163–70.

8. Labhasetwar, V., Underwood, T., Gallagher, M. *et al.* (1994) Epicardial controlled release ibutilide: effects on defibrillation threshold and electrophysiologic parameters. *J. Cardiovasc. Pharmacol.*, **24**, 826–840.

9. Stokes, K. B., Kriett, J. M., Gornick, C. A. *et al.* (1983) Low threshold cardiac pacing electrodes. *Proc., Annual Conference IEEE Engineering in Medicine and Biology*, **5**, 100–3.

10. Stokes, K. B., Graf, J. E. and Wiebusch, W. A. (1982) Drug eluting electrodes – improved pacemaker performance. *Proc., Annual Conference IEEE Engineering in Medicine and Biology*, **13**, 499–502.

11. Mond, H. G. and Stokes, K. B. (1992) The electrode–tissue interface: the revolutionary role of steroid elution. *Pacing Clin. Electrophysiol.*, **15**, 95–107.

12. Labhasetwar, V., Underwood, T., Gallagher, M. *et al.* (1994) Sotalol controlled-release systems for arrhythmias: *in vitro* characterization, *in vivo* drug disposition, and electrophysiologic effects. *J. Pharm. Sci.*, **83**, 157–64.

13. Labhasetwar, V., Kadish, A., Underwood, T. *et al.* (1993) The efficacy of controlled release *d*-sotalol–polyurethane epicardial implants for ventricular arrhythmias due to acute ischemia in dogs. *J. Controlled Release*, **23**, 75–86.

14. Levy, R. J., Johnston, T. P., Sintov, A. and Golomb, G. (1990) Controlled release implants for cardiovascular disease. *J. Controlled Release*, **11**, 245–54.

15. Sintov, A., Scott, W. A., Siden, R. and Levy, R. J. (1990) Efficacy of epicardial controlled-release lidocaine for ventricular tachycardia induced by rapid ventricular pacing in dogs. *J. Cardiovasc. Pharmacol.*, **16**, 812–17.

16. Sintov, A., Scott, W. A., Gallagher, K. P. and Levy, R. J. (1990) Conversion of ouabain-induced ventricular tachycardia in dogs with epicardial lidocaine: pharmacodynamics and functional effects. *Pharm. Res.*, **7**, 28–33.

17. Siden, R., Kadish, A., Flowers, W. *et al.* (1992) Epicardial controlled-release verapamil prevents ventricular tachycardia episodes induced by acute ischemia in a canine model. *J. Cardiovasc. Pharmacol.*, **19**, 798–809.

18. Villa, A. E., Guzman, L. A., Chen, W. *et al.* (1994) Local delivery of dexamethasone for prevention of neointimal proliferation in a rat model of balloon angioplasty. *J. Clin. Invest.*, **93**, 1243–9.

19. Faidutti, B., von Segesser, L., Velebit, V. and Leuenberger, A. (1986) Implantation of antibiotic-releasing carriers for treatment of recurrent prosthetic endocarditis. *J. Thorac. Cardiovasc. Surg.*, **92**, 159–61.

20. Heller, J. (1993) Modulated release from drug delivery devices. *Crit. Rev. Therapeut. Drug Carrier Syst.*, **10**, 253–305.

21. Hsieh, D., Langer, R. and Folkman, J. (1981) Magnetic modulation of release of macromolecules from polymers. *Proc. Natl Acad. Sci. USA*, **78**, 1863–7.

22. Kost, J., Leong, K. and Langer, R. (1989) Ultrasound-enhanced polymer degradation and release of incorporated substances. *Proc. Natl Acad. Sci. USA*, **86**, 7633–66.

23. Marliss, E. B., Caron, D., Albisser, A. M. and Zinman, B. (1981) Present and future expectations regarding insulin infusion systems. *Diabetes Care*, **4**, 325–7.
24. Petelenz, T. J., Buttke, J. A., Bonds, C. *et al.* (1992) Iontophoresis of dexamethasone: laboratory studies. *J. Controlled Release*, **20**, 55–66.
25. Yoshida, N. H. and Roberts, M. S. (1993) Solute molecular size and transdermal iontophoresis across excised human skin. *J. Controlled Release*, **25**, 177–95.
26. Schwendeman, S. P., Amidon, G. L. and Levy, R. J. (1993) Determinants of the modulated release of antiarrhythmic drugs by iontophoresis through polymer membranes. *Macromolecules*, **26**, 2264–72.
27. Avitall, B., Hare, J., Zander, G. *et al.* (1992) Iontophoretic transmyocardial drug delivery: a novel approach to antiarrhythmic drug therapy. *Circulation*, **85**, 1582–93.
28. Fernandez-Ortiz, A., Meyer, B. J., Mailhac, A. *et al.* (1994) A new approach for local intravascular drug delivery: iontophoretic balloon. *Circulation*, **89**, 1518–22.
29. Narebska, A., Koter, S. and Kujawski, W. (1985) Irreversible thermodynamics of transport across charged membranes. Part I. Microscopic resistance coefficients for a system with Nafion 120 membrane. *J. Membrane Sci.*, **25**, 153–70.
30. Wyllie, M. R. and Patnode, H. W. (1950) The development of membranes prepared from artificial cation-exchange materials with particular reference to the determination of sodium-ion activities. *J. Phys. Chem.*, **54**, 204–27.
31. Helfferich, F. (1962) *Ion Exchange*. New York: McGraw-Hill.
32. Schwendeman, S. P., Amidon, G. L., Meyerhoff, M. E. and Levy, R. J. (1992) Modulated drug release using iontophoresis through heterogeneous cation-exchange membranes: membrane preparation and influence of resin cross-linkage. *Macromolecules*, **25**, 2531–40.
33. Kobatake, Y., Yusasa, M. and Fujita, H. (1968) Studies of membrane phenomena. VI. Further study of volume flow. *J. Phys. Chem.*, **72**, 1752–7.
34. Barry, P. H. and Hope, A. B. (1969) Electroosmosis in membranes: effects of unstirred layers and transport numbers. *Biophys. J.*, **9**, 700–28.
35. Pikal, M. J. (1990) Transport mechanisms in iontophoresis. I. A theoretical model for the effect of electroosmotic flow on flux enhancement in transdermal iontophoresis. *Pharm. Res.*, **7**, 118–26.
36. Srinivasan, V., Higuchi, W. I., Sims, S. M. *et al.* (1989) Transdermal iontophoretic drug delivery: mechanistic analysis and application to polypeptide delivery. *J. Pharm. Sci.*, **78**, 370–5.
37. Reinauer, S., Neusser, A., Schauf, G. and Holzle, E. (1993) Iontophoresis with alternating current and direct current offset (a.c./d.c. iontophoresis): a new approach for the treatment of hyperhidrosis. *Br. J. Dermatol.*, **129**, 166–9.
38. Zakzewski, C. A., Amory, D. W., Jasaitis, D. K. and Li, J. K.-J. (1992) Iontophoretically enhanced transdermal delivery of an ACE inhibitor in induced hypertensive rabbits: preliminary report. *Cardiovasc. Drugs Ther.*, **6**, 589–95.
39. Schwendeman, S. P., Amidon, G. L., Labhasetwar, V. and Levy, R. J. (1994) Modulated drug release using iontophoresis through heterogeneous cation-exchange membranes. II. Influence of cation-exchanger content on membrane resistance and characteristic times. *J. Pharm. Sci.*, **83**, 1482–93.
40. Labhasetwar, V., Schwendeman, S. P., Underwood, T. *et al.* (1993) Epicardial iontophoretic delivery of antiarrhythmic agents. Proceedings of the 20th International Symposium on Controlled Release of Bioactive Materials. *J. Controlled Release*, **20**, 476–7.

19

Feedback Control of Antiarrhythmic Agents

John C. Wood
Marten Telting-Diaz
David R. Bloem
Tam Nguyen
Mark Meyerhoff
Robert Arzbaecher
Amnon Sintov
Robert J. Levy

Introduction

For centuries, physicians have employed feedback control implicitly. A therapy is prescribed, signs of efficacy and toxicity are noted and the therapy is modified accordingly. With the explosion in computer capabilities, microsensor technologies, drug-delivery systems, and control strategies in the past decade, the potential for explicit computer-assisted feedback control has never been greater. In this chapter, the motivation for computer-assisted drug delivery is discussed, followed by an outline of the control problem and a definition of terms. Automated drug delivery can be divided into two major problems: (1) rapidly achieving and maintaining a target serum drug level; and (2) tuning the target level according to physiologic and electrocardiographic measures of efficacy/toxicity. Here, these two feedback problems will be further subdivided and their major principles emphasized. To illustrate how the subcomponents interact in an integrated system, an experimental arrhythmia termination device will be presented in detail. Lastly, potential applications of feedback drug delivery to implantable and acute-care arrhythmia control are discussed.

Motivation for feedback control

In a perfect world, a drug-delivery system/control strategy would reach a therapeutic level rapidly, without overshoot, modulate the therapeutic level according to physiologic demands, be synergistic with defibrillator device technology, be non-invasive – and cost nothing. Reality, of course, forces compromise with clinical demands dictating the relative importance of different criteria. In the coronary care unit, for example, rapid response may be a higher priority than noninvasiveness, while the opposite is generally true in an outpatient setting. Although not yet harnessed, computer-assisted feedback drug delivery has many potential advantages over manually-controlled delivery with regard to realizing these 'ideal' properties.

Quicker response time

Interpatient pharmacokinetic variability requires conservative antiarrhythmic dosing to avoid toxicity. Consequently, a drug-delivery system employing online drug level or drug-effect feedback would allow more aggressive dosage trajectories than manual regimes. In the acute-care setting (e.g. following myocardial infarction or cardiac surgery) more rapid response might translate to improved clinical outcomes. In the inpatient wards or the electrophysiology laboratories, faster response time implies quicker assessment of drug efficacy and toxicity, reducing hospital costs. For example, inpatient initiation of antiarrhythmic agents for ventricular tachycardia prophylaxis typically requires an iterative sequence of dosage changes, serum drug levels after 3–5 half lives, followed by Holter monitoring, stress testing, or electrophysiological testing, to assess efficacy. A computer-driven infusion device, using serum levels and/or electrocardiographic feedback, could significantly shorten the cycle by facilitating rapid, controlled, serum level transitions and quicker convergence on therapeutic levels.

Decreased toxicity

In addition to improving response time, computer-assisted feedback control could decrease toxicity both by better drug-level control and by electrocardiographic 'effect' feedback. Effect feedback would be particularly beneficial when toxicity occurs within the therapeutic window, when unmeasured active drug metabolites are present, or when unexpected drug interactions occur.

Customized dosing

If an individual's pharmacokinetics were known exactly, a priori drug-level measurements would be unnecessary. Unfortunately, interpatient variability is significant and experimental pharmacokinetics determination is clinically not feasible. However, automatic drug-level or drug-effect feedback could derive a patient's individual pharmacokinetic parameters simultaneously with therapeutic drug delivery. Feedback control would also be robust to parameter changes, such as changing renal function or distribution volume. Potentially, computer-assisted feedback control could also modulate the drug dosage according to clinical demand. For example, it is well known that arrhythmogenicity follows a diurnal variation, with lethal arrhythmias most common in the early morning.[1,2] Consequently, diurnally-varying serum levels might offer adequate arrhythmia protection with lower net drug delivered. Physical activity and stress also alter arrhythmogenicity. Just as rate-controlled pacemakers titrate heart rate to exertion, electrocardiographic feedback might be used to titrate antiarrhythmic drug delivery in response to changes in automaticity, QT interval or other prognostic indicators.

Implantable devices

Management of recurrent ventricular arrhythmias, once the mainstay of antiar-rhythmic therapy, is progressively turning toward automated implanted cardio-defibrillators (AICDs).[3] The reason is simple: non-efficacious medical therapy for ventricular arrhythmias often manifests itself as sudden death, making therapy optimization difficult. Even though therapy is initiated in a controlled environment, either in the electrophysiology laboratory or the inpatient ward, the initial assess-ment of treatment 'efficacy' is a limited statistical sampling that is prone to error. AICDs offer a vital 'second chance' when medical therapy has failed, or even primary therapy in individuals with infrequent arrhythmias. Because the conse-quences of failed medical management are so high, AICDs will likely remain a dominant force even in the face of major pharmacologic advances. However, device and medical therapy are synergistic. Appropriate medical management decreases the number of shocks a patient receives, improving quality of life and device life expectancy. In addition, antiarrhythmic therapy also lower defibrillation thresholds, decreasing battery size requirements. Consequently, it is not surprising that 60–80% of AICD patients receive concomitant medical therapy.[4–6]

Given the synergism of device and medical therapy, the prospect of coupling a feedback drug-delivery system with AICD placement is exciting. The AICD already provides the computer and electrophysiologic transducers, and polymer-based local drug delivery is advancing at an explosive pace; successful chronic dog models for iontophoretic sotalol administration have already been accomplished (see Chapter 18). Iontophoretic membrane power requirements are approximately 4–10 μW for sotalol and ibutilide, well within the capability of pacemaker or AICD batteries.[7] Furthermore, the high potency of ibutilide and other new agents makes drug reservoir sizes realizable. Since the rate of iontophoretic drug release is linearly proportional to the membrane current, iontophoresis has potential as a low-power, implantable, programmable pump.

Outline of the clinical problem – general control strategies

Pharmacologic arrhythmia suppression is one of the most challenging tasks facing cardiologists. Antiarrhythmic agents have extremely low therapeutic indices, with unpleasant physical side effects and significant arrhythmogenicity. Complex drug interactions are not uncommon, particularly in the elderly. Prior to radioimmuno-assay development, toxicity was avoided only by cautious dosing schedules,

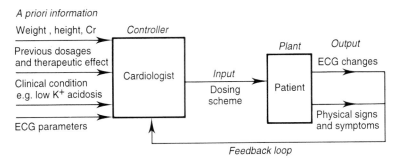

Figure 19.1   Simple control system for antiarrhythmic dosing consisting of a patient (plant), cardiologist (controller) and feedback loop (ECG and physical signs).

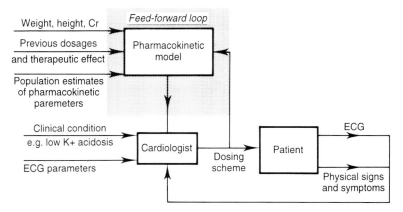

Figure 19.2   Strong feedforward, weak-feedback control system for antiarrhythmic dosing. The controller uses a plant model to adjust the input through a 'feed-forward' loop. Feedback correction occurs only through ECG and physical signs.

scrupulous attention to electrocardiographic changes, and careful documentation of physical signs and symptoms. This simple control system for drug delivery is shown schematically in Figure 19.1. The patient is the 'plant' to be controlled by 'input' of an antiarrhythmic drug. Electrocardiographic changes and physical signs represent the patient's 'output'. The 'controller' (cardiologist) integrates 'a priori information' about the 'plant' as well as plant 'feedback' to make intelligent input adjustments.

Initially, cardiologists had few guidelines for appropriate antiarrhythmic drug dosing. As pharmacokinetics advanced, the ability to predict a patient's serum drug level based upon their physical characteristics and drug 'input' improved markedly.[8-13] Simple one- and two-compartment pharmacokinetic patient models allowed the cardiologist to predict the drug dosage necessary to obtain a desired drug level in an 'average' patient of the given height, weight and renal function.[14,15] Drug dosage based upon a priori information alone is an example of 'feedforward', or open loop, control (Figure 19.2); the system shown might be described as

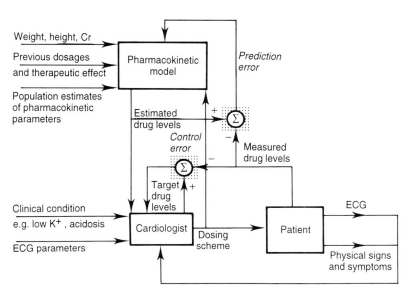

Figure 19.3 Scheme illustrating modern antiarrhythmic 'control' strategy. Measured serum levels are used to correct both the model and the drug dosing based upon the magnitude of the prediction and control errors, respectively.

'strongly' feedforward with 'weak' feedback control. For open-loop control to work well, the pharmacokinetic model structure must accurately describe drug dynamics and intersubject parameter variation must be small. While the first criteria is often satisfied, the second is not. That is, estimating an individual's pharmacokinetic parameters based solely upon physical observations and serum creatinine, has too much uncertainty for satisfactory, long-term, drug level control.[12,14,15]

Consequently, radioimmunoassay and ELISA (enzyme-linked immunosorbent assay) techniques revolutionized antiarrhythmic therapy. Differences between the targeted and the observed drug levels (control error), as well as the predicted and the observed drug levels (prediction error), were used to correct drug-level trajectories as well as the pharmacokinetic model (Figure 19.3). Although computer programs were developed for optimally updating drug delivery and pharmacokinetic models, feedback correction was generally performed implicitly rather than explicitly.[13,16,17]

Although Figure 19.3 may appear to be an overly formal schematic of clinical decision-making, it is a useful format for investigating automated feedback-control algorithms. The general problem represented in Figure 19.3 can be broken up into two major components: (1) rapidly achieving and maintaining a target serum drug level (or set point); and (2) modulating the 'set point' according to physiologic and electrophysiologic feedback (Figure 19.4). The first problem can in turn be broken down in four subcomponents: (1a) establishing an initial dosage trajectory; (1b) administering the antiarrhythmic agent in a controlled, reproducible manner; (1c) obtaining rapid, accurate estimates of serum drug concentration or drug effect; and (1d) correcting drug dosing and system models according to the control and prediction errors. Similarly, problem 2 can be subdivided into the following: (2a)

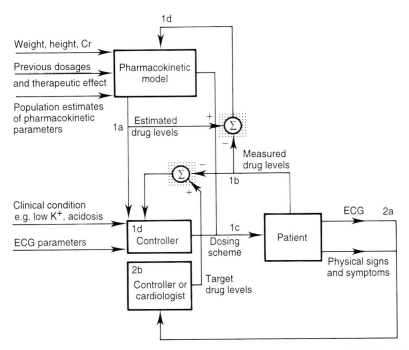

Figure 19.4 Scheme illustrating the general drug-delivery problem. Two general feedback loops are evident. The 'inner loop' achieves and maintains a given target drug level or effect, while the 'outer loop' adjusts the target level according to signs of efficacy/toxicity. The numerals (1a, 1b, etc.) indicate the problems noted in the text.

extracting relevant electrocardiographic and physiologic parameters; and (2b) adjusting the target drug level according to the extracted parameters. Each of these subcomponents will be discussed in detail, with regard to previous work, present capabilities/limitations and prospective developments.

Problem 1A: Choosing initial pharmacokinetic models, parameters, and dosage trajectory

Pharmacokinetic models and optimal dosage trajectories

One-compartment model

Antiarrhythmics, with the notable exception of amiodarone, have fairly simple pharmacokinetics. The simplest model, consisting of a single compartment, appropriately describes steady-state drug delivery by any route, as well as non steady-state kinetics of intramuscular or oral dosing (Figure 19.5). Infused agents reach the compartment immediately, while intramuscular and oral agents are stored in 'depots' which pass the drug to the compartment according to a first-order process.[18] Drug elimination occurs through first-order kinetics and no distinction is

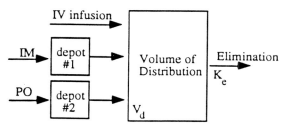

Figure 19.5 Open one-compartment pharmacokinetic model with intravenous (IV), intramuscular (IM) and oral (PO) inputs.

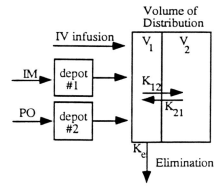

Figure 19.6 Open two-compartment model. Input and output occur only through the central compartment.

made between metabolism and excretion. The volume of distribution reflects the body's drug 'capacity'. Intuitively, greater capacity implies slower dynamics; it takes longer to achieve therapeutic drug levels (rise time) and longer to decline from toxic levels (decay time) for a given dose and elimination rate. One-compartment models have been used for open-loop and feedback control of digoxin levels.[8,9,11,15]

Two-compartment model

The single-compartment model is valid whenever changes in the input occur more slowly than drug redistribution within the body.[18,19] Oral or intramuscular dosing satisfy this assumption, but intravenous boluses and abrupt infusion rate increases will transiently elevate intravascular drug relative to peripheral tissues, necessitating a two-compartment model (Figure 19.6). The central compartment represents the intravascular compartment and blood-rich tissues whose drug concentration responds rapidly to intravenous drug concentration changes. The peripheral compartment represents the remainder of the drug's distribution volume, where drug

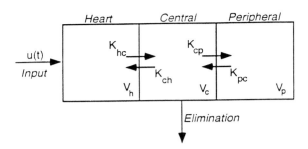

Figure 19.7 Three-compartment model representing local myocardial drug delivery. The heart, formerly included in the central compartment, now has important distinct pharmacokinetic properties. Elimination only occurs through the central compartment.

passage is slow. Drug redistribution between the peripheral and central compartments occurs as long as a gradient exists. Since the primary organs of elimination (kidney, liver) are blood-rich, net drug output occurs through the central compartment alone (input is directly into intravascular space).[19] Since the heart is blood-rich, the central compartment is assumed to represent the 'pharmacologically effective' compartment.

Local delivery pharmacokinetics

While local drug-delivery technologies have considerable therapeutic potential, the pharmacokinetics of local drug delivery must be characterized prior to clinical implementation. During local drug administration, myocardial pharmacokinetics can, in general, no longer be aggregated in the central compartment because the heart may act as a 'depot', analogous to an intramuscular injection.[18] Intuitively, a three-compartment model is a logical candidate as shown in Figure 19.7. The heart receives input from either an endocardial or epicardial source, and loses drug through redistribution to the 'central compartment'. The central compartment, consisting now of all blood-rich organs except the heart, loses drug to true elimination (metabolism, excretion), and redistribution to the peripheral compartment. This three-compartment model may reduce to a two-component model if the drug rate constants are well separated. For example, if the redistribution between central and peripheral compartments is much more rapid than the redistribution from heart to central compartment, the central and peripheral compartments may be effectively aggregated (Figure 19.8 left). If the converse is true, i.e. myocardial to serum exchange were rapid, then local delivery behaves like an intravenous infusion and a standard two-component model would be adequate (Figure 19.8, right).

As a model system for local delivery pharmacokinetics, serial peripheral blood samples were collected from six dogs following paired bolus intravenous (15–20 mg kg^{-1} over 5 min) and epicardial lidocaine (approximately 200 mg lidocaine delivered over 5 min from a polyurethane matrix) delivery. Intravenous and epicardial experiments were performed in random order, one week apart. Intravenous injection produced a classic biexponential (linear in log coordinates) curve with a steep initial redistribution and flatter elimination component, consistent with an

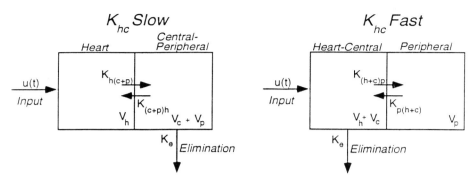

Figure 19.8 Reduced pharmacokinetic models for lidocaine local delivery. When K_{hc} is slow, the peripheral and central compartments behave as a single compartment because the transfer between cardiac and central compartments is limiting. When K_{hc} is fast, epicardial delivery is indistinguishable from a standard two-compartment model.

open two-compartment model with central elimination.[20] In contrast, epicardial kinetics encompassed the entire spectrum of proposed compartment models (Figure 19.9). Two animals (top panels) had slow cardiac–central-compartment transfer with delayed peak serum levels and monophasic decline. Two animals (middle panels) had rapid cardiac–central compartment flux with peak levels attained at patch removal, followed by readily distinguishable redistribution and elimination phases. For these four animals, biexponential fits adequately described the serum lidocaine profiles, supporting the reduced models in Figure 19.8. In contrast, the last two animals had intermediate cardiac–central compartment transfer rates; peak serum levels were slightly delayed but rapid redistribution phases were still evident. These animals required three exponentials to fit the serum level data, indicating the need for a full three-component pharmacokinetic model or a two-compartment model with first-order drug depoting. Table 19.1 summarizes the intravenous and epicardial bolus fit parameters.

In addition to reaching the central compartment more slowly than an intravenously-administered agent, an epicardially-delivered drug consistently achieves lower blood serum levels, despite comparable net weight of drug delivered (verified by lidocaine extraction from the epicardial patches). Based upon the total drug delivered and the area under the serum–time curves, the relative bioavailability of the epicardial lidocaine was estimated to be only 32.4%. Given the apparently rapid cardiac–central kinetics, a low bioavailability is quite surprising and suggests that epicardially-delivered lidocaine has a larger cardiac distribution volume than intravenously-administered drug. That is, epicardially-released drug must distribute simultaneously into central compartment-accessible and central compartment-inaccessible volumes. If so, characterization of the distribution volume, clearance, and 'effector' compartments for locally-delivered drugs will have profound efficacy and safety implications. However, while interstitial drug depoting is a possibility, direct myocardial homogenate assays will be required to verify that the 'missing' lidocaine is indeed contained in the heart. Furthermore, both the 'bioavailability' and pharmacokinetics of newer agents may be different and await characterization.

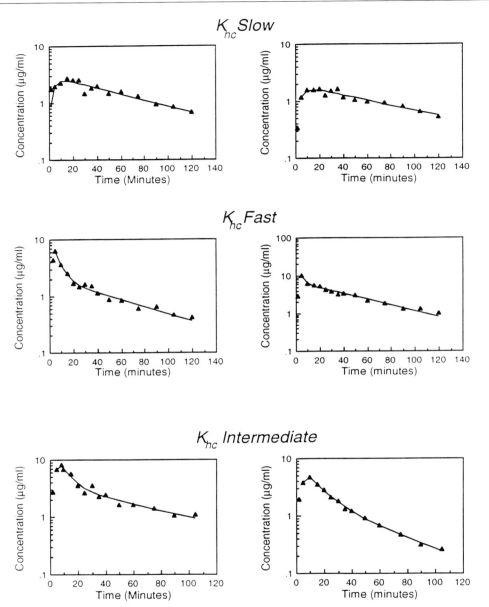

Figure 19.9 Peripheral serum lidocaine levels in six dogs following epicardial boluses, log concentrations versus time. Marks represent data points and solid line represents best fit to a sum of two or three exponentials. K_{he} was slow, relative to the other rate constants, in two animals (top), fast in two animals (middle), and intermediate in two animals (bottom).

Optimal dosage trajectories

Mathematically, the one-compartment model may be represented by a first-order differential equation:

Table 19.1 Serum level fit to a sum of exponentials*

Dog	Experiment	Compartments (n)	A1	λ1	A2	λ2	A3	λ3	MSE
53	IV	2	46.95	0.2430	5.4	0.0144	NA	NA	0.0678
	TE	2	NA	NA	6.97	0.0447	−120	0.831	0.0252
	TE	3	6.67	0.0876	2.39	0.0220	−177	0.832	0.0027**
52	IV	2	13.2	0.10	4.26	0.099	NA	NA	0.0724
	TE	2	NA	NA	3.00	0.0126	−3.58	0.2750	0.0454
	TE	3	3.99	0.0924	2.49	0.0102	−6.49	0.1533	0.0410
47	IV	2	25.1	0.0937	2.80	0.0007	NA	NA	0.290
	TE	2	10.8	0.182	2.09	0.0147	NA	NA	0.0135
	TE	3	20.2	0.2476	2.3	0.0094	−66.2	0.7278	0.0139
46	IV	2	77	0.256	6.17	0.0086	NA	NA	0.117
	TE	2	NA	NA	1.92	0.0104	−2.05	0.226	0.0123
	TE	3	3.64	0.228	1.91	0.010	−5.69	0.228	0.0139
34	IV	2	95.2	0.343	9.52	0.0216	NA	NA	0.1050
	TE	2	8.85	0.0482	0.755	−0.0034	NA	NA	0.365
	TE	3	18.9	0.226	3.67	0.0132	−67.8	0.7278	0.1099**
33	IV	2	39.8	0.116	5.25	0.0086	NA	NA	0.3761
	TE	2	25.0	0.363	6.71	0.0175	NA	NA	0.0628
	TE	3	15.1	0.223	6.73	0.0188	−67.1	0.728	0.193

Key: IV, intravenous; TE, transepicardial; MSE, mean squared error; NA, not applicable.
** = Significant improvement with three compartments.
*Summary of epicardial and intravenous parameter fit to the equation level = $A_1 e^{-k_1 t} + A_2 e^{-k_2 t} + A_3 e^{-k_3 t}$.
Only two exponentials were used for the intravenous data, while transepicardial data were fitted to both bi- and triexponentials.

$$\dot{C} = \frac{u}{V_d} - K_e C \tag{1}$$

where C is the compartment drug concentration, V_d is the volume of distribution, K_e is the elimination rate constant and u is the time-varying input (route-dependent). From this equation, the necessary input to achieve a desired output may be derived using a variety of techniques.[21–25] Using Laplace transforms, for example, the necessary infusion profile to cause an instantaneous increase to a desired steady-state level, C, can be shown to be.

$$u(t) = \mathscr{L}^{-1}\left[V_d\left(C\left(1 + \frac{K_e}{s}\right)\right)\right] = V_d C\{t = 0\} + V_d C K_e \quad (\text{for } t > 0) \tag{2}$$

where $\mathscr{L}^{-1}$ is the inverse Laplace transform. Consequently, the 'optimal' infusion protocol consists of a bolus coupled with a constant infusion, explaining the rationale behind conventional dosing of antiarrhythmic agents. The bolus loading dose produces an abrupt change in the serum drug level to the desired level, while the constant infusion exactly compensates drug elimination. Similarly, two-compartment models may be written

$$\dot{C}_1 = \frac{u}{V_1} - K_e C_1 - K_{12}(C_1 - C_2)$$

$$\dot{C}_2 = -K_{21}(C_2 - C_1) \tag{3}$$

where C_1 and C_2 are the central and peripheral compartment concentrations, V_1 is the central compartment volume of distribution, K_{12} and K_{21} represent the exchange kinetics and the other variables are defined as before. Using an identical approach to equation (1), the 'optimal' infusion regimen can be shown to be:[23]

$$u(t) = CV_1(\delta(t) + K_e + K_{12}\, e^{-K_{21}t}) \tag{4}$$

Notice that in addition to a bolus and a constant infusion, the 'optimal' infusion requires an exponentially tapering component. This extra component compensates for central compartment 'losses' to redistribution, having an infusion rate proportional to the gradient between the compartments. Using a conventional protocol, the serum level is initially therapeutic but falls rapidly with redistribution until the intravenous infusion saturates the peripheral compartment. In an attempt to compensate for redistribution, clinicians may attempt to emulate a tapering infusion component by administering multiple boluses, but this is less satisfactory.

Two-compartment open-loop control

While most intravenously infused antiarrhythmic agents can be described by two-compartment models, computer-assisted lidocaine dosing has attracted the most attention because of its widespread clinical applications in acute ventricular arrhythmic prophylaxis. Prior to widespread radioimmunoassay availability, conservative lidocaine dosing resulted in frequent rebolusing and a significant delay in achieving therapeutic levels.[26] Rodman *et al.*, in a prospective randomized study of 20 patients, demonstrated that computer-assisted population-based dosing, using a patient's height, weight and a clinical estimate of cardiac index (as a percentage of normal), achieved therapeutic drug levels more quickly than conventional therapy, without increased toxicity.[27] While the statistical power was insufficient to demonstrate any difference in clinical outcomes, computer-assisted open-loop lidocaine control delivered significantly more agent at all times during the first 8 hours of therapy, when postmyocardial infarction arrhythmias are most likely. Linear regression between observed and predicted levels produced a slope of 0.939 and a correlation coefficient of 0.795 ($P < 0.001$).

Open-loop intravenous antiarrhythmic delivery has also been proposed for paroxysmal atrial fibrillation/flutter conversion, both for acute-care settings and for recurrent arrhythmia termination.[23,28–31] In these systems, an atrial arrhythmia detector triggers an exponentially tapering infusion, based upon population pharmacokinetic parameters, until the arrhythmia is converted or a predetermined time has elapsed, e.g. 30 minutes. Figure 19.10 demonstrates the resulting blood serum levels in 12 patients receiving exponentially tapering procainamide infusions.[28] The target level, 8 mg ml^{-1}, was attained within 5 minutes and levels were therapeutic and stable over 30 minutes. Beyond 30 minutes, serum levels begin to climb because of a mismatch between estimated and true pharmacokinetic parameters. Therefore, pure feedforward control, based solely upon population pharmacokinetics, appears adequate for the short-term infusions required for arrhythmia termination devices.

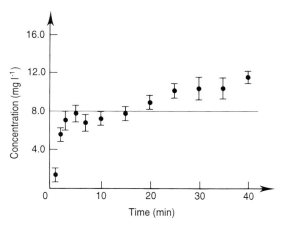

Figure 19.10 Mean plasma levels of procainamide during exponentially tapering infusions in 12 patients. (Reprinted with permission from Arzbaecher, R. and Bump, T. E. (1988). Development of an automatic implanted drug infusion system for the management of cardiac arrhythmias. *IEEE Proc.*, **76**, 1204–9. © 1988 IEEE.)

Longer intravenous infusions, however, will require drug or effect level feedback and dose corrections.

Deriving initial pharmacokinetic parameters

Given a chosen pharmacokinetic model for a drug, derivation of appropriate initial parameters may be achieved by direct individual measurement, or by population statistics. Derivation of individual pharmacokinetic parameters can be achieved by serial serum measurements following bolus injection. Applying this technique to alfentinyl (two-compartment) infusion, Martin *et al*. attained correlation coefficients between predicted and observed serum levels of 0.98 and 0.94 for dogs and humans, respectively.[21] Others have also noted markedly improved steady-state error when pharmacokinetic parameters were individually measured.[23,28,31] While these results demonstrate the capabilities of well-tuned open-loop control, this approach is clinically impractical for acute-care settings because it is too slow, and impractical for chronic dosing because pharmacokinetic parameters are nonstationary. In contrast, population-based statistics are suboptimal because of inherent unpredictable inter-individual parameter variation, but are quite easy to exploit clinically. Calculation of population statistics can be achieved through complete pharmacokinetic profiles on a small index population, or from incomplete profiles on a large index population; the relative merits of the two approaches are discussed in a review paper by Sheiner.[14] Drug trials often produce limited data of the first type, while conventional arrhythmia management produces large volumes of the latter data type. Either approach, or some combination of the two, should be adequate for initial parameter estimation. However, as observed in both the digoxin and lidocaine examples, population-based estimates cannot be expected to yield adequate parameter estimates for pure open-loop control.

Both 'effect' compartments, and metabolites can be modeled by a simple extension of the mathematical principles illustrated; open-loop control of third- and higher-order compartment models is discussed by Jacobs and others.[32–35] In general, one wants the lowest complexity model that adequately explains the drug kinetics. Programs such as NONMEM, allow statistical comparison of different pharmacologic models for a given set of data.[36]

Problem 1B: Drug administration

Routes of administration

Classically, antiarrhythmic drugs are delivered orally or intravenously. However, recent advances in drug delivery using magnetic, ultrasonic and iontophoretic modulation of drug-embedded polymer are particularly exciting because these modalities are well suited to feedback drug delivery.

Oral

Oral dosing yields the most uncertain changes in serum concentration; drug bioavailability and the rate constant between the gastrointestinal 'depot' and the central compartment depend upon both the drug (e.g. solubility, lipophilicity, formulation) as well as gastrointestinal factors (e.g. intestinal length, motility, gastric pH, mucosal disease).[37] Consequently, oral dosing is generally only suitable for steady-state chronic arrhythmic suppression where relatively constant serum levels are desired.

Intravenous

Many automatic infusion devices are currently available but most do not have programmable computer interfaces suitable for continuously varying infusion protocols. However, nonprogrammable pumps can simulate graded infusion regimes through automatic starting and stopping at a fixed infusion rate, or so-called 'pulse-code modulation'; satisfactory results have been demonstrated in both animal models and man with a nominal pump accuracy of $\pm$ 5%.[28,29,38–41] Implantable micropumps have improved considerably with recent applications toward endocrinology, chronic pain management and chemotherapy.[42–47] While these units appear suitable for arrhythmia termination applications, their power consumption may be prohibitively high for arrhythmia prophylaxis.

Magnetic modulation of controlled-release implants

Pioneering studies by Edelman _et al._ demonstrated that magnetic particles distributed throughout a nondegradable polymer implant could significantly perturb the implant during changes in magnetic field so as to vary release kinetics.[48] The rapid response and efficacy of this system had been well established _in vitro_ and _in vivo_.[49] However, this system has drawbacks in terms of the size and proximity of the variable magnetic field to the fixed polymer implant.[50] Although rapid response and sensitivity should be hypothetically possible, magnetic field strength falls off as an inverse function of the square of the distance from the source magnet. Therefore, both power, size and the position of the variable magnetic field for modulation are critical and limiting.

Ultrasound modulated controlled-release systems

Kost and his colleagues demonstrated that high-energy ultrasound transmitter implants placed in close proximity to nondegradable polymers could generate sufficient energy to accelerate drug-release kinetics.[51–53] The mechanism of drug release under these circumstances is incompletely understood, but may be due to simple thermal perturbation or perhaps heat-induced polymer phase changes. This system has been useful for modulating transdermal drug delivery, as well as during the drug-delivery kinetics for polymer matrix implants. As yet, this system has not been reduced to practice for clinical trials.

Iontophoretic implants

The use of transmembrane electrical currents to vary the transport of charged compounds has been investigated extensively for transdermal drug delivery. This technique has also been used for transmyocardial drug delivery. A novel approach to iontophoresis involves the authors' use of synthetic membranes consisting of cationic exchange beads combined with silicone rubber films, known as hetero-geneous cationic membranes (HCM). These HCMs represent the most energy-sensitive and energy-efficient iontophoretic systems and modulated systems devised thus far.[7] They are covered extensively in Chapter 18, and therefore will not be further dealt with here.

Types of dosage profiles

Since the initially estimated pharmacokinetic parameters may differ significantly from reality, parameter revision based upon system input and output relationships is necessary. While an exponentially tapering infusion is the optimal 'control' input to a two-compartment pharmacokinetic model, it is not the optimal 'interrogating' input for parameter estimation. The two most practical 'interrogating' inputs are boluses and the pseudo-random binary sequence (PRBS). The use of boluses for pharmacokinetic parameter estimation is well established; the system response to a bolus (impulse-response) completely characterizes any linear system. However, boluses are an unphysiologically powerful stimulus and may provoke nonlinearities not present for more gentle stimuli. An alternative approach is to use PRBS, which may be simulated by turning an infusion pump on and off randomly at fixed intervals. By itself, the PRBS is unsatisfactory for system control because it can produce significant variance about the desired target level. However, superimpos-ing a small amplitude PRBS on top of an exponentially tapering infusion provides an excellent compromise; the PRBS provides broadband excitation that facilitates parameter estimation without significantly perturbing the desired drug trajectory.[54–56]

Problem 1C: Online estimation of serum levels

Currently, antiarrhythmic-drug serum levels are measured offline through a variety of methods, most antibody-based, that provide accurate results in a few hours. Coefficients of variation may vary with concentration, but generally average around 3–5% for commercial assays. While conventional techniques are ideally suited for outpatient monitoring, the sample processing delay is a significant barrier to aggressive intravenous dosing in acute-care scenarios because toxicity may develop while awaiting laboratory results.

Ideally, one would like to be able to monitor drug levels in blood on a continuous basis and thus provide continuous feedback control of drug-delivery systems. Considerable progress has been made over the past decade in the development of chemical- and biosensor-type devices that may be used to measure the levels of many physiologically important species directly in whole blood.[57] In some cases, these sensors have been miniaturized for direct and continuous *in vivo* measurements. Indeed, blood gases (oxygen, carbon dioxide, pH),[58,59] electrolytes (potassium, calcium, sodium)[60] and certain metabolites (glucose, lactic acid, urea),[61,62] may be monitored continuously with devices based on either electrochemical or optical transducers. Such sensors can be fabricated in relatively small sizes (25–500 μm) which enables placement at the tip of an appropriate catheter than can be guided to a selected intravascular site or be implanted subcutaneously in tissue. No sampling, addition of reagents, or dilution is required to obtain accurate results with such self-contained probes.

Although the possibility of continuous drug monitoring with similar self-contained devices that respond reversibly to the concentration/activity of organic drug species has long been anticipated, success in developing drug sensors for *in vivo* applications has not yet been realized. A major problem associated with the design of indwelling sensors is the need for highly selective chemistry that would allow the transducer to discriminate one particular drug molecule in the presence of the many biochemicals found in physiological fluids. Further, the relatively low concentration of drugs *in vivo* demands that sensors exhibit extreme chemical sensitivity (i.e. 1.0–10 mg ml^{-1}, for most antiarrhythmic drugs). In addition, interactions which may occur between the sensor and the biologic milieu (i.e. biocompatibility) almost always have an adverse effect on the analytical performance of the device and in some cases may even jeopardize patient safety (e.g. thrombus formation). Add to this the requirements for rapid response times, reliable calibration procedures and long-term stability, and it is quite apparent why progress in this area has been relatively slow.

In this section, a concise and critical overview of the various electrochemical and optical chemical/biosensor schemes that have been investigated as potential *in vivo* drug monitoring systems is provided. While no single approach has yet been demonstrated to function reliably *in vivo* for extended periods, the prospects of achieving success in this direction with the available sensor technologies will be addressed.

Available chemical sensor technologies

Ion-selective electrodes

Ion-selective electrodes (ISEs) are relatively simple membrane-based potentiometric devices that are capable of accurately measuring the activity of ions in solutions including whole blood. The most successful ion-selective electrodes are cation-selective devices that are now used routinely within high-volume clinical chemistry analyzers as well as in highly portable point-of-care test units placed near the patient's bedside. These sensors may be employed for the direct measurement of electrolytes (K^+, Na^+, Ca^{2+}, Li^+, Cl^-) as well as pH and PCO_2 in undiluted physiological samples.[63]

Highly selective ion-complexing agents such as mobile, lipophilic ion carriers (ionophores) and various ion exchangers are typically used as the membrane active components of ion-selective sensors. The ionophore serves as a reversible and reusable binding reagent that selectively extracts the analyte ion into an organic membrane phase, typically a thin-film polymer matrix, e.g. PVC, thereby creating a charge separation or phase boundary potential at the membrane–sample interface. The sensing membrane, which also contains an appropriate plasticizer and lipophilic counterion sites, detects the difference in ion activity between an internal reference solution and the external sample solution (see Figure 19.11). Since the inner ion activity is held constant, the overall electrical potential of the cell (ISE vs appropriate reference electrode) may be expressed, for ions of the same charge, by an extended form of the well-known Nernst equation:

$$E_{cell} = E^0 + RT/z_i F \ln (a_i + K_{ij}a_j) \tag{5}$$

where E_{cell} is the measured potential for the electrochemical cell in volts, E^0 is the standard cell potential, R is the universal gas constant, T is the absolute temperature, F is Faraday's constant, a_i is the activity of the desired analyte ion with charge z_i, K_{ij} is the potentiometric selectivity coefficient and a_j is the activity of an interfering ion j. Clearly, to measure a_i accurately in the presence of large excess of j ions, then K_{ij} must be a small number, indicating that the membrane is highly selective for i over j ions.

The desire to perform pharmaceutical analysis with such polymer membrane-based ISEs has led to the development of a large number of sensors that can quantitate specific cationic and anionic organic drugs in commercial pharmaceutical preparations.[64] The principle behind the design of these ISEs is quite simple. To fabricate a membrane-electrode responsive to an anionic drug (D^-), the salt R^+D^- is incorporated into the organic membrane phase (at about 1 wt%), where R^+ is a very lipophilic cation such as a tridodecylmethylammonium ion. Similarly, for an electrode responsive to a cation drug (D^+), the salt D^+R^- is incorporated into the membrane, where the R^- is now a very lipophilic anion, such as tetraphenylborate. Anion drug sensors respond to given anions based on free energies of anion hydration, where the more lipophilic drug anions (least negative free energy of hydration) are preferred (i.e. organic drug anions > perchlorate > thiocyanate > iodide > nitrate > bromide > chloride). This order of decreasing hydrophobicity is known as the Hofmeister series. For example, a phenytoin electrode has been prepared by using tricaprylmethylammonium as a membrane anion exchanger.[65] Such an electrode responds well to phenytoin over the concentration range of 2.5×10^{-2} to 25.2 mg ml^{-1}; however, K_{ij} values with respect to many common blood anions may be too high ($K_{Ph^-,Cl^-} = 3.2 \times 10^{-3}$, $K_{Ph^-}, NO_3^- = 6.3 \times 10^{-1}$) to allow the use of this electrode to measure phenytoin levels accurately in physiological fluids (due, for example to high levels of chloride).

In an analogous manner, various tetraphenylborate derivatives have been widely used within polymer membranes to develop sensors responsive to cationic drug species. Indeed, sensors for antiarrhythmic cationic drugs such as bretylium,[66] mexiletine,[67] lidocaine,[68] propranolol[69] and verapamil[70] have all been reported. Typical selectivity coefficients for the drug cation over Na$^+$ and K$^+$ tend to be on the order of 1×10^{-3}. Thus, as in the case of the anionic drug sensors, the selectivity toward the antiarrhythmic agents may not be adequate to measure the targeted drug species as therapeutic levels in undiluted blood, limiting the application of such devices to measurements in relatively cleaner pharmaceutical preparations (see below).

Amperometric/voltammetric sensors

A second major class of electrochemical sensors involves measurement of current, not potential, resulting from the oxidation or reduction of a target analyte at the surface of an inert electrode (e.g. carbon, platinum, gold). The measured current at a given applied potential is linearly related to the concentration of analyte. Such heterogeneous electron transfer at an electrode surface has already been used in the development of several drug sensors for *in vitro* and *in vivo* monitoring applications.[57] The most commonly used three-electrode amperometric configuration consists of a working electrode where the primary redox process occurs, a reference electrode (used to control the potential of the working electrode) and an auxiliary electrode which carries the cell current. In voltammetric measurements, the potential of the working electrode is scanned continuously as a function of time through a potential region of interest and the resulting current is measured as a function of this potential. Solid microelectrodes (e.g. carbon fibers) have been employed for *in vivo* detection of certain neurotransmitters (dopamine, epinephrine) in the brain, and such methods illustrate how the implantation of solid electrodes allows for the direct monitoring of drug species.[71] It should be noted, however, that amperometric/voltammetric sensing can only be used to detect drug species that can readily undergo oxidation or reduction at a solid electrode without applying excessive voltage.

One significant advantage of amperometric techniques over potentiometric methods is the inherent improvement in the limits of detection (1–100 nmol l^{-1}) achieved by the various ways of generating the faradaic current response.[72] Solid microelectrodes work relatively well for detecting endogenous compounds in extracellular brain fluid; however, the implantation of bare electrodes into the vascular system to measure low concentration of drugs creates significant problems. First, there must exist some electrochemical potential for a given electrode at which the drug of interest is electroactive. Secondly, the current response must occur in a potential range where the many endogenous electroactive biologic components do not respond. In most cases this is difficult to achieve because electroactive biologic compounds will be present at higher concentrations than the drug, and this creates a background current that masks the response of the electrode to low drug levels. Furthermore, severe matrix effects originating from organic species, in particular proteins, adsorbing onto electrode surfaces may lead to electrode fouling, which slows the rate of heterogeneous electron-transfer process, thus leading to lower currents. Indeed, while *in vivo* voltammetric response for a series of electroactive antibiotic drugs (e.g. cefsulodin, chloramphenicol, nimorazole) with a small bare carbon rod (0.5-mm diameter) electrode in the bloodstream was shown to perform adequately for at least 30 min,[73] extended monitoring showed complete loss of sensor drug response due to increasing residual currents and electrical artifacts. Consequently, a common approach in the development of voltammetric sensors has been to use appropriate semipermeable membranes to cover and protect the electrode surface (see Figure 19.12). For example, one sensor being developed targets $Re(DMPE)_3CF_3SO_3$, a nonradioactive technetium (Tc) radiopharmaceutical analog often used for heart imaging.[74] The carbon electrode is coated with a thin layer of Nafion gel (a highly sulfonated polytetrafluoroethylene material) into which the radiopharmaceutical partitions to enable its detection by voltammetry. This potentially adds more selectivity to the voltammetric measurement and at the same time provides an exclusion barrier to biologic materials that may poison the active electrode surface. Cellulose acetate membranes supported on polycarbonate,[75] controlled photopolymerization of organic substrates to form net-like structures on electrode surfaces[76] as well as other approaches have been proposed to enhance selectivity and decrease *in vivo* electrode fouling. Despite the use of some barriers that may render a drug nonelectroactive (i.e. the drug cannot get close enough to electrode to undergo oxidation or reduction), this problem can be overcome by mediating the electron transfer chemically through the use of a smaller redox couple that undergoes electron transfer in the same potential range as the drug.[77] Finally, because dynamic flow characteristics of the blood can change the diffusion layer properties near the electrode surface, resulting in current fluctuations, ideally, any implantable amperometric/voltammetric electrode requires isolation from these hydrodynamic effects. Often, the outer membrane coating can serve simultaneously to diminish such effects.

With respect to sensing antiarrhythmic agents using the amperometric/ voltammetric approach, based on their known structures, it is unlikely that all such drugs will in fact be electrochemically active in the potential window available for *in vivo* measurements. Indeed, a detailed assessment of the electrochemistry of such agents would be required before attempting to develop amperometric/voltammetric sensors. However, one would expect that is should be possible to electrochemically oxidize the amino group of procaine at a potential similar to the oxidation potential of aniline (i.e. +0.6 V vs SCE). If so, it may be possible to develop a sensor for procaine using Nafion-coated electrodes to preconcentrate the procaine at the electrode surface and, at the same time, the Nafion film would help eliminate background signals from endogenous ascorbate and uric acid.

Fiberoptic sensors

The small size and flexibility of optical fibers make them attractive for use as transducers in the design of implantable chemical sensors. In fact, optical fibers can be used for microscale measurements of absorption or fluorescence *in vivo* in extremely small volumes of body fluids. Excitation with an external radiation source is essential with these techniques, with proper optics and filters, allowing a beam of light to be efficiently focused onto the distal tip of a single optical fiber. The intensity of light that comes back up the same fiber either at the same wavelength (absorbance) or at longer wavelength (fluorescence and phosphorescence) provides the analytical signal.

The simplest sensing scheme involves detecting an optical property of the analyte itself. For example, experimental *in vivo* measurements of the anticancer drug doxorubicin have been carried out in the interstitial fluids of tumors within animals by direct fluorescence methods.[78] The general utility of such fluoroprobe measurements is obviously limited to the unique fluorescence properties of the doxorubicin drug. Consequently, in an effort to expand the range of species that can be detected via the optical sensing methods, specific chemical reagents are usually immobilized at the end of the optical fibers to gain some element of selectivity. For example, implantable blood gas and electrolyte sensors have been prepared by immobilization of suitable indicator reagent dyes. The reagents can be retained at the fiber tip by polymerization in a gel attached to the glass fiber, or by incorporation within semipermeable membranes.[79] In the simplest case, pH measurements can be made by either absorbance or fluorescence using a wide range of immobilized pH indicators. The partial pressure of oxygen in blood can be determined *in vivo* by using immobilized fluorophores whereby the fluorescence (or phosphorescence) is quenched by oxygen. The specificity of enzyme and immunochemical reactions has also been adapted to optical fibers and such strategies will be discussed further in the section on biosensors.

The use of thin PVC films containing appropriate extraction and indicator chemistries can also be exploited to design optical sensors. In such systems, simultaneous coextraction of both an analyte ion (e.g. drug) and a counterion into the film deposited at the tip of an optical fiber is required to obtain an analytically useful optical signal. For example, penicillins in pharmaceutical preparations[80] have been determined optically with a film consisting of the anion exchanger tridodecyl-methylammonium chloride (TDMAC) and the pH chromoionophore *N*-octadecanoyl nile blue (ODNB). In a solution pH range 5.3–6.0, the penicillin carboxylate anion is extracted into the PVC membrane as the couteranion of TDMA$^+$. At the same time, a proton is coextracted, protonating the lipophilic pH indicator. Upon protonation, the indicator undergoes a significant change in fluorescence intensity. The optical response function can be related to the activity:concentration ratio of the two ions. The signal depends only on the activity:concentration of the pencillin if the pH value of the sample solution is kept constant via a buffer. Using the same basic approach, an optical sensing polymer film responsive to the antiarrhythmic agent propranolol has also been suggested recently.[81] In this sensor, the polymer film contains a lipophilic anionic site (i.e. di-*tert.*-butyl tartrate) that serves to extract the drug, and a lipophilic pH indicator dye that is deprotonated when the cationic drug is extracted into the film. As in the case of ion-selective polymer membrane electrodes that sense ionic drugs (see above), these optical sensors will exhibit selectively toward the drug in proportion to its lipophilicity relative to common inorganic and organic ions found in a given test sample.

Fiberoptic chemical sensors offer certain inherent advantages over the electrochemical sensors discussed above. They can be more easily miniaturized since they use optical fibers on the order of 100–150 mm o.d. and do not require the use of a reference electrode. In addition, they have better signal-to-noise ratios and do not need transduction wires. Furthermore, the use of ratiometric measurements at two wavelengths (one at the analytical wavelength and one at an isobestic point in the spectrum of the indicator) can enhance output signal stability by reducing sensitivity to numerous artifacts (optical source fluctuation, drift, temperature, quenching and ionic strength).

Biosensors

Biocatalytic probes

A biocatalytic type biosensor is configured with a biocatalyst immobilized at the tip of an electrochemical or optical transduction element (see Figure 19.13). Several types of biocatalytic materials such as isolated enzymes, subcellular fractions and whole-cell preparations can be used for the construction of functional biosensors. By far the most widely used approach in the fabrication of drug-based biosensors are enzyme probes. They are comprised of a thin enzyme layer immobilized on the surface of an appropriate chemical sensor and are used to detect the given substrate of the immobilized enzyme. Diffusion of the substrate into the enzyme layer results in an enzyme-catalyzed reaction with the liberation of a product toward which the underlying sensor responds optically or electrochemically. A steady-state analytical signal is observed when the rate of product formation (from the enzyme reaction) is equal to the rate of product escape from the immobilized layer. Selectivity, pH dependency, and useful lifetime are response characteristics that depend directly on the properties of the immobilized enzyme. Many enzymes are highly selective in the reaction they catalyze (glucose oxidase, urease) while others are more class specific, working on a group of structurally related compounds (e.g. β-lactamase for penicillins).

Enzyme electrodes exhibit many of the features of the underlying chemical sensor used to fabricate these probes. A biosensor based on an ion-selective electrode, for example, will generate a logarithmic response to a change in substrate concentration and will be subject to all the interferences that affect the underlying sensor.

Alternatively, an amperometric enzyme electrode produces a linear response to substrate, but high selectivity is difficult to achieve owing to the wide range of redox active species that can be present in blood or other physiologic samples.

Various methods are available to immobilize enzymes at surfaces of chemical sensors.[82] Immobilization procedures that involve covalent attachment, physical entrapment in an inert gel (e.g. polyacrylamide) or chemical crosslinking of the enzyme to a protein matrix (e.g. albumin) are commonly employed. Immobilization serves to improve not only storage stability but also the resistance of an enzyme to inhibitors, extremes of pH and elevated temperatures. Furthermore, with an immobilized enzyme, activity shows less dependence on pH and temperature than is the case with the corresponding soluble enzyme; this is an important factor when long-term stability is required. The concentration profiles of substrate and product within the enzyme layer depend upon both the rate of substrate mass transfer and on the rate of the enzyme reaction. In the case of an ion-selective electrode-based biosensor, the maximum concentration of product is obtained at the enzyme–sensor interface, where the product is being detected. In an amperometric device the electrochemical degradation of product (by oxidation or reduction) produces a near-zero concentration at the enzyme–sensor interface, but there is a diffusional concentration gradient further into the immobilized enzyme layer. For each substrate concentration in a test sample, a different steady state will develop, and it is the ability to attain substrate steady state which enables the enzyme sensor to be used for continuous monitoring. One disadvantage of coupling enzymes with chemical sensors is that the additional enzyme layer present adds an additional diffusion barrier which slows the response time. Indeed, typically at low substrate concentrations, 2–10 min may be required to obtain a complete steady-state response.

Shorter response times (40–60 s) have been reported for enzyme-based fiberoptic sensors. For example, a sensor for detecting penicillin has been reported in which the enzyme penicillinase is immobilized at the surface of an optical pH probe.[83] The enzyme catalyzes the cleavage of the β-lactam ring of penicillin to penicilloic acid which dissociates into penicilloate and a proton thus producing a pH change in the vicinity of the enzyme layers. The pH change at the surface is monitored by a pH-dependent fluorescent dye which is covalently bound to a polymer and intermixed with the enzyme, thus eliminating the diffusional barrier between the enzyme and the dye.

Immunochemical sensors

The high specificity and affinity of antibody–antigen interactions have prompted considerable efforts to use these immunochemical reactions to design biosensors. Indeed, many of the current therapeutic drug assays (e.g. digoxin) used in clinical laboratories employ highly selective antidrug antibodies as reagents. In designing biosensors with antibodies or other ligand specific receptors, the goal is to immobilize these binders at the surface of a suitable transducer such that reversible binding of the target analyte will lead to a measurable change in the output signal of the device. Ideally, such response should occur without the need to add external reagents. These types of direct-sensing schemes may include detecting a change in the spectral properties (e.g. fluorescence) of the immobilized antibody (or other receptor) upon binding the target species, detecting a mass change at the surface of an appropriate transducer (i.e. piezoelectric device), measuring a change in heat generated or consumed by the heat of reaction (via a thermistor-based sensor), quantitating a change in the surface refractive index due to the selective reaction (i.e. surface plasmon resonance technique)[84] or detecting changes in the surface properties of electrodes, such as capacitance, due to antibody–ligand interactions. Although such direct-sensing arrangements are the most desirable, there have only been a handful of literature reports in which this approach has been applied successfully to the development of biosensors that can function effectively in real biologic samples. For example, at a recent international meeting on biosensors, Pharmacia Inc. described a new surface plasmon system that can be used to measure various drugs (e.g. theophylline) directly in undiluted plasma at about micromolar levels via the use of immobilized antidrug antibodies. Of course, this system is rather complex (and costly) in terms of instrumentation and is thus probably restricted to *in vitro* use only.

The vast majority of immunosensors reported to date have been indirect, not direct, sensing systems. Here, the antibody–antigen binding reaction is detected by following a secondary reaction process. Sensors in this category can be further divided into two subclasses: those that use specific labels (e.g. enzymes, fluorophores) to follow the binding reaction, and those that rely on modulation of signals (usually electrochemical) arising from background ionic components within the sample. In the case of labeled assays, sensing is normally accomplished by using a competitive binding approach, whereby the degree of binding between a fixed amount of immobilized antibody and a second labeled form of the analyte is perturbed by the unlabeled analyte in the sample. Typically, such an approach can only be used for discrete sample measurements and not for continuous monitoring. To devise truly reversible biosensors based on this principle, both the labeled ligand and antibody/receptor must be immobilized or retained in a region adjacent to the detection element. An elegant example of such an approach was suggested by Anderson and Miller[85] who developed an optical immunosensor that responds reversibly to phenytoin (discussed later in the examples section).

Indirect immunosensors based on modulation of the secondary ionic process are typically electrochemical devices in which potentials, currents, capacitances or resistances are the measured parameters. Changes in these parameters can occur when the antibody/receptor interacts with its target species. The best example of this biosensing scheme may be found in nature. Many chemoreceptors in cell membranes function by altering the permeability of the cell membranes to ions as a result of the receptor–ligand binding reaction. When ion permeabilities change, the measurement of cell-membrane potentials or conductivities provides a means of detecting this binding reaction. However, reliable detection is critically dependent on bathing ion activities/concentrations in the sample medium. Rechnitz and Rechnitz designed an artificial ion-selective membrane based system that functions in an analogous manner[86] (see current status: examples).

The main problem with adapting antibodies or other receptors to the design of biosensors is the fact the most antibodies/receptors have relative high binding

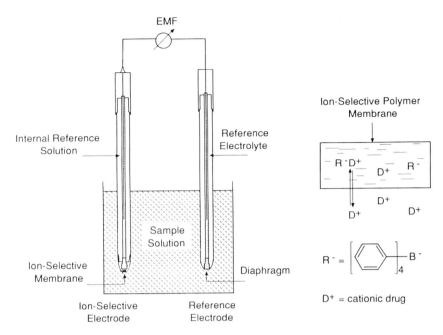

Figure 19.11 Prototypical ion-sensitive electrode. (Left) ISE cell demonstrating recording and reference electrodes. (Right) Scheme illustrating electrochemical concentration of cationic drug by polyanionic membrane.

affinities (in the order of 10^9 mol l^{-1}). Therefore, the selective reactions tend to be relatively irreversible (slow 'off' rate constants), making it difficult to envision sensors that will be able to respond on a continuous basis to changes in analyte levels (increasing and decreasing concentrations). Only by using selected monoclonal antibodies that exhibit much lower overall affinity, but maintain high specificity, can this inherent limitation be overcome. However, one should recognize that lower affinity also tends to degrade sensitivity, and thus some tradeoff with regard to reversibility versus sensitivity will be required when designing immunosensors for drug species.

Current status: some examples for the literature

The determination of the antiarrhythmic drug mexiletine in pharmaceutical preparations with a polymer membrane ISE illustrates the capabilities and limitations of these type of sensors. The electrode consists of a PVC matrix material in which a mexiletine–tetraphenylborate ion-pair complex is dissolved in dioctyl phthalate solvent plasticizer and incorporated into a PVC film. The ion formation of the protonated mexiletine with the negative ionophore, as depicted in Figure 19.11, yields a Nernstian response of 57.6 mV decade^{-1} and a linear response range from 2.7×10^{-3} to 17.9 mg ml^{-1}. The electrode shows only negligible interference from substances found in blood.[67] This is because mexiletine is a rather lipophilic species,

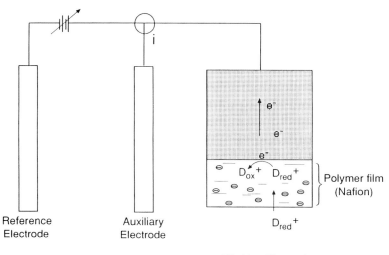

Figure 19.12 Schematic of voltammetric drug sensor employing semipermeable dialysis membrane to preselect for target agent.

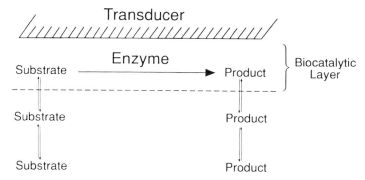

Figure 19.13 Schematic of biocatalytic drug sensor. The bound enzyme converts substrate to product within a restricted 'biocatalytic' layer.

making its extraction into the membrane far more favorable than small inorganic cations such as sodium and potassium. The major interferences observed with this sensor are other lipophilic cationic drugs. Since PVC membranes appear attractive because of their potential for very simple construction merely by depositing the active membrane on a semiconductor chip or by dip-coating a very thin reference wire with the membrane solution, there is no reason why the electrode could not be miniaturized. Also, assuming that appropriate protection from macromolecular interference could be devised, the electrode could come close to meeting the requirements for *in vivo* monitoring. The difficulty, however, is that the envisioned range of interest approaches the limit of detection, at which values the response

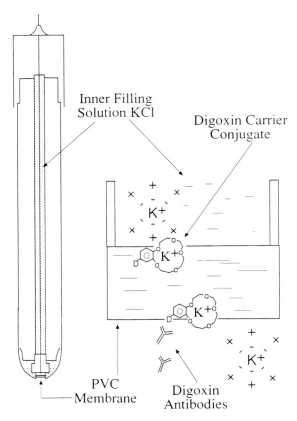

Figure 19.14   Digoxin drug sensor based upon the potentiometric ionophore-mediated immunoassay (PIMIA) scheme. Ligand binding alters the ability of the ionophore to complex cations, e.g. K^+ or Na^+, in the sample, leading to a large potentiometric change.

becomes nonlinear. Thus it would be very difficult to calibrate the electrode in this region, and subsequently to determine whether a potential response was due to a change in drug activity or to a change in liquid junction potential, ionic strength, pH or simply drift. This leveling of the potential response in the low concentration range is typical in ISE measurements and the problem is more pronounced at higher levels of interfering substances.

The electrochemical system reported by Keating and Rechnitz[86] can be employed to detect antibodies to given drugs, and thus, via competitive binding, it could be adapted for detecting drug levels. In their so-called potentiometric ionophore-mediated immunoassay (PIMIA) scheme, ionophores (e.g. benzo-18-crown-6) normally used to devise cation-selective electrodes were derivatized with digoxin. When incorporated into thin polymer membranes, the derivatized ionophore still serves as a selective ion-binding reagent, rendering the electrical potential across the membrane dependent on the activities of ions bathing both sides of the membrane. As depicted in Figure 19.14, when antibodies to the ligand or drug are added to one

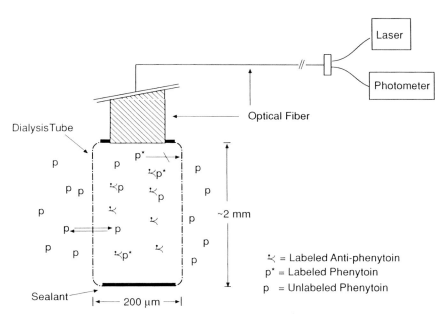

Figure 19.15 Sensor based upon homogeneous fluorescence energy-transfer immunoassay. Drug displaces a fraction of the β-phycoerythrin-labeled phenytoin with subsequent fluorescence signal perturbation measured through a fiberoptic fluorometer.

side of the membrane, a large potential change occurs due to the binding of the antibody to the derivatized ionophore at the membrane–sample interface (altering the ability of the ionophore to complex cations, e.g. K^+ or Na^+, in the sample). If the antibodies are immobilized behind a semipermeable membrane but still accessible to the surface of the membrane, then the modulation of ion response can be reversed when the free ligand/drug passes through the membrane and with appropriate antibody affinity constants, continuous monitoring of the target analyte may be possible.

As even more elegant immunosensor concept for detecting given drugs was suggested by Anderson and Miller.[85] These researchers developed a clever fiberoptic sensor that can be used to reversibly measure levels of phenytoin. The sensor was based on the principles of a homogeneous fluorescence energy-transfer immunoassay (see Figure 19.15). In this system a β-phycoerythrin–phenytoin conjugate and a Texas Red-labeled antibody to phenytoin were entrapped within a short length of cellulose dialysis fiber and the fiber was attached to the distal end of the optical fiber. Thus, when the sensor is placed in solution containing free phenytoin, the drug enters through the walls of the dialysis tubing and displaces a fraction of the β-phycoerythrin–phenytoin from the antibody. The resulting change in fluorescence signal can be measured with an associated fiberoptic fluorometer. Typical competitive binding calibrations curves for phenytoin concentrations ranging from 1.26 to 126 μg ml^{-1} were obtained.

While the semipermeable dialysis membrane plays an important role in the functioning of this sensor by forming a minireaction chamber, it also excludes large unwanted molecules such as albumin and allows only the nonprotein-bound (i.e. pharmacologically active) form of the drug to enter into the viewing region of the optical sensor. This design places a constraint in that labeled antibody and labeled hapten must be larger than the molecular weight cut-off of the dialysis membrane employed. Further, this design is generic in that it has the potential to measure any low-molecular-weight drug for which an antibody is available. Given its small size (200 μm o.d.) this type of sensor has the potential to be conveniently inserted through a small gauge intravascular needle for continuous monitoring applications. However, as stated above, to achieve lower limits of detection (i.e. for ng ml^{-1} range measurements), it would be necessary to use monoclonal antibodies that have higher affinity, and thus, this would compromise the reversibility of such a sensor (i.e. slow response time when level of the drug goes from high to low values).

Conclusions: Chemical biosensors

Although the design of chemical and biosensors that can detect specific drugs is gaining increased attention among scientists involved in sensor research, at present there are no approaches that offer adequate stability, selectivity, sensitivity and biocompatibility for chronic implantation. With respect to drug monitoring and feedback control of drug delivery, it would appear that the best hope for the immediate future will be the development of sensors that may operate external to the body. For example, a new approach to blood gas/electrolyte/metabolite sensing for critically ill patients has recently been introduced in which an array of appropriate sensors are actually mounted in series within the fluid path of radial artery catheters.[87] At preprogrammed times, a sample of arterial blood can be withdrawn back through the sensor array to obtain test results. Since the sensors are external to the patient, issues such as size and biocompatibility are greatly reduced. Furthermore, periodic automated calibration of the sensors is possible by diverting appropriate calibrating solutions through the sensor array. One can thus envisage similar intermittent sensing systems that could be employed to monitor drugs levels for patients undergoing drug therapy within the confines of the hospital. In the case of antiarrhythmic agents, there is no clear-cut choice as to the preferred sensor technology. Certainly, if improvements in chemical selectivity can be achieved for drug sensors based on ion-selective membrane electrode technology, this would be the most attractive avenue to pursue since this technology has already been proven to function effectively for blood gas and electrolyte measurements in undiluted blood samples. The more complex biosensor schemes, while capable of high selectivity, may not have the reversibility and simplicity required to be readily adapted for reliable online monitoring applications.

   Limitations of serum drug levels. Although one- and two-compartment models adequately describe serum levels of many antiarrhythmic agents, serum levels may not always parallel clinical effect. For example, QT prolongation by procainamide lags serum drug concentration changes with a half-time of approximately 7 minutes following rapid intravenous infusion.[88] This delay has been postulated to represent a transport phenomenon to the 'effect' compartment, i.e. drug uptake by the myocardial tissue (although rapid relative to the 'peripheral' compartment) is slower than other elements in the 'central' compartment.

The relationship between clinical effect and central compartment serum levels may also deviate if a given agent has active metabolites. With procainamide, for example, the primary metabolite *N*-acetyl procainamide (NAPA) has comparable potency to the parent agent but different kinetics and electrophysiologic action.[89] The relationship between QT prolongation and plasma procainamide levels may vary significantly as NAPA levels fluctuate. While the pharmacokinetics of procainamide–NAPA transfer are fairly well characterized and modeled, the pharmacokinetics and electrophysiologic activity of most other agents are poorly understood.

Serum drug levels are particularly suspect when using local delivery devices such as iontophoretic membranes or micropumps. Effect tissue concentrations will have an uncertain relationship to peripheral levels and may be an order of magnitude greater. Furthermore, the minute serum levels of the newer high potency antiarrhythmic agents such as ibutilide will be below the detection threshold of standard assay techniques.

Serum level estimates by ECG proxy

Continuous 'effect' feedback

Since pharmacokinetic drugs are defined by their electrophysiologic effects, it may be possible to use ECG statistics, particularly QRS and QT durations, as a surrogate for drug serum levels. Pure class I drugs lengthen action-potential duration by decreasing conduction velocity, simultaneously lengthening QRS and QT durations, while pure class III drugs lengthen QT alone by delaying ventricular repolarization.[90] QRS duraction is an easy parameter to estimate from either endocardial, epicardial or peripheral leads, making it an attractive candidate for feedback control for type I agents. Figure 19.16 demonstrates the change in QRS duration as a function of plasma quinidine level for a group of 20 patients.[91] Although a clear dose–response is evident, the correlation is only 0.56, limiting its predictive power. Platia *et al.* demonstrated similar results for procainamide.[92] However, Figure 19.16 does not distinguish interindividual versus intraindividual variation, nor does it control for use-dependent blockade.[93,94] Type I agents produce greater channel blockade at higher heart rates; the magnitude of this effect is determined primarily by the drug-channel unbinding rate constant (Ib < Ia < Ic). Figure 19.17 demonstrates the QRS duration as a function of heart rate, during treadmill, for 51 patients taking disopyramide, mexiletine and pilsicainide.[95] Significant use-dependent blockade was observed in 61%, 53% and 70%, respectively. Consequently, correction for interindividual sensitivities and for rate dependencies may significantly improve the predictive power of QRS broadening over that suggested by Figure 19.16.

Following the Cardiac Arrhythmia Suppression Trials, interest in type III agents as an alternative to type I therapy has escalated.[96–98] Consequently, measuring drug effect through QT prolongation has been proposed as a surrogate for drug plasma

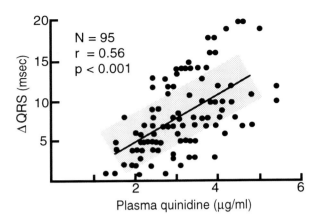

Figure 19.16 Change in QRS duration as a function of plasma quinidine level for 20 patients. (Reprinted with permission from Heissenbutal, R. H. and Bigger, J. T. (1970) The effect of oral quinidine on intraventricular conduction in man: correlation of plasma quinidine with charges in QRS duration. *Am. Heart J.*, **80**, 453–62.)

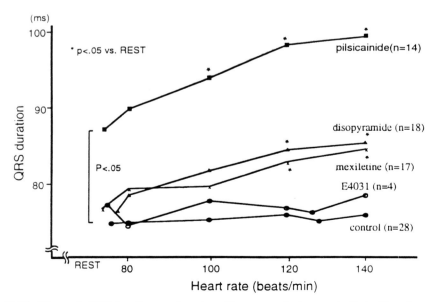

Figure 19.17 Change in QRS duration as a function of heart rate, during treadmill, for 51 patients taking disopyramide, mexiletine, pilsicainide and E4031 (type III agent). All three type l agents demonstrate use-dependence. (Reprinted with permission from Sadanga, T., Ogawa, S. Okada, Y. *et al.* (1993) Clinical evaluation of the use-dependent QRS prolongation and the reverse use-dependent QT prolongation of class I and class III antiarrhythmic agents and their value in predicting efficacy. *Am. Heart J.*, **126**, 115–21.)

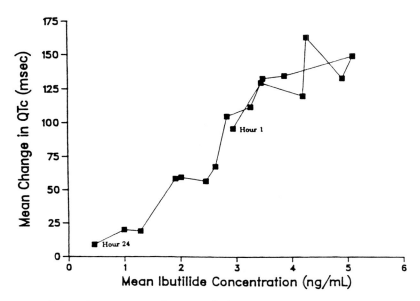

Figure 19.18 QT_c prolongation as a function of plasma ibutilide concentration for a single human volunteer during an 8-hour infusion at $0.1\ \mu g^{-1}\ kg^{-1}\ min^{-1}$. (Reprinted with permission from DiMarco, J. P., VanderLugt, J. T., Lee, K. S. and Gibson, J. K. (1994) Ibutilide. In: Singh, B. Wellens, H. and Hiroka, M. (ed.) *Electropharmacological Control of Cardiac Arrhythmias*. Mount Kisco, NY: Futura Publishing.

levels.[99,100] While many drugs have multiple electrophysiological effects, for example quinidine, the newer type III agents yield fairly selective and predictable QT prolongation. Figure 19.18 demonstrates QT_c prolongation as a function of plasma ibutilide concentration for a single human volunteer during an 8-hour infusion.[101] Similar dose–response effects are seen in Figure 19.19 for infusions at three different rates.[99] Notice that the QT_c curve, with an exponential decay following infusion cessation, is strikingly similar to the drug concentration predicted from a two-compartment pharmacokinetic model, suggesting that QT_c may be an effective and noninvasive surrogate for serum levels of ibutilide.

Unfortunately QT-interval measurement, unlike QRS duration, is fraught with technical difficulties. Superposition of the T and U wave may mislead computer algorithms and cardiologists alike as to the proper fiducial point, particularly if only a few ECG leads are examined.[99,102] Multilead recordings are helpful for resolving superpositions, but QT duration can vary considerably with recording site. Lead variation arises because ventricular repolarization is a complicated, three-dimensional phenomenon, that may be particularly inhomogeneous following myocardial damage. Subsequent projection onto individual leads produces 'dispersion' of the QT interval.[103–105] Since small changes in repolarization axis can produce significant changes in any single limb lead, some have argued for three-dimensional ECG measurements using the Frank lead system, or at least approximating orthogonal leads by lead I, AVF, V2.[99]

QT accuracy and reliability also vary with recording technique. Christiansen *et al.* compared QT intervals in V1 and V5 measured simultaneously on Holter and standard electrocardiographic equipment.[102] Relative to the standard ECG machine,

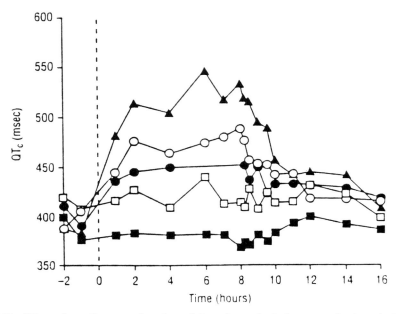

Figure 19.19 QT$_c$ prolongation as a function of time for a single human volunteer during 8-hour infusions at four infusion rates, 0.01 mg kg^{-1} (□), 0.03 mg kg^{-1} (●), 0.06 mg kg^{-1} (○) and 0.1 mg kg^{-1} (▲) versus placebo (■). (Reprinted with permission from Woosley, R. L. M S (1993) QT interval: a measure of drug action. *Am. J. Cardiol.*, **72**, 36B–43B.)

the Holter measurements -24 ± 32.5 ms and $+13 \pm 26$ ms for leads VI and V5, respectively. Intratechnique variability was not reported. The authors speculate that the surprisingly large discrepancies may be due to differences in high pass filtering (to reject baseline wander, ambulatory monitors typically have more stringent filter requirements) which can distort the low-frequency QT termination. Based upon these preliminary results, a more extensive and systematic evaluation of recording system bandwidth on QT values is warranted.

Even when accurately measured, QT interval is a complicated function of heart rate, sympathetic tone and serum drug level. QT correction for heart rate changes is nontrivial; the widely-use Bazett's square-root correction may actually increase QT$_c$ variance relative to uncorrected QT interval.[96,106] Multiparameter models, fit to individual rather than population-based data, yield better results. The relative superiority of linear, semilog or logarithmic regressions is currently unresolved. For manual QT measurements, Frieberg's cube-root correction yields better results than Bazett's correction, particularly at prolonged cycle lengths.[106]

QT variation with heart rate results from a combination of intrinsic myocardial rate-repolarization properties and autonomic modulation.[107,108] Both parasympathetic and sympathetic activity increase the QT interval. In healthy resting individuals, parasympathetic tone appears to dominate while sympathetic tone appears to be more prominent following myocardial infarction.[107] Since diurnal QT$_c$ fluctuations are abolished in postcardiac transplant patients and in diabetics having autonomic neuropathy, autonomic tone is thought to drive circadian QT$_c$ changes.

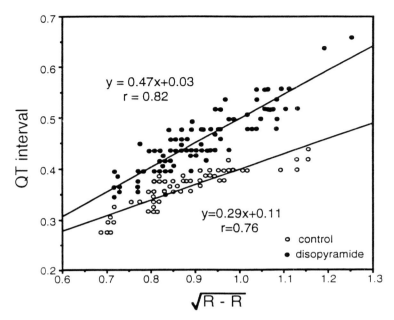

Figure 19.20 QT interval versus $(RR)^{\frac{1}{2}}$ for 28 control patients and 20 patients taking disopyramide; disopyramide steepened the QT rate dependence upon R–R interval. (Reprinted with permission from Sadanga, T., Ogawa, S., Okada, Y. *et al.* (1993) Clinical evaluation of the use-dependent QRS prolongation and the reverse use-dependent QT prolongation of class I and class III antiarrhythmic agents and their value in predicting efficacy. *Am. Heart J.,* **126**, 115–21.)

Twenty-four hour Holter recordings in 23 healthy subjects revealed a $4.2 \pm 2.1\%$ increase in QT60 at night compared with $-1.5 \pm 4.0\%$ ($P < 0.001$) for patients with diabetes mellitus.[108] Comparable changes have been seen by others, with peak effect between 12 p.m. and 3 a.m.[107] Although circadian fluctuation is a small effect, noncircadian autonomic fluctuations may have larger magnitude. Morganroth *et al.* reported an average 76 ± 19 ms QT_c fluctuation during three consecutive 8-hour recording intervals in 20 healthy volunteers.[109] The subjects had been admitted to an inpatient unit to control for activity-related changes. The relative contributions of measurement instability versus physiologic variability to these relatively large QT-interval fluctuations remains unclear.

In addition to intrinsic variability, QT intervals have a rate-dependent response to some type III antiarrhythmic agents.[110] Reverse use-dependent effects may also be observed with some type I agents.[93] Figure 19.20 demonstrates QT interval versus $(RR)^{\frac{1}{2}}$ for 28 control patients and 20 patients taking disopyramide. Sadanya *et al.*[95] showed that patients taking disopyramide demonstrated a significantly ($P < 0.01$) stronger linear relationship between QT interval and $(RR)^{\frac{1}{2}}$.

Given the technical difficulties recording QT intervals, assessing repolarization through monophasic action potentials (MAPs) may be advantageous.[111,112] MAP electrodes approximate intracellular action-potential shape by measuring the potential difference between normally depolarizing/repolarizing myocardium and myocardium whose voltage swings have been blunted by pressure or suction.[113,114]

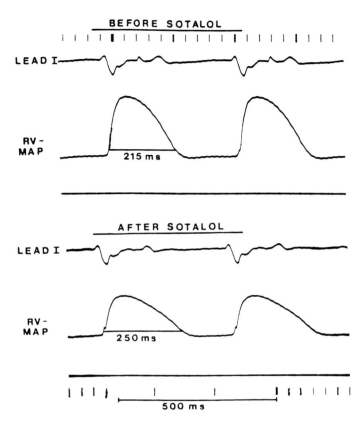

Figure 19.21 Monophasic action potentials recorded from paced human right ventricle prior to and following sotalol (0.60 mg kg^{-1}) administration. (Reprinted with permission from Echt D. S., Berte, L. E., Clusin, W. T. *et al.* (1982) Prolongation of the human cardiac monophasic action potential by sotalol. *Am. J. Cardiol.*, **50**, 1082–9.)

Figure 19.21 demonstrates MAPs recorded from human right ventricle prior to, and following, sotalol (0.60 mg kg^{-1}) administration.[115] The 90% repolarization point, MAPD$_{90\%}$, is a robust and reproducible measure of action-potential duration. Sotalol increased MAPD$_{90\%}$ from 215 ms to 250 ms in this example, indicative of sotalol's modest type III effect. Propranolol, in doses having comparable β-blockade, did not. The repolarization effects of type I agents can also be assessed through MAPs. Figure 19.22 demonstrates a dose–response of canine right-ventricular apical MAPs to quinidine infusion.[116] Although serum levels were not measured, a striking dose–response is seen.

Since the Vaughn-Williams antiarrhythmic classification is based upon intracellular voltage changes, MAPs potentially offer a very powerful and versatile assay of drug effect.[111] In particular, MAPs might be helpful as a feedback signal for implantable drug-delivery devices; the circuitry required for MAPD$_{90\%}$ measurement is trivial and could be easily miniaturized. However, MAPs are not without their limitations. First, absolute measures of phase 0 velocity cannot be accurately

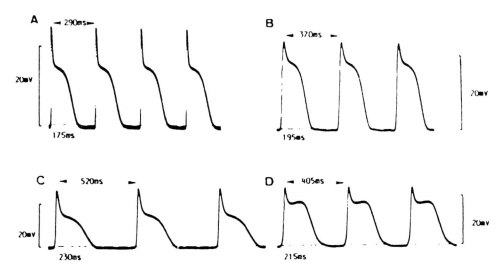

Figure 19.22 Response of monophasic action potentials recorded from canine apical right ventricle: (A) after 5 mg kg^{-1} i.v. quinidine, (B) after 10 mg kg^{-1} i.v. quinidine, (C) after 15 mg kg^{-1} i.v. quinidine, (D) 15 minutes later. (Reprinted with permission from Brugada, J., Sassine, A., Escande, D. *et al.* (1987) Effects of quinidine on ventricular repolarization. *Eur. Heart J.*, **8**, 1340–5.)

assessed using MAPs, although relative changes may still be useful. Second, while MAP measurements are stable over periods of hours, chronic, indwelling MAP recordings may be difficult.[113] Signal coupling problems similar to those encountered in pacemakers may also be problematic. Lastly, MAP recordings, by their nature, record focal phenomena rather than aggregate behavior. In the event of focal pathology, for example myocardial infarction, MAP measurements may be a poorer indicator of drug effect than surface ECG. All of these problems could be ameliorated, however, by recording MAPs from multiple sites and by simultaneous monophasic and biphasic recordings.

Problem ID: Optimally steering drug delivery and updating model coefficients

Feedback data availability dictates optimal feedback strategies. A continuous variable, such as QT interval, allows drug titration without a priori knowledge of the pharmacokinetics, just as visual feedback allows one to drive without having a road map. Previous examples of continuous feedback drug-delivery systems include applications toward automated nitroprusside blood pressure titration as well as anesthetic induction and maintenance. In contrast, feedback control based upon serum drug levels inherently requires an accurate 'road map' because serum samples are drawn infrequently and encounter significant processing delays.

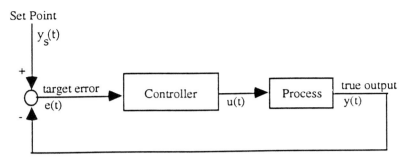

Figure 19.23   Schematic of a simple continuous feedback system. The controller adjusts the system input
to eliminate the difference between the true and the desired process ('plant') outputs.

Continuous feedback

The fundamental building blocks of a continuous feedback control system consist of
a controller, a plant and feedback measurements (Figure 19.23). The controller is just
an algorithm to optimally (according to predefined criteria) drive the difference
between the desired and actual outputs to zero. The simplest scheme consists of
setting the input proportional to difference between the set point and the measured
output, $u(t) = -K_p[y_{set}(t) - y(t)]$, or so-called proportional control.[117] Consider a
simple drug-delivery example. When the pump is first turned on, $y_{set}(t) - y(t)$ is large
and drug is infused rapidly, but as the true output approaches the set point, the
input slows down. Intuitively, a proportional controller will produce an appropriately tapering infusion for pharmacokinetic models. Unlike open-loop control,
however, the pharmacokinetics do not have to be known. In fact, unlike open-loop
control, the feedback controller would reduce the input appropriately if the patient
suddenly became anuric. Thus feedback control improves the robustness of drug
delivery to inter- and intrapatient variability while producing comparable response
time to 'optimal' open-loop delivery.

PID control

Simple proportional control has limitations. A large K is desirable for quick system
response but may cause the output to transiently overshoot and oscillate about the
target output. Consequently, it is common to add two additional terms to the
controller to form a so-called PID (proportional integral derivative) controller as
follows:

$$u(t) = K_p e(t) + K_i \int_0^t e(\tau)\, d\tau + K_d \frac{de}{dt} \qquad (6)$$

Intuitively, the integral term represents the error accumulation over time; a large K_i
coefficient improves long-term accuracy. The derivative part indicates the error
speed and direction; a large K_d helps the controller 'anticipate' how to best change
the input in the short term and quickens system response. Note that the derivative
term contributes nothing at steady state. The PID coefficients may be constant, but

are often updated as the dynamics of the process change to achieve a smooth transient (short term) as well as a stable steady state (long term). Various combinations of P-, PI- and PID-based controllers have been used for automated blood-pressure control as well as anesthetic induction.[118–120] The advantages of PID control are that it is simple, can be implemented directly with hardware, and requires no a priori knowledge of the system or its properties. The primary disadvantage is that the coefficients may be difficult to tune and the controller structure is not very robust to system disturbances. For example, in blood-pressure monitoring, routine arterial line flushing would produce huge proportional and derivative terms if the feedback signal were not properly preconditioned. In practical implementations, considerable modifications must be made in the integral and derivative terms to prevent static buildup (integral windup) and to avoid excessive impulse behavior (from the derivative term.)

Minimum variance controller and analogs

From equation (6), the PID controller can be viewed as a second-order filter that transforms the error signal $e(t)$ into an input $u(t)$, with frequency characteristics determined by the values of K_i, K_d and K_p. Perfect PID 'prefiltering' exactly compensates for the plant open-loop input/output characteristics, or transfer function, such that plant output, $y(t)$ exactly matches the set point $y_s(t)$. Another way to accomplish this 'prefiltering' is to abandon preconceived notions about the plant-transfer function and to search for a filter that best compensates the plant. Based upon the (measured) values of $e(t)$ and $u(t)$, a least-squares 'optimal' filter equation relating the two can be solved. The least-squares optimal 'filter' converts $e(t)$ into the $u(t)$ such that $|e(t)|^2$ is minimized, and hence is called the 'minimum variance controller'. In this controller, parameter estimation and process control are the same problem. Minimum variance controllers have also been applied to blood-pressure regulation, both simulations and animal experimentation.[121,122] The key advantages are their relative simplicity and flexibility as well as their ability to track wandering plant parameters. Unfortunately, simple minimum variance controllers achieve tight output regulation at the expense of large drug-input swings. Since no penalty is made for switching infusion rate, the controller general calls either for maximum or minimum infusion rates, often oscillating rapidly between them. While this so-called 'bang-bang modulation' may produce optimal output control, it is hard on infusion apparatus and power supplies, as well as exacerbating system nonidealities. As a result, it may be necessary to condition the input to the pump, for example with a moving average window or a median filter to prevent undesirable input oscillation.

   Another technique to prevent undue input oscillation is to solve for a controller that minimizes a weighted sum of $e(t)$, $u(t)$ and $u'(t)$ through a user-specified 'cost' function rather than simply minimizing the output error. That is,

$$\text{Min}_{u(t)} [J = K_e|y_s(t) - y(t)|^2 + K_u|u(t)|^2 + K_{u'}|u'(t)|^2] \qquad (7)$$

Equation (7) implies that it is undesirable to differ from the target effect, to supply drug unnecessarily, or to change the drug delivery rate. The coefficients determine

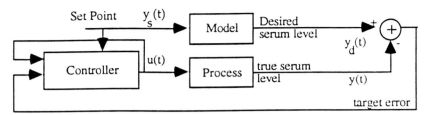

Figure 19.24 Schematic of a model reference feedback system. The controller adjusts the system input such that the plant 'behaves' like an idealized model.

the relative 'cost' for each of the terms. If K_u is high, the controller will sacrifice response time to prevent repeated pump cycling. Because the controller must minimize over past and present input, as well as the output error signal, the estimation and control problems are no longer identical. The prediction error generates a least-squares optimal model of the plant and the controller subsequently uses the model to minimize equation (7). Although equation (7) looks mathematically intractable, efficient, iterative techniques exist as well as direct analog implementations and have been applied to prototypical blood-pressure regulation systems.[121–126]

Excessive pump cycling reflects preoccupation with the present error rather than a longer term perspective; imagine trying to drive by looking at the road directly beneath the car. Consequently, input oscillation can be further decreased by 'extended horizon' techniques such as control advance moving average controllers (CAMAC).[127] Instead of trying to minimize the current output error, CAMAC controllers try to minimize the difference between the set point and the projected output at some future time, e.g. 1 minute in the future, given that the input is maintained constant. By minimizing over future behavior, CAMAC controllers tend to call for reasonable drug-delivery profiles, and are quite robust to unanticipated system perturbations.[125,126] In addition, the look-ahead properties of CAMAC controllers stabilize their performance in the presence of system 'dead time'.

Model reference adaptive systems (MRAS)

The previous feedback techniques have all striven to instantaneously match the input and output, i.e. a unity closed-loop transfer function. In contrast, the goal of a Model Reference Adaptive System (MRAS), is to make the output react to the input in a controlled and desirable manner, i.e. the MRAS forces the closed-loop transfer function to emulate a user-specified 'reference model' (Figure 19.24). For example, one could demand that a feedback antiarrhythmic drug-delivery system behave like a specific one-compartment pharmacokinetic model, regardless of the true drug pharmacokinetics. Obviously, the disparity of the true and the reference systems influences control accuracy. For example, the reference drug elimination rate should not be faster than determined by patient physiology because the controller cannot actively remove drug. The controller is generally adjusted to quadratic cost functions like equation (7) to balance output trajectory error with input restrictions.[128,129] Advantages of MRAS controllers are their stability, their robustness to plant parameter changes, and their ability to standardize very different plant behaviors. Disadvantages include uncertain handling of system nonlinearities and sensitivity to rapidly changing dynamics. In most drug-delivery cases, the process is linear, low order and dynamically slow, making them well suited to MRAS techniques. MRAS controllers have demonstrated promising results during simulations and animal models of arterial blood-pressure regulation.[130,131]

Multiple model techniques

In the Multiple Model Adaptive Control (MMAC) approach,[132] a finite set of patient pharmacodynamic models, based upon population estimates, are prestored in the computer. At any instant, only a few of these models approximate reality, as reflected by their prediction errors. Once the 'accurate' models have been selected, a weighted sum of their *predicted* outputs is compared to the set point and the error signal fed into a controller. Notice that the true output only selects a model, but is not directly used in the error signal. Consequently, when the output is contaminated by artifact, for example electrocautery interference in the operating room, or arterial line flushes during blood-pressure monitoring, multiple model techniques feedback is constrained to physically realizable values. The primary disadvantage of multiple model techniques is their computational overheads which increase geometrically with the number of varying parameters (degrees of freedom). The feasibility and robustness of arterial blood-pressure MMAC have been demonstrated in computer simulations as well as in a pulsatile-flow model of human blood pressure.[133,134]

System nonlinearities

Although pharmacokinetic equations are linear, drug delivery is inherently non-linear because a drug can be actively delivered but not removed. Yet most controllers assume physical realizability of negative system inputs, and often call for negative drug-delivery rates when the set point is exceeded. Similarly, drug pumps usually have a maximum delivery rate, either through physical constraints or for safety reasons. The simplest solution to this problem is to place a limiting device between the controller and the pump such that the input is clipped at zero, saturated above some maximum and passed unchanged otherwise. Unfortunately, this produces faster convergence toward the set point when the error is positive than when it is negative and may lead to oscillation about the set point (limit cycling). To combat this problem, hysteresis may be added to better match the positive and negative error convergence. As an example, the limiter might use a unity slope if the error term is increasing but a smaller slope if the error is decreasing.

A second approach to avoid negative infusion rates is to bias the input with an open-loop control signal. In drug delivery, for example, an a priori estimate of the steady-state infusion rate is generally available. Although the controller may generate negativity, the superposition of the controller and open-loop inputs will rarely, if ever, be negative. This approach essentially linearizes the fundamentally asymmetric drug delivery about an operating point. An advantage of this approach is that it eliminates limiter influence near the set point (although saturation nonlinearities are

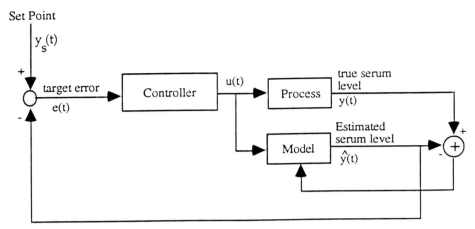

Figure 19.25 Schematic of a feedback system relying upon 'state estimation'. Except for model correction by measurements of the true output, this system represents open-loop control.

still present). The primary disadvantages of this approach are slower dynamics and propensity to steady-state error. However, steady-state error can be eliminated by an integral term in the controller or adaptively tuning the open-loop infusion rate according to prediction error.

Other nonlinear elements beside limiters are often included into system design, generally for safety considerations. In blood-pressure control, for example, drug delivery may be held if the pressure or its derivative drop outside some range.[131,133] These nonlinear elements are rarely included in the preliminary modeling and design procedures. While steps must always be provided for transient anomalies and system artifact, it is well known that the nonlinearities can introduce steady-state oscillations under unpredictable conditions. Hence, care must be taken as these safeguard features may introduce surprises of their own.

Sporadic feedback

With continuous feedback, modeling deficiencies are quickly corrected. However, sparse feedback demands an accurate underlying model because the output trajectory is observed so infrequently. Imagine trying to drive a car by looking at the road every four hours. Fortunately, pharmacokinetics are easily modeled by well-behaved, low-order differential equations whose dynamics are fairly slow. By incorporating a model, or 'state estimator', sporadic feedback systems can emulate continuous feedback; continuous correction of the drug delivery device occurs through estimated, rather than measured, serum levels. When available, true serum levels serve to correct the pharmacokinetic model. In their absence, Figure 19.25 simply represents open-loop control.[40] As a result, sparse feedback drug delivery is vulnerable to changing pharmacokinetics and drug interactions, because these changes will go unnoticed until the next 'true' feedback occurs.

The three basic methods for correcting the pharmacokinetic model based upon the prediction error are least squares, minimum prediction error and maximum likelihood estimation.[124] The first two techniques are analogous to linear regression except that they are applied over multiple variables, i.e. a vector, instead of a single parameter. Although they differ slightly in the error minimized, they are qualitatively similar and may be efficiently solved recursively with each new observation.[124] Both rely exclusively upon measured plasma values to derive the pharmacokinetic coefficients and have high variance until sufficient observations are available. Ideally, however, one would like to incorporate a priori knowledge about the patient's pharmacokinetics in addition to measured values. Maximum likelihood, or Bayesian, techniques attempt to optimally combine a priori pharmacokinetic information with incoming new serum-level information. Essentially, the Bayesian estimation methodologies treat the pharmacokinetic parameters as random variables with a priori distributions determined from population measurements. Bayesian techniques calculate the 'most likely' set of parameters that explain the a priori distribution and measured data together. These techniques can also be exploited to predict optimal blood sampling intervals for pharmacokinetic model determination.[135,136] Unfortunately, the nonlinear relationship between the compartmental coefficients and patient physical characteristics greatly increases the computational complexity of Bayesian techniques relative to least squares methods.

Because of superior predictive capability with sparse data, Bayesian forecasting techniques have been used almost exclusively for updating pharmacokinetic models.[11,12,15,137,138] In controlled human studies of digoxin and lidocaine dosing, computer models equaled or outperformed physician control. For example Vozeh *et al.* demonstrated comparable mean plasma lidocaine levels in patients receiving computer-guided and physician-guided dosing; however, computer-dosing resulted in significantly less variance about the mean level.[137] Although the sample size was too small to demonstrate significant clinical outcome differences, increased variance implies greater incidence of toxicity as well as subtherapeutic dosing. Peck *et al.* noted only a very modest improvement with computer dosing.[12] They attributed their results to significant physician motivation to 'beat the computer' and to the fact that 'simple systems lend themselves as readily to intuition as to automation'. Unfortunately, neither of the two lidocaine studies employing Bayesian feedback used an exponentially tapering infusion protocol, despite previously demonstrated efficacy and safety, in which automated control would be distinctly advantageous.

The relative importance of the a priori and the a posteriori information in predicting eventual serum levels was investigated by Sheiner *et al.* in a series of inpatients and outpatients on digoxin therapy.[15] Adjusting initial dosing based upon physical characteristics was indeed beneficial, but the benefit completely disappeared after the second serum sample. That is, after two serum samples, the a priori assumptions were worthless and comparable accuracy could be obtained from the serum samples alone. Consequently, while Bayesian techniques are superior to least-squares estimators for single-sample measurements, the added complexity of Bayesian techniques may be unwarranted as additional samples become available.

Problem 2: Titrating drug levels to physiologic/electrical/toxic effect

ECG assessment

For the past decade, electrophysiologic testing has represented the gold standard for the assessment of postmyocardial infarction arrhythmia risk as well as drug efficacy.[139–141] However, inducibility elimination through drug therapy may simply reflect more benign underlying disease rather than true drug effect; recent large randomized trials have not confirmed electrophysiologic measures of drug efficacy.[143] Furthermore, electrophysiologic testing is invasive and costly; consequently, noninvasive measures of drug efficacy continue to be investigated. Although cardiologists integrate all pertinent clinical data when assessing antiarrhythmic agent efficacy and toxicity, electrocardiography represents the single most important tool. Since decision-making is only as accurate as the data from which it is derived, reliable extraction of pertinent electrophysiologic parameters remains an active research area. Parameters can either be continuous (e.g. ECG intervals and durations) or discrete (e.g. arrhythmia present or not); however, discrete parameters can also be treated as a pseudocontinuous variable by counting occurrences per time interval (for example, PVC rate).

PVC rate

Premature ventricular contractions (PVC), representing ectopic ventricular pacemaker activity, are present at low frequency in many normal individuals. Although PVCs themselves are harmless, they are correlated with increased risk of serious ventricular arrhythmias following acute myocardial infarction.[143] Consequently, intravenous lidocaine or other type I agents have classically been given to suppress ventricular ectopy in the postmyocardial infarction period.[144,145] Since lidocaine plasma levels and PVC frequency tend to be inversely related, several experimental automated lidocaine and disopyramide drug delivery systems have used PVC rate as a single feedback variable.[56,137,146] Unfortunately, PVC rate within an individual fluctuates considerably, even at a fixed drug serum level.[143] Furthermore, while PVC suppression reflects drug effect, it fails to improve survival.[97] While complex ectopy and nonsustained ventricular tachycardia may be more predictive of potentially lethal arrhythmias, their relative infrequency on 24-hour Holter recordings limits the ability to distinguish spontaneous variation versus drug effect.[1,143]

QT dispersion

Surface ECG QT recordings represent one-dimensional projections of a complicated three-dimensional repolarization vector; inhomogeneous repolarization produces interlead differences in QT interval that have been termed dispersion.[103] While 'dispersion' complicates QT measurement, it may be an important clinical marker in its own right. Increased dispersion, as a marker of either asynchronous repolarization or early afterdepolarizations (EADs), appears to correlate with the incidence of ventricular tachyarrhythmias in long QT syndrome, postmyocardial infarction and drug-induced torsades de pointes.[104,147–151] QT prolongation without increased dispersion, for example during amiodarone therapy, is associated with less sudden death than more modest, inhomogeneous QT changes.[150,152] Similarly, patients who develop torsades de pointes during type Ia administration demonstrated significantly higher dispersion than patients who did not, despite comparable QT prolongation in both groups.[150] Since QT measurement is strongly lead-dependent, indices based upon body-surface potential maps have been proposed to improve diagnostic accuracy.[149] De Ambroggi *et al.* defined a similarity index, using principal component analysis of multisite QT waveforms, that identified patients having long QT syndrome with 87% sensitivity and 96% specificity.

While dispersion appears to be a harbinger of ventricular arrhythmias, dispersion changes with antiarrhythmic therapy have been inconsistent. In patients with congenital QT syndrome, symptom relief with β-blockade was not associated with reduced QT dispersion.[151] In contrast, decreased dispersion accompanied treatment success during sotalol therapy following myocardial infarction. One explanation is that dispersion may result from an anatomic or functional susceptibility, while therapies can act to reduce either susceptibility (by homogenizing repolarization) or by preventing initiating events (β-blockade). If so, QT dispersion (or some other measure of repolarization inhomogeneity) might be a useful feedback variable for type I or type III antiarrhythmic therapies, but of little prognostic value for β-blockade.

Signal-averaged ECG late potentials

Impaired conduction through infarcted tissue introduces small 'late potentials' superimposed upon the main QRS complex than can be detected through signal-averaged ECG (SAECG). Since myocardial regions of impaired conduction can serve as foci for re-entrant ventricular tachycardias, it is not surprising that late potentials have high sensitivity for predicting postmyocardial infarction arrhythmias.[153] But while late potentials identify potential anatomic substrates for re-entrant loops, they have poor specificity, i.e. many of the lesions are not prone to spontaneous arrhythmogenesis.

Signal averaged ECG has also been proposed for assessment of type I antiarrhythmic effect. Kulakowski *et al.* compared SAECG parameters in 15 patients that responded to procainamide (VT became noninducible in five patients, VT cycle length prolonged >100 ms in ten patients) therapy for monomorphic ventricular tachycardia versus 12 patients that failed to respond.[154] Responders had a total QRS prolongation of $24 \pm 16\%$, while nonresponders had a prolongation of only $10 \pm 11\%$ ($P < 0.014$). Changes in the low-amplitude signal and the RMS of the QRS terminal 40 ms were not significant. From these data they concluded that a fractional QRS prolongation >15% predicted responders with a sensitivity of 87% and specificity of 81%. In contrast, Hopson *et al.* found that while QRS prolongation was predictive of cycle-length slowing, it was not predictive of inducibility.[155] However, patients whose VT was rendered noninducible had significantly greater prolongation of effective refractory period and QT_c. In fact, the ratio of the QT_c increase (in milliseconds) to the SAECG QRS duration increase was >6 in all noninducible patients and <6 for those in whom VT cycle length was only slowed. This suggests that the type III effects of quinidine and procainamide were responsible for noninducibility, while type I effects resulted in cycle-length prolongation. A particularly good correlation was noted between VT cycle length and the low-amplitude signal prolongation. Taken together, these studies suggest that SAECG yields important information regarding type I antiarrhythmic effects but that repolarization parameters such as QT_c are more predictive of VT inducibility.

Use and reverse-use dependence

Both type I and type III antiarrhythmic agents demonstrated rate-dependent blockade determined by their individual kinetics. Classically, type I agents are 'use-dependent' in that greater blockade occurs at faster stimulation frequencies according to the agent subtype (type Ib < Ia < Ic).[94] Similarly, type III blockade generally manifests reverse-use dependence, with greater blockade at lower cycle lengths.[156] Figure 19.20 demonstrates steepening of the $QT/(RR)^{\frac{1}{2}}$ relationship for a single patient before and after disopyramide initiation, consistent with reverse-use blockade. Sadanga *et al.* proposed that since use and reverse-use dependence are known drug effects, their presence or absence might be predictive of drug efficacy complementary to the changes in QRS duration and QT interval.[95] For example, reverse-use blockade might distinguish QT_c prolongation secondary to increased sympathetic tone compared with type III drug effect. Alternatively, significant reverse-use blockade, by creating a marked sensitivity to bradycardia, may signal potential vulnerability to initiation of torsades de pointes.[157] However, a better fundamental understanding of the interplay between intrinsic repolarization rate dependencies, the autonomic nervous system, and the class I and class III drug effects, is necessary before conclusions can be made regarding drug efficacy/toxicity.

Heart-rate variability

Both the mean and variance of heart rate are regulated in part by the push–pull balance between the parasympathetic and sympathetic nervous system.[158,159] Heart-rate fluctuations occur on different timescales; high-frequency fluctuations are hypothesized to represent vagal influence, medium-frequency fluctuations to represent sympathetic stimulation and low-frequency fluctuations are not well understood. Decreased heart-rate variability, perhaps secondary to increased sympathetic tone, is strongly associated with lethal arrhythmias for patients with myocardial infarction or heart failure.[160,161] In fact, decreased heart variability following myocardial infarction is a poorer prognostic sign than late potentials, Killup class >2, ejection fraction <40, repetitive ventricular forms or a positive stress test,[161] with patients having <20 ms variability, having a relative risk of 6.67. Heart-rate variability is gradually restored in the months following infarction, paralleling the fall in arrhythmogenesis.[162] Consequently, heart-rate variability measures have been proposed for risk stratification of lethal arrhythmias.[161,163]

However, while decreased heart-rate variability is correlated with a poor outcome, its usefulness as a feedback variable for drug delivery is uncertain. β-Blockers increase heart rate variability and are protective, type Ic agents decrease heart rate variability and are deleterious; however these observations must be considered mere coincidence until proven otherwise.[164,165] Consequently, the potential role of heart rate variability in antiarrhythmic therapy appears to be as screening tool, i.e. identifying a high-risk patient subset warranting aggressive therapy and monitoring, rather than as a measure of treatment efficacy.

Arrhythmia detection

In contrast to electrocardiogram intervals and durations, cardiac rhythm is primarily a 'discrete' or 'Boolean' process. Automated ECG processing has an extensive history; good reviews on the subject may be found.[166–169] Commercially available systems perform better than many internists but still require double-reading by cardiologists for subtle arrhythmias. For some practical tasks, however, subtlety is not an issue. AICDs, for example, only need to recognize malignant ventricular tachycardias. Simple, fast algorithms that reliably identify atrial or ventricular fibrillation/flutter are widely available for implantable devices.[170–172]

Automated arrhythmia detection for more complicated rhythm disturbances, e.g. intermittent AV block, accessory pathway conduction, ectopic or escape beats, have also made significant recent advances.[173,174] Diagnostic accuracy has been improved through atrial monitoring, using esophageal electrodes, allowing reliable A-A, A-V, and V-A cycle length measurement. Using a simple classification scheme based upon A-V intervals and ECG morphology, DiCarlo *et al.* reported better than 99.2% classification accuracy in 21 patients with one to 28 supraventricular or ventricular arrhythmias.[174] Atrial and ventricular ECG morphologies were coded as normal or abnormal, and A-A, A-V and V-A cycle lengths were coded as normal, short, or increased. Contextual information, achieved by examining eight consecutive cardiac cycles, captured complex arrhythmias such as bradycardias, tachycardias and multigeminy patterns. Combined with individual beat analysis, contextual analysis improved detection to better than 99.5%

Using ECG parameters to modify target drug level

Given a set of electrocardiographic parameters, e.g. QT interval, dispersion and rate dependence, number of episodes of NSVT in the last 24 hours, presence of U waves, how does one use the data to modify therapy? The answer depends on the model relationship between the electrographic variable and the drug. If the variable is being used as a surrogate for plasma drugs level, for example the QT interval might be used instead of plasma ibutilide levels, then feedback occurs on the 'inner' loop of Figure 19.4. This scenario is becoming plausible as potency and specificity of type III agents simultaneously increase (serum levels are below conventional assay detection) or as local drug delivery devices become a clinical reality.

Alternatively, variables like QT dispersion or the number of NSVT episodes in 24 hours are markers of efficacy, while AV block and U waves may be early signs of drug toxicity. In this scenario, feedback occurs at the outer loop of Figure 19.4, i.e. the drug target level is inappropriate and must be adjusted. Incorporating such information into clinical decision-making is the most difficult part of feedback control, whether performed by a human or by a computer. Computer decision-making, or artificial intelligence (AI), has not been widely applied to antiarrhythmic drug administration.[175–179] A discussion of AI is beyond the scope of this chapter (see refs 180–182). Simplistically, AI relies upon hierarchical sets of explicit rules and decision trees to emulate the physician thought process. Unfortunately, while many clinical decisions can be transcribed into a flow chart, with predictable outcomes for various interventions, an even greater number of clinical decisions rely upon intangibles; intuition is a particularly difficult human trait to capture algorithmically. However, newer adaptive decision-making strategies, which are better suited for generalizing to the presentation of novel data, are improving rapidly. The terms 'fuzzy' logic, 'genetic' algorithms, 'neural networks', are becoming household words as well as the subject of entire scientific journals. Such techniques do not need explicit rules; they infer the rules based upon the input (therapy) and output (physiologic variables, clinical outcome). The key limitations with these algorithms is that they need large amounts of preliminary data to 'infer' the underlying rule structure, i.e. a large 'training set' is required. Well-controlled, prospective clinical data tend to be very expensive. Retrospectively compiled data, while much cheaper, are often much sparser and have many confounding variables.

Hybrid rules-based and non-rule systems also exist; an example is the ECG postprocessing arrhythmia detector, HOBBES.[183] HOBBES uses three basis rules, combined with ECG properties inferred from uncorrupted data, to resolve complex superpositions in noise and artifact corrupted data. A similar combination of rule-based and non-rule based methods will probably be necessary for successful computer titration of antiarrhythmic drug level.

Although computers may never perform the 'outer' feedback loop independent of human supervision, they can certainly aid the cardiologist at several levels in the decision-making process. First, by preprocessing electrocardiographic data, computers can compute, summarize and present in a rapidly-interpretable manner electrocardiographic statistics that would be too tedious and time-consuming to perform manually. Secondly, drug-administration histories and estimated pharmacokinetic profiles could be made available to assist in appropriate dosage modification. Lastly, by presenting a ranked list of probable diagnoses, their justification and recommended therapy, computers might remind the cardiologist of forgotten data or diagnoses (AF).

Example of practical implantable drug-delivery system

Introduction

As a specific example of the applicability of the various feedback techniques discussed so far, consider the use of accurate pharmacokinetic modeling and ECG-derived measures of efficacy to an implantable infusion system for the long-term treatment of paroxysmal atrial fibrillation (AF).

In clinical practice, atrial fibrillation is the most common,[184,185] least understood and most difficult arrhythmia to consistently manage. Paroxysmal atrial fibrillation warrants aggressive therapy, as it can severely reduce cardiac output and create an unacceptably high risk of stroke.[186] Present strategies for treating paroxysmal atrial fibrillation are centered on the use of prophylactic oral administration of anti-arrhythmic agents to prevent onset of the arrhythmia. Preventing atrial fibrillation by oral therapy introduces difficulties involving lack of efficacy,[187] poor patient compliance, inadequate control over plasma levels, long-term toxicity[188] and ex-cessive increases in mortality rates in patients with other cardiovascular complications.[97–189] In the event that atrial fibrillation develops despite prophylaxis, conventional treatment dictates a trip to the emergency room for cardioversion,[190] a procedure which can inadvertently damage cardiac tissue.[191,192] Electrical conver-sion of atrial fibrillation by existing implantable devices is also problematic, as antitachycardia pacemakers are incapable of conversion and the ability of implan-table defibrillators to convert fibrillation has not yet been demonstrated.[193–196] Surgical approaches for prevention of atrial fibrillation are experimental and limited in application.[197]

As an alternative to the limited efficacy of conventional therapies, which have been described as 'inconsistent, inefficient, and in some cases, inappropriate',[198] aggressive antiarrhythmic infusion immediately upon onset of fibrillation has been shown to greatly increase the chances of a successful conversion to sinus rhythm.[199–206] Therefore, an experimental implantable system has been developed, capable of providing long-term, round-the-clock outpatient arrhythmia monitoring as well as an on-demand infusion to produce rapid conversion.[28,30,41] The implan-table system approach is justified in patients who cannot hemodynamically tolerate AF for even short periods. Aggressive oral dosing protocols can take up to an hour to show any effect – much longer than the immediate arrhythmia control possible in 5 minutes with an implanted system. A conservative estimate of the fraction of the atrial fibrillation population for which this delay in efficacy is significant is 5%. Thus, of the one million patients in the USA alone who suffer from atrial fibrillation, 50 000 could potentially be treated with such a system.

System description

The Pharmacologic Atrial Defibrillator (PAD), shown in Figure 19.26(A), is based on a commercially available dual chamber pacemaker (Ela CHORUS) with 1500 bytes of RAM and a modified insulin pump (Infusaid Model 1000). The pacemaker's atrial lead senses atrial activity and its microprocessor is programmed to automatically detect atrial fibrillation. The ventricular lead is not used to sense ventricular activity but is used as a control wire with ventricular 'pacing' pulses activating the pump valves and delivering microboluses of drug.

The CHORUS is a multiprogrammable DDD pulse generator utilizing two custom integrated circuits. An 8-bit integer arithmetic microprocessor is used for control of the operating system and telemetry functions in addition to data manipulation and storage. The second integrated circuit processes analog signals from the heart and telemetry antenna, provides clocking for the microprocessor, converts electrogram

(A)

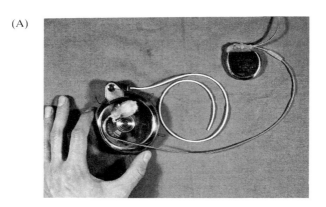

(B)

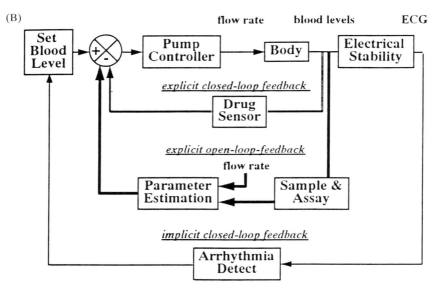

Figure 19.26 **A.** The implantable Pharmacologic Atrial Defibrillator (PAD) system based upon a CHORUS pacemaker and an Infusaid infusion pump. The atrial sensing lead (top right), delivery catheter (center), and ventricular control lead (bottom to top right) are also shown. **B.** PAD control loop. PAD utilizes implicit closed-loop feedback, assessing cardiac electrical stability via the ECG for antiarrhythmia detection. Detection of fibrillation sets the target blood level and operates the pump open-loop according to a predetermined pharmacokinetic model. Incorporation of a drug sensor would allow the pump to operate with explicit closed-loop feedback and eliminate the need for pharmacokinetic modeling. Alternatively, several serial blood samples taken during infusion could be used to adaptively update the preprogrammed model.

features to measurements usable by the processor and converts control outputs from the processor into cardiac pacing pulses. The 1.5k of RAM available on-board the CHORUS was originally intended for storage of Holter histographic data. However, the ROM program can be bypassed in order to allow the operating system to reside in the Holter RAM. The PAD system software operates the device in AAI mode with on-demand ventricular pacing for pump control. Upper and lower rate intervals, atrial refractory period, and stimulation level/pulse width are programmable via an external telemetry head. A marker channel output from the telemetry head allows sensed activity and paced responses to be displayed.

The Infusaid Model 1000 pump is a programmable rate device employing a reciprocating accumulator mechanism to approximate continuous infusion. A 25-ml capacity drug reservoir is enclosed by a compartment containing a liquid producing constant vapor pressure at body temperature. Two solenoid valves control drug flow between the drug reservoir/accumulator and accumulator/catheter. Valve hold-open time is programmable and controls the volume of drug transferred to the accumulator (nominal value: 35 μl). The pump has been customized allowing direct access to the valve activation circuitry via an externalized contact. Connection to the CHORUS through a unipolar ventricular control lead allows ventricular pacing pulses at CMOS logic levels to open the accumulator valves and deliver drug.

Program control

The control algorithm encompasses fibrillation detection, infusion control and standard demand pacing functions. When fibrillation is detected on the atrial electrogram, the on-board microprocessor begins delivery of an optimum pharmacokinetically-based infusion to rapidly terminate the arrhythmia. Upon conversion to sinus rhythm, the infusion is shut down and the pacemaker is returned to the state where pacing will occur if necessary. It should be noted that this system is an example of closed-loop effect feedback: the arrhythmia detector's assessment of physiological state (AF/SR), influenced by infusion efficacy, provides automatic control of pump status (on/off); however, the pump itself operates open-loop according to a predetermined pharmacokinetic model rather than closed loop in the sense of direct drug level measurement. Figure 19.26(B) illustrates the system along with examples of how other types of feedback can be incorporated.

The CHORUS is an interrupt-driven device. When operating from RAM, the ROM program is maintained for nominal operating functions with control passing back to RAM upon execution of an interrupt. The interrupt structure is shown in the top half of Figure 19.27. Note that clock access is not continuous. The system clock can be indirectly accessed after an interrupt via the time since last interrupt (TSLI) counter. This counter allows elapsed time measurements in 1/64-second increments. In order to avoid multiple triggering during sinus rhythm, there is a programmable atrial refractory period following atrial sensing or pacing. Four possible events can generate interrupts: atrial sensing (ASENSE), atrial pacing (APACE), end of a refractory period (ERP) and atrial sensing during a refractory period (RAS). The nonrefractory interrupts, ASENSE and APACE, are generated, respectively, dependent upon atrial sensing or TSLI equal to the lower rate interval. During a refractory period, an ERP interrupt (if TSLI equals the atrial refractory period) or RAS interrupt (dependent on atrial sensing) is possible.

Once an interrupt has been generated, it must be handled accordingly to measure the current interbeat interval (AANOW), update the record of recent A-A intervals (AAREC), update the elapsed time clock required for infusion control (ETIME), detect fibrillation and control infusion. The bottom half of Figure 19.27 describes

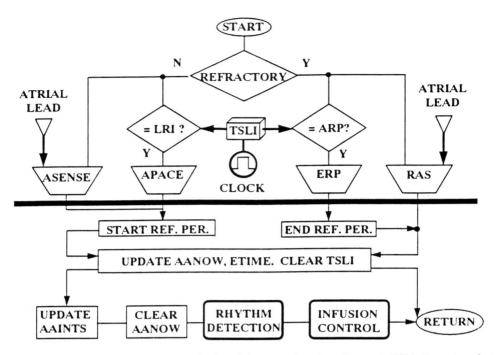

Figure 19.27 PAD interrupt structure (top) and interrupt handlers (bottom). TSLI, time since last interrupt; ASENSE, atrial sensing interrupt; ERP, end refractory period interrupt; RAS, refractory sense interrupt; ARP, programmed atrial refractory period; LRI, programmed lower rate interval; AANOW, current interbeat interval; ETIME, elapsed clock time. ASENSE and RAS interrupts depend upon atrial sensing, APACE and ERP interrupts depend upon TLSI.

how these functions are handled based on interrupt type. All interrupts update the current A-A interval and elapsed time clock. However, only the nonrefractory interrupts update the interval record and execute the rhythm detection and infusion control subroutines. The interval record is updated in a first-in, first-out manner with the current A-A interval becoming the most recent entry. This record is used later for the construction of a robust rate estimator.

Fibrillation detection

Achieving reliable sensing of atrial fibrillation is difficult with existing pacemaker systems. The large variations in signal amplitude during atrial fibrillation are a significant obstacle to consistent event detection. Additional difficulties are introduced by inappropriately designed sensing amplifiers and the imposition of long refractory periods.

Atrial electrograms show a large degree of amplitude variation even in normal sinus rhythm in spite of the additional difficulties imposed by atrial fibrillation. The largest degree of variation is typically between electrograms measured at rest and after exercise-induced hemodynamic stress. The fusion wave (F wave) associated with atrial fibrillation is characterized by even greater variations in morphology, amplitude, and cycle length. The atrial rate is 400–650 bpm in humans, with rates of up to 1000 bpm in canines. The amplitude of the F wave is less than that of the P wave, nominally 58% for unfiltered signals.[207] The morphology of atrial fibrillation ranges from coarse waves typical of atrial flutter to waves so fine that they are difficult to distinguish from baseline.[208]

Detection of atrial fibrillation is also complicated by hardware limitations imposed by the frequency response of pacemaker sense amplifiers. This problem was addressed by Arzbaecher in a canine study.[209] Typical high-pass cutoff frequencies for pacemakers are 15 and 30 Hz. Cutoff points at these frequencies allow differentiation of the normal P wave in order to accentuate the amplitude and slew rate of the initial atrial depolarization and remove low-frequency baseline fluctuations. However, this arrangement often fails to detect atrial fibrillation since 71% of the signal power during atrial fibrillation is in the 6–30 Hz band, as opposed to only 19% for sinus rhythm. Figure 19.28 illustrates relative sinus rhythm and atrial fibrillation amplitudes as a function of filtering. The poor filtering arrangement and reduced amplitude often combine to produce severe undercounting during fibrillation.

Software refractory periods also contribute to poor event sensing during atrial fibrillation. In the original designs for dual-chamber pacing systems, the purpose of the atrial refractory period (ARP) and postventricular atrial refractory period (PVARP) was to allow the pulse generator to ignore far-field QRS events because of the lack of an effective method to discriminate between atrial and ventricular

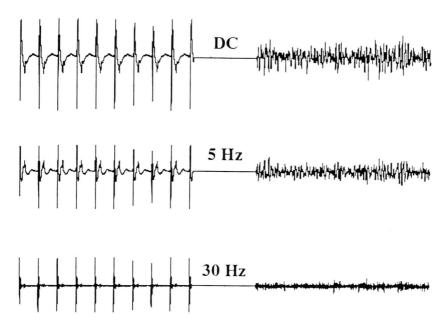

Figure 19.28 Amplitudes of sinus rhythm and atrial fibrillation as a function of cut-off frequency for single-pole high-pass filters.

activity. In order to avoid inappropriate ventricular pacing after atrial beats caused by retrograde atrial activation of premature ventricular contractions, the manufacturers extended ARP and PVARP to an even longer period. Thus, the answer to difficulties with atrial sensing has been to increasingly limit the allowable time during which atrial sensing is permitted.[210] During fibrillation, these excessive refractory periods handicap discrimination algorithms by removing a significant fraction of the valid atrial fibrillation events from consideration. For example, a typical pacemaker in AAI mode imposes a minimum 360 ms ARP after an atrial event, while a device in DDD mode uses a minimum PVARP value of 140 ms. With an upper-rate interval of 500 ms (120 bpm), the result is inhibition of 64% or 28% of the valid atrial events during AAI and DDD mode, respectively. Clearly, this is a significant disadvantage when trying to detect atrial fibrillation.

Median filtering

The CHORUS has a sense-amplifier low-frequency cutoff of 30 Hz, making it susceptible to sporadic undersensing during fibrillation. Attempts at identifying fibrillation by simply counting sensed atrial beats are often unsuccessful as undersensing prevented the accumulation of enough detections to diagnose fibrillation. To improve the robustness of the atrial fibrillation detection scheme, a record of the most recent A-A intervals is stored and a median filter applied.

Undersensing during fibrillation produces artificially long A-A intervals, 'outliers' in the A-A interval array. The robustness of an estimator to outliers is determined by its 'breakpoint', which is the smallest number of outliers needed to corrupt the estimate. The median possesses the best possible breakpoint since at least half the data must be outliers to the median. Hence, if at least $N/2$ of the last N observed A-A intervals are shorter than the detection threshold (in milliseconds), atrial fibrillation will be diagnosed.

In the PAD detection algorithm, median filtering is done by bubble-sorting the A-A interval record. The bubble-sort is implemented in such a way as to minimize the number of comparisons. The median element of the sorted array is used as the rate estimate. Atrial fibrillation is diagnosed and infusion started if the rate estimate is less than an arbitrary threshold AF_THRESH. Infusion is terminated by either a rate estimate greater than a sinus rhythm detection SR_THRESH or failure to detect conversion within 30 minutes. Typical values used for AF_THRESH and SR_THRESH were 200 and 330 ms, respectively.

Figure 19.29 illustrates the superior rate-estimation performance of the running median as compared to simple beat counting and the running average. The top trace shows an atrial electrogram, the middle trace shows pacemaker sense markers while on the bottom are the estimated A-A intervals. The sense markers tend to either cluster together quite nicely, as shown on the top trace at about the 6-s mark, or they occur sporadically with long pauses when the atrial amplitude drops off, as seen at in the 10–16 s band. Approximately one-third of the A-A intervals in this trace are outliers. On the bottom trace, the left-hand side corresponds to initialization 21 point filters. The lower curve represents the running median, the upper curve the running average. Following initialization and using an AF_THRESH value of 200 ms, the

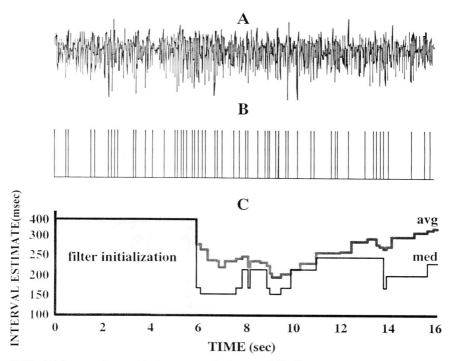

Figure 19.29 (A) Intracardiac atrial electrogram during atrial fibrillation. (B) Sensed atrial events (C) Interbeat interval estimator performance: 21-point median filter versus 21-point moving average filter (bold).

median correctly diagnoses fibrillation, then rises a little as the effect of the outliers becomes stronger. However, notice how the outliers cause the running average to produce an estimate which is always larger than the running median since the outliers are always large. The running average fails to reach the detection threshold.

It should be noted that the median is also superior to simple beat counting. An earlier CHORUS system using simple beat counting for rate estimation required 50 beats in 10 s to diagnose fibrillation. In this 16-s trace, only 54 beats have been detected, and no 10-s interval within this trace contains 50 beats. Thus, it can be seen that simple beat-counting produces excessive delays in diagnosis of fibrillation, an unacceptable situation if the dectection scheme is to quickly recognize the onset of fibrillation.

Infusion control

Antiarrhythmic drugs employed in the treatment of atrial fibrillation, such as procainamide and disopyramide, typically follow two-compartment kinetics described earlier in equation (3). The protocol for achieving and maintaining a desired target concentration consists of a bolus followed by an exponentially tapering drip, as shown in equation (4). The major drawback to implementing this infusion is that the exponentially-tapering term in equation (4) requires a variable-speed pump capable of continuous flow rate adjustment. Additionally, the system must also deliver the initial loading bolus $C_{1d}V_1$, where C_{1d} is the desired target level. However, on/off control of a constant speed pump via pulse-frequency modulation can provide an excellent approximation to the exponentially tapering infusion. The Euler approximation of an on/off control scheme can be easily derived by substituting the derivative operators in equation (3) with finite difference operators and replacing the continuous rate term involving $u(t)$ with a switching function which allows for discrete concentration increases. The resulting equations are

$$C_1[n] = C_1[n-1][1 - (K_e + K_{12})T] + K_{12}TC_2[n-1] + S(\Delta C) \tag{8}$$

$$C_2[n] = C_2[n-1][1 - K_{21}T] + K_{21}TC_1[n-1] \tag{9}$$

where n is the discrete time index, T is the discrete time increment, ΔC is the increase in central compartment concentration due to a single pumping pulse, and $S(\Delta C)$ is a switching function controlling the discrete concentration increase. The simplest function for $S(\Delta C)$ is given by:

$$S(\Delta C) = \begin{cases} M_{\text{pulse}}/V_1 & C_1[n-1] \leqslant C_{1d} \\ 0 & \text{otherwise} \end{cases} \tag{10}$$

where M_{pulse} is the drug mass delivered per pumping pulse.

Constraints on the discrete time increment. Implementation of equations (8) and (9) depends on an appropriate choice of calculation interval T. Selection of T is constrained by five factors: the magnitudes of the pharmacokinetic time constants, desired bolus delivery time T_b, target concentration level C_{1d}, pulse concentration ΔC and maximum pumping rate. Eigenvalue analysis of the numerical stability of the discrete time equations[211] places an upper bound on T of:

$$T_{\text{maxPK}} = \frac{2}{\alpha} \tag{11}$$

where

$$\alpha = K_e + K_{12} + K_{21} \tag{12}$$

Choice of calculation interval must also take into account the time required to deliver the loading bolus and the number of pump strokes this will require. This bolus constraint, T_{bc}, can be expressed as:

$$T_{bc} = \frac{T_b}{I\left(\dfrac{C_{1d}}{\Delta C}\right)} \tag{13}$$

where $I(X)$ is the roundup function and $I(C_{1d}/\Delta C)$ is the number of strokes required to deliver the bolus. Finally, consistent stroke volume delivery is contingent on pumping at intervals longer than those dictated by the hardware-limited maximum pumping rate. All of these constraints are summarized by the inequality:

$$T_{\text{mpr}} \leqslant T \leqslant \min(T_{bc}, T_{\text{maxPK}}) \tag{14}$$

where T_{mpr} is the inverse of the maximum pumping rate.

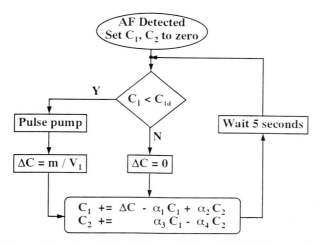

Figure 19.30 Integer arithmetic on/off infusion controller. ΔC is the increase in central compartment concentration due to a single pumping pulse, m is the drug mass delivered per pulse, V_1 is the central compartment volume, and α_i are the integer ratio approximations to the real number coefficients in equations (8) and (9).

Constraints on the discrete time increment. When designing an infusion using the on/off control scheme, the value of ΔC must be balanced by consideration of two factors: desired bolus delivery time and maximum acceptable overshoot. The infusion system must be capable of delivering drug as quickly as possible in order to approximate the ideal bolus infusion $C_{1d}V_1\mathrm{d}(t)$. As discussed above, this delivery time is given as $t_{bolus} = T*I(C_{1d}/\Delta C)$. The maximum percentage overshoot is equal to $\Delta C/C_{1d}$. Thus, a trade-off exists between maximum percentage overshoot and bolus delivery time, and must take into account the aforementioned constraint on T as well as any possible physiologic effects of rapid bolus infusion.

Implementation. Integer arithmetic microprocessors, such as that used by CHORUS, are limited to the operations of two's complement addition and arithmetic shifts. Solving equations (8) and (9) with these operations requires numerical approximations involving ratios of integers as well as appropriate quantification of ΔC and C_{1d}. While a discussion of the approximation process is beyond the scope of this text, the interested reader is referred to the article by Bloem and Arzbaecher.[30] A simplified flowchart of the integer arithmetic infusion control scheme is shown in Figure 19.30.

Results

The experimental procedure for *in vivo* canine testing of the PAD system employs an acetylcholine infusion followed by rapid atrial pacing to induce fibrillation, followed by an antiarrhythmic infusion of disopyramide. Modeling of the pharmacokinetics of disopyramide under these conditions has yielded the population parameter set $V_1 = 0.08 \text{ l kg}^{-1}$ (central compartment volume / kg total mass), $K_e = 0.120 \text{ min}^{-1}$,

$K_{12} = 0.460$ min^{-1} and $K_{21} = 0.028$ min^{-1}. A target level of 8 mg l^{-1} is desired in a 35-kg test subject with no more than 11.2% overshoot, and the bolus must be delivered in 45 s. The minimum time between consecutive pumping pulses for consistent stroke volume is 4 s. With these constraints, ΔC was set to 0.896 mg l^{-1} and T at 5 s.

The infusion trajectory obtained with the integer arithmetic on/off controller is shown in Figure 19.31(A). The target level of 8 mg l^{-1} is quickly achieved and then maintained. The maximum overshoot is 7.7%, less than the maximum theoretical overshoot of 11.2%. For a 30-minute infusion, the cumulative dosage delivered is 9.6% above that obtained via an exact solution of equations (8) and (9).

Figure 19.31(B) demonstrates the on/off controller's pulse-frequency modulation of the pumping intervals. During the course of the infusion, the on/off controller has changed the pumping interval 68 times in order to maintain the desired central compartment level. This degree of control over plasma level is not possible with a simple table lookup method, as the number of table entries required becomes prohibitive given available memory. Additionally, direct online solution of the two-compartment equations is superior to a simple table lookup since extension of the infusion to an arbitrary duration requires no additional memory. Finally, the direct

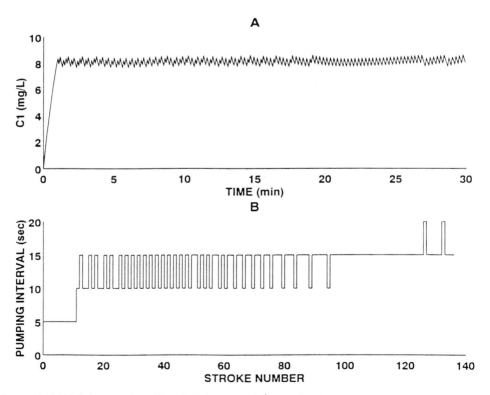

Figure 19.31 (A) C_1 for equations (8) and (9) for a 8 mg l^{-1} target level. (B) Pulse-frequency modulation of pumping intervals. Cumulative dosage delivered by the integer solution is 9.6% below that delivered by a floating-point solution for a 30-minute simulated infusion. The desired level is quickly achieved and then maintained for the infusion duration.

solution method is capable of tracking postconversion blood levels. In the event of recurring fibrillation, infusion can be restarted taking into account initial conditions for C_1 and C_2.

Experimental procedure

Implantation

Following the hardware and software development described above, a chronic dog model was used to validate the overall system. Observing the guidelines set down in the PHS *Guide for the Care and Use of Laboratory Animals*, the animal is anesthetized with pentobarbitol and actively ventilated with a Harvard respirator. A lateral thoracotomy performed in the fifth intercostal space exposes the heart.

Two unipolar electrodes with active fixation helical screws are than attached to the atrial appendage with 1-cm spacing. A differential (bipolar) signal is obtained using a unipolar/bipolar bifurcation adapter. Signal amplitude during sinus rhythm is measured in the frequency bands 2–300 Hz and 30–300 Hz. The latter band has the same frequency response as the CHORUS atrial lead sense amplifier. Electrode position and spacing is adjusted until the signal amplitude is satisfactory and QRS artifacts are minimal. A third unipolar electrode is attached to the atrial appendage for the delivery of rapid electrical stimulation to induce atrial fibrillation. This lead is tunneled to a subcutaneous location on the back of the animal so that it can be easily exposed for atrial fibrillation induction during subsequent experiments.

The pump is placed in a submuscular pouch on the high lumbar spine. Submuscular placement ensures mechanical stability superior to that possible using a subdermal pouch. The depth of the pouch is such that there is easy access to the accumulator port.

The drug catheter is subdermally tunneled from the pouch to a position allowing access to the right femoral vein. A cutdown performed on the femoral vein allows introduction of the catheter tip to a position in the inferior vena cava. A medical grade silicone-rubber catheter with antithrombogenic properties is used to impede clot formation. A pouch for the pacemaker is made subdermally in the lower right abdominal area. The pump control lead is tunneled to the pacemaker pouch and attached to the ventricular lead of the pacemaker. Finally, the bipolar cardiac lead is tunneled subdermally to the pacemaker's atrial lead input. Incisions are closed and the chest evacuated following confirmation of system operation.

On each subsequent experiment day, the dog is anesthetized with Brevitol and the atrial fibrillation induction lead is exposed. Atrial fibrillation is induced by a 1-s burst of atrial pacing while maintaining an acetylcholine infusion at 0.2 ml kg^{-1}. In our experience, atrial fibrillation so induced will persist until the acetylcholine is stopped or the antiarrhythmic drug is delivered.

Experimental results

Nine experiments were performed on two animals implanted with the PAD system. Table 19.2 provides a summary of the fibrillation detection times, conversion times,

Table 19.2 Summary of experimental results with PAD system

Experiment	ARP (ms)	AF_THRESH (ms)	Detection time (s)	Time of conversion (min)/ blood levels (mg l^{-1})
A1	78	125	3.5	1:10/1.7
A2	155	200	54	5:36/3.08
B1	155	200	NA*	NA*, converted
B2	155	200	54	2:28/NA*
B3	155	200	NA*	3:41/4.7
B4	187	250	66	3:52/5.0
B5	187	250	64	0:48/4.7
B6	187	250	66	1:09/2.8
B7	187	250	61-74	1:08/2.9

*NA = not available.

and blood levels at the time of conversion. Target level for these experiments was 5 mg l^{-1}, and a 21-point median filter was used for arrhythmia detection. The ARP was adjusted to prevent farfield QRS detection during sinus rhythm, with corresponding adjustments of the atrial fibrillation detection threshold.

The first, Dog A1, experiment resulted in an extremely fast detection time. However, extremely fast detection is a liability rather than an asset when fibrillation is not sustained. A more desirable method of diagnosing fibrillation is to detect the onset of fibrillation, wait a suitable length of time, and then confirm that fibrillation has been sustained. Thus, a DWC (detect–wait–confirm) algorithm was incorporated into the arrhythmia detector. The DWC algorithm waits 255 beats after the first detection of atrial fibrillation before making a decision to infuse. DWC was used in the second Dog A experiment and all of the Dog B experiments. The resulting detection times were on the order of 1 minute, sufficient to confirm sustained fibrillation, and within 30% of the minimum theoretical detection time (minimum detection time = 266* ARP, 11* ARP for median filter delay plus 255* ARP 'wait-and-confirm' period).

A major justification for the development of the PAD system is capability of rapidly producing therapeutic blood levels and quickly converting fibrillation. This capability has clearly been achieved with Dog B, whose longest conversion time was about 4 minutes. All experiments demonstrated blood levels at time of conversion well within the therapeutic range of disopyramide. Finally, Figure 19.32 illustrates the maintenance of a constant target level. While the desired target level was 5 mg l^{-1}, the constant deviation from target level represents underestimation of the volume of distribution.

Conclusion

We conclude from these experiments that an implantable system for automatic detection of cardiac arrhythmia and infusion of antiarrhythmic drug is technically feasible based on existing components. The technical difficulties experienced with these first implants are minor and the concept has been well demonstrated in a realistic experimental model of atrial fibrillation. Some obvious improvements can be made: the onboard microprocessor needs more sophistication, the two devices

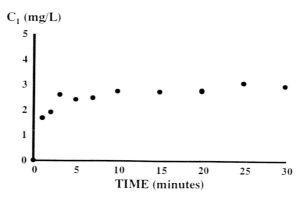

Figure 19.32   Measured blood levels for experiment A1, demonstrating maintenance of a constant plasma level.

should be combined into one package for ease in implantation, with a smaller total size and fewer interconnections. With these improvements, one can foresee clinical testing of the system.

Examples of potential applications for feedback drug delivery

If reliable online drug or disease activity sensors were available, feedback drug delivery would be trivial and widely utilized. Since development of online drug sensors remains distant, feedback devices must rely primarily upon pharmacokinetic models or upon electrocardiographic drug effect estimates. Nevertheless, significant progress can be made toward clinically feasible devices with present technology, or with technology that could reasonably developed in the next ten years.

Implantable devices

As previously discussed, combination implantable drug-delivery and cardiodefibrillating devices may represent the best of both worlds. One hypothetical system is demonstrated in Figure 19.33; the top panel illustrates physical components while the bottom panel illustrates functional elements. Physically, the device consists of a defibrillator, a drug pump (in this example an iontophoretic membrane is employed), and a computer to drive them both, according to ECG feedback and remote physician programming. Since serum drug levels are meaningless in a local drug delivery system, the ECG must serve as the sole feedback variable, functioning both as a proxy for 'target' drug levels and as a measure of efficacy/toxicity.

Functionally, the device computer has several distinct tasks, input control, arrhythmia detection, efficacy/toxicity assessment, pharmacokinetics estimates and ECG signal processing. To demonstrate task interactions, consider a hypothetical

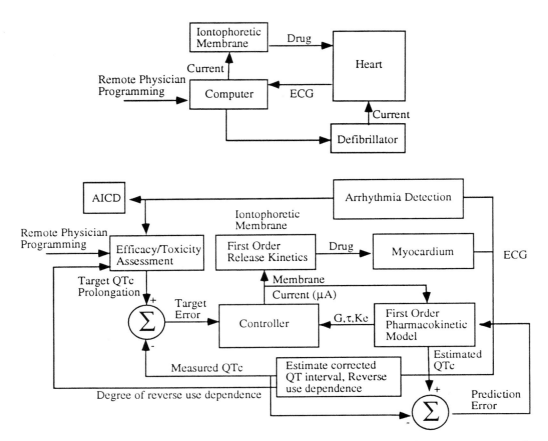

Figure 19.33 Proposed implantable class III drug-delivery system. (Top) Physical components consist of a microcomputer, power supply, iontophoretic membrane, defibrillating electrodes and monophasic or bipolar electrocardiogram electrodes. (Bottom) Functional components consist of arrhythmia detection, input control, efficacy/toxicity assessment, pharmacokinetics estimates and ECG signal processing.

clinical scenario. Ibutilide is to be used for postmyocardial infarction ventricular tachycardia suppression; electrophysiological studies using intravenously administered ibutilide demonstrate decreased inducibility when the patient's QT_c was prolonged an average of 10% from baseline. Consequently, the physician initially programs the device to maintain a 10% 'target' QT_c prolongation. The controller decides upon an appropriate current signal to apply to the iontophoretic membrane to eliminate the difference between the desired and observed QT_c values. If one assumes that the QT_c is roughly proportional to effector tissue level (for example, $QT_c = k[\text{ibutilide}] + \text{random fluctuations}$), then a pharmacokinetic model can be used to derive the appropriate current change. A single-compartment model characterized by a volume of distribution, and elimination rate constant, K_e, is a logical choice for local drug-delivery systems. On the other hand, the controller could completely ignore model-based information and use conventional PID control on the error signal. However, since QT_c will not be a perfect surrogate for local effect (because of autonomic modulation, rate-correction errors, etc.), and pharmacokinetic models will not perfectly represent drug dynamics, a reasonable controller would balance the two contributions.

The iontophoretic membrane responds to the controller by first-order kinetics described by a 'gain' and a rise time, τ.[7] By aggregating the iontophoretic and pharmacokinetics models, the entire 'transfer function' between the iontophoretic current, I, and the change in QT_c could be described in three variables, G τ and K_e (again assuming QT_c proportional to effector tissue level). The value of G can be deduced experimentally; it is simply the steady-state ratio of the average change in QT_c divided by the change in iontophoretic current. Obviously G might fluctuate as the membrane ages or as patient drug sensitivity alters, but the difference in predicted QT_c and observed QT_c (prediction error) could be used to track these changes. The release constant, t, is an intrinsic membrane property that can be measured *ex vivo* prior to implantation. As discussed in the pharmacokinetics section, the drug elimination rate constant, K_c has not been well characterized for local drug-delivery systems. It represents the half-time of QT_c changes following a step decrease in iontophoretic current (minus the known delay effects of the membrane) and could be estimated experimentally. In general, K_c will be a function of membrane placement, local blood flow and individual differences in drug metabolism. Consequently, it is unclear whether population estimates would be adequate or whether K_c would have to be derived experimentally.

To close the inner feedback loop, QT measurements and RR intervals must be converted into QT_c measurements. While the optimal algorithm is controversial, a linear regression in linear, or log coordinate systems would be performed initially to establish the conversion coefficients. Because of use and reverse-use effects, these coefficients would have to be updated for significant changes in estimated drug level; however, calibration every 1–2 hours would probably be adequate. Changes in the regression coefficients will provide information regarding rate-dependent drug effects as well as sympathetic tone. Since QT_c fluctuates at a faster rate than tissue drug-level changes, low-pass or median-filtering would be appropriate prior to comparison with the 'target' QT_c

The 'outer', or efficacy feedback loop, might be as simple as the cardiologist's clinical judgment and AICD's arrhythmia detector. That is, based upon patient symptomatology, 24 hour Holter monitor and the stress test, the cardiologist might decide that the QT_c 'set point' was ineffective or approaching toxicity. Similarly, AICD triggering indicates medical therapy failure; local delivery is either subtherapeutic or toxic (e.g. torsades de pointes).

Automated feedback could help distinguish between inadequate therapy and toxicity (which is rarely trivial). The pharmacokinetic model provides estimates of tissue drug concentration (which may differ from QT_c in acute situations). The presence or absence of significant rate dependence might also be inferred by the strength of the QT–RR interval coupling (regression coefficients) with low rate dependence supporting subtherapeutic dosing. Similarly, a powerful rate dependence in conjunction with higher than projected QT_c would support a torsades proarrhythmic event.

Although the computational tasks may appear too formidable for the primitive implantable computers currently available, the slow system dynamics dictate otherwise. Arrhythmia detection is the only component that must respond in seconds; the rest of the system can operate on the scale of minutes to hours and still be significantly faster and more appropriately responsive than manual drug delivery. The computational burden of QT postprocessing (smoothing and rate dependence), pharmacokinetic modeling (using fixed parameters or recursive linear updates) and controller output, has smaller magnitude than the tachyarrhythmia detection routines already implemented on devices. QT-interval measurement represents the greatest technological barrier because of limited on-chip memory and A/D converter capability, and because it is intrinsically difficult. On the other hand, $MAPD_{90\%}$ contains the same information as QT interval, but is much easier to quantitate. In fact, $MAPD_{90\%}$ and RR interval could probably be measured through analog preprocessing (comparator with self-tuning threshold and a counter) and digital inputs. If so, the implanted computer would only have to process two data points per heart beat, instead of thousands. However, at present, this technique is only speculative. Furthermore, the reliability and robustness of chronically recorded MAPs remains to be demonstrated.

Acute-care intravenous delivery

Postoperative and postmyocardial infarction arrhythmia suppression are important clinical problems. As discussed previously, computer-controlled intravenous antiarrhythmia-agent delivery has many potential advantages including faster response, decreased toxicity and the ability to adapt to changing physiology/pharmacology. The chief barrier to both manual and computer dosing has been the burden, expense and delay of obtaining serum drug levels. While an intravenous drug sensor is unlikely to occur within the next few decades, rapid, commercial, *ex vivo*, use-once drug assays are becoming commonplace. Conventional glucose monitoring for diabetics is a perfect example. Consequently, one could easily envision an intensive-care unit based system that would withdraw a small venous or arterial sample, perform a use-once assay of the desired agent and correct the infusion rate based upon the information. This approach has precedence; many prototypical automated arterial blood gas systems use serial *ex vivo* measurements instead of an implantable transducer.[58] Since the pharmacokinetic time constants associated with most drugs are fairly slow, sampling requirements are low. During the loading phase, samples might be drawn once an hour, with declining frequency thereafter. From the predicted and observed serum levels, the computer would be able to estimate that patient's individual pharmacokinetic parameters, facilitating subsequent titration of the target serum level. Schematically, this approach was shown previously in Figure 19.5.

If the intravenously infused agent is extremely potent, reproducible, rapid assays may be difficult to develop commercially. In this case, an intensive-care unit based feedback drug delivery system would be functionally identical to the implantable device, except the iontophoretic membrane would be replaced by a programmable infusion pump. Even if serum levels are readily attainable, a hybrid feedback scheme integrating QT_c and serum level feedback may be more robust than either alone. For example, an unexpected drug interaction might be missed until the next blood draw, except that QT_c prolongation would be significantly higher than the established 'set point'. Hence, in addition to alerting the clinician to the model mismatch, the controller would attempt to decrease QT_c prolongation by lowering drug input. In general, agreement between the two feedback 'arms' suggests appropriate modeling and good controllability, whereas deviation might be an early clue for drug toxicity, drug interactions, unexpected or nonlinear physiological response or device malfunction.

As with the implantable-device example, assessment of efficacy/toxicity would probably receive contributions from both computer and physician. The ECG monitoring could be fairly sophisticated because it would be *ex vivo*; accurate estimates of intervals and durations (and their rate dependence) would not be difficult, nor would arrhythmia detection and characterization. Multilead recordings would allow measurement of QT dispersion. Currently, efficacy assessment is still the exclusive domain of the cardiologist, but automated techniques could make significant contributions toward establishing objective criteria.

Summary

In this chapter, antiarrhythmia drug delivery, manual or automated, has been divided into two different feedback loops. The first loop involves rapid agent delivery and stable maintenance at a desired serum level or 'set point'. Although *in vivo* drug sensors would trivialize this task, development of such devices is distant. Fortunately, since antiarrhythmic pharmacokinetics are slow, and cheap, reliable, fast *ex vivo* commercial assay kits may soon be readily available, automated serial *ex vivo* assays may obviate the need for an *in vivo* drug inducer.

Drug levels, however, may not always be available, or interpretable for feedback. For example, local drug-delivery devices may produce nearly undetectable amounts peripherally, whose values may or may not correlate well with effect tissue concentrations. Hence, electrocardiographic changes, e.g. QRS, QT_c or $MAPD_{90\%}$ durations, might be used as a proxy for effector tissue concentrations. Although antiarrhythmic agent classes are defined by their electrophysiologic effects, correlations between serum level and ECG intervals have typically been poor. Many factors have contributed, including intersubject variability, autonomic nervous system influences, mixed-class pharmacologic effects, active metabolites and use/reverse-use effects. Newer class III agents, however, appear to have more selective action and much better dose–electrophysiologic response. Preliminary experiments with ibutilide, for example, show very promising potential for QT_c or $MAPD_{90\%}$ feedback. Correlations between serum level and interval prolongation might be further improved by more reliable measurement of drug intervals, better rate-correction algorithms (including use-dependent blockade) and the use of intraindividual rather than interindividual relationships. However, whether ECG or MAPD intervals can yield effective feedback remains an open question.

The second feedback loop involves set point titration according to the electrophysiologic assessments of efficacy/toxicity, either by a clinician, a computer or both. Efficacy is difficult to quantitate because it is defined by the absence of a rare event; electrophysiologic studies, Holter monitoring, heart rate variability and QT dispersion have significant prognostic power for arrhythmia risk stratification but no technique to date has consistently predicted drug efficacy in large randomized, controlled, clinical trials. For patients with AICDs, changes in shock frequency may be the most accurate measure. While drug efficacy assessment remains problematic, drug effect has many electrocardiographic correlates, include changes in QRS and QT durations (including use/reverse-use dependence), QT dispersion, as well as PVC rate and morphology. Furthermore, while efficacy represents absence of symptoms, drug toxicity is marked by characteristic electrocardiographic changes, making toxicity easier to assess by computer. Automated ECG analysis, although still not as good as a cardiologist, can capture most abnormal rhythms associated with toxicity. As arrhythmogenesis and its electrocardiographic correlates become better understood, automated ECG efficacy/toxicity assessment will likewise improve.

Acknowledgments

This work was supported by NIH Grants R01 HL41663, USPHS Grants R01 HL35554 and R01 HL32131 and by the Upjohn Company. The contributions of the surgical team of Todd Guynn and Michael Haklin at Rush-Presbyterian-St. Luke's Hospital, Chicago, IL, are also gratefully acknowledged.

References

1. Raeder, E. A., Hohnloser, S. H., Graboys, T. B. *et al.* (1988) Spontaneous variability and circadian distribution of ectopic activity in patients with malignant ventricular arrhythmia. *J. Am. Coll. Cardiol.,* **2**, 656–61.
2. Muller, J. E., Tofler, G. H. and Stone, P. H. (1989) Circadian variation and triggers of onset of acute cardiovascular disease. *Circulation,* **79**, 733–43.
3. Cannom, D. S. (1993) Current indications and contraindications for ICD implantation. In: Naccarelli, G. V. and Veltri, E. P. (eds) *Implantable Cardioverter–Defibrillators.* Oxford: Blackwell Scientific Publications.
4. Winkle, R. A., Fain, E. S., Sweeney, M. B., Senelly, K. M. and the Cadence investigators (1992) Survival in patients with ventricular tachyarrhythmias treated with programmable tiered therapy implantable defibrillators. *J. Am. Coll. Cardiol.,* **19**, 209.
5. Harwin, R. M., Ruder, M. A., Gaudini, V. A. *et al.* (1989) Long-term outcome with the automatic implantable cardioverter–defibrillator. *J. Am. Coll. Cardiol.,* **13**, 1353–61.
6. Echt, D. S., Armstrong, K., Schmidt, P. *et al.* (1985) Clinical experience, complications and survival in 70 patients with the automatic implantable cardioverter–defibrillator. *Circulation,* 291–6.
7. Schwendeman, S. P., Amidon, G. L. and Levy, R. J. (1993) Determinants of modulated release of antiarrhythmic drugs by iontophoresis through polymer membranes. *Macromolecules,* **26**, 2264–72.
8. Jelliffe, R. W. (1968) An improved method of digoxin therapy. *Ann. Int. Med.,* **69**, 703–17.

9. Jelliffe, R. W., Buell, J. and Kalaba, R. (1972) Reduction of digitalis toxicity by computer-assisted glycoside dosage regimens. *Ann. Int. Med.,* **77**, 891–906.
10. Jelliffe, R. W., Buell, J. and Kalaba, R. *et al.* (1972) An improved method of digitoxin therapy. *Ann. Int. Med.,* **72**, 453–64.
11. Sheiner, L. B., Halkin, H., Peck, C. *et al.* (1975) Improved computer-assisted digoxin therapy: a method using feedback of measured serum digoxin concentrations. *Ann. Int. Med.,* **82**, 619–27.
12. Peck, C. C., Sheiner, L., Martin, C. M. *et al.* (1973) Computer assisted digoxin therapy. *N. Engl. J. Med.,* **289**, 441–6.
13. Sheiner, L. B., Rosenberg, B. and Melmon, K. L. (1972) Modelling of individual pharmacokinetics for computed-aided drug dosage. *Comp. Biomed. Res.,* **5**, 441–59.
14. Sheiner, L. B., Rosenberg, B. and Marathe, V. V. (1977) Estimation of population characteristics of pharmacokinetic parameters from routine clinical data. *J. Pharm. Biopharm.* **5**, 445–79.
15. Sheiner, L. B., Beal, S., Rosenberg, B. and Marathe, V. V. (1979) Forecasting individual pharmacokinetics. *Clin. Pharmacol. Therapeut.* **25**, 294–305.
16. Jelliffe, R. W. (1987) Clinical applications of pharmacokinetics and adaptive control. *IEEE Trans. Biomed. Eng.,* **34**, 624–32.
17. D'Argenio, D. Z. and Schumitzky, A. (1979) A program package for simulation and parameter estimations in pharmacokinetics systems. *Comp. Progr. Biomed.,* **9**, 115–34.
18. Wagner, J. G. (1971) *Biopharmaceutics and Relevant Pharmacokinetics,* 1st edn. Hamilton, IL: Drug Intelligence.
19. Schwartz, S. L., Wellstein, A. and Woosley, R. L. (1994) Significance of pharmacokinetic principle. In: Singh, B. N., Dzeu, V. J., Vanhoutte, P. M. and Woosley, R. L. (eds) *Cardiovascular Pharmacology and Therapeutics.* New York, NY: Churchill Livingstone.
20. Rowland, M., Thompson, P. D., Guichard, A. and Melmon K. L. (1971) Disposition kinetics of lidocaine disposition in normal subjects. *Ann. NY Acad. Sci.,* **179**, 383–98.
21. Martin, R. W., Hill, H. F., Yee, H. S. *et al.* (1987) An open-loop computer-based drug infusion system. *IEEE Trans. Biomed. Eng.,* **34**, 642–9.
22. Kruger-Themer, K. (1968) Continuous intravenous infusion and multicompartment accumulation. *Eur. J. Pharmacol.,* **4**, 317–24.
23. Collins, S. and Arzbaecher, R. (1977) Automated intravenous antiarrhythmic intravenous drug infusion. *Computers in Cardiology,* pp. 55–60.
24. Jacobs, J. R. (1990) Algorithm for optimal linear model-based control with application to pharmacokinetic model-driven drug delivery. *IEEE Trans. Biomed. Eng.,* **37**, 107–9.
25. Takada, K., Yoshikawa, H. and Muranishi, S. (1985) Optimal dosage regimen calculation program based on the remaining drug concentrations in plasma. *Int. J. Biomed. Comput.,* **16**, 267–75.
26. Wyman, M. G., Lalka, D., Hammersmith, L. *et al.* (1978) Multiple bolus technique for lidocaine administration during the first hours of an acute myocardial infarction. *Am. J. Cardiol.,* **41**, 313–17.
27. Rodman, J. H., Jelliffe, R. W., Kolb, E. *et al.* (1984) Clinical studies with computer-assisted initial lidocaine therapy. *Arch. Int. Med.,* **144**, 703–9.
28. Arzbaecher, R. and Bump, T. E. (1988) Development of an automatic implanted drug infusion system for the management of cardiac arrhythmias. *IEEE Proc.,* **76**, 1204–9.
29. Arzbaecher, R., Ripley, R., Guenneguez, J. *et al.* (1991) A combined monitor and pump controller for management of atrial arrhythmias in postsurgical patients. *Am. Assoc. Med. Instn,* S2:49.
30. Bloem, D. and Arzbaecher, R. (1993) Use of a microprocessor-based pacemaker to control an implantable drug delivery system. *Computers in Cardiology,* pp. 1–4.
31. Bump, T., Brown, J., Yurkonis, C. *et al.* (1987) Optimal control of antiarrhythmic drug infusion. In: Ensminger, W. D. and Selam, J. L. (eds) *Infusion Systems in Medicine,* pp. 249–61. Mount Kisco, NY: Futura Publishing.
32. Jacobs, J. R. (1988) Analytical solution to the three-compartment pharmacokinetic model. *IEEE Trans. Biomed. Eng.,* **35**, 763–5.

33. Jacobs, J. R., Sheppard, L. C. and Reves, J. G. (1988) Simulation of compartment models. *IEEE 8th Int. Conf. Eng. Med. Bio. Soc.*, 702–4.
34. Alvis, J. M., Spain, J. A. and Sheppard, L. C. (1985) Computer-assisted continuous infusion of the intravenous analgesic fentanyl during general anesthesia – an interactive system. *IEEE Tran. Biomed. Eng.*, **32**, 323–9.
35. Brown, R. F. (1980) Compartmental analysis: state of the art. *IEEE Trans. Biomed. Eng.*, **27**, 162–6.
36. Vozeh, S., Wenk, M. and Follath, F. (1984) Experience with NONMEM: analysis of serum concentration data in patients treated with mexiletine and lidocaine. *Drug Metab. Rev.*, **15**, 305–15.
37. Notari, R. E. (1987) *Biopharmaceuticals and Clinical Pharmacokinetics: An Introduction.* New York, NY: Marcel Dekker.
38. Connor, S. B., Quill, T. J. and Jacobs, J. R. (1992) Accuracy of drug infusion pumps under computer control. *IEEE Trans. Biomed. Eng.*, **39**, 980–2.
39. Pioger, G., Jenkins, J., Guezennec, A. *et al.* (1988) Feasibility of computerized exponential infusion of disopyramide in cardiac patients. *J. Electrophysiol.*, **2**, 207–14.
40. Yurkonis, C. and Arzbaecher, R. (1987) Computer simulation of adaptive drug infusion. *IEEE Trans. Biomed. Eng.*, **34**, 633–5.
41. Bloem, D., Arzbaecher, R. and Remy, M. (1993) Microprocessor-based automatic drug infusion system for treatment of paroxysmal atrial fibrillation. *J. Electrocardiogr.*, **26S**, 60.
42. Blackshear, P. J., Dorman, F. D., Blackshear, P. L. J. *et al.* (1970) A permanently implantable self-recycling low flow constant rate multipurpose infusion pump of simple design. *Surg. Forum*, **21**, 136–7.
43. Coombs, D. W., Saunders, R. L., Gaylor, M. and Pagesu, M. G. (1982) Epidural narcotic infusion reservoir; implantation techniques and efficacy. *Anesthesiology*, **56**, 469–73.
44. Erickson, D. L., Backlock, J. B., Michaelson, M. *et al.* (1985) Control of spasticity by implantable continuous flow morphine pump. *Neurosurgery*, **16**, 215–17.
45. Kemeny, N., Cohen, A., Bertino, J. R. *et al.* (1989) Continuous intrahepatic infusion of floxurident and leucovorin through an implantable pump for the treatment of hepatic metastases from colorectal carcinoma. *Cancer*, **65**, 2446–50.
46. Onofrio, B. M., Yaksh, T. L. and Arnold, P. G. (1981) Continuous low-dose morphine administration in the treatment of chronic pain of malignant origin. *Mayo Clin. Proc.*, **16**, 215–17.
47. Penn, R. D. and Kroin, J. S. (1987) Long-term intrathecal baclofen infusion for treatment of spasticity. *J. Neurosurg.*, **66**, 1981–5.
48. Edelman, E. R., Brown, L., Taylor, J. and Langer, R. (1987) *In vitro* and *in vivo* kinetics of regulated drug released from polymer matrices by oscillating magnetic fields. *J. Biomed. Mater. Res.*, **21**, 339–53.
49. Edelman, E. R., Fiorino, A., Grodzinsky, A. and Langer, R. (1992) Mechanical deformation of polymer matrix controlled release devices modulates drug release. *J. Biomed. Mater. Rest.*, **26**, 1619–31.
50. Edelman, E. R. and Langer, R. (1993) Optimization of release from magnetically controlled polymeric drug release devices. *Biomaterials*, **14**, 621–6.
51. Kost, J., Noecker, R., Kunica, E. and Langer, R. (1985) Magnetically controlled release systems: effect of polymer composition. *J. Biomed. Mater. Res.*, **19**, 935–40.
52. Kost, J., Wolfrum, J. and Langer, R. (1987) Magnetically enhanced insulin release in diabetic rats. *J. Biomed. Mater. Res.*, **21**, 1367–73.
53. Kost, J., Leong, K. and Langer, R. (1989) Ultrasound-enhanced polymer degradation and release of incorporated substances. *Proc. Natl Acad. Sci. USA*, **86**, 7663–6.
54. Slate, J. B. and Sheppard, L. C. (1979) A model for design of a blood pressure controller for hypertensive patients. *IEEE Proc. Eng Med. Biol. Soc.* Denver, 285–9.
55. Sheppard, L. C. and Sayers, B. M. (1977) Dynamic analysis of the blood pressure response to hypotensive agents studied in postsurgical patients. *Comp. Biomed. Res.*, **10**, 237.

56. Jannett, T. C. and Sheppard, L. C. (1987) Modeling the rate of premature ventricular contractions and its response to lidocaine infusion. *IEEE Trans. Biomed. Eng.,* **34**, 636–41.
57. Junter, G. A. (1988) *Electrochemical Detection Techniques in the Applied Biosciences: Analysis and Clinical Applications.* Vol. 1. New York: John Wiley.
58. Meyerhoff, M. E. (1993) *In vivo* blood-gas and electrolyte sensors: progress and challenges. *Trends Analyt. Chem.,* **12**, 257–66.
59. Telting-Diaz, M. W., Collison, M. E. and Meyerhoff, M. E. (1994) Simplified dual-lumen catheter design for simultaneous potentiometric monitoring of carbon dioxide and pH. *Anal. Chem.,* **66**, 576–83.
60. Haase, E. A. Spichiger, U. E., Schlatter, K. J. *et al.* (1992) Continuous monitoring of electrolytes during hemodialysis. *GIT Labor-Medizin,* **15**, 84–7.
61. Kyrolainen, M., Hakanson, H., Ekroth, R. and Mattiasson, B. (1993) Biosensor monitoring of blood lactate during open-heart surgery. *Anal. Chim. Acta,* **279**, 149–53.
62. Reach, G. and Wilson, G. S. (1992) Can continuous glucose monitoring be used for the treatment of diabetes? *Anal. Chem.,* **64**, 381A–6A.
63. Meyerhoff, M. E. (1990) New *in vitro* analytical approaches for clinical chemistry measurements in critical care. *Clin. Chem.,* **36**, 1567–72.
64. Cosofret, V. V. and Buck, R. P. (1993) Recent advances in pharmaceutical analysis with potentiometric membrane sensors. *Crit. Rev. Anal. Chem.,* **24**, 1–58.
65. Cosofret, V. V. and Buck, R. P. (1986) A poly(vinyl chloride) membrane electrode for the determination of phenytoin in pharmaceutical formulations. *J. Pharm. Biomed. Anal.,* **4**, 45–51.
66. Eppelsheim, C., Brauchle, C. and Hampp, N. (1992) Ion-selective electrodes for the determination of the antiarrhythmic drug bretylium. *Analyst,* **117**, 1609–12.
67. Leng, Z. Z. and Hu, X. Y. (1989) PVC membrane mexiletine selective electrodes. *Fenxi Huaxue,* **17**, 854.
68. Satake, A., Miyata, T. and Kaneshina, S. (1991) Coated wire electrodes sensitive to local anesthetic cations and their application to potentiometric determination. *Bull. Chem. Soc. Jap.,* **64**, 3029–34.
69. Takisawa, N., Hall, D. G., Wyn-Jones, E. and Brown, P. (1988) The construction and characterization of drug-selective electrodes. *J. Chem. Soc. Faraday Trans.,* **84**, 3059–70.
70. Bo, Z. G. and Lu, X. H. (1990) Poly(vinyl chloride) membrane electrode for the determination of verapamil. *Anal. Chim. Acta,* **235**, 461–4.
71. Adams, R. (1990) *In vivo* electrochemical measurements in the CNS. *Progr. Neurobiol.,* **35**, 297–311.
72. Osteryoung, J. G. and Schreiner, M. M. (1988) Recent advances in pulse voltammetry. *Crit. Rev. Anal. Chem.,* **19**, S1–S27.
73. Meulemans, A. (1987) Measurement of electroactive antibiotic drugs in the blood stream of rats with a catheter electrode. *Anal. Chem.,* **59**, 1872–4.
74. Heineman, W. R., Swaile, B. H., Blubaugh, E. A. *et al.* (1993) Chemical sensors for radiopharmaceuticals. *Radiochim. Acta,* **63**, 199–203.
75. Johnson, J. M., Halsall, H. B. and Heineman, W. R. (1982) Potential dependent enzymatic activity in an enzyme thin layer cell. *Anal. Chem.,* **54**, 1377–83.
76. Pace, S. J. (1981) Surface modifications and commercial application. *Sens. Actuat.,* **4**, 475–525.
77. Heineman, W. R. and Kissinger, P. T. (1980) Analytical electrochemistry: methodology and applications of dynamic techniques. *Anal. Chem.,* **52**, 138R–51R.
78. Sepaniak, M. J., Tromberg, B. J. and Eastham, J. F. (1983) Optical fiber fluoro-probes in clinical analysis. *Clin. Chem.,* **29**, 1678–82.
79. Wolfbeis, O. S. and Koller, E. (1991) Sensor chemistry. In: Wolfbeis, O. S. (ed.) *Fiber Optic Chemical Sensors and Biosensors,* Vol. 1, pp. 330–58. Boca Raton: CRC Press.
80. He, H., Li, H., Uray, G. and Wolfbeis, O. S. (1993) Non-enzymatic optical sensor for penicillins. *Talanta,* **40**, 453–7.
81. He, H. and Wolfbeis, O. S. (1990) An enantioselective optode for the β-blocker propranolol. *Proc. Int. Soc. Optical Eng.,* **1368**, 175–81.

82. Guilbault, G. G. (1984) *Analytical Uses of Immobilized Enzymes*. New York, NY: Marcel Dekker.
83. Kulp, T. J., Camins, I., Angel, S. L. *et al.* (1987) Polymer immobilized enzyme optrodes for the determination of penicillin. *Anal. Chem.*, **59**, 2849–53.
84. Jonsson, U. (1992) Real time biospecific interaction analysis. *Proceedings of the Second World Congress on Biosensors*, pp. 260–6. Geneva.
85. Anderson, F. P. and Miller, W. G. (1988) Fiber optic immunochemical sensor for continuous, reversible measurement of phenytoin. *Clin. Chem.*, **34**, 1417–21.
86. Keating, M. Y. and Rechnitz, G. A. (1984) Potentiometric digoxin antibody measurements with antigen-ionophore based membrane electrodes. *Anal. Chem.*, **34**, 801–6.
87. Wong, D. K. and Jordon, W. S. (1992) Microprocessor-based near real-time bedside blood chemistry monitor. *Int. J. Clin. Monit. Comp.*, **9**, 95–102.
88. Galeazzi, R. L., Benet, L. Z. and Sheiner, L. B. (1976) Relationship between the pharmacokinetics and pharmacodynamics of procainamide. *Clin. Pharm. Therapeut.*, **20**, 278–89.
89. Koch-Weser, J. (1971) Pharmacokinetics of procainamide in man. *Ann. NY Acad. Sci.*, **179**, 370–82.
90. Franz, M. R., Koller, B. and Woosley, R. L. (1994) Pharmacologic therapy in cardiac arrhythmias: principles and background. In: Singh, B. N., Dzeu, V. J., Vanhoutte, P. M. and Woosley, R. L. (eds) *Cardiovascular Pharmacology and Therapeutics*, New York, NY: Churchill Livingstone.
91. Heissenbutal, R. H. and Bigger, J. T. (1970) The effect of oral quinidine on intraventricular conduction in man: correlation of plasma quinidine with changes in QRS duration. *Am. Heart J.*, **80**, 453–62.
92. Platia, E. V., Wisfeldt, M. and Franz, M. R. (1988) Immediate quantitation of antiarrhythmic drug effect by monophasic action potential recording in coronary artery disease. *Am. J. Cardiol.*, **61**, 1284–7.
93. Zaza, A., Malfatto, G., Ravelli, F. and Schwartz, P. J. (1994) Rate dependence of cardiac repolarization: autonomic modulation and interference with antiarrhythmic drug action. In: Singh, B., Wellens, H., Hiroka, M. (eds) *Electropharmacological Control of Cardiac Arrhythmias*. Mount Kisco, NY: Futura Publishing.
94. Hondeghem, L. M. (1987) Antiarrhythmic agents: modulated receptor applications. *Circulation*, **75**, 514.
95. Sadanga, T., Ogawa, S., Okada, Y. *et al.* (1993) Clinical evaluation of the use-dependent QRS prolongation and the reverse use-dependent QT prolongation of class I and class III antiarrhythmic agents and their value in predicting efficacy. *Am. Heart J.*, **126**, 115–21.
96. Roden, D. M. (1993) Current status of class III antiarrhythmic drug therapy. *Am. J. Cardiol.*, **72**, 44B–9B.
97. The Cardiac Arrhythmia Suppression Trial (CAST) investigators (1989) Preliminary report: effect of encainide and flecainide on mortality in a randomized trial of arrhythmia suppression after myocardial infarction. *N. Engl. J. Med.*, **321**, 406–12.
98. Singh, B. N. (ed.) (1988) *Control of Cardiac Arrhythmias by Lengthening Repolarization*. Mount Kisko, NY: Futura Publishing.
99. Woosley, R. L. M S (1993) QT interval: a measure of drug action. *Am. J. Cardiol.*, **72**, 36B–43B.
100. Roden, D. M. (1988) Role of the electrocardiogram in determining electrophysiologic end points of drug therapy. *Am. J. Cardiol.*, **62**, 34H–8H.
101. DiMarco, J. P., VanderLugt, J. T., Lee, K. S. and Gibson, J. K. (1994) Ibutilide. In: Singh, B., Wellens, H. and Hiroka, M. (eds) *Electropharmacological Control of Cardiac Arrhythmias*. Mount Kisco, NY: Futura Publishing.
102. Garson, A. J. (1993) How to measure the QT interval – what is normal? *Am. J. Cardiol.*, **72**, 14B–16B.
103. Cowan, J. C., Hilton, C. J. and Griffiths, C. J. (1988) Sequence of epicardial repolarization and configuration of the T wave. *Br. Heart J.*, **60**, 424.

104. Day, C. P., McComb, J. M. and Campbell, R. W. F. (1990) QT dispersion: an indication of arrhythmia risk in patients with long QT intervals. *Br. Heart J.*, **63**, 342–4.
105. Moore, E. J. (1993) Mechanisms and models to predict a QT_c effect. *Am. J. Cardiol.*, **72**, 4B–9B.
106. Funck-Bretano, C., and Jaillon, P. (1993) Rate-corrected QT interval: techniques and limitations. *Am. J. Cardiol.*, **72**, 17B–22B.
107. Ahnve, S. and Vallin, H. (1982) Influence of heart rate and inhibition of autonomic tone on the QT interval. *Circulation*, **65**, 435–9.
108. Murakawa, Y., Inoue, H., Nozaki, A. and Sugimoto, T. (1992) Role of sympathovagal interaction in diurnal variation of QT interval. *Am. J. Cardiol.*, **69**, 330–43.
109. Morganroth, J., Brozovich, F. V., McDonald, J. T. and Jacobs, R. A. (1991) Variability of the QT measurement in healthy men, with implications for selection of an abnormal QT value to predict drug toxicity and proarrhythmia. *Am. J. Cardiol.*, **67**, 774–7.
110. Schmitt, C., Beyer, T., Karch, M. *et al.* (1992) Sotalol exhibits reverse use-dependent action on monophasic action potentials in normal but not in infarcted canine ventricular myocardium. *J. Cardiovasc. Pharmacol.*, **19**, 487–92.
111. O'Donoghue, S. and Platia, E. (1991) Monophasic action potential recordings: evaluation of antiarrhythmic drugs. *Progr. Cardiovasc. Dis.*, **34**, 1–14.
112. Patterson, E., Jackman, W. M., Scherlag, B. J. and Lazzarfa, R. (1991) The monophasic action potential in clinical cardiology. *Clin. Cardiol.*, **14**, 505–10.
113. Franz, M. R. (1983) Long-term recording of monophasic action potentials from human endocardium. *Am. J. Cardiol.*, **51**, 1629–34.
114. Ino, T., Karagueuzian, H. S., Hong, K. *et al.* (1988) Relation of monophasic action potential recorded with contact electrode to underlying transmembrane action potential properties in isolated cardiac tissues: a systematic microelectrode validation study. *Cardiovasc. Res.*, **22**, 255–64.
115. Echt, D. S., Berte, L. E., Clusin, W. T. *et al.* (1982) Prolongation of the human cardiac monophasic action potential by sotalol. *Am. J. Cardiol.*, **50**, 1082–9.
116. Brugada, J., Sassine, A., Escande, D. *et al.* (1987) Effects of quinidine on ventricular repolarization. *Eur. Heart J.*, **8**, 1340–5.
117. Dorf, R. (1983) *Modern Control Systems*, 3rd edn. Reading, MA: Addison-Wesley.
118. Packer, J., Mason, D. G., Cade, J. F. and McKinley, S. M. (1987) An adaptive controller for closed-loop management of blood pressure in seriously ill patients. *IEEE Trans. Biomed. Eng.*, **34**, 612–16.
119. Sheppard, L. C., Kouchoukas, N. T., Schotts, J. F. and Wallace, E. D. (1978) Regulation of mean arterial pressure by computer control of vasoactive agents in postoperative patients. *IEEE Proceedings of Computers in Cardiology*.
120. *Jaklitsh, R. R. and Westenkow, D. R. (1987) A model-based self-adjusting two-phase controller for vecuronium-induced muscle relaxation during anesthesia. IEEE Trans. Biomed. Eng., 34, 583–94.*
121. Stern, K. S., Walker, B. K. and Katona, P. G. (1981) Automated blood pressure using a self-tuning regulator. *IEEE Proceedings on Frontiers of Engineering in Health Care*, pp. 255–8. Houston, TX.
122. Arnsparger, J. M., McInnis, B. C., Glover, J. R. and Normann, N. A. (1983) Adaptive control of blood pressure. *IEEE Trans. Biomed. Eng.*, **30**, 168–76.
123. Koivo, A. J. (1980) Automatic continuous-time blood pressure control in dogs by means of hypotensive drug injection. *IEEE Trans. Biomed. Eng.*, **27**, 574–81.
124. Ljung, L. and Soderström, T. (1987) *Theory and Practice of Recursive Identification*. Cambridge, MA: MIT Press.
125. Voss, G. I., Chizeck, H. J. and Katona, P. G. (1988) Self-tuning controller for drug delivery systems. *Int. J. Controls*, **47**, 1507–20.
126. Voss, I. G., Katona, G. P. and Chizek, J. H. (1987) Adaptive multivariable drug delivery: control of arterial pressure and cardiac output in anesthetized dogs. *IEEE Trans. Biomed. Eng.*, **34**, 617–23.
127. Voss, G. I., Chizeck, H. J. and Katona, P. G. (1987) Regarding self-tuning regulators for non-minimum phase plants. *Automatica*, **23**, 405.

128. Sobel, K., Kaufman, H. and Yekutile, O. (1980) Direct discrete model reference adaptive control: the multivariable case. *Proc. 19th IEEE Conference on Decision and Control*, pp. 1152–7.
129. Goodwin, G. C. and Sin, K. S. (1984) *Adaptive Filtering, Prediction, and Control*. Englewood Cliffs, NJ: Prentice-Hall.
130. Kaufman, H., Roy, R. and Xu, X. (1984) Model reference adaptive control of drug infusion rate. *Automatica*, 205–9.
131. Pajunen, G. A., Steinmetz, M. and Shankar, R. (1990) Model reference adaptive control with constraints for postoperative blood pressure management. *IEEE Trans. Biomed. Eng.*, **37**, 679–87.
132. Lainiotis, D. G., Upadhyay, T. N. and Deshpande, J. G. (1971) A nonlinear separation thereom. *Proc. Symp. Nonlinear Estimation Theory, San Diego, CA*, pp. 184–7.
133. Martin, J. F., Schneider, A. M. and Smith, N. T. (1987) Multiple model adaptive control of blood pressure using sodium nitroprusside. *IEEE Trans. Biomed. Eng.*, **34**, 603–11.
134. He, W. G., Kaufman, H., Roy, R. (1986) Multiple-model adaptive control procedure for blood pressure control. *IEEE Trans. Biomed. Eng.*, **33**: 10–19.
135. Cobelli, C., Ruggeri, A., Distefano, J. J. and Landaw, E. M. (1985) Optimal design of multioutput sampling schedules – software and applications to endocrine–metabolic and pharmaceutic models. *IEEE Trans. Biomed. Eng.*, **32**, 249–55.
136. D'Argenio, D. Z. (1981) Optimal sampling times for pharmacokinetic experiments. *J. Pharm. Biopharm.*, **9**, 739–56.
137. Vozeh, S., Uematsu, T., Ritz, R. *et al.* (1987) Computer-assisted individualized lidocaine dosage: clinical evaluation and comparison with physician performance. *Am. Heart J.*, **113**, 928–33.
138. Beach, C. L., Farringer, J. A., Peck, C. C. *et al.* (1988) Clinical assessment of a two-compartment Bayesian forecasting method for lidocaine. *Ther. Drug Monitor.*, **10**, 74–9.
139. Richards, D. A. B., Byth, K., Ross, D. L. and Uther, J. B. (1991) What is the best predictor of spontaneous ventricular tachycardia and sudden death after myocardial infarction? *Circulation*, **83**, 756–63.
140. Mason, J. W. and Winkle, R. A. (1980) Accuracy of the ventricular tachycardia – induction study for predicting long-term efficacy and inefficacy of antiarrhythmic drugs. *N. Eng. J. Med.*, **303**, 1073–77.
141. Mitchell, L. B., Duff, H. J., Manyari, D. E. and Wyse, D. G. (1987) A randomized clinical trial of the noninvasive and invasive approaches to drug therapy of ventricular tachycardia. *N. Engl. J. Med.*, **317**, 1681–7.
142. Mason, J. and the ESVEM investigators (1993) A comparison of electrophysiologic testing with Holter monitoring to predict antiarrhythmic drug efficacy for ventricular tachyarrhythmias. *N. Engl. J. Med.*, **329**, 445–51.
143. Podrid, P. J., Bilazarian, S. D. and Fuchs, T. (1993) Prognostic importance of ventricular premature beats. In: Kapoor, A. S. and Singh, B. N. (eds) *Prognosis and Risk Assessment in Cardiovascular Disease*, pp. 367–402. New York, NY: Churchill Livingstone.
144. Wyman, M. G. and Hammersmith, L. (1974) Comprehensive treatment plan for the prevention of primary ventricular fibrillation in acute myocardial infarction. *Am. J. Cardiol.*, **33**, 661–7.
145. Greenblatt, D. J., Koch-Weser, J. *et al.* (1976) Pharmacokinetic approach to the clinical use of lidocaine intravenously. *JAMA*, **236**, 273–7.
146. Collins, S. M. and Arzbaecher, R. C. (1979) Feedback control in the management of cardiac arrhythmias. *ISA Trans.*, **18**, 95–100.
147. Carlsson, L., Abrahamsson, C., Anderson, B. *et al.* (1993) Proarrhythmic effects of the class III agent almokalant: importance of infusion rate, QT dispersion, and early afterdepolarisation. *Cardiovasc. Res.*, **27**, 2186–93.
148. Day, C. P., McComb, J. M. and Campbell, R. W. F. (1991) Reduction in QT dispersion by sotalol following myocardial infarction. *Eur. Heart J.*, **12**, 423–7.
149. De Ambroggi, L., Negroni, M. S., Monza, E. *et al.* (1991) Dispersion of ventricular repolarization in the long QT syndrome. *Am. J. Cardiol.*, **68**, 614–20.

150. Hii, J. T. Y., Wyse, D. G., Gillis, A. G. *et al.* (1992) Precordial QT interval dispersion as a marker of torsades de pointes: disparate effects of class IA antiarrhythmic drugs and amiodarone. *Circulation,* **86**, 1376–82.
151. Linker, N. J., Colonna, P., Kekwick, C. A. *et al.* (1992) Assessment of QT dispersion in symptomatic patients with congenital long QT syndromes. *Am. J. Cardiol.,* **69**, 634–8.
152. Dritsas, A., Gilligan, D., Nihoyannopoulos and Oakley, C. M. (1992) Amiodarone reduces QT dispersion in patients with hypertrophic cardiomyopathy. *Int. J. Cardiol.,* **36**, 345–9.
153. Winters, S. L., Stewart, D., Targonski, A. and Gomes, J. A. (1988) Role of signal averaging of the surface QRS complex in selecting patients with nonsustained ventricular tachycardia and high grade ventricular arrhythmias for programmed ventricular stimulation. *J. Am. Coll. Cardiol.,* **12**, 1481–7.
154. Kulakowski, P., Bashire, Y., Heald, S. *et al.* (1992) Prediction of antiarrhythmic efficacy of class I and III agents in patients with ventricular tachycardia by signal-averaged ECG analysis. *PACE,* **15**, 2116–21.
155. Hopson, J. R., Kienzle, M. G., Aschoff, A. M. and Shirkey, D. R. (1993) Noninvasive prediction of efficacy of type IA antiarrhythmic drugs by the signal-averaged electrocardiogram in patients with coronary artery disease and sustained ventricular tachycardia. *Am. J. Cardiol.,* **72**, 288–93.
156. Funck-Brentano, C. (1993) Rate-dependence of class III actions in the heart. *Fund. Clin. Pharmacol.,* **7**, 51–9.
157. Fontaine, G. (1992) A new look at torsades de pointes. *Ann. NY Acad. Sci.,* **644**, 157–77.
158. Akselrod, S., Gordon, D., Ubel, F. A. *et al.* (1981) Power spectrum analysis of heart rate fluctuation: a quantitative probe of beat-to-beat cardiovascular control. *Science,* **213**, 220–2.
159. Malik, M. and Camm, A. L. (1990) Heart rate variability. *Clin. Cardiol.,* **13**, 570–6.
160. Odemuyiwa, O., Malik, M., Farrell, T. *et al.* (1991) Comparison of the predictive characteristics of heart rate variability index and left ventricular ejection fraction for all-cause mortality, arrhythmic events and sudden death after acute myocardial infarction. *Am. J. Cardiol.,* **68**, 434–9.
161. Farrell, T. G., Bashire, Y., Cripps, T. *et al.* (1991) Risk stratification for arrhythmic events in postinfarction patients based on heart rate variability, ambulatory electrocardiographic variables and the signal-averaged electrocardiogram. *J. Am. Coll. Cardiol.,* **18**, 687–97.
162. Bigger, J. T., Fleiss, J. L., Rolnitzky, L. M. *et al.* (1991) Time course of recovery of heart period variability after myocardial infarction. *J. Am. Coll. Cardiol.,* **18**, 1643–9.
163. American College of Cardiology Cardiovascular Technology Assessment Committee (1993) Heart rate variability for risk stratification of life-threatening arrhythmias. *J. Am. Coll. Cardiol.,* **22**, 948–50.
164. Zuanetti, G., Latini, R., Neilson, J. M. M. *et al.* (1990) Heart rate variability in patients with ventricular arrhythmias: effect of antiarrhythmic drugs. *J. Am. Coll. Cardiol.,* **17**, 604–12.
165. Hohnloser, S. H., Klingenheben, T., Zabel, M. and Just, J. (1993) Effect of sotalol on heart rate variability assessed by Holter monitoring in patients with ventricular arrhythmias. *Am. J. Cardiol.,* **72**, 67A–72A.
166. Ligtenberg, A. and Kunt, M. (1983) A robust-digital QRS-detection algorithm for arrhythmia monitoring. *Comp. Biomed. Res.,* **16**, 273–86.
167. Pahlm, O. and Sornmo, L. (1984) Software QRS detection in ambulatory monitoring – a review. *Med. Biol. Eng. Comput.,* **22**, 289–97.
168. Thakor, N. V., Webster, J. G. and Tompkins, W. J. (1984) Design, implementation and evaluation of a microcomputer-based portable arrhythmia monitor. *Med. Biol. Eng. Comput.,* **22**, 151–9.
169. Jenkins, J. M. (1983) Automated electrocardiography and arrhythmia monitoring. *Progr. Cardiovasc. Dis.,* **25**, 367–408.
170. Throne, R. D., Jenkins, J. M. and Di Carlo, L. A. (1991) A comparison of four new time-domain techniques for discriminating monomorphic ventricular tachycardia from sinus rhythm using ventricular waveform morphology. *IEEE Trans. Biomed. Eng.,* **38**, 561–70.

171. Chiang, C. M. J., Jenkins, J. M., DiCarlo, L. A. *et al.* (1993) Real-time arrhythmia identification from automated analysis of intraatrial and intraventricular electrograms. *PACE*, **16**, 223–7.
172. DiCarlo, L. A., Jenkins, J. M., Winston, S. A. and Kriegler, C. (1992) Differentiation of ventricular tachycardia from ventricular fibrillation using intraventricular electrogram morphology. *Am. J. Cardiol.*, **70**, 820–2.
173. Greenhut, S. E., Jenkins, J. M. and DiCarlo, L. A. (1991) Computerized interpretation of the paced ECG. *J. Electrocardiogr.*, **24**, 147–52.
174. DiCarlo, L. A., Lin, D. and Jenkins, J. M. (1993) Automated interpretation of cardiac arrhythmias. *J. Electrocardiogr.*, **26**, 53–67.
175. Windyga, P., Almeida, D., Passariello, G. *et al.* (1991) Knowledge-based approach to the management of serious arrhythmia in the CCU. *Med. Biol. Eng. Comput.*, **29**, 254–60.
176. Pryor, A., Goldberg, R., Brown, W. F. and Anderson, J. (1984) Computerized arrhythmia management of patients in a coronary care unit. *Computers in Cardiology*, pp. 25–30. IEEE Computer Society.
177. Porenta, G., Peahringer, B., Binder, T. *et al.* (1988) A decision support system for selecting and assessing antiarrhythmic therapies. *Computers in Cardiology*, pp. 137–40. IEEE Computer Society.
178. Hulstaert, F., De Jonghe, D., Bouckaert, A. *et al.* (1987) The design of an expert system for the management of cardiac arrhythmias. *Computers in Cardiology*, pp. 231–4. IEEE Computer Society.
179. Guarino, N., Bortolan, G., Cabaggion, C. and Degan, I. R. (1985) Rhythm analysis and clinical management of arrhythmias using AI techniques. *Computers in Cardiology*, pp. 181–4. IEEE Computer Society.
180. Levine, R. (1990) *Artificial Intelligence and Expert Systems: A Comprehensive Guide*, 2nd edn. New York, NY: McGraw Hill.
181. Williams, B. T. (1982) *Computer Aids to Clinical Decisions*. Boca Raton: CRC Press.
182. Winston, P. H. (1992) *Artificial Intelligence* 3rd edn. Reading, MA: Addison-Wesley.
183. Greenwald, S. D., Patil, R. S. and Mark, R. G. (1992) Improved detection and classification of arrhythmias in noise-corrupted electrocardiograms using contextual information within an expert system. *Biomed. Inst. Tech.*, **26**, 124–32.
184. Bialy, D., Lehman, M. H., Schumacher, D. N. *et al.* (1992) Hospitalization for arrhythmias in the United States: importance of atrial fibrillation. *J. Am. Coll. Cardiol.*, **19**, 41A.
185. Katz, L. and Pick, A. (1956) *Clinical Electrocardiography. Part I. The Arrhythmias*. Philadelphia: Lea and Febiger.
186. Stroke Prevention in Atrial Fibrillation Study Group Investigators (1991) Stroke prevention in atrial fibrillation study: final results. *Circulation*, **84**, 527–39.
187. Rawles, J. M., Metcalfe, M. J. and Jennings, K. (1990) Time of occurrence, duration and ventricular rate of paroxysmal atrial fibrillation: the effect of digoxin. *Br. Heart J.*, **63**, 225–7.
188. Coplen, S. E., Antman, E. M., Berlin, J. A. *et al.* (1990) Efficacy and safety of quinidine therapy for maintenance of sinus rhythm after cardioversion: a meta-analysis of randomized control trials. *Circulation*, **82**, 1106–16.
189. Falk, R. H. (1989) Flecainide-induced ventricular tachycardia and fibrillation in patients treated for atrial fibrillation. *An. Int. Med.*, **111**, 107–11.
190. Lown, B., Perlroth, M. G., Kaidbey, S. *et al.* (1963) 'Cardioversion' of atrial fibrillation: A report on the treatment of 65 episodes in 50 patients. *N. Engl. J. Med.*, **269**, 325–31.
191. Pansegrau, D. G. and Abboud, F. M. (1970) Hemodynamic effects of ventricular defibrillation. *J. Clin. Invest.*, **49**, 282–97.
192. Dahl, C. F., Ewy, G. A., Warner, E. D. and Thomas, E. D. (1974) Myocardial necrosis from direct current countershock: effect of paddle size and time interval between discharge. *Circulation*, **50**, 956–61.
193. Kumugai, K., Yamanouchi, Y., Tashiro, N. *et al.* (1990) Low energy synchronous transcatheter cardioversion of atrial flutter/fibrillation in the dog. *J. Am. Coll. Cardiol.*, **16**, 497–501.

194. Kalman, J. M. and Tonkin, A. M. (1992) Atrial fibrillation: epidemiology and the risk and prevention of stroke. *PACE*, **15**, 1332–46.
195. Cooper, R. A. S., Alferness, C. A., Smith, W. M. and Ideker, R. E. (1993) Internal cardioversion of atrial fibrillation in sheep. *Circulation*, **87**, 1673–86.
196. Powell, A. C., Garan, H., McGovern, B. A. *et al.* (1992) Low energy conversation of atrial fibrillation in sheep. *J. Am. Coll. Cardiol.*, **20**, 707–11.
197. Cox, J. L., Boineau, J. P., Schuessler, R. *et al.* (1991) Successful surgical treatment of atrial fibrillation. *JAMA*, **266**, 1976–80.
198. Roberts, S. A., Diaz, C., Nolan, P. E. *et al.* (1993) Effectiveness and costs of digoxin treatment for atrial fibrillation and flutter. *Am. J. Cardiol.*, **72**, 567–73.
199. Lewis, T. (1992) The value of quinidine in cases of auricular fibrillation and methods of studying the clinical reaction. *Am. J. Med. Sci.*, **163**, 781–94.
200. Viko, L. E., Marvin, H. M. and White, P. D. (1923) A clinical report on the use of quinidine sulfate. *Arch. Int. Med.*, **31**, 345–63.
201. Sokolow, M. and Ball, R. E. (1956) Factors influencing conversion of chronic atrial fibrillation with special reference to serum quinidine concentration. *Circulation*, **14**, 568–83.
202. Halpern, S. W., Ellrodt, G., Singh, B. N. and Mandel, W. J. (1980) Efficacy of intravenous procainamide infusion in converting atrial fibrillation to sinus rhythm. *Br. Heart J.*, **44**, 589–95.
203. Fenster, P. E., Comess, K. A., Marsh, R. *et al.* (1983) Conversion of atrial fibrillation to sinus rhythm by acute intravenous procainamide infusion. *Am. Heart J.*, **106**, 501–4.
204. Suttorp, K. J., Kingma, J. H., Jessurun, E. R. *et al.* (1990) The value of class IC antiarrhythmic drugs for acute conversion of paroxysmal atrial fibrillation or flutter to sinus rhythm. *J. Am. Coll. Cardiol.*, **16**, 1722–27.
205. Campbell, T. J., Gavaghan, T. P. and Morgan, J. J. (1985) Intravenous sotalol for the treatment of atrial fibrillation and flutter after cardiopulmonary bypass: comparison with disopyramide and digoxin in a randomized trial. *Br. Heart J.*, **54**, 86–90.
206. Margolis, B., DeSilva, R. E. and Lown, B. (1980) Episodic drug treatment in the management of paroxysmal arrhythmias. *Am. J. Cardiol.*, **45**, 621–5.
207. Jenkins, J., Noh, K., Guezennec, A. *et al.* (1988) Diagnosis of atrial fibrillation using electrograms from chronic leads: evaluation of computer algorithms. *PACE*, **11**, 622–31.
208. Wells, J., Karp, R., Kouchoukos, N. *et al.* (1978) Characterization of atrial fibrillation in man: studies following open heart surgery. *PACE*, **1**, 426–38.
209. Arzbaecher, R., Bump, T., Yurkonis, C. and Bloem, D. (1991) Pacemaker sensing during atrial fibrillation. *13th Int. Conf. IEEE Eng. Med. Biol. Soc.*, **13**, 730–1.
210. Goldreyer, R. (1985) Atrial sensing in permanent pacing systems. In: Barold, S. (ed.) *Modern Cardiac Pacing*, pp. 121–36. Mount Kisco, NY: Futura Publishing.
211. Collins, S. (1977) *A Computer-Based Integrated System for Intravenous Antiarrhythmic Drug Management*. PhD Thesis, University of Illinois at Chicago Circle.

Index

(*Italic* page numbers refer to figures and tables)

Accelerated arteriopathies 2, 79–101
  atherosclerotic lesions 81, *82*
  extracellular matrix 83
  immune/inflammatory cells recruitment 83
  pathogenesis 84–6
    vessel trauma 53
  pathology 79–84
  targeted therapies 53–5
    antisense technology 86–101
    cell-adhesion molecules 60–5
    extracellular matrix 66–9
    monoclonal antibodies 65–6
    proliferating smooth muscle cell selective
      ablation 55–60
  vascular injury surface markers 54
  see also Restenosis
ACCORD trial 216
Acebutolol, iontophoretic delivery 393
Acetylcholine
  endothelial cell nitric oxide stimulation 215
  endothelium-dependent vasodilator function 204
    atherosclerosis 206, 207
    endothelial damage 204–5
Acidic fibroblast growth factor (aFGF)
  cardiomyocyte growth regulation 277
  injury-associated release, targeted therapies 55
Adenovirus vectors
  duration of gene expression *185*, 185, 192, 317
  hepatic gene transfer
    apolipoprotein A1 (Apo A1) 192
    LDL-receptor deficiency 189–90, *190*
  myocardial gene transfer *194*, 194, *195*, 316–18
    local therapy 317, 318
  toxicity 192
  vessel wall gene transfer 179, 181–2, *182*, *185*,
    185
    efficiency of transfer 181, *182*
    hirudin expression 188
    level of recombinant gene expression 181,
      182, *183*
    safety 186
ADP
  endothelial cell nitric oxide stimulation 215
  restenosis pathophysiology 3
Adult respiratory distress syndrome (ARDS) 251
  endogenous NO production impairment 250
  nitric oxide inhalation 251, 254–6, *255*, *256*
  pulmonary hypertension 251
  pulmonary vascular changes 251
  systemic vasodilators 251

aFGF-PE40 60
aFGF-PE4E-KDEL 60
AIMS trial 113, 149
Alfentinyl, pharmacokinetic parameters
  estimation 411
Almitrine 255
Alpha-1 adrenergic receptors, cardiomyocyte
  growth regulation 275
Amiodarone
  clinical trials 332–4
  QT prolongation 440
  side effects 333, 334
  structure *333*
Amperometric sensors 416–19
  enzyme biosensors 420
Amyl nitrite 216
Angiogenesis
  myocardial gene transfer 193, 314, 320–1
  polymer-based controlled drug delivery 35, 42
Angiogenic factors, myocardial gene transfer 193
  coronary collateral circulation promotion 314,
    320–1
Angiopeptin 86
  local therapies 223
    porous balloon catheter release 33
  restenosis prevention 10
Angiotensin II 233–44
  AT-1 receptor 238
  AT-2 receptor 237–8
  cardiac myocyte production 276
  endothelin expression regulation 277
  extracellular matrix production 239
  hypertension 242–3
  local tissue systems 234–5
  myocardial infarction 276
  pathogenic role 235–40
    atherosclerosis 235–6
  smooth muscle cells (SMC) growth response
    86, 238–9
  smooth muscle cells (SMC) migration 86, 239
  thrombosis 240
  vascular remodelling 237–40, 276
Angiotensin II receptors 276
Angiotensin-converting enzyme (ACE) 234
  atherosclerotic plaque expression 239
  carotid artery vascular pathology 235
  gene deletion polymorphism 235
  myocardial infarction risk 235
  plasma level variation, associated pathology
    235

Angiotensin-converting enzyme (ACE) (*cont.*)
  vessel wall expression
    antisense oligonucleotide inhibition 242
    enhancement 243
Angiotensin-converting enzyme (ACE) inhibitors
    780
  antihypertensive effects 234–5
  congestive heart failure 313
  myocardial infarction 120–1, 240
  restenosis 10, 242
  tissue angiotensin system inhibition 235
  vasculoproliferative disease 29
Angiotensinogen 234
  genetic linkage to essential hypertension 236
  myocardial infarction-associated expression 276
Anisoylated plasminogen streptokinase activator
    complex *see* APSAC
Anistreplase *see* APSAC
Antiarrhythmic agents
  administration problems 401–2
  automated delivery *see* Feedback controlled
    automated drug delivery
  automated serum concentration estimation
    ECG characteristics 427–33
    monophasic action potential responses *432*,
      432–3, *433*
  Class I 345
    clinical trials 331–2
    heart rate variability effect 442
    serum level estimation from QRS duration
      427, *428*
    signal-averaged ECG late potentials 441–2
    use dependence 442
  Class III 345
    clinical trials 332–5
    controlled release polymer matrix delivery 344
    implanted cardiac defibrillator adjunctive
      therapy 334, 345, 401
    newer agents 339–43
    reverse-use dependence 442
    serum level estimation from QT prolongation
      427, *429*, 429
    structure–activity relationships 344
  classification
    Sicilian gambit 331
    Vaughan Williams *330*, 330, 345
  ion-selective electrode sensors 416
  iontophoretic epicardial/endocardial delivery
    390–6
    feedback delivery systems 390–1, 396
    see also Heterogeneous cation-exchange
      membranes (HCMs)
  Lambeth conventions 337 *337*, 338
  local application 343–4
  myocardial infarction
    associated arrhythmic death 331–2
    postinfarction ventricular fibrillation/sudden
      death 333–4
  preclinical models 335–9
Antibody targeted agents 149–66
  antibody–protein chemical cross-linkage 151–2
  bifunctional antibodies 152–3

fibrin-specific antibody generation 150–1
hirudin–antifibrin bifunctional antibody 165
plasminogen activator–platelet receptor
    antibody conjugate 164–5
recombinant fusion protein production 153–64
    59D8 monoclonal antibody–scuPA fusion
      protein 156–64
    59D8 monoclonal antibody–tPA fusion
      protein 154–6
  vascular function restoration 216
Antigen presentation 296
  MHC class I molecules 296
  MHC class II molecules 296
  xenografting 301
Anti-inflammatory drugs
  polymer-based local delivery 45
  restenosis prevention 6, 9–10
Antilymphocyte antibodies
  antilymphocyte globulin (AlG) 288, 289
  antithymocyte globulin (ATG) 289
  initial post-transplant rejection (induction
    therapy) 289
  OKT3 290–1
  side effects 288, 289
  transplantation rejection prevention 288–94,
    302
Antilymphocyte globulin (AlG) 288, 289
  acute rejection treatment 289
  initial post-transplant rejection (induction
    therapy) 289–90
  repeated administration 289
Antimitotic agents, catheter-based local vascular
    release 33
Antiplatelet agents, restenosis prevention 5, 7–9
Antiproliferative agents, restenosis prevention 6,
    10–11
Antisense technology 86–101
  accelerated arteriopathy 86, 91–7
    non-specific effects 97
    oligonucleotide delivery 97, 99–100
    oligonucleotide toxicity 97, 100
    problems 97–100
  cell cycle protein targets *91*, 91, 92–3
  cell-adhesion molecule suppression 96–7
  evaluation of antisense effect 88–90, *91*
    controls *90*, 90
    unintended effects 89
  HVJ-liposome transfer to vessel wall 241
  oligonucleotide delivery methods 93–4, *96*, 97,
    99–100
    extravascular 93, 94, 95
    intravascular 93
    polymeric implants local delivery 42–4, *43*
  oligonucleotides 88
    chemical modification 88, *89*, 97–9, 100
  primary atherosclerotic plaques *84*
  protein synthesis interruption *87*, 87–8
    anti-DNA strategy 87–8
    anti-RNA strategy 87
  smooth muscle cells (SMC) proliferation effect
    in vivo *91*, 93–7, *98*, *99*
    long-term efficacy 96, *101*

target gene selection 90
  message abundance 90
  target protein half-life 90–1
  vascular function restoration 216
Antithrombotic drugs
  coronary angioplasty adjunctive treatment 136
  local delivery systems *137*
    perivascular EVA copolymer 139, *140*
    stents 138–41
    transluminal methods 137–8
  myocardial infarction 119, 134
  restenosis prevention 5, 6, 7–9
Antithymocyte globulin (ATG) 289
  initial post-transplant rejection (induction
    therapy) 289
Apolipoprotein A1 (Apo A1) hepatic gene transfer
  191–2
APSAC, myocardial infarction thrombolytic
  therapy 113, *115*, 115, 149
Arterial thrombotic disease, local therapy 131–42
  anatomical targeting 131
  biochemical targeting 131
Aspirin
  delivery modulation 225
  myocardial infarction 118
  platelet inhibition 225
  prostacyclin synthesis inhibition 225
  restenosis prevention 7, 8
  thrombolytic therapy adjuvant treatment 118,
    150
  unstable angina 123, 135
Aspirin–dipyrimadole combination 7, 8
ASSETT trial 113
Atenolol 360
Atherectomy tissue 81, *82*
  molecular analysis 81
  molecular markers 83, *84*
  smooth muscle cell proliferative potential 83
Atherosclerosis 123, 123–4
  accelerated *see* Accelerated arteriopathies
  angiotensin II 237, 239–40
    pathogenic role 235–6
  endothelial gene expression abnormalities
    172
  endothelin elevation 224
  endothelium-dependent vasodilator function
    impairment 206, 215
    risk factor associations 205, 213
  gene transfer for antithrombotic/fibrinolytic
    agent delivery 187
  L-arginine supplementation 217
  myocardial infarction 108
  primary/restenotic lesions 81, *82*
  vascular dysfunction 206–9
    abnormal constriction 206, 207
    epicardial artery stress responses 207
    experimental studies 206
    treatment 207–9
  vascular remodelling 237, 239
Atrial fibrillation *see* Paroxysmal atrial fibrillation
Atrial natriuretic peptide (ANP), ventricular
  remodelling 269

Atrial pacing 361
Autoimmune disease
  oral antigen administration 299
  T cell thymic clonal selection 298
Automated arrhythmia detection 443–4
  HOBBES detector 445
Automated drug delivery *see* Feedback controlled
  automated drug delivery
Automated ECG analysis 462
Automated implanted cardio-defibrillators
  (AICDs) 401
  antiarrhythmic agents adjunct treatment 334,
    345, 401
  atrial fibrillation 446
  automated arrhythmias detection 444
  feedback drug-delivery device coupling 401,
    457–60, *458*, 462
Automated infusion pumps 412
Autonomic effector pathways, cardiac failure
  272–3

B lymphocyte recruitment, accelerated
  arteriopathy 83
Basic fibroblast growth factor (bFGF)
  angiotensin II induction 238
  cardiac myocyte growth regulation 277
  collateral circulation promotion in ischaemic
    myocardium 320
  heparin-like compounds binding 39
  inhibition 55, 57
    antisense oligonucleotides 96
    monoclonal antibody blockade 66
  myocardial gene transfer 193
  necessity for controlled release 39
  polymeric device local delivery 39–42, *141*, 141
    effects in culture *41*, 41
    effects *in vivo* 41–2, *42*
    heparin encapsulated alginate microspheres
      preparation 39–41, *40*
  restenosis pathophysiology 3
  smooth muscle cells (SMC) proliferation 57,
    85
  stent-based local delivery 140, *141*, 141
  vessel injury-induced release 39, 85
  targeted therapies 55
BASIS trial 333, 334
Bazett correction 329, 361, 430
Benestent trial 13
Beta-adrenergic kinase (βARK) expression,
  cardiac failure 273, *274*
Beta-adrenergic pathway, cardiac failure 272
Beta-adrenergic receptor gene
  myocardial contractility-associated expression
    321–2
  myocardial transfer 314
Beta-blockers
  heart rate variability effect 442
  long QT syndromes 356, 359–60, *360*
  myocardial infarction 109, 119–20
bFGF-PE40 60
bFGF-PE4E-KDEL 60

bFGF-saporin
  hepatotoxicity 60
  intimal hyperplasia inhibition 58, *59*, 60
  smooth muscle cell selective ablation 57–8, *58*
Biocatalytic probes 419–20, *423*
Bioresorbable stent drug delivery, restenosis
    prevention 18, *19*
Blood gases monitoring 414, *415*, 426
  fiberoptic sensors 418
BMA031 291
Bone marrow mixed chimerism 300, 301
Bradykinin 215
Brain natriuretic peptide (BNP) 269
Bretylium, ion-selective electrode sensors 416

c-myb
  antisense oligonucleotides SMC proliferation
      suppression 43, *91*, 93, 94–5, 96, *97*
    delivery methods 93–4
    polymer gel local delivery *43*, 43–4
  cell cycle regulation 92
c-myc
  antisense oligonucleotides SMC proliferation
      suppression *91*, 93, 95, 96
  cell cycle regulation 92
Cadherins 54
Calcineurin 287
  cyclosporine/FK-506 mode of action 287, *288*,
      302
Calcium channel blockers
  myocardial infarction 121
  restenosis prevention *5*, 7
  vasculoproliferative disease 29
Calcium regulation, cardiac failure 270–1
  calcium handling proteins expression 270
Calcium release channel (CRC) 270
Calsequestrin 270
CAMIAT trial 334
CAMPATH-1 291
CAPS trial 331
Captopril 121
Cardiac arrhythmias 327–45
  antiarrhythmic agents *see* Antiarrhythmic
      agents
  automated implanted cardio-defibrillators
      (AICDs) 401
  device-related therapies 335
  ECG automated detection 443–4
    HOBBES detector 445
  genesis 327–9
    re-entrant cardiac conduction 328
    ventricular repolarization 328–9
  heart rate variability 442
  interventional ablation therapies 335
  preclinical models
    experimental design 337–8
    in vitro models *336*, 336
    in vivo models 336–8
    Lambeth conventions 337 *337*, 338
  QT interval 329
  torsades de pointes 338–9

Cardiac failure
  adult/fetal gene expression changes *269*, 269,
      277
  autonomic effector pathways 272–3
    β-adrenergic kinase (βARK) expression 273,
        274
    β-adrenergic pathway 272
    β_1-adrenergic receptor reduction 273, *274*, 274
  calcium regulation 270–1
    calcium handling proteins expression 270
  contractile apparatus 271–2
  extracellular matrix 270, 277–9
  growth signaling pathways 273–7
    catecholamines 275–6
    endothelin 276–7
    mechanical stresses 275
    myocyte second messengers 273–4
    peptide growth factors 277, *278*
    renin–angiotensin system 276
  myocardial remodelling 267–8, *269*, 269, 270
    fibroblast hyperplasia 270
    myocyte hypertrophy 270
    myocyte signaling pathways 274
    ventricular remodelling 268–70
  myocyte action potential 270, *271*
  secondary molecular alterations *267*, 267–79
  sympathetic nervous system activity 275
  see also Congestive cardiac failure
Cardiac myocytes
  angiotensin II production 276
  endothelin responses 276–7
  gene transfer *see* Myocardial gene transfer
  signaling pathways 273–4
  transplantation 314, 322–3
Cardiac myosin antibodies 65
Cardiac transplantation
  clinical follow up 284
  clinical outcome 283
  congestive cardiac failure 283–303
  immunosuppression *see* Immunosuppression,
      cardiac transplantation
  rejection
    antisense oligonucleotide ICAM-1
        suppression 97
    endothelial cell ICAM-1 expression 62–3
    leukocyte recruitment pathway 62
Cardiopulmonary bypass surgery, nitric oxide
    inhalation 258
Cardiovascular controlled release systems 383
CARPORT study 8
CASCADE trial 333, 334
CAST trial 329, 331–2, 345, 427
CAST II trial 331, 332
Catecholamines, cardiac myocyte growth
    regulation 275–6
Cathepsins 234
Cationic lipids, antisense oligonucleotide delivery
    100
CAVEAT trial 16
CCAT trial 16
CD4 T cells, MHC class I molecule interaction
    296, 298

CD8 T cells, MHC class I molecule interaction 296
CD11a/CD-18
    leukocyte–endothelium adhesion 62
    monoclonal antibodies 63
cdc2
    antisense oligonucleotides
        liposomes delivery 44
        SMC proliferation suppression 95, 96, *101*
    cell cycle regulation 93
cdk2 kinase
    antisense oligonucleotides
        liposomes delivery 44
        SMC proliferation suppression 95, 96, *101*
        vessel wall expression inhibition 241
    cell cycle regulation 93
cDNA library direct screening 372–4
Cefsulodin, voltammetric sensors 417
Cell cycle proteins, smooth muscle cells (SMC)
        proliferation *92*, 92
    antisense technology suppression *91*, 93
    targets *91*, 91, 92–3
Cell-adhesion molecules
    antisense technology suppression 96–7
    endothelial cells expression 215
    leukocyte recruitment 61–2, 63
    leukocyte–endothelial cell adhesion *61*
    smooth muscle cells (SMCs) 54
        targeted therapies 60–5
Channel balloon catheters 33
Chloramphenicol, voltammetric sensors 417
Chloroaluminum-sulfonated phthalocyanine
        photosensitization 46
Cholesterol plasma level 208
Cholesterol-lowering agents 11
CHORUS pacemaker
    fibrillation rate estimation 450, 451
    Pharmacologic Atrial Defibrillator (PAD)
        system *443*, 446, 447
Chronic obstructive pulmonary disease
    endogenous NO production impairment 250
    pulmonary hypertension, nitric oxide
        inhalation 258
Chymase 234
Cilazapril 10
Ciprostene 8
Cis element oligonucleotides, transfer to vessel
        wall 241
Colchicine
    porous balloon catheter local release 33
    restenosis prevention 10
Collagen, extracellular matrix 83
Collagen matrices, local cyclosporine delivery
        45
Computer-driven infusion devices *see* Feedback
        controlled automated drug delivery
Congenital heart disease, pulmonary
        hypertension 258
Congestive cardiac failure 283–303
    angiotensin-converting enzyme (ACE)
        inhibitors 313
    cardiac transplantation 283–303
    cardiomyocyte transplantation 314, 322–3

endothelin elevation 224
    gene therapies 313, 314–22
CONSENSUS trial 313
CONSENSUS II trial 121, 332
Continuous drug monitoring sensors 414
Control advance moving average controllers
        (CAMAC) 436
Cor pulmonale, endogenous NO production
        impairment 250
Cordis stent 13
Coronary angioplasty 135–6
    excimer laser (ELCA) 15, 17
    intracoronary thrombolytic agents 135–6
    laser balloon angioplasty (LBA) *14*, *15*, 17
    localized antithrombotic therapy 8–9, 136
    nitric oxide donor adjuvant therapy 216
    restenosis following *see* Restenosis
    unstable angina 135, 136
Coronary artery disease
    endothelial gene expression abnormalities 172
    gene transfer 171–96
        congestive cardiac failure management 320–1
        see also Vessel wall gene transfer
    risk factor management 207–9
        cholesterol 207–8
        hormone replacement therapy 208
        L-arginine supplements 208–9
        oxygen free radicals 208
    see also Myocardial infarction
Coronary artery spasm 224
Corticosteroids
    restenosis prevention 9–10
    vasculoproliferative disease 29
Cyclophilin 286
    cyclosporine binding 286, 288
    enzymatic activity 286
Cyclosporine 284, 295
    actions on T lymphocytes 284–6
    calcineurin activity blockade 287, 288
    cardiac transplantation 283, 284–8, 302
    cyclophilins activity inhibition 287
    cyclophilins binding 286
    low dose in immediate post-transplant period
        289
    mode of action 286–8
    nephrotoxicity 289
    polymer-based local delivery 45
    structure *285*
    transdermal iontophoretic delivery 389

59D8 monoclonal antibody
    antibody–plasminogen activator chemical
        cross-linkage 151–2
    generation/fibrin binding 150–1
    tissue-type plasminogen activator (t-PA)
        conjugate 152
    urokinase plasminogen activator conjugate
        152
59D8 monoclonal antibody–scuPA fusion protein
        156–64
    cloning 157

59D8 monoclonal antibody–scuPA fusion protein
    (*cont.*)
    expression plasmid construction *155*, 157
    expression plasmid transfection 157
    functional properties 159–64
        clot lysis assay 161, *162*
        fibrin-binding activity *160*, 160–1
        in vivo thrombolytic potency 160–4
        kinetic properties 159, *160*, 160
        specific amidolytic activity 160
    heavy chain loss variant selection 157
    plasmid modification to increase protein
        secretion *158*, 158–9
    production in large quantities 159
    protein expression levels 157–8
59D8 monoclonal antibody-tPA fusion protein
    expression plasmid transfection 156
    expression vector construction 154, *155*
    fusion protein purification 156
    heavy-chain loss variant cell line selection 156
    immunoglobulin gene cloning 154
    plasma clot lytic activity 156
    recombinant fusion protein production 153–64
DAB$_{389}$ EGF 56
Dacron grafts, cell-based vascular gene transfer
    175
Dexamethasone
    cardiac pacing catheter release 383
    polymer-based local delivery 45
    transdermal iontophoretic delivery 389
Diabetes mellitus
    polymer-based controlled drug delivery 35
    vasomotor function disturbance 205, 213, 215
Digoxin
    feedback control of delivery 405
    immuno assay-based sensor 420, *424*, 424–5
    pharmacokinetic parameters estimation 411
Dilantin 360
Diltiazem 121
Diphtheria toxin
    mitogen combinations 56
    monoclonal antibody conjugates 294
Dipyrimadole–aspirin combination, restenosis
    prevention 7, 8
Directional coronary atherectomy (DCA) *14*, *15*,
    16
Disopyramide 329, 333
    automated delivery
        Pharmacologic Atrial Defibrillator (PAD) *in
            vivo* testing 453
        premature ventricular contractions (PVC) as
            feedback variable 440
    QRS duration at higher heart rates 427, *428*
    reverse use-dependent QT prolongation *431*,
        431, 442
    two-compartment kinetics 451
DNA direct injection
    myocardial gene transfer 194, *195*, 314–16
        angiogenesis promotion 321
        efficiency of gene transfer 315
        inflammatory response 315
    vessel wall gene transfer 177

Dofetilide 340–1
    structure *340*
Double balloon catheter
    antisense oligonucleotide delivery 93
    iloprost local delivery 222
Doxorubicin
    fiberoptic sensors 418
    porous balloon catheter delivery 33
Duchenne muscular dystrophy 319
    dystrophin gene mutations 319
    dystrophin gene transfer 314, 319–20
    myocardial gene transfer 314, 318, 319–20
Dystrophin gene
    mutations 319
    myocardial gene transfer 314, 319–20

7E3 monoclonal antibody 65
E-4031 339–40
    structure *339*
    structure–activity relationships 344
E-selectin 61
    endothelial trauma-associated expression 63
    heart transplant rejection 63
ECG
    automated antiarrhythmic drug serum level
        estimation 427–33
        Class I estimation from QRS duration 427,
            428
        Class III estimation from QT prolongation
            427, *429*, 429, *430*
        QT-interval measurement problems 429–31
    automated arrhythmia detection 443–4
        HOBBES detector 445
    automated drug delivery feedback parameters
        440–4, 461
        heart rate variability 442–3
        premature ventricular contractions (PVC)
            440
        QT dispersion 440–1
        signal-averaged ECG late potentials (SAECG)
            441–2
        use/reverse-use dependence 442
    automated target drug level modification 444–5
    QT prolongation
        Bazzet correction for heart rate 329, 361, 430
        Frieberg's cube-root correction 430
ECSG-6 trial 115, 119
E2F transcription factor inhibition 241
Electrolyte monitoring 414, 415, 426
    fiberoptic sensors 418
EMERAS trial 113
EMIAT trial 334
Enalapril 121, 313
Encainide 331, 332, 333
Endothelial cells
    activation 61–2
    adhesion molecule expression 61–2, 204, 215
    extracellular matrix production 67
    functions 203–4
    gene expression abnormalities in
        atherosclerosis *81*, 81, 172

gene transfer 182, 183, 187–8
  cell-based 174, 176
  u-PA expression on cell surface 187–8
hormone/neurotransmitter responses 204
leukocyte adhesion *61*, 61–2
nitric oxide synthetase targeted delivery 221–2
second messenger systems 204
selectins surface presentation 61–2
surface receptor functions 204
vascular injury surface markers 54
vasomotor tone control 214
  see also Endothelium-dependent vasodilator
    function
vasoregulatory mediators production 204, 214
Endothelin 223–4
  angiotensin II regulation of expression 239, 277
  cardiac myocyte growth regulation 276–7
  disease-associated elevation 224
  endothelial cells production 204
  local delivery of antagonists 224
  smooth muscle cell (SMC) vasoconstriction 204
Endothelin-1 239
Endothelium 204–5
  smooth muscle cell (SMC) interactions 203–4
  vasoreactive disease 203–9
Endothelium-dependent vasodilator function
    204–5
  atherosclerosis 206
    experimental studies 206
    risk factor-associated impairment 205, 213
  coronary artery disease risk factor management
    207–9
    cholesterol 207–8
    hormone replacement therapy 208
    oxygen free radicals 208
  disease-associated impairment 215
  endothelial damage-associated impairment
    205
  forskolin local therapy 222–3
  nitric oxide replacement
    endogenous 221–2
    exogenous 221
    L-arginine supplementation 208–9, 217
    nitric oxide adducts/S-nitrosothiols 217–22
    nitric oxide donors 216–17
  prostacyclin (PGI_2) local therapy 222
  pulmonary arteries 250
Endothelium-derived relaxation factor (EDRF) *see*
    Nitric oxide
Endotoxin
  endothelial cell activation 61
  platelet nitric oxide synthetase activation 221
  pulmonary hypertension, nitric oxide
    inhalation 252, 253
Enzyme biosensor probes 419–20
EPIC trial 65
Epidermal growth factor (EGF)
  angiotensin II induction 239
  injury-associated release 55
  targeted therapies 55, 56
    diphtheria toxin combinations 56
17β-Estradiol 208

Estrogens, endothelium-dependent vasodilatory
    function 208
Ethylene–vinyl acetate copolymer (EVAc)
  basic fibroblast growth factor (bFGF) release 39,
    40
  c-myb antisense oligonucleotides delivery 44
  heparin local delivery 35, *36*, 139–40
EVESM trial 334
Excimer laser coronary angioplasty (ELCA) *15*, *17*
Exon amplification method 371, *373*
Extracellular matrix 67, *69*
  accelerated arteriopathies 4, 79, 83
    targeted therapies 66–9
  angiotensin II-induced production 239
  cardiac failure 277–9
  collagen 83
    fibrils contraction 68
  early provisional matrix 66, 67
  fibronectin 83
  heparin actions 68
  metalloproteins in leukocyte recruitment 62
  proteoglycans 83
  smooth muscle cells (SMC) production 4, 66
  tenascin *67*, 67, 84
  thrombospondin 67, *68*
  transforming growth factor-β_1 (TGF-β_1)
    stimulation 86
  vascular injury surface markers 54
  ventricular remodelling 270

Factor VIII-related antigen 54
Familial hypercholesterolaemia, LDL-receptor
    hepatic gene transfer 189, *191*, 192, 196
Feedback controlled automated drug delivery
    339, 399–462
  acute-care intravenous delivery 460–1
  atrial fibrillation long-term treatment *see*
    Paroxysmal atrial fibrillation
  continuous feedback *434*, 434–8
    control advance moving average controllers
      (CAMAC) 436
    minimum variance controllers 435–6
    model reference adaptive systems (MRAS)
      436, 436–7
    multiple model techniques 437
    PID control 434–5
    system nonlinearities 437–8
  control system for dosing 402
    feedforward/open loop *402*, 402–3
    simple feedback loop *402*, 402
  customized dosing 400–1
  drug administration 403, 412–14
    intravenous 412
    iontophoretic implants 413
    magnetic modulated contolled-release
      implants 412–13
    oral 412
    ultrasound modulated contolled-release
      systems 413
  drug delivery optimization 403, 433–8
  drug dosage profiles 413–14

Feedback controlled automated drug delivery
    (*cont.*)
  ECG feedback parameters 440–4
    arrhythmia detection 443–4
    heart rate variability 442–3
    premature ventricular contractions (PVC) 440
    QT dispersion 440–1
    signal-averaged ECG late potentials (SAECG)
      441–2
    target drug level modification 444–5
    use/reverse-use dependence 442
  efficacy/toxicity modulation 403, *404*, 462
    ECG assessment 404, 440–4
    target drug level adjustment 404, 444–5
  ideal properties of system 399–400
  implantable devices 401, 457–60, *458*
  initial dosage trajectory 403, *404*, 404–11, 461
    local delivery pharmacokinetics 406–9, *407*,
      408
    one-compartment pharmacokinetic model
      404–5, *405*, 409
    optimal trajectories 409–10
    three-compartment model *406*, 406–8, *407*,
      408
    two-compartment open-loop control 410–11
    two-compartment pharmacokinetic model
      405, 405–6, 409–10
  initial pharmacokinetic parameters 411–12
  pharmacokinetic coefficient updating 439
  potential applications 457–61
  response time improvement 400
  sensor devices 414–15, 426–7
    amperometric/voltammetric sensors 416–19,
      423
    biocatalytic probes 419–20, *423*
    biosensors 419–22, 426
    chemical sensors 415–19
    fiberoptic sensors 418–19
    immunochemical sensors 420–2, *424*, 424–6
    ion-selective electrodes 415–16, *422*, 426
  serum level online estimation 403, 414–33
    chemical-/biosensor devices 414–27
    current examples 422–6
    ECG proxy 427–33, *428*, *429*, *430*, *431*, *432*, *433*
    serum level-clinical effect relationship 426–7
  sporadic feedback *438*, 438–9
  toxicity reduction 400
Feedback controlled non-automated drug dosing
    402
  clinical decision-making process *403*, 403
  drug level control error/prediction error *403*,
    403
  feedforward/open loop *402*, 402–3
  simple feedback loop *402*, 402
Fiberoptic sensors 418–19
  immunosensor 421, *425*, 425–6
Fibrin-specific antibody
  bifunctional antibodies
    hirudin-antifibrin 165
    plasminogen activator conjugates 152
    somatic cell fusion product 152–3
  generation 150–1

    plasminogen activator chemical cross-linkage
      151–2
    recombinant fusion protein production 153–64
      59D8 monoclonal antibody–scuPA fusion
        protein 156–64
      59D8 monoclonal antibody–tPA fusion
        protein 154–6
      immunoglobulin gene cloning 154
Fibroblast growth factor-5 (FGF-5) 321
Fibroblast growth factors (FGFs)
    extracellular matrix proteoglycan binding 83
    myocardial angiogenesis gene therapy 321
    restenosis pathophysiology 4
Fibroblasts, gene transfer targets 183
Fibronectin 83
FK-506 286, 302
    actions on T lymphocytes 286
    calcineurin activity blockade 287, 288
    cytosolic binding protein (FKBP) 286
    FKBP activity inhibition 287
    mode of action 286–8
    structure *285*
FKBP 286
    enzymatic activity 286
    FK-506 binding 286, 288
    rapamycin binding 286, 288
Flecainide 331, 332, 333
Flow-mediated coronary dilation 204
Fluoroprobe fiberoptic sensors 418
Forskolin
    coated stent delivery 221, 223
    platelet inhibition 222–3
    platelets nitric oxide synthetase activation 221
    smooth muscle relaxation 222–3
Fosinopril 10
Frieberg's cube-root correction 430

G_1 proteins 92
G_1/S cyclins 93
G_2/S cyclins 93
72kD Gelatinase, leukocyte recruitment 62
Gene targeting 301
Gene transfer
    liver *see* Hepatic gene transfer
    local therapy 172
    myocardium *see* Myocardial gene transfer
    pre-transplant MHC Class I genes 299
    vascular *see* Vessel wall gene transfer
Gianturco–Roubin stent 13
GISSI trial 149
GISSI-1 trial 110, 113
GISSI-2 trial 113, 119
GISSI-3 trial 120, 121
GP IIb/IIIa inhibition
    monoclonal antibody 64, 65
    restenosis prevention 8
GPIIb/IIIa antibody 64, 65
    thrombin blocking action 150
    thrombolytic therapy adjuvant treatment 150
    urokinase plasminogen activator (uPA)
      antibody conjugate 164–5

GR32191B 8
GUSTO trial 115–17, 119, 123, 133, 149

H-*ras*–1 locus
  genetic mapping *367*, 367
  physical mapping 369–71, *370*
  Romano–Ward syndrome
    candidate gene 368
    linkage 353, 361, 363, 364, 366
HART trial 115, 119
HDL level enhancement, hepatic gene transfer
  191–2
Heparin
  coated stent delivery 34, 138, *139*, 139, 141
  coronary angioplasty adjunct treatment 136
  extracellular matrix effects 68
  hydrogel-coated balloon catheter delivery 33
  myocardial infarction 134
    thrombolytic therapy adjuvant treatment 115,
    116, 119
  polymer-based local delivery 35–8, *36*, *38*
    non-anticoagulant preparations 35, *36*, 37
    perivascular delivery 37, 38, 139, *140*
    polymer-bound stent delivery 34
    stent-induced arteriosclerosis 37
  porous balloon catheter delivery 31–2, 137
    intravascular half-life 35
  restenosis prevention 9, 29, 30
    complications of treatment 30
    intermittent versus continuous therapy 30, *31*
    local therapy 30, 31–47
    long-acting preparations 30
  smooth muscle cell (SMC) growth inhibition
    29–30
  unstable angina 123, 135
  vasculoproliferative disease 29
Hepatic gene transfer 172, 189–93
  hypercholesterolaemia 189–93
    familial 189, *191*, 192, 196
    HDL level enhancement 191–2
    LDL-receptor deficiency 189–90, *190*
    plasma LDL reduction 189
Heterogeneous cation-exchange membranes
  (HCMs) 384–90
  cation-exchange resin conditioning 391
  design criteria 384–5
  design equations 388
  formulation 391
  iontophoretic drug delivery 384, 413
    cardiac implant design 391, *392*
    conditioning to drug form 391–2
    drug transport *393*, 393–6, *394*, *395*
    epicardial/endocardial antiarrhythmic agents
    390–6
    in vitro modulation of antiarrhythmic drugs
    392
    in vivo cardiac implant study 392–3
    steady-state bi-ionic transport 386–8
Hirudin 123
  antifibrin bifunctional antibody 165
  balloon catheter local delivery systems 137

coronary angioplasty adjunct treatment 136
  iontopheretic delivery 34, 137, 390
  myocardial infarction local therapy 134
  restenosis prevention 9
  smooth muscle cells (SMC) antiproliferative
    activity 86
  unstable angina 135
  vessel wall gene transfer 188
Hirulog 123
  myocardial infarction local therapy 134
  polymer-based local delivery 45
  smooth muscle cells (SMC) antiproliferative
    activity 86
Histamine, endothelial cell activation 61
HOBBES automated arrhythmia detection 445
Homologous recombinaton (gene targeting)
    technique 301
  xenografting 301
Hormone replacement therapy 208
HVJ-liposomes
  vessel wall antisense/cis element
    oligonucleotides delivery 44, 240–1
    angiotensin system modulation 242
  vessel wall gene transfer 179, 180–1
    efficiency of transfer 180
    nitric oxide synthase expression 243
Hydrogel-coated balloon catheters 31, 33–4
  antithrombotic drug delivery 137
5-Hydroxytryptamine (5-HT) *see* Serotonin
Hypercholesterolaemia
  endothelium-dependent vasodilator function
    impairment 205, 206, 213, 215
  hepatic gene transfer 172, 189
    apolipoprotein A1 (Apo A1) overexpression
    191–2
    familial hypercholesterolaemia 189, *191*, 192
    LDL-receptor deficiency 189–90, *190*
  L-arginine supplementation 217
Hyperglycaemia, endothelium-dependent
    vasodilator function impairment 205
Hyperpolarizing factor 204
Hypertension
  angiotensin II 242–3
    local tissue system activation 234, 236
  animal models 236
  endothelin elevation 224
  endothelium-dependent vasodilator function
    impairment 205, 213, 215
  genetic aspects 236
  myocardial infarction risk 235
  vascular remodelling 237, 242–3
Hypolipidemic agents, restenosis prevention 6, 11

Ibutilide 342–3
  automated delivery feedback parameters 461
  iontophoretic delivery system 396, 401
    feedback-controlled with implantable
    defibrillator 458
  polymer matrix cardiac implantation 344
  serum level estimation from QT prolongation
    429, 429, *430*

Ibutilide (*cont.*)
    serum level-tissue effect relationship 427
    structure *342*
    structure–activity relationships 344
Iloprost, local delivery 222
Imipramine 335
Immune response
    accelerated arteriopathy 83
    polymer-based controlled drug delivery 35
Immunochemical sensors 420–2, *424*
    optical immunosensor 421, *425*, 425–6
    potentiometric ionophore-mediated
        immunoassay (PIMIA) 424–5
Immunoglobulin genes, 'humanized' monoclonal
    antibody modification 293
Immunosuppression, cardiac transplantation 283,
    284
    antilymphocyte antibodies 288–94
    cyclosporine 283, 284–8, 302
        local delivery 45
    FK-506 286, 302
    monoclonal antibodies 290–4
        antibody–toxin conjugates 294
        CD4/CD8 T cell targeting 292
        constant region removal 293–4
        'humanized' antibody 293
        ICAM-1 292–3
        IL-2 receptor 292
        LFA-1 292–3
        OKT3 290–1
        T lymphocyte receptor/CD3 complex target
            290, *291*, 291
    pre-transplant blood transfusion effect 294–6,
        298, 299–300
    problems 283
    rapamycin 286, 302
    tolerance induction 294–302
        bone marrow mixed chimerism 300, 301
        homologous recombinaton (gene targeting)
            techniques 301
        intrathymic alloantigen inoculation 299
        oral antigen administration 299
        peristence of tolerance 299–300
        pre-transplant MHC Class I gene transfection
            299
    transplantation complications 283
    xenotransplantation 301
IMPACT study 8
Implantable defibrillators, *see* Automated
    implanted cardio-defibrillators (AICDs)
Implantable micropumps 412
Infusaid Model 1000 pump 446–7
Insulin, transdermal iontophoretic delivery 389
Insulin-like growth factor-1 (IGF-1)
    angiotensin II induction 239
    injury-associated release 85
        targeted therapies 55
    smooth muscle cells (SMC) production 80, 85
    smooth muscle cells (SMC) proliferation
        85–6
Integrelin 8
Integrin $\alpha V \beta 3$ inhibition 64

Integrins
    endothelial VCAM-1/ICAM-1 binding 62
    leukocyte–endothelial cell high affinity
        adhesion 62
    monoclonal antibody inhibition 64, 65
    polymer-based local antagonism 45
    subendothelial collagen 62
    thrombotic cascade activation 62
Intercellular adhesion molecule-1 (ICAM-1)
    accelerated arteriopathy 63–4, 83
    leukocyte–endothelial adhesion 62
    T-lymphocyte recruitment 62–3
Intercellular adhesion molecule-1 (ICAM-1)
    inhibition 63
    antisense oligonucleotide 96, 97
    leumedins 64
    monoclonal antibody immunosuppressive
        therapy 63, 292–3
    T-lymphocyte recruitment inhihition 63
    vascular graft injury 63–4
Interferon-gamma (IFN-gamma)
    endothelial cell activation 61
    recruited T-lymphocyte release 62
    smooth muscle cell antiproliferative effect 62,
        64
Interleukin-1 (IL-1)
    accelerated arteriopathy 84
    endothelial cell activation 61
    platelets nitric oxide synthetase activation 221
Interleukin-1 (IL-1) receptors, antisense
    oligonucleotide suppression 96
Interleukin-2 (IL-2)
    cyclosporine/FK-506 blockade of transcription
        286, 287, 288
    transplant rejection 65
Interleukin-2 (IL-2) receptor monoclonal antibody
    65
    cardiac transplantation immunosuppressive
        therapy 292
Interleukin-6 (IL-6) 84
Interleukin-8 (IL-8) 84
Intimal hyperplasia
    antisense oligonucleotides 43, 44
    basic fibroblast growth factor (bFGF) *42*, 42
    bFGF-saporin inhibition 58, *59*, 60
    extracellular matrix proteins 67
    heparin 36, *38*
        chronic subcutaneous delivery 32
        continuous versus intermittent therapy 30
        non-anticoagulant preparations 36, 37
        perivascular release 38
        polymer-based delivery 35, *36*, 37
    leukocyte recruitment 62
    local therapies 29–50
    photodynamic therapy 46
    platelet-derived growth factor (PDGF)
        monoclonal antibody blockade 65
    platelet-induced effects 3
    polymer-based drug delivery 35, *36*, 37, 45
    porous balloon catheter local drug delivery 32,
        33
    restenosis 1, 2

smooth muscle cells (SMC) proliferation rates 81, 83
stent-based drug release 34
Intracoronary stents, restenosis prevention 12–13, *14*, *15*
Intravascular catheters
  double balloon 31
  hydrogel-coated 31, 33–4
  iontophoresis catheters 31, 34
  local drug delivery 31–4, *32*
  porous balloon 31–3
Ion transport equations 385–6
  steady-state bi-ionic transport through heterogeneous cation-exchange membranes (HCMs) 386–8
Ion-selective electrodes 415–16, *422*, 426
  biosensors 419, *420*
Iontophoresis catheters 31, 34
Iontophoretic drug delivery 389–90
  antithrombotic drugs 137
  automated implanted cardio-defibrillator (AICD) coupled therapy 401, 458–9
  definition 384
  electro-osmotic aspects 388–9
  epicardial/endocardial antiarrhythmic agents 390–6
  heterogeneous cation-exchange membranes (HCMs) 390–6, 413
    cardiac implant design 391, *392*
    conditioning to drug form 391–2
    design criteria 384–5
    design equations 388
    drug transport *393*, 393–6, *394*, *395*
    equilibrium swelling 391–2
    in vitro antiarrhythmic drug modulation 392
    in vivo cardiac implant study 392–3
    steady-state bi-ionic transport 386–8
  ion transport equations 385–6
  serum level-tissue effect concentration relationship 427
  transarterial 390
  transdermal 389–90, 413
  transmyocardial 390, 413
Ischaemic heart disease *see* Coronary artery disease
ISIS trial 149
ISIS-2 trial 113, 118, 119
ISIS-3 trial 115, 119
ISIS-4 trial 120, 121, 216

Jervell–Lange–Nielsen long QT syndrome 353, 354, *359*
  β blockade 360
  gene therapy approach 376
  left cardiac sympathetic ganglionectomy (LCSG) 360
  linkage analysis 366
  ventricular arrhythmias 358–9

Ketanserin, restenosis prevention 11

L-691,121 344, *345*
L-706,000 (MK-499) 344, *345*
L-arginine
  coronary artery disease risk factor management 208–9
  nitric oxide production 221
  supplements 208–9, 217
Lambeth conventions 337 *337*, 338
Laser balloon angioplasty (LBA), restenosis prevention *14*, *15*, 17
LATE trial 113, 119
LDL oxidation inhibition 208
LDL plasma elevation
  endothelium-dependent vasodilation impairment 205
  therapeutic reduction 208
LDL-receptor hepatic gene transfer 189–90, *190*
  familial hypercholesterolaemia 189, *191*, 192, 196
Left cardiac sympathetic ganglionectomy (LCSG) 356, 357, 359, *360*, 361
Leukocyte activation 61
  endothelial cell adhesion *61*, 61, 62
  restenosis pathophysiology 3
Leukocyte recruitment 61, 62
  accelerated arteriopathies 4, 60, 79
  adhesion molecules 61–2, 63
    blockade 63–4
  endothelial cell activation 61
  high affinity adhesion 61, 62
  labile adhesion/rolling 61, 62
  selectins 61–2
  steps in process *61*, 61
  transmigration to subendothelial space *61*, 62
Leukocyte rolling 61, 62
Leukotrienes, restenosis pathophysiology 3
Leumedins 64
Leuprolide acetate, transdermal iontophoretic delivery 389
LFA-1 monoclonal antibody inhibition 63
  immunosuppressive therapy 292–3
Lidocaine
  computer-assisted open-loop dosing 410
  ion-selective electrode sensors 416
  iontophoretic modulated delivery 393
  local myocardial delivery pharmacokinetics 406–9, *407*, *408*
  myocardial infarction 123
  pharmacokinetic parameters estimation 411
  polymer matrix cardiac implantation 343
  premature ventricular contractions (PVC) as feedback variable 440
Lidocaine analogs 329
Lidoflazine 121
Lignocaine, transdermal iontophoretic delivery 389
LIMIT-2 trial 121
Linkage analysis
  long QT syndromes 362–6
    presymptomatic patient identificaton 366
  microsatellite marker allele detection with PCR *363*, *365*

Linkage analysis (*cont.*)
  polymorphic markers 363, *364*
  recombination events 363, *366*
Lipofection
  antisense oligonucleotide delivery 100
  efficiency of transfer 178, *180*
  vessel wall gene transfer 177, 178
Lipopolysaccharide *see* Endotoxin
Liposomes
  antisense oligonucleotides delivery 44, 93, 100
  vessel wall gene transfer 177, 178
    duration of expression 184–5, *185*
    efficiency of transfer 178
    toxicity 185–6
  see also HVJ-liposomes
Lisidomine 216, 217
Lisinopril 121
Long QT syndromes 353–76
  acquired *359*
  definition of phenotype 361–2
    Bazett's correction for heart rate 361
    range of corrected QT intervals 361, *362*
  diagnostic criteria *356*, 356–7
  historical background 354–7
  Jervell–Lange–Nielsen syndrome *see* Jervell–
      Lange–Nielsen long QT syndrome
  linkage analysis 362–6
    genetic heterogeneity 363–4
    LOD score 363
    microsatellite marker allele detection with
        PCR 363, *365*
    polymorphic markers 363, *364*
    presymptomatic patient identificaton 366
    recombination events 363, *366*
  molecular biology 362–75
  mortality 354, 356, 361, 362
  pathophysiology 357–9
    myocardial repolarization defect 358, 359
    stellate ganglion sympathetic innervation
        imbalance 357–8
  positional cloning techniques 353, *354*
  QT dispersion as ventricular tachyarrhythma
      marker 440, 441
  Romano–Ward syndrome *see* Romano–Ward
      long QT syndrome
  sporadic/idiopathic form 354, *359*
    management 360
  therapy 359–61
    atrial pacing 361
    β blockade 356, 359–60, *360*
    implantable defibrillators 361
    left cardiac sympathetic ganglionectomy
        (LCSG) 356, 357, 359, *360*, 361
    torsades de pointes 354, *355*, 358, 360, 362
    ventricular arrhythmias 358–9
Lovastatin 208
  restenosis prevention 11
Lovastatin Restenosis Trial 11

M-CSF, accelerated arteriopathy 84
M-HEART study 10

M-HEART II study 8
Macrophage–monocyte recruitment 62
  accelerated arteriopathy 60, 62, 83
Magnesium sulfate
  myocardial infarction 121–2
  torsades de pointes 339
Magnetic bead capture technique 371
Magnetic modulated controlled-release implants
    412–13
Major histocompatibility complex (MHC) 296
  T cell receptor repertoire restriction 298
  tolerance induction
    oral antigen administration 299
    pre-transplant blood transfusion 298
Major histocompatibility complex (MHC) class I
    molecules 296, *297*
    antigen presentation 296
    T cell receptor interaction 296
  pre-transplant gene transfection of organ
      recipient 299
Major histocompatibility complex (MHC) class II
    molecules 296, *297*
    accelerated arteriopathy 84
    antigen presentation 296
    T cell receptor interaction 296, 298
Marfan's syndrome, fibrillin gene positional
    cloning 368
MERCATOR study 10
Metalloproteases, smooth muscle cells (SMC)
    migration 66
Methotrexate
  coated stent delivery 34
  porous balloon catheter delivery 33
8-Methoxypsoralen photodynamic therapy 46
Methylprednisolone, restenosis prevention 9–10
5-Methylurapidil 275
Mexiletine 333, 334, 335, 360
  ion-selective electrode sensors 416, 422–4
  QRS duration at higher heart rates 427, *428*
Microporous balloon catheters 33
Microsatellite marker allele detection 363, *365*
Minimum variance controllers 435–6
Mitogen–toxin combinations
  diphtheria toxin 56
  non-specificity 65
  Pseudomonas endotoxin 56, 60, 294
  saporin 57–60, *58*, *59*
  SMC proliferating cell selective ablation 55–60
Model reference adaptive systems (MRAS) *436*,
    436–7
Molsidomine 216, 217
Monoclonal antibodies
  accelerated arteriopathy targeted therapy 65–6
  anti-antibody antibody development 64, 66, 293
    genetic alterations for reduction 293
    inhibition 66
  antibody–toxin conjugates 294
  constant region removal 293–4
  immunochemical sensors 422, 426
  immunosuppressive therapy 290–4
    CD4/CD8 T cell targeting 292
    ICAM-1 292–3

IL-2 receptor antibodies 292
LFA-1 292–3
OKT3 290–1
modifications 293–4
Moricizine 331, 332, 333
Multiple Model Adaptive Control (MMAC) 437
Myocardial gene transfer 172, 193–5, 314–22
 cardiomyocyte delivery system 323
 congestive cardiac failure 313, 314–22
 candidate genes 318–22
 Duchenne muscular dystrophy 318, 319–20
 duration of gene expression 317
 ischaemic cardiomyopathies 320–1
 myocardial angiogenesis 320–1
 myocyte troponin C isoform expression 321
 long QT syndromes 375, *376*, 376
 myocardial contractility modification 321–2
 vector/delivery systems 314–18
 adenovirus vectors *194*, 194, *195*, 316–18
 direct plasmid DNA injection 194, *195*, 314–16
 efficiency of gene transfer 315, 316, 318
 local delivery systems 317, 318
Myocardial infarction 107–24
 angiotensin II
 local tissue activation 234
 receptor expression 276
 arrhythmia-associated death 331–2
 classification 109
 collateral circulation 193
 gene therapy promoting development 320
 coronary vascular dysfunction 207
 endothelin elevation 224
 heart rate variability 442
 infarct size determinants 111–12
 management 109–22, *110*
 angiotensin converting-enzyme (ACE)
 inhibitors 120–1, 240
 anticoagulants 119, 134
 aspirin 118
 beta blockers 109, 119–20
 calcium channel blockers 121
 effects on mortality *111*
 gene transfer therapy 171–96, 320
 lidocaine 123
 local therapy 131–42
 magnesium 121–2
 nitrates 120, 216
 primary revascularization 117
 reperfusion therapy 111–17, 123
 thrombolytic therapy 109, 111–17, *114*, 132–4, 149
 time variables 111–12, 122–3, 149
 mortality rates *107*, 107, 109, *111*, 113, *114*
 artery patency at hospital discharge 113
 early artery patency *116*, 116, 117, 123, 149
 patients excluded from thrombolytic therapy *117*, 117
 pathophysiology 108–9
 atherosclerotic plaque disruption 108
 coronary artery atherosclerosis 108, *123*, 123–4
 thrombus formation 108

platelets aggregation 225
Q wave/non-Q wave 109
QT dispersion as ventricular tachyarrhythmia
 marker 440, 441
risk stratification 109–11
 Killip classification *110*
 TIMI classification *110*
unstable angina 123
ventricular remodelling 268
wave front of ischaemic cell death 111, *112*
Myocyte transplantation 322–3
Myosin, cardiac failure 271
 isoform alterations 271–2

N-acetylcysteine 217
Nadolol 360
NE-10064 341–2
 structure *341*
Nernst–Planck equation 385
Niguldipine 275
Nimorazole, voltammetric sensors 417
Nipedipine 121
Nitinol temporary stents 139
Nitrates 120
Nitric oxide 249–51
 actions 216, 250
 atherogenesis reduction 204
 adducts 217–22
 atmospheric 258–9
 breakdown pathway 259
 biosynthesis 249
 donor adjuvant therapy 216–17
 endogenous in inhaled/expired air 250
 endothelial cell adhesion molecule expression 215
 endothelial cells production 204, 214
 endothelium-dependent vasodilator function 204, 215, 249
 atherosclerosis-associated impairment 206
 gene expression in ischaemic heart disease 172
 haemoglobin binding 249, 259
 inhalation 249–61
 acute pulmonary hypertension models 252–4, *253*
 adult respiratory distress syndrome (ARDS) 254–6, *255*, *256*
 chronic pulmonary hypertension 258
 persistent pulmonary hypertension of newborn (PPHN) 256–7
 pulmonary hypertension reduction 250–1
 technical aspects 260–1
 toxicity 258–60
 local therapy 216–17
 L-arginine substrate provision 208–9, 217
 nitric oxide donor adjuvant therapy 216–17
 platelet responses 215, *220*, 220–1
 pulmonary vascular resistance 250
 smooth muscle cells (SMC)
 proliferation response 215
 vasodilatory response 204, 215
 thiols adduct formation 217

Nitric oxide synthase 250
  activation in platelets 221
  endothelial cell activity 204
  HVJ-liposome-mediated vessel wall expression 243
  isoforms 221, 250
    constitutive calcium-dependent form 221, 250
    inducible calcium-independent form 221, 250
    targeted delivery in altered endothelial cells 221–2
Nitrogen dioxide (NO_2) toxicity 259, 260
Nitroglycerin 120, 216, 249
Nitroprusside 249
  adult respiratory distress syndrome (ARDS) 251
Nitrosothiol
  endothelial cells production 204
  smooth muscle cell (SMC) vasodilation 204
Nitrovasodilators 216
NONMEM program 412
Nonmuscle myosin
  antisense oligonucleotide suppression *91*, 93, *94*
  cell cycle regulation 93
Norepinephrine, cardiac myocyte growth regulation 275
NPC15669 64

OKT3
  'humanized' antibody 293
  mode of action 290–1
  side effects 291
  transplantation immunosuppressive treatment 65, 290–1
Omega-3 fatty acids 11
Optical sensors 418–19
  immunosensor 421, *425*, 425–6
Osteopontin 80
Oxygen free radicals
  endothelial cells production 204
  nitric oxide inactivation 208, 215
  smooth muscle cell (SMC) vasoconstriction 204
  therapeutic inhibition 208

P-selectin 61
  accelerated arteriopathies 63
Palmaz–Schatz stent 13
PAMI trial 117
Pancreatic islet graft 299
PARK study 11
Paroxysmal atrial fibrillation
  antiarrhythmic agent infusion therapy 446
  electrical cardioversion 445–6
    implantable devices 446
  implantable feedback controlled drug-delivery system 445–57
    fibrillation detection 448–51, *449*, *451*
    implantation procedure 455
    in vivo test results 453–5, *454*, *456*, 456, *457*
    infusion control 451–3, *453*
    program control *443*, 447–8
    system description *443*, 446–8

open-loop antiarrhythmic agent delivery 410
oral preventive therapy 445
Penicillins
  biocatalytic probes 420
  fiberoptic sensors 418–19
Persistent pulmonary hypertension of newborn (PPHN) 251–2
  endogenous nitric oxide production impairment 252
  nitric oxide inhalation 252, 256–7
PET stents, local drug delivery 19
pH monitoring 415
  fiberoptic sensors 418
Pharmacologic Atrial Defibrillator (PAD) *443*, 446–8
  CHORUS pacemaker *443*, 446, 447, 450, 451
  fibrillation detection 448–51, *449*
    median filtering 450–1, *451*
  implantation procedure 455
  in vivo test results 453–5, *454*, *456*, 456, *457*
  Infusaid Model 1000 pump 446–7
  infusion control 451–3, *453*
  program control 447–8
Phenylethylamine, transdermal iontophoretic delivery 389
Phenytoin
  ion-selective electrode sensors 416
  optical immunosensor 421, *425*, 425–6
Phospholamban, expression in cardiac failure 270
Photodynamic therapy 46
Pilsicainide, QRS duration 427, *428*
Pirmenol 335
Plasminogen activator inhibitor-1, expression in ischaemic heart disease 172
Platelet-derived growth factor (PDGF)
  angiotensin II induction 238
  cardiac myocyte growth regulation 277
  injury-associated release 85
    targeted therapies 55
  isoforms
    PDGF-AA 85, 86
    PDGF-AB 85
    PDGF-BB 85
  monoclonal antibody blockade 65
  restenosis pathophysiology 3, 4
  smooth muscle cells (SMC)
    migration 225
    proliferation 85
    secretion 80, 85
  trapidil inhibition, restenosis prevention 7–8
Platelet-endothelial cell adhesion molecule-1 (PECAM-1)
  leukocyte recruitment 62
  monoclonal antibody inhibition 64
Platelets
  aggregation
    endothelial response 204, 205
    monoclonal antibody blockade 65
  aspirin effects 118
  drug delivery vehicles (plateletosomes) 225
  forskolin inhibition 222–3

nitric oxide
  injury-associated release 221
  responses 215
nitric oxide synthetase activation 221
platelet-derived growth factor (PDGF) isoforms
    85
prostacyclin (PGI_2) inhibition 222
restenosis pathophysiology 3
S-nitrosothiols inhibition 217
  S-nitroso serum albumin adduct (S-NO-BSA)
    220, 220–1
unstable angina 123
vasomotion mediation 224–6
Pluronic gel
  antisense oligonucleotides delivery 43, 44, 93–4
  cyclic integrin antagonist (RGD peptide)
    delivery 45
Polymer membrane based ion-selective electrodes
    415, *422*
  mexiletine determination 422–4
Polymeric implants
  antiarrhythmic agent local delivery 343, 390
  antisense oligonucleotide delivery 42–4, 93–4,
    95
  antithrombotic drug delivery 139, *140*, *141*, 141
  basic fibroblast growth factor (bFGF) delivery
    39–42
  cardiac implantation 343
  cardiovascular controlled release systems 383
  dexamethasone local delivery 45
  heparin local delivery 35–8, *36*, *38*
  hirulog local delivery 45
  local delivery of drugs 34–5, *45*
  magnetic modulation of drug release 412–13
  polyurethane matrices 343
  silicone polymer matrices 45
  ultrasound modulation of drug release 413
Polymeric stents
  antithrombotic drug delivery 138
  restenosis prevention 18, 19
Polyurethane matrix implants 343
Porous balloon catheters 31–3, *32*
  antisense oligonucleotide delivery 93
  antithrombotic drug delivery 137
  channel balloons 33
  intravascular half-life 35
  low pressure drug infusion modification 33
  microporous balloons 33
  tissue injury 33
Positional cloning techniques 353, *354*
Potentiometric ionophore-mediated
    immunoassay (PIMIA) *424*, 424–5
PPACK
  balloon catheter local delivery systems 137
  hydrogel-coated balloon delivery 33, 138
Prednisolone, restenosis prevention 10
Prednisone, cardiac transplantation 283
Premarin 208
Probucol 208
Procainamide 329, 333, 335
  exponentially tapering infusion 410, *411*
  serum level estimation from QRS duration 427

serum level-clinical effect relationship 426–7
signal-averaged ECG late potentials (SAECG)
    441
transmyocardial iontophoretic delivery 390
two-compartment kinetics 451
Procaine, amperometric/voltammetric sensors
    417–18
Procollagen 80
Proliferating cell nuclear antigen (PCNA)
  antisense oligonucleotides
    SMC proliferation suppression 95, 96, *161*
    vessel wall expression inhibition 241
  cell cycle regulation 93
  primary/restenotic atherosclerotic lesions 81
Propafenone 333, 335
Proportional integral derivative (PID) control 434–
    5
Propranolol 360
  ion-selective electrode sensors 416
Prostacyclin (PGI_2)
  adult respiratory distress syndrome (ARDS)
    251, 254
  aspirin inhibition of synthesis 225
  endothelial cells production 204, 222
  endothelium-dependent relaxation function
    204, 222
  local delivery therapeutic approach 222
  platelet inhibition 222
  restenosis prevention 8
  vessel wall gene transfer 188
Prostaglandin H synthase gene transfer 188
Prosthetic heart valve calcification 35
Proteoglycans, extracellular matrix 83
Pseudomonas endotoxin
  mitogen–toxin combinations 56, 60
  monoclonal antibody conjugates 294
Pulmonary hypertension, nitric oxide inhalation
    249–61
  acute models 252–4, *253*
  adult respiratory distress syndrome (ARDS)
    254–6, *255*, *256*
  chronic hypertension 258
  persistent pulmonary hypertension of newborn
    (PPHN) 256–7
  pulmonary vascular resistance 250
  technical aspects 260–1
  toxicity 258–60
Pump-based local delivery 35

QT interval *355*
  Bazzet correction 329, 361, 430
  cardiac arrhythmias 329
  congenital prolongation *see* Long QT
    syndromes
  dispersion 440–1
  Frieberg's cube-root correction 430
  measurement problems 429–31
  prolongation
    amiodarone 440
    Class III antiarrhythmic agent serum level
      estimation 427, *429*, 429

QT interval (*cont.*)
    disopyramide *431*, 431, 442
    ibutilide *429*, 429, *430*
    torsades de pointes 338
Quinidine 333, 334, 335
    mode of action 328–9
    monophasic action potential responses *433*
    serum level estimation from QRS duration 427, *428*
    syncope 329

Rapamycin 286, 302
    actions on T lymphocytes 286
    FKBP activity inhibition 287
    FKBP binding 286
    mode of action 286–8
    structure *285*
Recombinant fusion protein production
    59D8 monoclonal antibody-scuPA 156–64
    59D8 monoclonal antibody-tPA 154–6
Renal allograft rejection
    HLA sensitization 293
    pre-transplant blood transfusions 294–5
Renal failure 224
Renin 234
Renin–angiotensin system 234
    cardiac failure-associated activation 276
    restenosis pathophysiology 3
Reperfusion therapy 111–17, 123
    infarct size limitation 111–12
    primary revascularization 117
    rationale 111
    thrombolysis *see* Thrombolytic therapy
Restenosis 1–20
    incidence 1
    local preventive therapies 18–19, 30, 31–47
        catheter-based intravascular drug delivery 18, 31–4
        drug-impregnated stents 18, 19, 34
        gene therapy 19
        genetically-primed cellular elements on stents/grafts 18
        polymeric implants 34–5
    mechanical prevention 11–13, *14*, *15*, 16–18
        directional coronary atherectomy (DCA) *14*, *15*, 16
        excimer laser coronary angioplasty (ELCA) *15*, 17
        intracoronary stent 12–13, *14*, *15*
        laser balloon angioplasty (LBA) *14*, *15*, 17
        rotational atherectomy (RA) *15*, 17–18
        transluminal extraction-endarterectomy catheter (TEC) *15*, 18
    pathophysiology 2–4
        endothelial denudation 3–4
        extracellular matrix production 4, 83
        late SMC proliferative phase 2, 4
        leukocyte recruitment 2, 4, 62
        neointimal response 1, 2
        platelet activation 2, 3–4
        thrombus formation 2, 3–4

pharmacological prevention 4, 5, 6, 7–11
    angiotensin-converting enzyme (ACE) inhibitors 10, 242
    anti-inflammatory drugs 6, 9–10
    anticoagulants 5, 6, 7–9
    antiplatelet agents 5, 7–9
    antiproliferative agents 6, 10–11
    calcium antagonists 5, 7
    cholesterol-lowering agents 11
    colchicine 10
    heparin 9
    hypolipidemic agents 6, 11
    omega-3 fatty acids 11
    platelet glycoprotein IIb/IIIa inhibitor 8
    platelet-derived growth factor (PDGF) inhibitor 7–8
    prostacyclin 8
    serotonin antagonist 10–11
    somatostatin analogue 10
    specific antithrombin agent 9
    thromboxane A$_2$ inhibition 8
    warfarin 8–9
    photodynamic therapy 46
    residual stenosis 12
    SMC elastic recoil 12
    vascular remodelling 237
    see also Accelerated arteriopathies
Retroviral vectors
    hepatic gene transfer, LDL-receptor deficiency 189, 190
    vessel wall gene transfer 178
        antithrombotic/fibrinolytic agent delivery 188
        duration of expression 184
        efficiency of transfer 178
        hirudin 188
        prostaglandin H synthase 188
        tissue-type plasminogen activator (t-PA) 187, 188
        urokinase plasminogen activator (u-PA) 187–8, *188*
RGD peptide, polymer-based local delivery 45
Ricin A monoclonal antibody conjugates 294
Ro 46–2005 224
Romano–Ward long QT syndrome 353, 354, *359*
    β blockade 360
    clinical features 354, 356
    detection of new genes 371–4, *372*
        cDNA library direct screening 372–4
        exon amplification 371, *373*
        magnetic bead capture technique 371
        sequencing strategies 374
    diagnosis 356–7
    gene locus 353
    gene therapy approach 375, *376*
    H-*ras*–1 candidate gene 368
    H-*ras*–1 locus
        genetic mapping *367*, 367
        physical mapping 369–71, *370*
    left cardiac sympathetic ganglionectomy (LCSG) 360

linkage analysis 363, 367
   genetic heterogeneity 363–4
   H-*ras*–1 locus linkage 353, 361, 363, 364, 366
   LOD score 363, 366
   microsatellite marker allele detection with
      PCR 363, *365*
   polymorphic markers 363, *364*
   recombination events 363, *366*
   mutations identification 374–5
   positional cloning approach 353, 362–3, 367–75
   presymptomatic patient identificaton 366
   torsade de pointes 354, *355*
   ventricular arrhythmias 358–9
Rotational atherectomy (RA) *15*, 17–18

S-nitroso serum albumin adduct (S-NO-BSA)
      217–18
   local NO delivery to injured vessel 218–20, *219*,
      220
   platelet inhibition *220*, 220–1
S-nitrosoproteins, vasodilatory/platelet inhibitory
      properties 217
S-nitrosothiols
   duration of action 217–18
   endothelium-dependent vasodilator function
      217
   exogenous NO replacement 221
   local delivery to injured vessels 218–20, *219*
   plasma 259
   platelet inhibition 217, *220*, 220–1
Saporin–mitogen combinations 57–60, *58*, *59*
Sarcoplasmic reticulum Ca^{2+}-ATPase (SERCA2)
   expression in cardiac failure 270
   ventricular remodelling-associated expression
      269
SAVE trial 240, 244, 332
SCATI trial 119
Selectins, leukocyte recruitment pathway 62
Sensors, whole blood monitoring 414, 426–7
   amperometric/voltammetric 416–19, *423*
   biocatalytic 419–20, *423*
   biosensors 419–22, 426
   chemical 415–19
      enzyme coupled 419–20
   continuous drug monitoring 414
   externally mounted arrays 426
   fiberoptic 418–19
   immunochemical 420–2, *424*, 424–6
   ion-selective electrodes 415–16, *422*, 426
   self-contained probes 414
Serotonin
   endothelial cell nitric oxide stimulation 214
   endothelial response 204
      damaged endothelium 205
   restenosis pathophysiology 3
      effects of antagonists 10–11
   vasoactivity 204, 224–5
Serum metabolites monitoring 414, 426
Shear stress
   endothelial cell nitric oxide stimulation 215
   thiols potentiation 217

Silicone polymer matrices 45
SIN-1 nitric oxide donor 216
Smooth muscle cells (SMC)
   adhesion molecules expression 62, 63
   balloon dilatation responses 3–4
   endothelial cell interactions 204
   endothelium-dependent vasodilator function
      204
      atherosclerosis-associated impairment 205
      endothelial damage-associated impairment
         205
   extracellular matrix production 4, 66
      early provisional matrix 66, 67
   gene transfer 183
      cell-based 174, *175*, 176
      nitric oxide synthetase 222
   injury-associated mitogen release 55, 85
   insulin-like growth factor-1 (IGF-1) secretion 80
   leucocyte recruitment 62
   nitric oxide-mediated relaxation 204, 214
   osteopontin secretion 80
   phenotype
      intimal lesions *80*, 80
      primary atherosclerotic lesions *81*, 81
   platelet-derived growth factor (PDGF) secretion
      80
   procollagen secretion 80
   restenosis pathophysiology 4
   tropoelastin secretion 80
Smooth muscle cells (SMC) migration 66, 79
   angiotensin II 86, 239
   monoclonal antibody inhibition 64, 65
   platelet-derived growth factor (PDGF) 65
Smooth muscle cells (SMC) proliferation 81
   angiotensin II 86, 238–9
   anti-inflammatory drugs, local delivery 45
   antisense oligonucleotides 42, 43, 93–4, *96*, *97*,
      99
      in vitro 91, 93
      in vivo 91, 93–7, *98*, *99*
      non-specific effects 93
   basic fibroblast growth factor (bFGF) 85
      controlled release in culture 41
      monoclonal antibody blockade 66
   cell cycle proteins *92*, 92
      antisense technology suppression *91*, 93
   cell-adhesion molecule targeted therapies 60–5
   heparin 29–30, 38
      continuous versus intermittent therapy 30
      polymer-based delivery 35
   insulin-like growth factor-1 (IGF-1) 85–6
   mitogen–toxin combinations 55–60
   nitric oxide 215
   photodynamic therapy 46
   platelet-derived growth factor (PDGF) isoforms
      85
   post-traumatic stimulating factors 57, 85
   proliferating cell selective ablation 55–60
   proliferation rates 81, 83
   restenosis 2, 3, 79
      late proliferative stage 4
   thrombin 85, 86

Smooth muscle cells (SMC) proliferation (*cont.*)
  transforming growth factor-β_1 (TGF-β_1) 86
  vascular endothelial growth factor (EGF) 85
  vascular injury surface markers 54
  VCAM-1/ICAM-1 expression 63
Soluble complement receptor 1 (sCR1), graft heart
    survival 64
SOLVD trial 313, 332
Somatostatin analogue 10
Sotalol 441
  clinical trials 334–5
  iontophoretic modulated delivery *393*, 393–6,
    394, *395*, 401
    in vitro 392
    in vivo cardiac implant 392–3
  iontophoretic transdermal delivery 389
  monophasic action potential responses *432*
  polymer matrix cardiac implantation 343
  structure *335*
  structure–activity relationships 344
STARC study 8
Stent Restenosis Study (STRESS) 13
Stent-induced arteriosclerosis, local heparin
    delivery 37
Stents, drug-releasing 18, 19, 34
  antisense oligonucleotide delivery 93
  antithrombotic drug delivery 138
  cell-based vascular gene transfer 175, *176*
  drug-eluting biodegradable polymer 34, *37 38,*
    38
  forskolin 221, 223
  heparin 37, *38*, 38
  temporary 139
  vascular function restoration 216
Stents, endovascular 34
  antithrombotic regimens 34
  restenosis prevention 12–13, *14*, *15*
  thrombosis/intimal hyperplasia limiting efficacy
    34
Streptokinase
  hirulog adjuvant therapy 134
  intracoronary during coronary angioplasty 135,
    136
  myocardial infarction thrombolytic therapy 113,
    115, 115, 116, 132, 133, 134, 149
    aspirin therapy combination 118
    coronary artery catheter delivery 132
  unstable angina 135
Stromelysin, leukocyte recruitment 62
Substance P
  coronary endothelium-dependent vasodilation
    204
  endothelial cell nitric oxide stimulation 215
Sulotroban 8

T10B9 291
T12 antibody 291
T lymphocyte receptor/CD3 complex *291*
  genomic repertoire 298
    restriction by thymic selection 298
  MHC class I molecule interaction 296
  MHC class II molecule interaction 296, 298

monoclonal antibody immunosuppressive
    therapy target 291
  OKT3 mode of action 290
T lymphocytes
  cyclosporine effects 284–6
  FK-506 effects 286
  graft rejection 298
  monoclonal antibodies immunosuppressive
    therapy 292
  rapamycin effects 286
  recruitment
    accelerated arteriopathies 60, 62, 83
    adhesion molecule monoclonal antibody
      inhibition 63–4
    endothelial cell damage 62
    graft acceptance 65
    intercellular adhesion molecule-1 (ICAM-1)
      62–3
    SMC proliferation stimulation 62
  thymic clonal selection 298
    intrathymic alloantigen in tolerance
      induction 299
Temporary stents, antithrombotic drug delivery
    139
Tenascin *67*, 67
  extracellular matrix 84
TGFα-KDEL 56
TGFα-PE40
  hepatotoxicity 56
  smooth muscle cell (SMC) selective ablation 56
Theophylline, immunochemical sensors 421
Thrombin
  endothelial cell activation 61
  endothelial cell nitric oxide stimulation 214
  myocardial infarction 119
  smooth muscle cells (SMC) proliferation 85, 86
  vasoconstrictor response 204, 213
Thrombolytic therapy 109, 111–17, 123, 132–4, 149
  adjuvant treatments 115, 116, 119, 134, 150
  anatomical targeting 132
  aspirin combination 118, 119
  biochemical targeting 133
  clinical trials 113, 114, *115*, 116, 149
  early artery patency *116*, 116
  heparin 115, 116, 119
  intracoronary administration 112–13, 132, 133
    during coronary angioplasty 135–6
  intravenous administration 113, 132
  myocardial infarction mortality
    reduction 113, *114*
    subgroup analysis *114*
  new agents development 150
    antibody-targeted approach 150–66
  rationale 111–12
  systemic lytic state 133
  treatment availability 113, *116*
  unstable angina 123, 135
Thrombosis
  angiotensin II 240
  drug release from stents 34
  gene transfer drug delivery 186–9
  myocardial infarction 108

Thrombospondin 67, *68*
Thromboxane A$_2$
  aspirin inhibition of synthesis 118
  inhibition, restenosis prevention 8
  restenosis pathophysiology 3
  vasoconstriction 204, 224–5
Thromboxane A$_2$ receptor antagonists 225
Thromboxane A$_2$ synthase inhibitor 225
Thrombus
  fibrin-specific antibody 150–1
  imaging 65
  restenosis pathophysiology 2, 3–4
    neoendothelialization 4
  smooth muscle cells (SMC) proliferation 85
  unstable angina 123
Thyrotropin releasing hormone, transdermal
    iontophoretic delivery 389
Ticlopidine, restenosis prevention 7
TIMI Phase I trial 133
Tissue factor expression, ischaemic heart disease
    172
Tissue-type plasminogen activator (t-PA)
  anti-fibrin antibody conjugate 152
  anti-fibrin bispecific antibodies 152–3
  anti-fibrin recombinant fusion protein
    production 153–64
  desulfatohirudin adjuvant therapy 134
  intracoronary during coronary angioplasty 135,
    136
  myocardial infarction thrombolytic therapy 113,
    115, 115, 116, 117, 123, 133, 134, 149
    accelerated regimen 115–16
    adjuvant heparin 115, 116, 119
    fibrin specificity 113, 115, 133, 134
  unstable angina 135
  vessel wall gene transfer 187, 188
Tocainide 333
Tolerance induction 294–302
  bone marrow mixed chimerism 300, 301
  homologous recombinaton (gene targeting)
    techniques 301
  intrathymic alloantigen inoculation 299
  oral antigen administration 299
  peristence of tolerance 299–300
  pre-transplant blood transfusion effect 294–6,
    298
  pre-transplant MHC Class I gene transfection
    299
  xenotransplantation 300–1
Torsades de pointes 338–9, 343
  drug-induced 339
    QT dispersion as ventricular tachyarrhythma
      marker 440, 441
  electrophysiologic cause 338–9
  long QT syndromes 360, 362
    Romano–Ward syndrome 354, *355*
  management 339
  QT interval prolongation 338
Toxins
  mitogen combinations *see* Mitogen–toxin
    combinations
  monoclonal antibody conjugates 294

Transforming growth factor-a$_1$ (TGF-a$_1$)
  Pseudomonas endotoxin combination 56
  restenosis pathophysiology 4
Transforming growth factor-β_1 (TGF-β_1)
  angiotensin II induction 238
  cardiac myocyte growth regulation 277, *278*
  extracellular matrix production 86
  injury-associated release 55, 56
  restenosis pathophysiology 3, 4
  smooth muscle cells (SMC) proliferation 85, 86
Transfusion effect 294–6
Transluminal extraction-endarterectomy catheter
    (TEC) *15*, 18
Transplant rejection
  adhesion molecule monoclonal antibody
    inhibition 63–4
  antilymphocyte antibody therapy 288–94, 302
  antisense oligonucleotide ICAM-1 suppression
    97
  E-selectin 63
  endothelial cell ICAM-1 expression 62–3
  HLA sensitization 293
  interleukin-2 (IL-2) monoclonal antibody
    blockade 65
  leukocyte recruitment pathway 62
  monoclonal antibody therapy 65
  pre-transplant blood transfusion effect 294–6
Trapidil, restenosis prevention 7–8
Triazolopyrimidine *see* Trapidil
Tropoelastin 80
Troponin C
  myocardial gene transfer 314, 315
  skeletal isoform expression in myocardium 321
Troponin T, cardiac failure 272
Tumour necrosis factor α (TNFα)
  cardiac myocyte growth regulation 277
  endothelial cell activation 61

UK-68,798 344
Ultrasound modulated contolled-release systems
    413
Unstable angina 123
  aspirin 123
  atherosclerotic plaque disruption 134
  coronary angioplasty 135, 136
  coronary vascular dysfunction 207
  heparin anticoagulation 123
  intracoronary thrombus 123
  local therapy 134–5
  nonfatal MI risk 123
  platelet activation 225
  thrombolytic therapy 123
  thromboxane A$_2$ 225
  thrombus formation 134–5
Urokinase
  intracoronary during coronary angioplasty 135,
    136
  myocardial infarction thrombolytic therapy
    113
  smooth muscle cells (SMC) migration 66
  unstable angina 135

Urokinase plasminogen activator (uPA)
  anti-fibrin antibody conjugates 152
  anti-fibrin cell fusion bispecific antibody 153
  fibrin-specific antibody fusion protein *see* 59D8
    monoclonal antibody–scuPA fusion
    protein
  GPIIb/IIIa receptor antibody conjugates 164–5
  vessel wall gene transfer 187, *188*
    expression at cell surface 177–8

Vascular adhesion molecule-1 (VCAM-1)
  accelerated arteriopathy 84
  inhibition, T cell recruitment blockade 63
  leukocyte–endothelial adhesion 62
  monoclonal antibody 63
Vascular endothelial growth factor (VEGF)
  extracellular matrix proteoglycan binding 83
  myocardial collateral circulation promotion 320
  restenosis pathophysiology 4
  smooth muscle cells (SMC)
    post-traumatic production 85
    proliferation 85
Vascular endothelial growth factor (VEGF)
    receptors 54
Vascular remodelling
  angiotensin II 237–40
  atherosclerosis 237, 239
  hypertension 237, 242–3
  restenosis 237
  vein bypass graft 237
Vasomotion
  endogenous mediators *214*, 214
  local therapy restoration 215–26
  molecular control 214–15
Vasoreactive disease
  angiotensin II 233–44
  endothelial function 203–9
  molecular approach 213–26
Vein bypass graft 237
Ventricular assist surgery 258
Ventricular remodelling 268–70
  adult/fetal gene expression changes *269*, 269
  angiotensin II 276
  catecholamines 275–6
  extracellular matrix overproduction 270
  fibroblast hyperplasia 270
  mechanical stress stimuli 275
  myocyte hypertrophy 270
  peptide growth factors 277
Verapamil 121
  ion-selective electrode sensors 416
  polymer matrix cardiac implantation 343

Vessel wall gene transfer 171, 172, 173–89
  antithrombotic/fibrinolytic agent delivery
    186–9
    hirudin expression 188
    prostacyclin expression 188
    tissue-type plasminogen activator (t-PA) 187,
      188
    urokinase plasminogen activator (u-PA) 187–
      8, *188*
  cell-based transfer 173–7
    implanted devices 174–6, *176*
    limitations 176–7
    retroviral transduction effiency 176
    transformed endothelial cells 174, 176
    transformed smooth muscle cells (SMC) 174,
      175, 176
  cellular targets 182–4
    in diseased arteries 184
    gene expression histochemical markers 183
  duration of expression 184–5
  ischaemic heart disease therapy 171–96
  nitric oxide synthetase 222
  restenosis prevention 19
  safety 185–6
  vascular function restoration 216
  vector-based transfer 174, 177–82, *179*
    adenoviral vectors 179, 181–2, *185*, 185, 186
    detection of gene transfer 178, *180*
    efficiency of transfer 178, 180, 181, 182
    HVJ-liposome complexes 179, 180–1
    level of transgenic protein expression 178,
      181, 182
    liposomes 178, 184–5
    non-viral methods 177
    retroviral vectors 178, 184
    viral methods 177–8
Voltage-dependent Ca^{2+} channels (VDCC) 270
Voltammetric sensors 416–19, *423*

Wallstent 12
Warfarin, restenosis prevention 7, 8–9
Wiktor stent 13
WT32 291

Xenotransplantation 300–1, 302
  homologous recombinaton (gene targeting)
    technique 301
  tolerance induction/bone marrow mixed
    chimerism 301